Applied Anatomy
& Physiology

An Interdisciplinary Approach

Applied Anatomy & Physiology

An Interdisciplinary Approach

EDITED BY

ZERINA TOMKINS

BAppSc (Med. Lab. Sci.), BAppSc (Hons), MNSc (Nurs) PhD (Cell Biology), Grad Cert (University Education)

Degree Coordinator, Senior Researcher
Department of Nursing & Department of Paediatrics
University of Melbourne
Parkville, Victoria, Australia

ELSEVIER

ELSEVIER

Elsevier Australia. ACN 001 002 357
(a division of Reed International Books Australia Pty Ltd)
Tower 1, 475 Victoria Avenue, Chatswood, NSW 2067

ISBN: 978-0-7295-4319-4

Notice

National Library of Australia Cataloguing-in-Publication Data

 A catalogue record for this book is available from the National Library of Australia

---

Content Strategist: Natalie Hunt
Content Project Manager: Kritika Kaushik
Edited by Caroline Hunter
Proofread by Tim Learner
Cover by Georgette Hall
Internal design: Standard (SD 40)
Index by SPi Global
Typeset by Toppan Best-set Premedia Limited
Printed in China by RR Donnelley

Last digit is the print number: 9 8 7 6 5 4 3 2 1

Contents

Foreword

In my many years of experience in teaching anatomy and physiology to first-year allied health students undertaking nursing, midwifery, paramedic or occupational therapy degrees I have found that they are all very eager to learn the clinical skills associated with these professions but when it comes to anatomy and physiology they often ask, 'Why do I need to know this?' Early on in their studies, they do not always make the connection between having a solid foundational understanding of anatomy and physiology and improved clinical outcomes once they are practising their chosen profession. This textbook helps students to make that link, to appreciate that the more they understand how the body normally works, the better able they are to provide care and treatment when it does not work normally.

In addition to providing an overview of the structure and functions of each organ system, this textbook emphasises the functional integration of these systems in maintaining homeostatic processes and how the breakdown of homeostatic processes leads to malfunction and disease. Clinical application of this knowledge is elucidated through the use of case studies, written by academics and clinicians with a wide range of expertise in various health-related disciplines, helping students to consolidate and assess their understanding. Clinical application of anatomy and physiology is further supported with highly relevant online materials, sourced from Australian sites such as healthcare providers that may proffer future employment.

Applied Anatomy & Physiology: an interdisciplinary approach provides an invaluable resource to help students understand anatomy and physiology and to make the meaningful connections to clinical practice that are essential for the best possible clinical outcomes.

Natalie Bennett
B.Sc. Honours (Immunology), PhD (Immunology), Grad. Cert. Ed. (Professional Development Studies)
Lecturer
School of Biomedical Sciences
Monash, University Peninsula Campus
Frankston, Victoria, Australia

Preface

Students commencing a nursing degree to become enrolled nurses or registered nurses through Diploma of Nursing, Bachelor of Nursing or Graduate Entry Nursing (GEN) programs (Masters) come from a variety of educational backgrounds. Many have never studied human anatomy, the study of body structure, or physiology, the study of how the body functions. Thus, when first encountering anatomy and physiology, a key challenge is to determine how much theoretical content you must understand to effectively navigate through the fundamental processes underpinning healthy human function. This challenge may be exacerbated if the subject content is delivered intensely over a short period, as is often the case in GEN programs. At the same time, you must overcome the challenge of acquiring the scientific language. Compounding this is a lack of accessible clinical case studies that you can go through in your own time to understand how anatomy and physiology relate to person-centred care. It may help to know that this feeling is temporary.

As a subject coordinator and degree coordinator for the GEN program at The University of Melbourne, I teach a significant cohort of students who do not have a science background and am acutely aware that a different resource is needed, rather than the standard anatomy and physiology textbook. My aim in producing this textbook was to fill this gap. The intent was to produce a simpler textbook with essential cellular and mechanistic information that allows you to build a foundation for understanding fundamental anatomy and associated physiological processes. This information is then linked to clinical practice through case studies. The underlying drive to this approach is a strong focus on the homeostatic mechanisms governed by each body system, aiming to help you understand what is 'normal' and how 'normal' works, so that it is easier to understand why and when a person is no longer able to compensate and enters into a disease state. My vision was supported and shared by colleagues from nursing, midwifery, medicine, physiotherapy, visual science and audiology. We are all educators, but also maintain our clinical roles.

What is different about this textbook is that there is a comprehensive chapter on pain, as I felt that it is important for nursing students to understand pain physiology as early as possible since a large proportion of our clinical time is spent on pain management. Given the close link between nursing and midwifery, a chapter on pregnancy, birth and lactation from the midwifery perspective is included to increase nursing students' awareness and appreciation of the midwifery speciality, but also to enhance awareness that knowledge of pregnancy, birth and lactation is important in providing nursing care to pregnant patients. Patient mobility after surgery, during illness recovery or as part of the patient's daily living activities is also an important nursing role. Thus I asked physiotherapy colleagues to write chapters on skeletal, joint and muscular systems while highlighting the importance of these systems in facilitating patient mobility.

This textbook was purposefully written to help you feel connected with the material. Wherever possible, case studies reflect everyday situations so that it is easier to visualise and think through logically what may be occurring at the cell, tissue, organ and system levels. Sometimes the same topic is covered from different angles to help you understand the interconnection of the body systems. I appreciate that some of this text may be too simple for those who have had a prior exposure to anatomy and physiology. However, from my experience, these students require transition and instruction on how to apply that existing knowledge to patient scenarios in a person-centred manner. It is my belief that the case studies presented in this textbook may assist this transition process, as they allow you to test your knowledge and skills while focusing on person-centred care. I am also aware that you will outgrow this textbook and move on to more complex theory and practice. This is exactly the way it should be as you master the content and are ready to learn more.

Provision of effective nursing care is driven by the depth of knowledge each of us has. Our capacity to help patients will heavily depend on how well we apply that knowledge to patient care in the moment of need. Subject coordinators understand that this depth of knowledge and our capacity to use it are built over time and through experience. You need to understand this too as your journey starts with understanding the normal structure and function of the human body and all of the processes allowing human existence. On behalf of the authors who helped in creating this textbook, and whose intent was to help start this voyage with ease, I wish you a wonderful journey.

Zerina Tomkins

Contributors

Amany Abdelkader, PhD
Scholarly Teaching Fellow
School of Nursing and Healthcare Professions
Federation University
Berwick, Victoria, Australia

Kim Allison, PhD
Lecturer
Department of Physiotherapy
The University of Melbourne
Carlton, Victoria, Australia

Michael Salvatore Barbagallo, PhD
Lecturer
School of Nursing & Healthcare Professions
Federation University
Berwick, Victoria, Australia

Nick Bridge, Master of Health Education
Teaching Specialist
Department of Nursing
Melbourne School of Health Sciences
The University of Melbourne
Carlton, Victoria, Australia

Bethany Carr, BMidwif, BClinMidwif
Nursing & Midwifery
Monash University
Frankston, Victoria, Australia

Clare Fenwick, PhD
Director of Nursing and Midwifery, Education and
    Research
Central Australia Health Service
Northern Territory, Australia
Lecturer
Nursing and Midwifery
James Cook University
Townsville, Queensland, Australia

Angela Fraser, MBBS, MPHTM, FACEM
Visiting Medical Officer
Royal North Shore Hospital
St Leonards, New South Wales, Australia

Peter Haywood, BNurs
Haematology
Wellington Hospital
Wellington, New Zealand

Susanne Kapp, PhD
Research Nurse
Department of Nursing
The University of Melbourne
Parkville, Victoria, Australia

Erin Laing, BNutDiet (Hons)
Clinical Dietitian
Nursing Department
The University of Melbourne
Parkville, Victoria, Australia

Michael Lee, BSc, MPhty, MChiro, PhD
Senior Lecturer
Faculty of Health, Graduate School of Health,
    Discipline of Physiotherapy
University of Technology Sydney
Broadway, New South Wales, Australia

Yeong Jer Lim, MBChB
Haematology Registrar
Royal Liverpool University Hospital
Liverpool, England

Rachel Macdiarmid, RN, BSc, MHSc, DHSc
Senior Lecturer
Nursing Department
Auckland University of Technology
Auckland, New Zealand

Elissa M McDonald, PhD
Senior Lecturer
Nursing Department
Auckland University of Technology
Auckland, New Zealand

Jed Montayre, RN, PhD
Senior Lecturer
Nursing Department
Auckland University of Technology
Auckland, New Zealand

Sonya Moore, DHealth
Sports Medicine Programs
The University of Melbourne
Physiotherapist
Alphington Sports Medicine Clinic
Melbourne, Victoria, Australia

Bryony A Nayagam, BSc (Hons), PhD
Associate Professor
Audiology and Speech Pathology
The University of Melbourne
Principal Research Fellow
The University of Melbourne
Carlton, Victoria, Australia

David AX Nayagam, BSc/BE (ElecEng) (Hons), PhD
Senior Research Fellow
Bionics Institute
East Melbourne, Victoria, Australia

Steven Nelson, GDCE
Clinical Nurse Educator
Nursing Education
The Royal Melbourne Hospital
Parkville, Victoria, Australia

Fiona Newall, PhD, RN
Professor
The Royal Children's Hospital Melbourne
Director, Nursing Education
The Royal Children's Hospital Melbourne
Clinical Nurse Consultant, Department of Clinical
   Haematology
The Royal Children's Hospital Melbourne
Parkville, Victoria, Australia

Wei Heng On, MBChB
Gastroenterology Registrar
Aintree University Hospital
Liverpool, England

Jane Phillips, BAppSc (Physio)
Lymphoedema Physiotherapist
Honorary Physiotherapist
The Royal Children's Hospital Melbourne
Parkville, Victoria, Australia

Padmapriya Saravanakumar, RN, PhD
Lecturer
Nursing Department
Auckland University of Technology
Auckland, New Zealand

Zerina Tomkins, BAppSc (Med Lab Sci), BAppSc (Hons), MNSc (Nurs), PhD, Grad Cert (University Education)
Degree Coordinator, Senior Researcher
Department of Nursing & Department of Paediatrics
The University of Melbourne
Parkville, Victoria, Australia

Kiryu Yap, BMedSc, MBBS
Research Fellow
Department of Surgery, University of Melbourne & St
   Vincent's Institute of Medical Research
Surgical Registrar
St Vincent's Hospital Melbourne & Epworth Hospital
Victoria, Australia

Reviewers

Rachel Ch'ng, MNursSc
The University of Melbourne
Parkville, Victoria, Australia
(Chapters 3, 4, 5, 8, 11, 13, 14, 21 and 22)

Julie Cooke, PhD
Senior Lecturer Anatomy & Physiology
Discipline Lead of Sport & Exercise Science
University of Canberra
Bruce, ACT, Australia

Angus A Cooper, MNursSc
The University of Melbourne
Parkville, Victoria, Australia
(Chapters 3, 4, 5, 8, 11, 13, 14, 21 and 22)

Ann Framp, PhD
Clinical Program Coordinator
University of the Sunshine Coast
Sippy Downs, Queensland, Australia

Justine Khamara, MNursSc
The University of Melbourne
Parkville, Victoria, Australia
(Chapters 3, 4, 5, 8, 11, 13, 14, 21 and 22)

Ellie Kirov, BSc (BiolSc) (Hons), PhD
Lecturer, Human Bioscience
School of Science
Edith Cowan University
Lecturer, Biomedical Science
Department of Health Studies
Edith Cowan College
Perth, Western Australia

Suzanne Reid, PhD
Professional Teaching Fellow
School of Biological Sciences
University of Auckland
Auckland, New Zealand

Mia Schaumberg, BExSS (Hons), GCHEd, PhD
Lecturer in Physiology
School of Health and Sport Sciences
University of the Sunshine Coast
Honorary Research Fellow
School of Human Movement and Nutrition Sciences
The University of Queensland
Queensland, Australia

Lena Shchreider, MNursSc
The University of Melbourne
Parkville, Victoria, Australia
(Chapters 3, 4, 5, 8, 11, 13, 14, 21 and 22)

Acknowledgements

I thank my husband Andy and my daughter Emma for their patience and unconditional support.

I would also like to thank Professor Marie Gerdtz, Head of Department, Nursing, The University of Melbourne, for her steadfast support of this project.

CHAPTER 1

Cellular response to injury

ZERINA TOMKINS, BAPPSC (MED LAB SCI), BAPPSC (HONS), MNSC (NURS), PHD, GRAD CERT (UNIVERSITY EDUCATION)

KEY POINTS/LEARNING OUTCOMES

1. Discuss how atoms and molecules participate in chemical reactions, and the importance of chemical reactions in cell function.
2. Describe the main components of cell structure and their function.
3. Discuss how mitochondria generate energy from glucose in the form of adenosine triphosphate (ATP) molecules.
4. Discuss cellular responses to repair cell injury and processes that occur when cells cannot repair injury—that is, programmed cell death (apoptosis) and autolysis (necrosis).
5. Link how failure to repair or adapt to injury leads to disease development.

KEY DEFINITIONS

- **Apoptosis:** programmed cell death that occurs with activation of enzymes called caspases.
- **Cell:** the smallest functional and structural unit of an organism.
- **Homeostasis:** a steady-state equilibrium that favours optimal cell function.
- **Inflammation:** an orchestrated sequence of tissue responses aimed at removing injurious stimuli and repairing injured tissue.
- **Necrosis:** a form of cell death characterised by cellular autolysis.

ONLINE RESOURCES/SUGGESTED READINGS

- **Biology: cell structure** available at www.youtube.com/watch?v=URUJD5NEXC8
- **A tour of the cell** available at www.youtube.com/watch?v=1Z9pqST72is
- **Everything you need to know about cells** available at www.youtube.com/watch?v=Ta_zGRHGaHw
- **Cell signals** available at www.youtube.com/watch?v=89W6uACEb7M

INTRODUCTION

Your body is composed of organ systems (Fig. 1.1) with different types of organs that function together to enable you to walk, breathe, think, pass urine and faeces, sit down and make conversation with other people. An example of an organ system is the urinary system, which includes the kidneys and urinary bladder that work together to form and excrete urine.

Each organ is built of different types of **tissues**, structures composed of different types of **cells** that collaborate with each other to enable your body to function. Cells are the basic functional unit of the living organism. **Cell communication** is based on a complex set of chemical reactions that only stop when a person dies. Many diseases are linked to dysfunction in these chemical reactions, so having knowledge of the main chemical reactions that take place in the body will help you to understand when something is no longer 'normal' and may be causing disease signs and symptoms.

Cells are made of different structural components organised into **organelles** comprised of different substances or compounds, more scientifically known as matter. The term '**matter**' refers to anything that occupies space and has mass. If you examine the composition

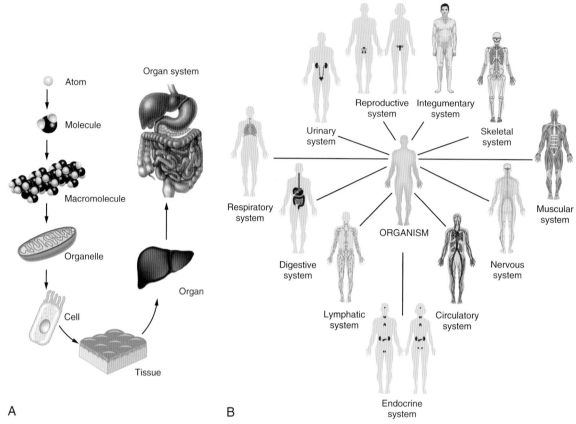

FIGURE 1.1 **Organisational levels of the human body. A** From atom to organ systems. **B** Organisation of organs into body systems.

of the matter, you will find that it is composed of **macromolecules**, a complex formation of different types of molecules, which in turn are made of atoms.

Your body depends on chemical reactions which drive processes to keep you alive. Those processes include: detecting and responding to changes within the body and the surrounding environment; obtaining food to derive the energy needed to drive the cellular processes that keep you alive and fully functional and to produce building materials to replace dead cells; the capacity to release energy from nutrients through a process known as **cellular respiration**; excreting waste products of the cellular processes, such as carbon dioxide; synthesising building materials to make or repair cell structures; movement; and reproduction. In some ways, cells are chemical factories that continuously use raw materials (food) to produce energy and metabolic waste. Through these tightly regulated processes, cells work constantly to achieve and maintain a steady state or equilibrium

inside the cells and surroundings that favours optimal cell function. This is known as **homeostasis**.[1,2]

Cells are continuously engaged in monitoring homeostasis by constantly checking that the composition of their immediate external environment and what is happening inside them (intracellular settings) remains within a narrow range of functional or physiological parameters.[1,2] This surveillance is needed because some changes in the cells' environment may induce **stress** or **injury**. The capacity to sense and immediately respond to these challenges is integral to cell survival and preservation of cell function if injury is to be avoided. Simple examples of these changes include fluctuations in temperature or oxygen availability and changes in the main source of energy, glucose, which is derived from the food we eat.

This chapter links how atoms become molecules; how atoms and molecules participate in chemical reactions to form different types of chemical compounds such as organic compounds, proteins, carbohydrates and fats; and how these compounds build cell structures responsible for cell function. Within the context of cell structure and function, the chapter addresses basic structural components, and how cells communicate with each other and respond to injury. Understanding basic cell structure and function and how this helps cells to respond to stress and injury should make it easier to understand why alterations at the cellular level lead to disease and how treatments address those alterations so that some form of homeostasis can be achieved.

BASIC CONCEPTS IN THE BIOCHEMISTRY OF LIFE

Atoms, molecules and compounds

All matter is composed of **elements**, the smallest parts of matter that cannot be further broken down into even smaller particles. **Atoms** are the basic unit of elements. An atom is made of a dense positively-charged **nucleus** surrounded by negatively-charged **electrons** that travel in a region referred to as an electron cloud (Fig. 1.2). Inside the atomic nuclei are **protons**, which are positively charged particles, and **neutrons**, which do not have an electric charge. Atoms of a single element contain the

same number of protons but the number of neutrons may differ. This means that atoms may have a different **atomic mass**. Atoms that have the same atomic number but differ in atomic mass are called **isotopes**. You may have heard about isotopes in carbon dating, a technique used to establish the age of fossils using the carbon isotope C-14.[3]

There are two main models proposed to describe how electrons are distributed in the electron cloud. **Bohr's model** (also known as the planetary model) describes electrons as neatly ordered in rings or shells where each ring represents different energy levels, and proposes that the electrons closest to the nucleus are those most strongly attracted to the nucleus. Each ring may contain a certain maximum number of electrons. **Schrödinger's model** proposes that electrons travel in the space designated as a 'cloud' and therefore cannot always be located in one location or region of that cloud.[4] In both models, electrons travel at high speed while orbiting the nucleus. This atomic structure is held together by the attraction that exists between protons and orbiting electrons. Electrons most distant from the nucleus are those more likely to react with another atom and participate in the creation of a **chemical bond**. Atoms that have unpaired electrons in the outermost cloud are those that are termed to be unstable and therefore likely to be chemically reactive, whereas those that are paired will not be chemically reactive. Atoms with unpaired electrons will gain, lose or share electrons with another atom to achieve atom stability.

The **periodic table of elements** (Fig. 1.3) presents the different types of elements known to date. Each element has a designated **chemical symbol**, which is usually a single capital letter or a combination of two letters. You may be familiar with some elements such as oxygen (O), carbon (C) and iron (Fe, from its Latin name *ferrum*). In the periodic table the elements are ordered sequentially but also allocated to groups and periods. The sequential order of increasing numbers reflects the increasing **atomic number**, which in turn reflects the number of protons in the nucleus. In contrast, the electrons associated with an element determine the type of chemical reaction that the atom can participate in. **Atomic mass** represents the mass of protons and neutrons in the nucleus of a single atom.[4]

The vertical columns in the periodic table are known as **groups**. Elements arranged in groups have similar properties to each other. Elements are also ordered in horizontal rows known as **periods** based on additional properties shared among the elements. The periodic table also reflects the increase in **atomic radius**, with the smallest atomic radius (Helium) found in the upper

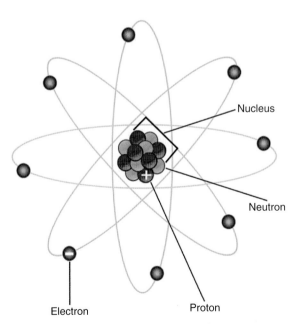

FIGURE 1.2 General representation of atom structure with a central nucleus containing protons and neutrons surrounded by electrons. (*Source:* https://wpclipart.com/energy/atom/atomic_diagram.png.html.)

Nucleus

Neutron

Electron

Proton

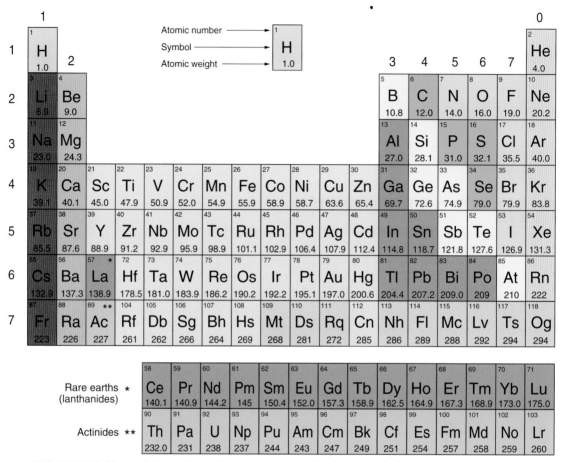

FIGURE 1.3 **The periodic table of elements is an organised representation of chemical elements grouped on their common properties.**

right-hand corner of the table and the largest atomic radius, francium (Fr), located in the far-left bottom corner.

Atoms usually react with each other to form **molecules** (Fig. 1.4). Atoms of an element can interact with other atoms of the same element or with atoms of another element to form a neutrally charged **compound**. This occurs by forming chemical bonds through sharing or exchange of electrons among the atoms. An example of a molecule is water, which is composed of two hydrogen atoms and one oxygen atom. Molecules then react with one another to form more complex forms of matter or, as we more commonly know them, **compounds** and **substances**. A **pure compound** contains atoms of only that element. Based on how those atoms interact with each other, the pure compound might be solid, liquid or gas.

Chemical bonds

When atoms react to form molecules, the resulting compound is held together by **chemical bonds**. Similarly, when a molecule is broken down into atoms, the chemical bonds are broken to release the atoms from their molecular state. Biologically important bonds include ionic (or electrovalent) bonds, covalent bonds, hydrogen bonds, metallic bonds, van der Waals forces and disulfide bonds.

Ionic bonds (Fig. 1.5A) are formed between an electropositive element and an electronegative element and involve a complete transfer of electrons from one atom to another. This is seen in metals, which tend to lose an electron to become positively charged cations, whereas non-metals accept the electron to become negatively charged anions. Ions with opposite charges are attracted to each other. Compounds that form ionic

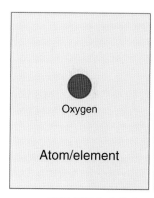

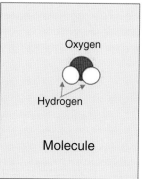

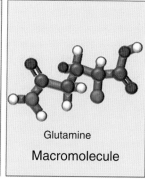

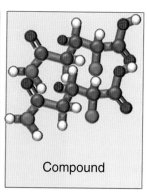

FIGURE 1.4 **Schematic representation of atoms, molecules, macromolecules and compounds.**

bonds and can be dissolved in water tend to separate into **cations** and **anions**. For example, salt is formed when sodium (Na) gives its only unpaired electron from the outer shell to chloride (Cl), which has three paired and one unpaired electron (totalling seven electrons). By donating the electron, sodium becomes positively charged sodium cations (Na^+), whereas chloride, by accepting the electron from sodium, becomes negatively charged chloride anions (Cl^-). As positive and negative charges attract, Na^+ and Cl^- will form NaCl **crystals**, which we see as salt. When salt is dissolved in water, it separates into sodium cations and chloride anions.

Covalent bonds are formed when two atoms share electrons (Fig. 1.5B). When two atoms share one pair of electrons, this is called a **single covalent bond**. This is presented graphically by a single line linking two atoms. When atoms share two pairs of electrons, this is known as a **double covalent bond**. Graphically, this is presented as two lines between the atoms. When the sharing of electrons in the covalent bond is equal, this is known as a **symmetrical covalent bond**. When the sharing of electrons is not equal, with one molecule attracting more of the electron pair than the other, an **asymmetrical bond** known as a **polar covalent bond** is formed. This means that there is a charge separation occurring with one atom slightly more positively charged and the other more negative. This forms a **dipole moment**, which is a measure of net molecular polarity.[5]

Hydrogen bonds, sometimes abbreviated as H bonds, represent a force of attraction formed between the positively polarised hydrogen atom from one molecule and the negatively polarised oxygen atom of another molecule (Fig. 1.5C). Hydrogen atoms forming hydrogen bonds must themselves already be attached to negatively charged atoms such as nitrogen and oxygen.

Metallic bonds are formed between metal atoms to form compounds with unique properties such as high melting points and malleable characteristics (Fig. 1.5D). These bonds have not been observed to occur in our bodies.

Van der Waals forces describe the attraction of intermolecular forces between molecules. They tend to attract neutral molecules to one another in gases, liquefied and solidified gases and most organic liquids and solids.[6]

Disulfide bonds are bonds formed between two sulfur (chemical symbol S) atoms. They have a significant role in human biology as they are important in the formation of two amino acids, cysteine and methionine, which are protein building blocks. Formation of disulfide bonds (S-S) is fundamental to correct protein assembly and structural folding to generate the final protein product.

Chemical reactions

Now that you are familiar with what atoms are and how they come together to form molecules through different types of chemical bonds, it is time to introduce some very basic chemical reactions that occur in our bodies. For a chemical reaction to occur, energy is either used or produced. When thinking about the concept of energy, you need to understand what is meant by the terms kinetic energy, potential energy and chemical energy. Energy is neither created nor destroyed. Instead, it is converted from one form to another. **Kinetic energy** is the energy of motion or movement and it is defined as the energy needed to accelerate an object or substance of a given mass from rest to its known speed or velocity. In terms of atoms and molecules, it refers to the motion of electrons and the energy absorbed that enables them to move to a higher energy level. **Potential energy** is

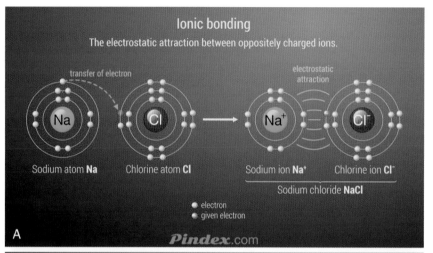

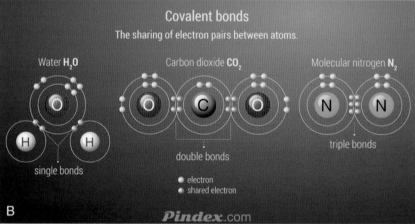

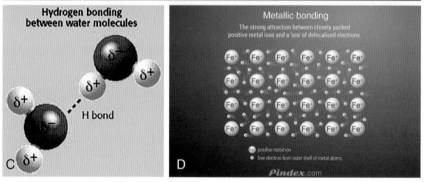

FIGURE 1.5 **Chemical bonds. A** Covalent bond. **B** Ionic bond. **C** Hydrogen bond. **D** Metallic bond. (Source: A, B, D, www.pindex.com/b/visual-science-/chemical-bonds.)

energy stored within an object or substance because of the object's position, arrangement or state (e.g. gas, liquid or solid). In terms of atoms and molecules, it describes what occurs when an electron moves to a higher energy orbit further away from the atomic nucleus. The further the electron is from the atomic nucleus, the greater the potential energy. When an electron releases that energy and returns to a lower energy level, that potential energy will be converted to kinetic energy—for example, in the form of visible light. **Chemical energy** is energy stored inside a chemical and is a form of potential energy.

In general, chemical reactions can be grouped as follows:

- A **synthesis reaction** (Fig. 1.6A) describes how a new product is formed through formation of new chemical bonds, a process that requires energy input. An example is the formation of protein molecules, where protein building blocks, the amino acids, are joined together via a synthesis reaction to form a protein.
- A **decomposition reaction** (Fig. 1.6B) occurs when a product is broken down into simpler forms as existing chemical bonds are broken down, thus releasing the energy stored in those bonds. An example is the breakdown of complex food molecules into smaller absorbable molecules. **Oxidation** and **reduction reaction** (**redox reaction**) are another example: they refer to reactions that involve a transfer of electrons between two reactants with the same chemical formula. This is evident during cellular respiration, where glucose is broken down (oxidised) to carbon dioxide and oxygen is reduced to water to generate energy for cell function.
- An **exchange reaction** (Fig. 1.6C) occurs when two different compounds or molecules are broken down (decomposed) to form (synthesise) two new molecules or compounds.[7]

Chemical reactions are described in a specific language that relies on using chemical elements and mathematical symbols to capture how substances, also known as reactants, interact with each other to form a specific product. A **reversible reaction** (denoted by an arrow pointing in both directions) outlines where reactants form products, which can then themselves react together; the individual reactants will be formed as a product in this case (Fig. 1.6D).

Several factors impact the rate of a chemical reaction. These include:

- the **properties of the reactants** (e.g. surface area; whether a reactant is a gas, liquid or solid; the number of bonds involved in the reaction; and the innate reactiveness of the chemical element)
- the **temperature** at which the chemical reaction occurs, with a faster rate occurring at increasing temperatures due to the increase in kinetic energy that is gained in response to increased temperature—some chemical reactions require high temperatures in order to take place; as the body's temperature is strictly regulated and kept at approximately 37° Celsius, these reactions would not take place if it weren't for **enzymes** (an enzyme is a substance composed of protein or a ribonucleic acid that acts as a catalyst, meaning that it lowers the level of energy needed for a chemical reaction to occur) (Fig. 1.7)
- the **concentration and pressure** at which the chemical reaction takes place, with higher concentrations and greater pressure increasing the rate of chemical reaction.[7]

Chemical reactions that occur in living organisms are collectively referred to as **metabolism**. A decomposition reaction, which involves the release of energy during the chemical reaction, may occur prior to a synthesis reaction. The energy formed through decomposition is used for the synthesis reaction. A defined sequence of chemical reactions is known as a **metabolic pathway**.

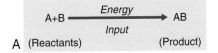

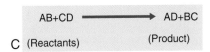

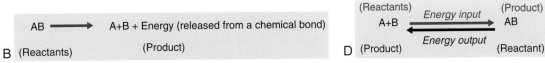

FIGURE 1.6 **Types of chemical reactions. A** Synthesis reaction. **B** Decomposition reaction. **C** Exchange reaction. **D** Reversible reaction.

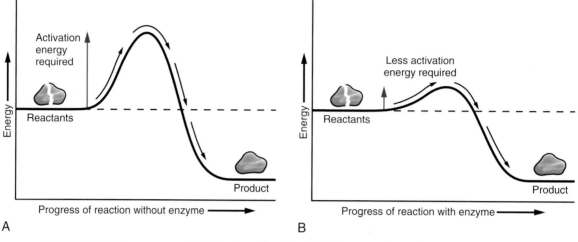

FIGURE 1.7 **Enzymes are catalysts whose function is to decrease the activation energy required for a given chemical reaction to occur. A** Without an enzyme, the energy input needed for a reaction to begin is high. **B** In the presence of an enzyme, less energy is needed for a reaction to begin. (*Source:* https://opentextbc.ca/anatomyandphysiology/chapter/2-3-chemical-reactions.)

Metabolic activity can be grouped into two types: catabolism and anabolism. **Catabolism** encompasses chemical reactions that break down complex molecules into smaller chemical units by breaking down existing chemical bonds; this process is accompanied by a release of chemical energy and involves the breakdown of a chemical bond by the addition of water molecules. This type of chemical reaction is known as **hydrolysis**. **Anabolism** encompasses chemical reactions that synthesise smaller chemical units to generate more complex structures such as carbohydrates, proteins and fats. During the chemical reaction, a water molecule is removed to fuse the smaller chemical units together. This chemical reaction is known as **dehydration** or **condensation** and the energy needed for the reaction comes in the form of adenosine triphosphate, which is generated during cellular respiration.

Energy created during catabolism can also be used to generate other forms of energy, such as **mechanical energy**, which powers movement such as muscles lifting an object. However, the body derives its own energy from nutrients absorbed from digested food. Other forms of energy such as radiant and electrical energy needed for body function are generated by different means. **Radiant energy** is derived from energy emitted and transmitted as waves, such as sunlight, and is needed for synthesis of molecules that will later be converted to vitamin D. The light rays that enter a human eye are responsible for the brain's capacity to see and interpret an image. **Electrical energy** drives the transmission of

nerve impulses and is generated from electrolytes present in the body.

Complex macromolecules

Atoms form molecules and molecules form bonds with other molecules to form complex macromolecules or compounds, which in cell biology are known as **biomolecules**. Biomolecules can be grouped into two groups: organic compounds and inorganic compounds. Both are equally important to human health. **Organic compounds** are compounds whose molecules contain carbon–carbon covalent bonds or carbon–hydrogen covalent bonds. Carbohydrates, proteins, lipids (fats) and nucleic acids are examples of organic compounds; we obtain these compounds through either diet or cell synthesis. **Inorganic compounds** are composed of all other elements and include biomolecules such as water, oxygen, carbon dioxide, acids, bases and salts.

Organic biomolecules contain a carbon backbone and specific group of atoms attached to that backbone. These groups of atoms are known as **functional groups** or **radicals**. The functional groups are responsible for unique properties of biomolecules as they define in which chemical reactions the biomolecule can participate, thus conferring a predictable chemical behaviour for that biomolecule in different environmental conditions. A **free radical** is a functional group that is not attached to the carbon backbone and contains unpaired electrons. This highly reactive and short-lived entity has been associated with the pathology of many diseases.

Carbohydrates contain carbon, hydrogen and oxygen where the carbon atoms link together in chains or rings. Carbohydrates are the main source of energy in cells. They also have a structural role as the building blocks of cell membrane components and nucleic acids and participate in immune functions. Carbohydrates are classified by the length of their chain (Fig. 1.8). The simplest form is a **monosaccharide**, which contains only one unit of saccharide, a term used to describe sugar. The most abundant monosaccharide is glucose, which is the main source of energy for all organisms. A **disaccharide** contains two units of saccharide formed through a dehydration synthesis reaction, which involves loss of a water molecule. The prefixes tri-, tetra-, penta- and hexa- denote three, four, five and six units of saccharide, respectively. An **oligosaccharide** has three to ten saccharide units linked together also through dehydration synthesis reaction. Examples are raffinose, a trisaccharide found in green vegetables such as cabbage, asparagus and broccoli; and stachyose, a tetrasaccharide made of four simple sugars found in soybeans and lentils.[8] A polysaccharide has 10 or more saccharide units. Examples include glycogen, starch and cellulose. **Glycogen** is a polymer of glucose and it is used in the body as a means to store excess glucose. Starch is commonly found in potatoes and it is a means of storing excess glucose in plants, whereas cellulose is a structural component of a plant's cell wall. Although you eat cellulose when you eat plant-based foods (e.g. spinach), your body cannot digest cellulose. Instead, cellulose is an important dietary fibre that helps keep the bowels healthy.

Proteins are composed of carbon, oxygen, hydrogen and nitrogen as their main building blocks. Other building elements include sulfur, iron, magnesium and zinc. Protein functions can be grouped into structural and functional roles. **Structural roles** include building cell organelles and tissues, including supportive connective structures. **Functional roles** include transport (e.g. the protein haemoglobin carries oxygen to cells), defence (antibodies are proteins), signalling (e.g. the hormone insulin is a small protein that signals to cells to take up glucose), digestion (where digestive enzymes break down food) and regulation of chemical reactions (where enzymes act as catalysts to reduce the temperature at which a chemical reaction takes place). All proteins are composed of amino acids, whose unique combination leads to diversity in the shapes and sizes of proteins.

An **amino acid** is a monomer (building block) of protein that is composed of a central carbon atom bonded to an amino functional group (NH_2), a carboxyl group (COOH) and a hydrogen atom. Every amino acid also contains additional molecules bonded to the central carbon atom, which is termed the **R group**. The R group determines the amino acid's identity (Fig. 1.9A). There

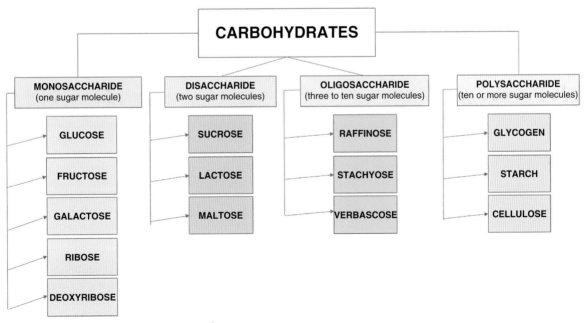

FIGURE 1.8 **Carbohydrate classification.**

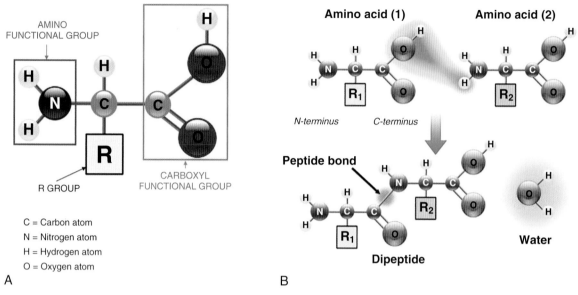

FIGURE 1.9 **Amino acids. A** Generalised structure of an amino acid. **B** Formation of a polypeptide bond. (*Source:* A, Adapted from https://en.wikipedia.org/wiki/Amino_acid. B, From https://en.wikipedia.org/wiki/Amino_acid#/media/File:Peptidformationball.svg)

are 21 naturally occurring amino acids; of these, eight are essential amino acids. This means that they cannot be made by the body and need to be ingested via food in the diet. The remaining 13 amino acids can be synthesised in the body. Amino acids join to one another by forming covalent bonds known as **peptide (amide)** bonds. In this case a covalent bond is formed between a carboxyl functional group of one amino acid (known as the **C-terminus**) and an amino functional group of another amino acid (known as the **N-terminus**) (Fig. 1.9B) through a condensation reaction to form a linear chain.[9] The shortest linear chain contains two amino acids and is called a **dipeptide**, whereas a very long linear chain is called a **polypeptide**. Proteins are built from one or more polypeptides. The sequence of amino acids, which is determined by your genes, gives rise to the primary (most primitive) protein structure. As peptide backbones interact with each other they form a secondary protein structure. These can be grouped into α-helix and β-pleated sheets. When α-helix and β-pleated sheets fold further, they form a **globular or tertiary protein** structure (Fig. 1.10). A **quaternary protein** structure is a three-dimensional aggregation of two or more polypeptide chains (subunits) that act together as a single unit. These dynamic structures often contain binding sites for metals such as iron. Correctly folded protein is essential to protein function, thus any exposure to

high heat, pH, radiation or denaturing chemicals will lead to undesirable changes in the protein structure and loss of function. When a person experiences high temperature (fever), for example above 40° Celsius, cellular proteins will start to denature and lose function. This is one of the reasons why it is important to reduce high body temperature.

Lipids are made of carbon, hydrogen and oxygen atoms. They can be broadly classified into triglycerides, phospholipids, steroids and prostaglandins (Fig. 1.11). **Triglycerides**, also known as triacylglycerols or **fats**, are made of two main molecules: a glycerol and a fatty acid. Each glycerol molecule contains three carbons, five hydrogens and three hydroxyl (OH) groups. This is a constant component in any triglyceride molecule, which is then linked to another three-fatty-acid molecule. The difference in fatty acid composition determines the chemical name and nature of any triglyceride. Fatty acids vary in the length of the carbon chain and in the number of hydrogen atoms bound to the carbon atoms, features which dictate whether a fatty acid is saturated or unsaturated.

A **saturated fatty acid** contains single bonds between carbon atoms in the hydrocarbon chain. If a hydrocarbon chain contains multiple double bonds, it is **unsaturated fatty acid**. If there is only one double bond in the hydrocarbon chain, the fatty acid is said to be a **monosaturated**

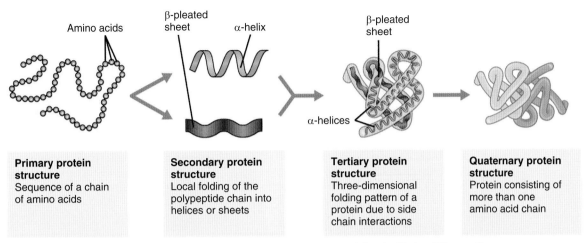

FIGURE 1.10 **Protein structures.** (*Source:* Modification of work by the National Human Genome Research Institute.)

fatty acid. Fatty acids can also be grouped into **essential and non-essential fatty acids**. Examples of essential fatty acids that your body cannot synthesise include omega-3 and omega-6 fatty acids, both of which are found in fish such as salmon, trout and tuna.

Phospholipids are made of a glycerol, two fatty acids and a phosphate group. The phosphate group is hydrophilic in nature and has a negatively charged polar head. The fatty acid chains are not charged and are hydrophobic in nature.

Steroids have a four-linked carbon ring and may contain a hydroxy functional group (OH group). An example of a steroid in the body is cholesterol, which is found in the plasma membrane of every cell and is also a building component of hormones that are steroid-based or lipid-soluble.

Prostaglandins are a family of lipid compounds composed of 20 carbon unsaturated fatty acids that contain five carbon rings. These physiologically active compounds are formed from the fatty acid known as

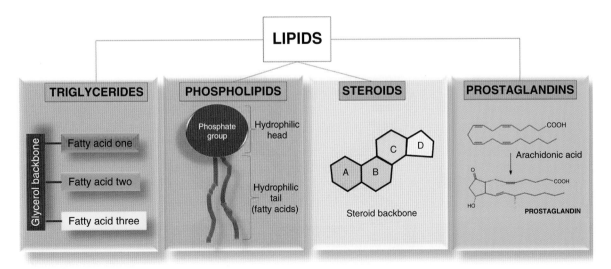

FIGURE 1.11 **Classification of lipids.** (*Source:* Prostaglandin chemical derivation adapted from www.chm.bris.ac.uk/motm/prostanoic/prostanoich.htm.)

arachidonic acid and are released from the cell membrane in response to stimuli such as an injury.

Nucleic acids (Fig. 1.12) are carriers of genetic material. **Deoxyribonucleic acid (DNA)** and **ribonucleic acid (RNA)** are made of many nucleotides joined together in a long chain. Each nucleotide has a sugar component, amine base and phosphate. The sugar component in RNA is **ribose** and in DNA it is **deoxyribose**. There are four amine bases in DNA: adenine, guanine, cytosine and thymine. RNA differs from DNA in that the thymine is replaced by uracil. Nucleotides are joined together by forming a covalent bond (termed a **phosphodiester bond**) between the phosphate component of the nucleotide and the hydroxyl (OH) component of another nucleotide. The sequence of nucleotides determines the structure of the nucleic acid. Adenine exclusively forms a hydrogen bond with thymine, whereas guanine and cytosine form strong hydrogen bonds only to each other. This means that DNA's two polynucleotide strands twist around each other in a double helix and are complementary to one

another. The biological significance of this will become apparent in Chapter 2, where genes are discussed in greater details.

Inorganic biomolecules are compounds that do not contain carbon-hydrogen (C-H). Examples include water, carbon monoxide, carbon dioxide, electrolytes such as sodium, potassium, chloride, magnesium, calcium, acids, bases and salts. Each of these plays a significant role in human health. For example, calcium, magnesium and potassium all play a role in muscle contraction.

Now that you are familiar with basic components of chemistry that are involved in forming complex compounds or biomolecules, it is time to examine how these components contribute to cell structure and function, including response to injury at the cellular level.

General cell structure and function

Tissue cells differ in appearance, size, shape and physiological function.[1,2,10] Despite this variation, eukaryotic cells (cells that contain a nucleus and organelles) are

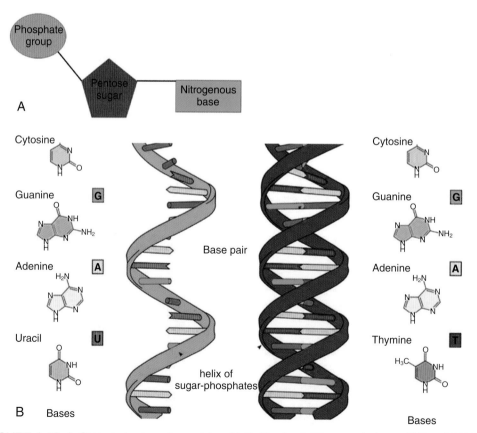

FIGURE 1.12 A, General structure of a nucleic acid. B, Structural differences between RNA and DNA. (*Source:* B, Modified from www.thoughtco.com/dna-versus-rna-608191.)

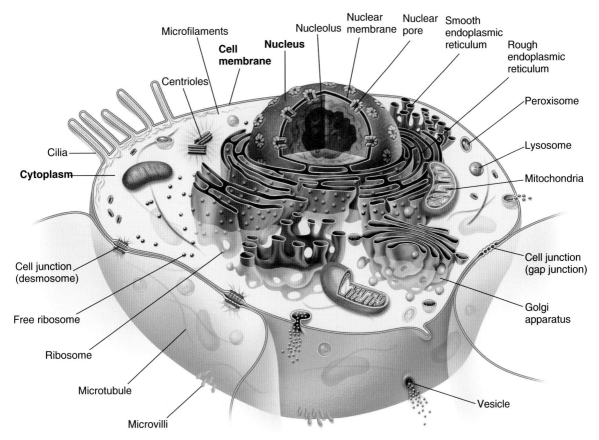

FIGURE 1.13 **Generalised structure of a human cell.** (*Source:* Craft JA, Gordon CJ, Huether SE, McCance KL, Brashers VL, Rote NS. Understanding pathophysiology, 3 ed. Sydney: Elsevier; 2019.)

generally composed of a cell membrane, cell nucleus, cytoplasm and organelles, such as mitochondria, ribosomes, endoplasmic reticulum, Golgi apparatus, lysosomes, proteasomes and peroxisomes (Fig. 1.13). Cells possess a cytoskeleton, which provides mechanical support needed to maintain cell shape, internal organisation and supports cell division and movement. Structures such as flagella, microvilli and cilia are not found in all cells. Instead, they are found in specialised cells; for example, flagella help sperm motility, cilia sweep the mucus of lung epithelial cells towards the trachea, while microvilli in the gastrointestinal tract aid in the absorption of nutrients.[10]

A **plasma membrane** (Fig. 1.14) separates the internal cell content from the external environment, such as neighbouring cells, the extracellular matrix, interstitial fluid or blood. It is composed of a phospholipid bilayer, cholesterol and proteins.[10] The **phospholipid bilayer** is composed of two layers of phospholipids, molecules that

have a hydrophobic (water-fearing) end composed of a fatty acid chain structure facing inwards and a hydrophilic (water-loving) structure (phosphate) facing outwards. This structural composition permits selective control of which molecules cross the phospholipid bilayer.[2,10] For example, a hydrophilic molecule will not easily cross the membrane due to the lipid nature of the interior of the plasma membrane. Transport of hydrophilic molecules is facilitated by specialised structures in the plasma membrane, called transporters, embedded inside the phospholipid bilayer that are predominantly composed of proteins. Molecules that are small and hydrophobic will cross more easily as they are lipid soluble. In clinical settings, this will affect how medications dissolve in the blood and access their cellular targets.

Depending on their structure, cell membrane proteins can:

- **transport water-soluble molecules** through the cell membrane—for example, medications that dissolve

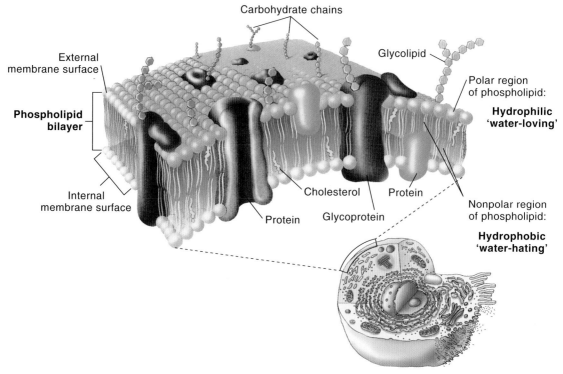

FIGURE 1.14 **Schematic representation of cell membrane structure.** (*Source:* Craft JA, Gordon CJ, Huether SE, McCance KL, Brashers VL, Rote NS. Understanding pathophysiology, 3 ed. Sydney: Elsevier; 2019.)

in water would otherwise remain within the blood and interstitial fluid

- **facilitate translation of signals** that cells receive from their external environment that trigger specific changes in cell function—for example, a growth hormone binds to a growth hormone receptor on the cell surface to initiate a cascade of signals to induce change, such as cell growth; this is known as signal transduction
- **act as cell identification markers or recognition sites** for other cells—for example, expression of specific cell surface markers enables immune cells to recognise what is self and what is foreign; this facilitates initiation of the correct immune response to destroy the foreign cell rather than the body's own cells
- **form connections** between cells
- **form support structures** with other cells, within the cell or with the extracellular matrix.[1,10,11]

Cell cytoplasm is a gel-like hydrophilic substance in which cellular organelles and molecules are suspended.[10] It is composed of five basic substances: water (accounting

for 70–85% of the content), proteins (10–20% of the content), electrolytes, lipids and carbohydrates. Many cellular chemicals are dissolved or suspended in water. **Electrolytes**—a type of chemical, predominantly minerals in your body such as sodium, potassium and bicarbonate—mediate cellular reactions needed for survival. A prime example is the electrochemical impulses in nerve and muscle fibres that are electrolyte-dependent. Maintaining this composition is clinically relevant and it is taken into consideration when infusing fluid replacement therapies or electrolyte replacement therapies due to the high potential to disturb this balance.

Proteins in cells have a structural or functional role.[2,10] Structural proteins form the **cell cytoskeleton**, whereas functional proteins are mainly enzymes, structures that catalyse intracellular chemical reactions. Lipids are predominantly found in cell membranes and intracellular structures that separate individual cell compartments. Carbohydrates are a source of cell nutrition as discussed in the section on mitochondria. The chemical composition of the cytoplasm is tightly regulated as it facilitates all biochemical processes required for cell function.[2] For example, any change in acidity inside the cell will affect how proteins in the cell are formed and how they function. Changes in the concentration of sodium or potassium will affect cellular membrane potential and therefore the ability to conduct electrical signals. For example, low levels of potassium impact on heart cell contractility, while sodium concentrations affect neuronal cell signalling. From a clinical perspective, incorrect administration of potassium or sodium intravenous therapy has a great capacity to disrupt this balance and can be life-threatening.

The **cell nucleus** (Fig. 1.13) is present in all but red blood cells.[2,10] It contains DNA, a genetic code necessary for life to form. The coding regions of DNA are blueprints for the formation of proteins.[10] The function of non-coding DNA is unresolved. During cell division, nuclear DNA is duplicated (discussed in Chapter 3) to allow DNA to be inherited from a parent cell by two daughter cells. Cellular DNA is organised in structures called **chromosomes**.[10] The cell nucleus is separated from the rest of the cell structures by a **nuclear membrane**. This membrane contains **nuclear pores**, which transport

molecules from the cell cytoplasm to the nucleus and from the nucleus to the cell cytoplasm.[2,10]

The **nucleolus** (Fig. 1.13) is housed in the cell nucleus where it assembles ribosomes (Fig. 1.15). Once synthesised, ribosomes are transported from the nucleolus via the nuclear membranes into the cytoplasm.[10] **Ribosomes** are composed of two subunits. The unit of measurement used to describe ribosomal subunits is the Svedberg unit (S), a measure of the rate of sedimentation in centrifugation. In humans, the larger unit is known as 60S and the smaller unit is known as 40S.[12] In bacteria the smaller unit is known as 30S and the larger unit is known as 70S.[13] The main function of ribosomes is to translate messenger RNA (mRNA) molecules that code for individual proteins. In simplest terms, the smaller unit reads the mRNA whereas the larger unit joins individual amino acids to form polypeptide chains. Transfer RNA (tRNA) brings amino acids from the cytoplasm into the cavity between subunits, where they are assembled into a strand. Additional enzymes are present to assist with the translational molecules. Ribosomes and the associated molecules involved in mRNA translation into the protein are called the translational **apparatus**.[10]

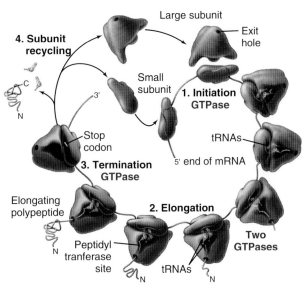

FIGURE 1.15 **Ribosome.** Ribosome is composed of a small subunit (30S) and a large subunit (60S), shown here from two different perspectives. After the small subunit attaches to a messenger RNA (mRNA) strand, which contains a code and instructions for synthesising a polypeptide strand, the subunits come together to form a complete ribosome. Transfer RNA (tRNA) brings amino acids into the cavity between subunits, where they are assembled into a strand according to the mRNA code. As the polypeptide strand elongates, it moves out through a tunnel and an exit hole in the large subunit. (*Source:* Pollard TD, Earnshaw WC, Lippincott-Schwartz J, Johnson GT. Cell biology, 3 ed. Elsevier; 2017.)

Mitochondria (Fig. 1.16) produce cellular energy in the form of **adenosine triphosphate (ATP)**, a fuel that drives all cell metabolic processes.[2,10] This energy is needed for cell survival, repair and division. Disruption of mitochondrial function leads to changes that precipitate early cell death, negatively impact on cell division or result in a cellular dysfunction that will eventually manifest itself through signs and symptoms of a disease.[1] Structurally, mitochondria are shaped like a rod, with an **outer membrane**, a highly convoluted **inner membrane** and a narrow **intermembrane space** in between them. The outer membrane selectively permits entry of molecules into the mitochondria. The inner membrane, which folds into **infoldings (cristae)** and surrounds the **mitochondrial (inner) matrix**, is also highly selective in permitting molecular transport into the mitochondria.[1,2,10]

The number of mitochondria in an individual cell depends on the function of that cell; the more metabolically active a cell is, the more mitochondria it will have. Mitochondria have their own DNA, which enables the mitochondria to replicate independently of cell division. That same DNA codes for the enzymes needed for the **oxidative phosphorylation process**,[1] a process regulating energy production in the cell. This is an important adaptive mechanism when the cell must increase the number of mitochondria to meet the increase in metabolic function.

ATP stores energy in its chemical bonds that can be released on demand.[1] Generation of ATP is a complex biochemical process that commences with the breakdown of the food we eat. For example, carbohydrates are broken down into their simplest format, glucose. Transformation of glucose into energy is achieved through three complex chemical reactions known as glycolysis, cellular respiration and anaerobic respiration. During **glycolysis**, in the presence of oxygen, glucose is processed in the cytoplasm to generate two molecules of pyruvate. Through the process of **cellular respiration**,[1,2] pyruvate molecules are converted to acetyl co-enzyme A (acetyl CoA) and carbon dioxide. Acetyl CoA enters reactions that comprise cellular respiration, which occur inside the mitochondria and comprises three pathways: pyruvate oxidation, the citric acid cycle and the electron transport chain.[1]

Via oxidative phosphorylation, energy is transferred to the maximum number of ATP molecules. In the event that a cell has run out of oxygen, pyruvate can be converted to lactic acid in a process known as **anaerobic respiration**.[1] This is often seen during intense physical exertion, for example where skeletal muscles have run out of oxygen to convert glucose to pyruvate and then to carbon dioxide. Instead, pyruvate is converted to lactic acid, which then builds up in the bloodstream and changes blood acidity (pH), leading to symptoms such as muscle cramps or pain.[14]

Other food molecules such as fats and proteins can also act as a source of energy, but only once they have been converted to glucose. Metabolic pathways involved in the utilisation of lipids, and amino acids and pathways involved in urea and haem molecule synthesis, are also located in the mitochondria.[1] In addition to the production of ATP, mitochondria regulate calcium concentrations in the cells and play a role in cell death.

The **endoplasmic reticulum (ER)** is a network of continuous interconnected channels and sacs arranged in parallel rows that span from the outer nuclear membrane into the cytoplasm, held together by cell cytoskeleton (Fig. 1.13).[10] There are two types of ER: **rough ER** and **smooth ER**. The difference in the appearance is due to ribosomes. ER facilitates the synthesis and transport of the protein and lipid components of most of the organelles, protein folding and sensing cell stress. ER can be interrupted by a multitude of factors both inside the cell and in its microenvironment. For instance, the availability of oxygen or glucose, hyperthermia, acidosis, calcium levels and energy levels (modulated by low levels of oxygen and glucose) negatively affect the function of ER, resulting in stress and impacting protein folding in the lumen of the ER.[1] Dysfunctional ER has been reported in a range of disorders, including Alzheimer's, Parkinson's and Huntington's diseases, multiple sclerosis, cerebral ischaemia, stroke, sleep apnoea and cancer.[15–17]

The **Golgi apparatus** or Golgi complex (Fig. 1.13) is a membranous organelle that receives proteins from rough ER, performs final protein modifications and then packages protein into membranous structures called vesicles for export from the cell.[10] This packaging format protects protein from degradation and facilitates transport to destinations such as cell membrane or the bloodstream. In Duchenne's muscular dystrophy, a disease characterised by the failure of the dystrophin protein to express, cells contain abnormal Golgi apparatus, which further impacts on the production and transport of defective proteins.[18]

Lysosomes (Fig. 1.13) are membrane-bound vesicles formed by pinching off the Golgi apparatus.[10] Their roles span participating in recycling of the dead intracellular components such as protein debris to chemical reactions that regulate cellular signalling, cellular metabolism and cellular repair.[1,10] Lysosomes contain a large repertoire of enzymes. Inborn genetic errors affecting these enzymes are responsible for a group of genetic disorders called

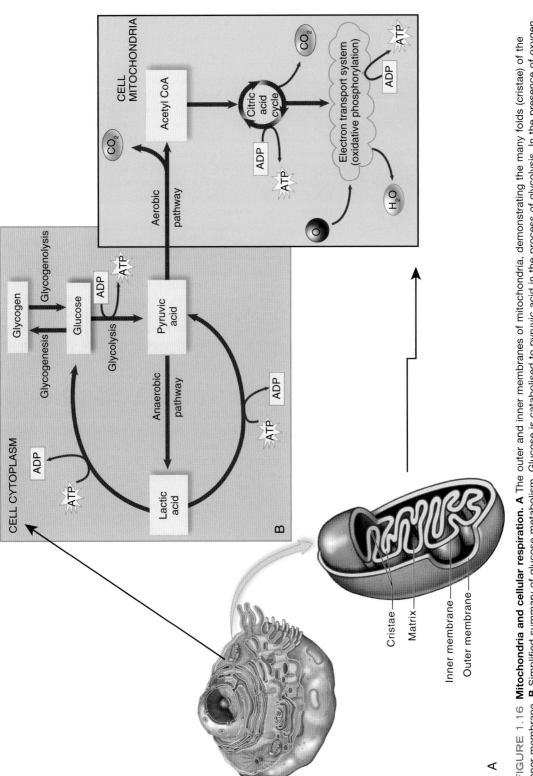

FIGURE 1.16 Mitochondria and cellular respiration. A The outer and inner membranes of mitochondria, demonstrating the many folds (cristae) of the inner membrane. **B** Simplified summary of glucose metabolism. Glucose is catabolised to pyruvic acid in the process of glycolysis. In the presence of oxygen, pyruvic acid is converted to acetyl coenzyme A (CoA) and enters the citric acid cycle, transferring energy to the maximum number of adenosine triphosphate (ATP) molecules via oxidative phosphorylation. In the absence of oxygen, pyruvic acid is converted to lactic acid. (*Source*: Patton KT, Thibodeau GA, editors. Anatomy and physiology. 10 ed. London: Elsevier Health Sciences; 2017.)

lysosomal storage disease, which are characterised by neurodegenerative processes.[19] Lysosomal enzyme, hydrolase, catalyses bonds in proteins, lipids, nucleic acids and carbohydrates to their basic units (i.e. breaks down proteins to amino acids). Due to its potency, this digestive enzyme is enclosed in lysosomal membrane. If this membrane is disrupted, enzyme leaks into the cell cytoplasm where it ultimately causes cellular self-digestion and death.[1]

Proteasomes act as a quality control centre ensuring that each newly synthesised protein is correct—if not, it is destroyed. Protein that has passed its 'use-by' date is also targeted for degradation by proteasomes. Failure to remove a faulty protein is one of the mechanisms thought to be responsible for the development of Parkinson's disease.[20]

Peroxisomes are membrane-enclosed organelles that contain many enzymes.[10] One of these enzymes oversees the breakdown of fatty acid chains, which are then transported to mitochondria for further metabolism to yield carbon dioxide and water. Peroxisomes play a role in bile synthesis and in immune defence, where the enzyme myeloperoxidase is released by neutrophils to kill the engulfed bacteria. Peroxisomes are fundamental to the neutralisation of reactive oxygen species, molecules thought to induce cell damage through non-specific damage to proteins, lipids and nucleic acids and dysregulation of cell signalling cascades. Peroxisome enzymes chemically neutralise poisons such as alcohol through a process that produces large amounts of toxic hydrogen peroxide (H_2O_2), which is then converted into water and oxygen.[1,10]

The **cytoskeleton** (Fig. 1.13) is a flexible framework that supports cell shape and internal organisation of cells.[10] It is composed of three major classes of filamentous proteins: microtubules, intermediate filaments and actin. Of these, microtubules are the largest and they are composed of a protein called tubulin. Intermediate filaments are twisted strands of mid-sized protein molecules. Actin is the smallest filament and is made of the protein actin. Cytoskeleton contains a centrosome, a region of the cytoplasm near the nucleus that manufactures and recycles microtubules in the cells. The centromere is particularly important during cell division when it organises replicated chromosomes and correctly pulls them apart into daughter cells.[10]

Cellular communication

Cells possess a complex machinery that involves the above-named structures and complex chemistry that collectively enable cells to rapidly respond to environmental changes. In addition to individual cell responses, cells also communicate with each other to achieve a uniform response to challenges by receiving and emitting signals.[11] **Signalling** can be thought of as a language of chemistry that cells use to get the work done. Different cell types respond differently to the same signalling molecule as the speed and selectivity with which signalling molecules are delivered to their receptors differs. This concept is important when considering how cells respond to injury. Cells' internal ability to respond to an external stimulus by activating internal mechanisms is known as **intracellular communication** (Fig. 1.17). Cells' ability to collaborate and coordinate their response with other cells is known as **intercellular communication**.[11]

The communication or signalling cascade commences when an extracellular signalling molecule, often called a **ligand**, binds to its receptor on the target cell.[11] Each ligand fits to the receptor like a key fitting into a lock. This **ligand–receptor binding** causes modification of the shape or activity of that receptor, which activates one or more signalling pathways downstream from that receptor. Relay of the message from the receptor through one or more signalling pathways leads to some change in the cell. Each cell is programmed to respond in a specific way to one extracellular signal or a combination of many specific extracellular signals.[11] An outcome of such a response could be cell growth, cell division, cell differentiation into a new cell type or cell death.

There are five basic forms of intercellular signalling (Fig. 1.18): paracrine, synaptic, autocrine, endocrine and contact-dependent:[11]

- **Paracrine signalling** occurs over a short distance as cells release chemical messengers that act on neighbouring cells. An example is release of transforming growth factor beta (TGF-β), which regulates the development of new blood vessels and connective tissue during tissue wound repair.[21]
- In **synaptic signalling** one neuronal cell releases chemical messengers (neurotransmitters) to cause a chemical change in muscle cells (target cells) to generate muscle contraction.
- In **autocrine signalling**, the cell releases chemical messengers that act on the cell from which the message was released. For example, when a T-cell is exposed to a foreign antigen, it releases a growth factor to which it responds by dividing many times to generate T-cell clones capable of eliminating that antigen.
- **Endocrine signalling** is an example of long-distance signalling as the chemical messengers released by specialised cells are released into the bloodstream and carried to the distant part of the body where the

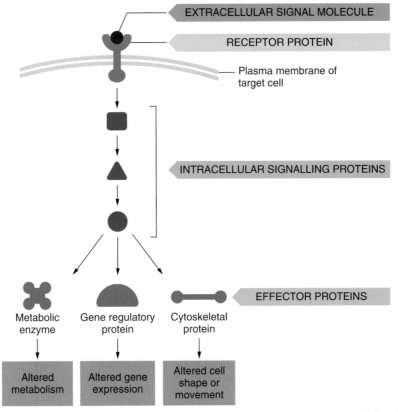

FIGURE 1.17 **A simplified intracellular signalling pathway activated by an extracellular signal molecule.** Binding of the signal molecule to the receptor located on the target cell modifies the receptor. This leads to activation of one or more intracellular signalling pathways, which predominantly involve protein molecules. The end of the signalling cascade is the activation of effector proteins, which modify cell behaviour according to the signal received. (*Source:* Alberts B, Johnson A, Lewis J, Morgan D, Raff M, Roberts K. Molecular biology of the cell, 6 ed. New York: Garland Science; 2014.)

target cells are located.[11] For example, the pancreas is an endocrine organ that releases the hormone insulin into the bloodstream. Once it reaches the target cells found throughout the body, insulin regulates glucose uptake by those cells.

- **Contact-dependent signalling**, also known as **juxtacrine signalling** or **cell–cell contact signalling**, is divided into three types.[11] The first is based on a ligand being expressed on the cell membrane of one cell and the receptor being present on the adjacent cell. The second mechanism involves communicating cell junctions that link two adjacent cells.[11] An example of this is **gap junctions** formed between cardiomyocytes that enable the conduction of the heart impulse from the source to the rest of the heart to generate heart contraction and relaxation. The third

mechanism involves **cell-extracellular matrix signalling**, where the cell interacts with the extracellular matrix via specialised receptors called integrins, which transmit information from the extracellular matrix to the cell.[11,22] This is evident during wound healing where the extracellular matrix composition provides the cell with a cue to move into the wound bed to repair the injured area.

Cellular responses to stress and injury

Any undesirable change in a cell's environment will lead to stress for the cell. If the stress is transient, the cell will most likely recover without any evidence of the challenge presented. However, when the stress exceeds the cell's capacity to respond and/or adapt to the changes to maintain homeostasis, the cell will show signs of

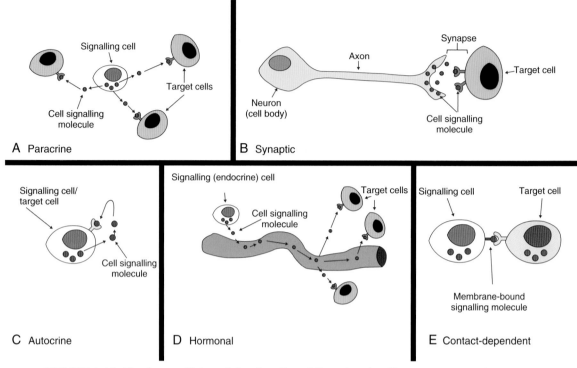

FIGURE 1.18 **Five forms of intercellular signalling. A** Paracrine signalling occurs over a short distance as cells release chemical messengers that act on the neighbouring cells. **B** Synaptic signalling is characterised by the release of chemical messengers (known as neurotransmitters) by a neuron to cause a chemical change on their target cells. **C** In autocrine signalling, the cell releases chemical messengers that act on the secreting cell itself. **D** Endocrine signalling is an example of long-distance signalling as the chemical messengers are released by the secreting cells into the bloodstream to reach a target cell in a distant part of the body. **E** Contact-dependent signalling, also known as cell–cell contact signalling, occurs when a signalling cell and target cell are in direct contact with one another via cell membrane. (*Source:* Modified from Alberts B, Johnson A, Lewis J, Morgan D, Raff M, Roberts K. Molecular biology of the cell, 6 ed. New York: Garland Science; 2014.)

injury and may die. If the stress is reversible or removed on time, the cell will recover and either adapt or return to its initial normal structure and function. Exposure to chronic levels of sub-lethal stress, such as exposure to tobacco smoke for lung cells, will lead to **adaptation** on the molecular, biochemical and structural cell level. In time the cells will start to fail to cope and show signs of chronic injury. This may result in the cells being replaced by another cell type that can cope better with the injurious stimuli. Sometimes the replacement may lead to undesirable consequences, such as the development of cancer cells.[1,23]

What this means is that all forms of disease start at the cellular level with genetic, molecular and structural changes in cells that can no longer maintain healthy homeostasis.[1] While initially not visible, failure in a cell's capacity to compensate in the presence of one or more injurious stimuli will culminate in extensive cellular injury that becomes clinically evident when a person shows early signs and symptoms of disease. At this stage, the initial cellular response to adapt to the external stimuli and return to a normal state is less likely. Unresolved injury in the form of poorly managed disease leads to continual insult on cells, leading to further changes in cellular structure and function so that the cells start to fail and die and more severe manifestations of disease become apparent.

Injury at the cell level

Cells constantly encounter physiological stress, whereas pathological stimuli are sporadic events resulting from exposure to injury. To survive physiological stress and

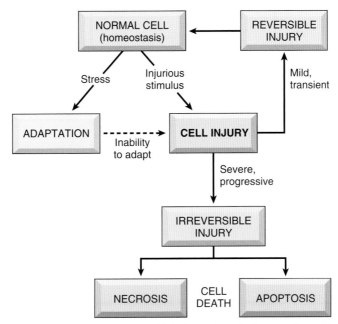

FIGURE 1.19 **Cellular response to stress and injurious stimuli.** (*Source:* Kumar V, Abbas A, Aster JC. Robbins and Cotran pathologic basis of disease, 9 ed. St Louis: Elsevier; 2015.)

some forms of pathological stimuli (Fig. 1.19), cells adjust by activating adaptive functional and structural responses. The aim is to either return to homeostasis or achieve a new steady state, which may differ from the initial homeostatic state but allows cell survival and function.[1] Stress that is mild and quickly removed is not likely to lead to major cellular changes. The cells will recover and return to pre-existing homeostasis. However, stress that exceeds the cells' capacity to adapt will result in cell injury.[1] Exposure to chronic levels of sub-lethal stress will progress from adaptation at the molecular, biochemical and structural level to transformation to other cell types, including progression to cancerous cells.[1,23] Severe and progressive stress leads to irreversible injury and cell death.

Injury can be reversible if the stimulus is removed on time, or irreversible, in which case the cell cannot recover and dies.[1] Causes of cell injury are many and include oxygen deficiency, mechanical impact, extremely low or high temperatures (burns or deep cold), rapid changes in atmospheric pressure, exposure to radiation and electric shock. Chemical agents, infectious agents, autoimmune conditions and inborn or acquired genetic abnormalities also induce cell damage, and nutritional imbalances remain a significant cause of cell injury in malnourished populations.[1] Each cause will elicit unique

cellular responses that will either result in survival or affect the cell so severely that the cumulative outcome is death.

It is usual to group causes of cell injury into **acquired** (e.g. infection, exposure to chemicals) or **inherited** (due to genetic abnormalities caused by inherited mutations or mutation developed after conception). An injury can be caused by a single agent (e.g. virus-induced flu) or have multifactorial causes. An example of this is cancer, which in general arises from a combination of genetic susceptibility and external stimuli such as poor diet and low exercise or exposure to pollutants.[1,23] The process of how injury leads to biochemical and molecular changes at the cellular level and then to clinical manifestation in terms of signs and symptoms, progression and end outcome of the disease process is called pathogenesis.[1]

Morphological changes and functional abnormalities following cell injury

Because each tissue undertakes a specialised function, the cells constituting that tissue have a characteristic structural appearance (morphology) when examined under the microscope.[1] Pathologists use changes in these unique features to diagnose disease and stage disease progression—for example, establishing whether cancer has metastasised. The earliest changes occur

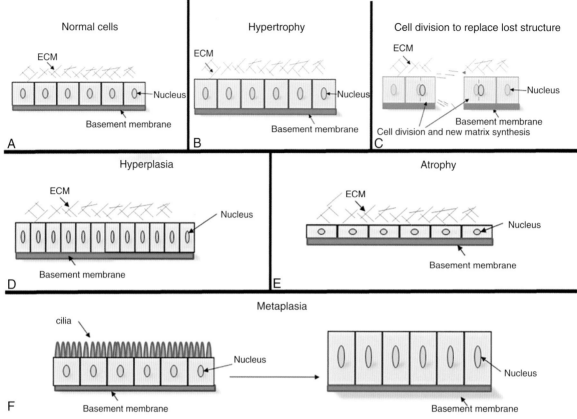

FIGURE 1.20 **Cell adaptation to reversible injury. A** Normal cells. **B** In response to injury normal cells can hypertrophy, **C** divide to replace lost structures such as cells and extracellular matrix, **D** undergo hyperplasia or **E** atrophy. **F** Cells can also be replaced by a different cell type through the process of metaplasia. An example of metaplasia is replacement of ciliated lung epithelial cells with non-ciliated squamous epithelial cells in smokers. (*Source:* http://images.slideplayer.com/24/6979080/slides/slide_4.jpg.)

at the biochemical level encompassing genetic and molecular changes and result in functional outcomes that culminate in visible structural alterations.[1] These alterations include **cellular swelling** due to changes in a cell's ability to maintain fluid homeostasis; plasma membrane alterations such as blebbing; blunting or loss of external structures like villi; changes in mitochondrial appearance such as swelling; and dilation of ER. The combined result of all these changes are functional abnormalities that in time lead to clinical manifestations of disease.[1]

Adaptation to stress and injury

A cell's response to an injurious agent depends on the cell's type, age and capacity to respond to the stimuli.

Initial exposure to injury that is not severe enough to cause disease leads to various adaptations, as outlined below (see also Fig. 1.20).

Adapting the function of cell organelles to respond to the stress. Cells sense stress and respond rapidly by activating mechanisms that may otherwise be dormant. For example, mechanical stress such as tension causes cells to alter their shape through changes in the cytoskeleton with the intent of preventing cell rupture. Sensing chronic demand for energy can cause mitochondria to increase in number through mitochondrial division. Similarly, lack of oxygen forces cells to bypass mitochondria and use the anaerobic mechanism if the cells are to survive. A mild increase in body temperature, such as observed in mild infections, results in cellular production of heat shock proteins, which have a protective effect on cells' capacity to survive.[1] Failure of this mechanism would lead to disastrous effects of increased temperature on the function of all proteins, including enzymes. Likewise, failure to correct errors in DNA replication result in dysfunctional cells destined to die prematurely.

Increasing cell size. Increased assembly of additional intracellular components such as an increased number of mitochondria or the increased surface area of the ER due to increased protein synthesis results in an increase in cell size, known as **hypertrophy**.[1] This process is characteristic of cells that have a very low capacity to divide and generate new cells (e.g. muscle cells). Hypertrophy can be classified as physiological or pathological. Examples of physiological hypertrophy are an increase in skeletal muscle size due to increased functional demand during weight-lifting, and the expanding uterus during pregnancy. An example of pathological hypertrophy is an increase in the size of cardiac muscle cells due to increased demand on a dysfunctional heart to pump blood more effectively. In this case, hypertrophy contributes to worsening of the condition as the overall effect is to increase the size of the affected organ, the heart.[1]

Replacing lost structure through cell division. Cells are either in close contact with other cells or embedded in the extracellular matrix. Some cells have their own specialised extracellular matrix called basement membrane that provides cues for cell orientation and instructions on what function to perform.[22] Absence of a neighbouring cell signals a cell to divide and close the gap. Absence of extracellular matrix signals a cell to synthesise new extracellular matrix to replace the missing matrix. In each case, the aim is to maintain tissue integrity. From a clinical perspective, the best example is that of a superficial cut, where neighbouring skin cells are lost and the matrix is damaged. Skin cells will simultaneously migrate across the clotted blood to close the wound gap and synthesise new matrix in the form of a scar to close the wound and prevent further breakdown.

Increasing cell numbers in the absence of cell loss. In response to a stimulus, cells can divide to increase their overall number. This process is called **hyperplasia**. It can be physiological or pathological in nature.[1] **Physiological hyperplasia** is observed in situations where there is a need to produce a new structure. For example, following removal of a liver lobe for transplantation, liver cells divide to grow a liver lobe of similar size. In cases of severe bleeding following trauma, bone marrow activates a system to grow progenitor red blood cells to replace lost cells. Another example is seen during puberty, where the effect of hormones on breast glandular tissue causes proliferation of glandular tissue to form the female breasts. **Pathological hyperplasia** can be seen in cases of abnormal menstrual bleeding where the lining of the uterus (the endometrium) proliferates due to abnormalities in hormone balance.[1] Hyperplasia and hypertrophy can occur as individual processes but can also overlap.

Decreasing cell size and number. When an external stress is removed and there is reduced functional demand on cells, the cells may respond by decreasing in size and/or decreasing in number, a process known as **atrophy**.[1] The underlying general mechanisms are thought to be due to a reduction in protein synthesis and accelerated protein degradation. Examples of **physiological atrophy** are loss of muscle tissue after ceasing weight-lifting exercises, loss of muscle mass due to ageing combined with reduced physical activity[1] and a decrease in the size of the uterus following birth. **Pathological atrophy** can be subdivided into localised and generalised. Localised pathological atrophy can be seen in skeletal muscle following prolonged leg immobilisation in a plaster cast following a bone fracture, and in senile atrophy (loss of brain tissue associated with decreased blood supply). Generalised pathological atrophy is seen in cases of severe malnutrition, which result in breakdown of muscle tissue as a source of energy after all other sources, such as fat tissue, have been depleted.[1]

Replacing an existing cell with a different cell type. When a cell is unable to respond to injurious stimuli, it may be replaced by a different cell type that is better able to cope. The process by which one cell type is replaced with another in the same tissue is called **metaplasia**.[1] During metaplasia, resident tissue stem (progenitor) cells differentiate to a tissue type that is suitable for the new function. Metaplasia is often seen in casual smokers whereby normal ciliated columnar epithelial cells that line the respiratory tract are replaced by stratified squamous epithelial cells. A negative consequence of metaplasia in this case is that mucus secretion and ciliary action of the columnar epithelium are lost, meaning that an important mechanism of protecting the lungs from infection is compromised.[1] Furthermore, metaplastic cells can transform into cancer cells if the injurious stimuli are not removed.[1,23]

Irreversible cell injury and cell death

When cells' capacity to manage stress is exceeded or if cells are subjected to persistent or severe injurious stimuli, the outcome is irreversible cell injury and eventually cell death. Cell death can also occur as part of healthy ageing and in tissue remodelling observed during development of an embryo into a fetus and then a baby.[24] It is also part of the normal development of organs, tissue repair and associated remodelling to form a scar where it maintains normal homeostasis. There are two main pathways of cell death: necrosis and apoptosis.[1] Each has distinct morphological features, as outlined below. While necrosis and apoptosis can occur independently, they can also occur together.[25] However, while apoptosis is an evolutionary protective process,[23] necrosis is viewed as detrimental and often fatal.

Necrosis

Following reversible cell injury, a cell swells and there will be some plasma alterations, such as blebbing, mitochondrial swelling, distended ER and nuclear alterations. When a cell is lethally injured, these changes are extremely rapid and beyond the cell's capacity to respond. **Necrosis** follows.[1] An equivalent would be the immediate death of a car passenger at an accident scene. This type of death occurs prematurely when considered in the context of the maximum age that the cell can live and is characterised by loss of cell membrane integrity, cellular self-digestion (autolysis) and uncontrolled release of cellular components into the extracellular space.[1,25] The enzymes that perform self-digestion are lysosomes, which are released by the dead cell itself (Fig. 1.21).

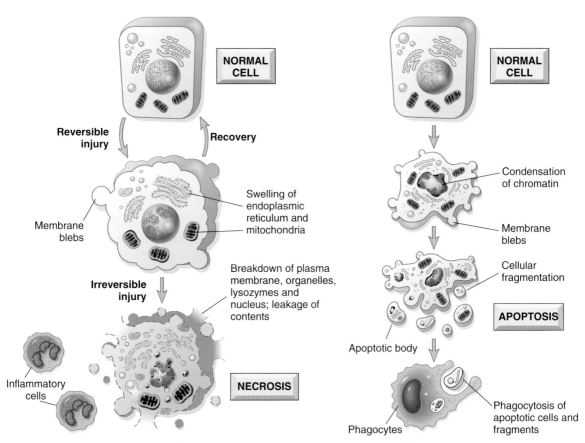

FIGURE 1.21 **Cell death.** Cellular changes following injury characteristic of necrosis and apoptosis (*Source:* Kumar V, Abbas A, Aster JC. Robbins and Cotran pathologic basis of disease, 9 ed. St Louis: Elsevier; 2015.)

Apoptosis

Apoptosis or programmed pathway (Fig. 1.21) is induced by the cell's own machinery, in which the cell suicides in a controlled and predictable manner.[1] It is part of normal embryonic development, throughout adulthood, during healing processes and as the end of cell life. In some ways, you can think of apoptosis as the equivalent of death that comes because of old age. The aim of apoptosis is to remove old dead cells but also to remove unwanted cells that may potentially turn into harmful cells, such as cancer cells.[23,25] In pathological conditions, apoptosis eliminates cells that cannot be repaired. For example, cells containing damaged DNA or misfolded proteins or those infected by a virus would be earmarked for apoptosis.

If a cell has a dysfunctional apoptotic pathway, it will become immortal, a hallmark feature of cancer cells.[23] The apoptotic pathway is characterised by activation of the cell's own biochemical processes involving enzymes that break down DNA, organelles and proteins. It can be initiated through one of two main pathways. The **intrinsic (mitochondrial) pathway** is characterised by the cell killing itself because of the increased permeability of the mitochondrial outer membrane, followed by the release of death-inducing molecules from the mitochondrial inner space into the cell cytoplasm.[1] The **extrinsic pathway** is characterised by engagement of the death receptor expressed on the surface of the plasma membrane, which then delivers signals to activate the death-inducing signalling pathway.[1] The intrinsic and extrinsic apoptotic pathways converge to activate a cascade of **caspases**, enzymes that degrade cellular proteins. The product is the formation of apoptotic bodies, which are further broken down for removal by immune cells that can ingest (phagocytose) those fragments.

INTEGRATION WITH OTHER BODY SYSTEMS

In the coming chapters, you will have the opportunity to see how nothing in the body functions in isolation. While cells may have evolved to meet the needs of individual organs, fundamentally their internal structures share many common features. They all have organelles, a cell membrane and complex machinery that drives chemical reactions that work constantly to achieve and maintain homeostasis.[1,2] Cells of one organ are connected to cells of another organ through extensive blood vessel supply, where often cells secrete chemical signals that act on a subgroup of cells or the whole body. This systemic response is covered more in Chapter 16.

AGE-RELATED CHANGES

Age-related changes at the cellular level affect cell structure, molecular and chemical processes, loss of capacity to maintain homeostasis and reduced capacity to recover from injury.[26] They occur in all cell types at a variable rate. Of interest is the age-related decline in mitochondrial function, a process that it is suggested may lead to increased formation of **reactive oxygen species** through cellular respiration. A key target of mitochondrial reactive oxygen species is mitochondrial DNA.[27] Damage to mitochondrial DNA leads to changes in the newly formed mitochondria that carry the damaged DNA. As mitochondria are involved in responses associated with inflammation and apoptosis, it is easily envisioned how each would be affected by age-related decline in mitochondrial function. Cell capacity to repair also decreases with age. Some of this decline is associated with wear and tear of cell machinery as it ages, as evidenced by increased functional decline in the heart, liver and brain and in repair capacity following injury in ageing populations.[27]

CONCLUSION

The integrity of cellular structure and function through complex cell machinery dictates cellular ability to maintain homeostasis. The capacity to maintain homeostasis depends on internal and external (environmental) factors and the cell's ability to sense these changes and activate appropriate adaptive mechanisms. These mechanisms include increase or decrease in cell size and cell number and replacement of one cell type with another. Inability to respond to irreversible cell injury leads to cell death. For example, failure to produce ATP (energy) results in lethal consequences for cells with necrosis or apoptosis as outcomes, which can further amplify the extent of injury. Knowledge of these concepts should better aid your understanding of inflammation (Chapter 16), an orchestrated process activated in response to injury with the aim to restore homeostasis.

CASE STUDY 1.1

When four-year-old Denis and his mum Lara were visiting his grandmother, Denis and his two cousins sneaked into their grandmother's bedroom where they bounced on her bed. On one of those bounces Denis flew off the bed and landed heavily on his left hand. He cried out in pain and Lara rushed to him. Concerned that Denis might have fractured his arm, Lara took Denis to the hospital. X-rays showed that Denis had fractured his left radius (the bigger forearm bone). A plaster cast was set to immobilise his hand. After the cast was removed, Lara noticed that Denis' healed arm was smaller than his other arm.

Q1. Which of the following statements best describes cellular adaptation to injury?

   a. It is a coordinated cellular response to injury aimed at achieving homeostasis.

   b. It is a response designed to maximise the impact of the injurious stimuli.

   c. It is a process of programmed cell death.

   d. It is the development of an altered state that cannot maintain homeostasis.

Q2. All the following are features of reversible cell injury except:

   a. complete loss of cell membrane integrity.

   b. cellular swelling.

   c. increase in endoplasmic reticulum size.

   d. cell autolysis.

Q3. Damage to mitochondria will result in loss of which of the following functions?

   a. Production of adenosine triphosphate (ATP), a fuel needed for cell survival, cell repair and cell division

   b. Synthesis of proteins

   c. Production of carbohydrates

   d. Production of phospholipids

Q4. Explain why Denis's left arm was smaller following cast removal.

Q5. Following bone fracture, local tissue will swell in response to injury to the cells. If a plaster cast is applied too tightly, what effect can this have on local tissue?

CASE STUDY 1.2

Karl was referred to a general surgeon after he complained of experiencing severe heartburn (acid reflux) for the past nine months. While Karl's doctor had prescribed oral medications to manage the heartburn, overall it had worsened. The surgeon performed a biopsy of oesophageal tissue and sent the tissue sample to pathology for diagnosis. The oesophagus is a muscular tube covered with epithelial cells that connects the mouth with the stomach. The biopsy showed that Karl had oesophageal metaplasia, meaning that his oesophagus lining contained gastric epithelial cells.

Q1. Metaplasia is:

   a. reversible change of one cell type to another that occurs after prolonged injury.

   b. irreversible change of one cell type to another that occurs after prolonged injury.

   c. cell death.

   d. swelling of mitochondria.

Q2. The injurious agent that has caused changes in oesophageal epithelial tissue is:

   a. chemical injurious stimuli that are a base compound.

   b. chemical injurious stimuli that are an acid compound secreted by the stomach cells.

   c. mechanical injury.

   d. medications that Karl was prescribed.

Q3. Homeostasis is a process of:

   a. cell adaptation to irreversible injury.

   b. differentiation of one cell type into another cell type.

   c. achieving a steady state or equilibrium in internal conditions that support optimal cell function.

   d. mitochondrial production of cell energy.

Q4. Suggest why metaplasia occurred in this case and what would happen if metaplasia had not occurred.

Q5. If the injurious stimulus is not removed, what is the likely consequence of metaplasia in Karl's case?

CASE STUDY 1.3

Sara had a skin biopsy done after she went to see her doctor worried about the appearance of a mole. The skin tissue was sampled by punch biopsy and sent to pathology for analysis. The biopsy report stated that the skin tissue contained occasional dead epidermal cells characterised by rounded cells with nuclei containing irreversible condensed chromatin (pyknosis). No other abnormalities were reported.

Q1. This form of cell death is known as:
    a. apoptosis.
    b. necrosis.
    c. hypertrophy.
    d. metaplasia.

Q2. Which of the following statements describes caspases?
    a. Caspases are enzymes that degrade carbohydrates.
    b. Caspases are enzymes that degrade fats.
    c. Caspases are enzymes that degrade intracellular proteins.
    d. Caspases are enzymes that build cell membrane.

Q3. Apoptosis can occur via two main pathways. These are:
    a. metaplastic and hypertrophy pathways.
    b. atrophy and necrosis pathways.
    c. necrosis and hyperplasia pathways.
    d. intrinsic and extrinsic apoptotic pathways.

Q4. What is the role of apoptosis in healthy skin tissue?

Q5. If apoptotic process was dysfunctional, what would you expect would be the consequences of this?

CASE STUDY 1.4

John is an 80-year-old farmer who has suffered lower back pain for the past four years. Last week John underwent four-hour-long spinal surgery to repair the damage to his spine. During surgery John was placed in the prone position (laid down on his stomach). Due to the nature of the procedure, it was not possible to reposition John's hips during surgery. Following his transfer to the intensive care unit it was noted that John has developed a pressure sore on both of his hip bones. On the fifth day after surgery, during skin assessment, the nurse documented that John's pressure sores were necrotic.

Q1. Which of the following statements are not suitable to describe necrosis?
    a. It is a tightly regulated process governed by activation of caspases.
    b. It is characterised by rapid self-lysis of cells.
    c. It is characterised by shrinking cytoplasm, chromosomal condensation in the nucleus that will lead to chromatin fragmentation.
    d. It occurs when a cell is lethally injured.

Q2. When viewed under the microscope, a necrotic cell would be characterised by:
    a. loss of plasma membrane, cell swelling, mitochondrial swelling, extended endoplasmic reticulum.
    b. the cell membrane rupture.
    c. chromatin condensation and fragmentation.
    d. mitochondrial swelling and chromatin fragmentation.

Q3. During necrosis, cell death is caused by:
    a. autolysis caused by lysosomal release.
    b. bacterial enzymes found in the injured tissue.
    c. uncontrolled cell growth.
    d. activation of caspases.

Q4. Suggest why tissue necrosis occurred in John's case.

Q5. Suggest what preventive strategies could have been implemented to avoid the formation of pressure sores in John's case.

REFERENCES

1. Kumar V, Abbas AK, Aster JC. Cellular responses to stress and toxic insults: adaptation, injury and death. In: Robins and Cotran pathologic basis of disease. 9th ed. Philadelphia: Saunders; 2015. p. 31–68.

2. Patton K, Thibodeau G. Cell function. In: Anatomy and physiology. 9th ed. St Louis: Elsevier; 2016. p. 98–119.

3. Peppe DJ, Deino AL. Dating rocks and fossils using geologic methods. The Nature Education Knowledge Project 2013;4(10):1.

4. What is an atom? Available from: www.livescience.com/37206-atom-definition.html.

5. Dipole moments. Available from: https://chem.libretexts.org/Bookshelves/Physical_and_Theoretical_Chemistry_Textbook_Maps/Supplemental_Modules_%28Physical_and_Theoretical_Chemistry%29/Physical_Properties_of_Matter/Atomic_and_Molecular_Properties/Dipole_Moments.

6. Encyclopaedia Britannica. Van der Waals forces. Available from: www.britannica.com/science/van-der-Waals-forces.

7. Covalent bond energies and chemical reactions. Available from: https://chem.libretexts.org/Bookshelves/General_Chemistry/Map%3A_Chemistry_%28Zumdahl_and_Decoste%29/08%3A_Bonding_General_Concepts/13.08_Covalent_Bond_Energies_and_Chemical_Reactions.

8. Avigad G, Dey PM. Carbohydrate metabolism: storage carbohydrates. Plant Biochemistry 1997;143–204.

9. Learn more about peptide bond. Available from: www.sciencedirect.com/topics/medicine-and-dentistry/peptide-bond.

10. Patton K, Thibodeau G. Cell structure. In: Anatomy and physiology. 9th ed. St Louis: Elsevier; 2016. p. 75–97.

11. Alberts B, Johnson A, Lewis J, et al. Cell signalling. In: Molecular biology of the cell. 6th ed. New York: Garland Science; 2015. p. 813–88.

12. Khatter H, Myasnikov AG, Natchiar SK, et al. Structure of the human 80S ribosome. Nature 2015;520(7549):640–5.

13. Schuwirth BS, Borovinskaya MA, Hau CW, et al. Structures of the bacterial ribosome at 3.5 A resolution. Science 2005;310(5749):827–34.

14. Andrews MAW. What causes leg cramps? Available from: www.scientificamerican.com/article/what-causes-leg-cramps.

15. Roussel BD, Kruppa AJ, Miranda E, et al. Endoplasmic reticulum dysfunction in neurological disease. Lancet Neurol 2013;12(1):105–18.

16. Schonthal AH. Endoplasmic reticulum stress: its role in disease and novel prospects for therapy. Scientifica (Cairo) 2012;857516.

17. Schonthal AH. Targeting endoplasmic reticulum stress for cancer therapy. Front Biosci (Schol Ed) 2012;4:412–31.

18. Bexiga MG, Simpson JC. Human diseases associated with form and function of the Golgi complex. Int J Mol Sci 2013;14(9):18670–81.

19. Ferreira CR. Lysosomal storage diseases. Transl Sci Rare Dis 2017;2(1–2):1–71.

20. Bentea E, Verbruggen L, Massie A. The proteasome inhibition model of Parkinson's disease. J Parkinsons Dis 2017;7(1):31–63.

21. Lokmic Z, Musyoka J, Hewitson TD, et al. Hypoxia and hypoxia signaling in tissue repair and fibrosis. Int Rev Cell Mol Biol 2012;296:139–85.

22. Lokmic Z, Lammermann T, Sixt M, et al. The extracellular matrix of the spleen as a potential organizer of immune cell compartments. Semin Immunol 2008;20(1):4–13.

23. Hanahan D, Weinberg RA. Hallmarks of cancer: the next generation. Cell 2011;144(5):646–74.

24. Elliott MR, Ravichandran KS. Clearance of apoptotic cells: implications in health and disease. J Cell Biol 2010;189(7):1059–70.

25. Samali A, Fulda S, Gorman AM, et al. Cell stress and cell death. Int J Cell Biol 2010;245803.

26. Fedarko NS. The biology of aging and frailty. Clin Geriatr Med 2011;27(1):27–37. doi:10.1016/j.cger.2010.08.006.

27. Poulose N, Raju R. Aging and injury: alterations in cellular energetics and organ function. Aging Dis 2014;5(2):101–8. doi:10.14336/AD.2014.0500101.

CHAPTER 2

Genes and genomics

ZERINA TOMKINS, BAPPSC (MED LAB SCI), BAPPSC (HONS), MNSC (NURS), PHD, GRAD CERT (UNIVERSITY EDUCATION)

KEY POINTS/LEARNING OUTCOMES

1. Understand the structure and function of a gene.
2. Discuss how genes regulate cell function and the inheritance of physical and behavioural characteristics.
3. Describe cell division, including the growth phase of the cell cycle and how genes are inherited during cell division.
4. Discuss how mutations in DNA can lead to genetic diseases and how environment influences your genome.
5. Explain the concept of genomics and personalised medicine.

KEY DEFINITIONS

- **DNA mutation:** a permanent change in DNA composition that results in a change in the gene in which the mutation is found. It can lead to a change in the structure and function of that gene.
- **Epigenetics:** the study of how environmental conditions (other than DNA sequence) affect gene expression and activity during development and therefore influence the development of that organism.
- **Gene:** a basic unit of heredity, composed of DNA; varies from small to quite large. Genes control cell development, behaviour and ability to respond to external challenges.
- **Genomics:** the study of human genome structure, function, evolution and inheritance, and how these processes can be mapped or edited to achieve an altered health state (e.g. cure a disease).
- **Heterozygous:** a gene that has two different alleles.
- **Homozygous:** a gene that has two identical alleles.

ONLINE RESOURCES/SUGGESTED READINGS

- **Genomics education websites** available at www.genome.gov/10000464/online-genetics-education-resources/
- **Genetics Home Reference** available at https://ghr.nlm.nih.gov/resources
- **An introduction to genetic mutations** available at www.khanacademy.org/test-prep/mcat/biomolecules/genetic-mutations/v/an-introduction-to-genetic-mutations
- **Regulatory genes** available at www.khanacademy.org/test-prep/mcat/behavior/behavior-and-genetics/v/regulatory-genes
- **So, what is epigenetics?** available at http://epialliance.org.au/what-is-epi

INTRODUCTION

Every nucleated cell in your body contains instructions on when and how to divide, when and how to migrate, how to respond to external pressures and when to die. These instructions are coded in your **DNA (deoxyribonucleic acid)**, which is packaged in genes housed in chromosomes in cell nuclei (Fig. 2.1).[1] Collectively, the genetic code that regulates cell behaviours and allows your body to function as one entity is what gives you your unique physical and behavioural characteristics and resistance or susceptibility to certain diseases such as heart disease, diabetes or cancer.

Errors arising in the DNA code during fetal development can result in genetic disorders or diseases that affect physical and/or mental development. These are diagnosed predominantly during pregnancy or within

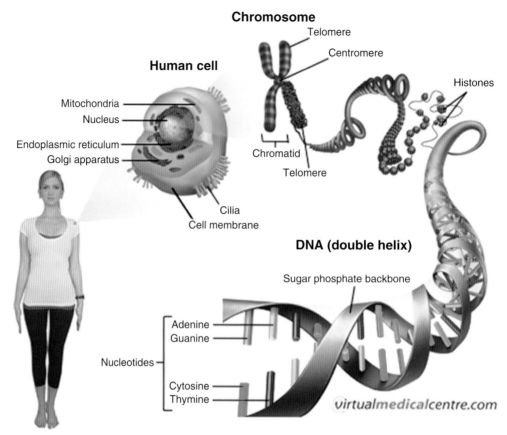

FIGURE 2.1 **From human body to DNA.** (*Source:* https://healthengine.com.au/info/dna-deoxyribonucleic-acid.)

the first few years of life. Depending on which gene is affected and how it is affected, these conditions can range from hardly noticeable to severe and incompatible with life. Genetic screening of maternal blood for detection of many fetal abnormalities constitutes part of prenatal care, as does the prenatal ultrasound. The non-invasive prenatal screening test (NIPT), abbreviated to NIPS in Australia, uses a sample of the mother's blood, collected around the 10th week of pregnancy, to isolate circulating cell-free DNA released from the baby's placenta into maternal blood circulation. Isolated fetal DNA is then subjected to complex genetic analysis to identify whether the baby may have common chromosomal abnormalities (Fig. 2.2).[2] This test is available in private obstetrics care centres and is currently not covered by Medicare. As the technology evolves, so will the power of this test to identify even more genetic abnormalities. Targeted prenatal screening for genetic abnormalities

to identify rare diseases also provides guidance to the best possible clinical and therapeutic management of the child once born. Knowing this information assists genetic counsellors to better understand the nature of the condition and the associated risks, and to translate that knowledge to inform the parents of the likely future for the child. This helps parents to make evidence-informed decisions regarding their child's care.

While genes are responsible for instructing the formation of all tissues and organs such as the heart or brain, genes are also susceptible to environmental influences, or what is commonly referred to as **nurture**. Thus, the development of a child's cognitive abilities will be shaped not only by the genes the child has inherited but also by the environment in which the child grows. For example, whether the child gets enough nutrition or loving care may determine the potential to which the

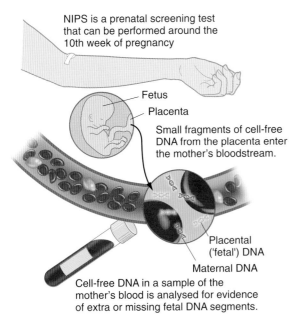

NIPS is a prenatal screening test that can be performed around the 10th week of pregnancy

Fetus

Placenta

Small fragments of cell-free DNA from the placenta enter the mother's bloodstream.

Placental ('fetal') DNA

Maternal DNA

Cell-free DNA in a sample of the mother's blood is analysed for evidence of extra or missing fetal DNA segments.

FIGURE 2.2 **Schematic representation of non-invasive prenatal screen testing.**

target the function of the defective gene or replace the gene with a functional copy. Such a targeted approach is known as **gene therapy**. Errors in DNA code are also possible as we age. As we get older, cancers are more likely to develop and our tissues and organs are affected by changes in structure and become less efficient in their function. If you want to trace your own ancestry or find your biological parents you may be directed towards commercial companies to find your relatives. Sometimes, information collected by these commercial companies can be searched by legal authorities to identify and arrest criminals.[3] Collectively, this information should help you realise that it is no longer possible to deliver person-centred care without understanding the basic biology of genetic and hereditary biology.

In this chapter, we examine what genes are and how genes function and code for protein synthesis and control mechanisms that give rise to traits that you have inherited from your ancestors. We also examine how errors, or mutations, in genes lead to genetic diseases and how a person's genetic makeup may lead to more personalised treatment and care.

child's genetically determined intellectual capacity will develop.

Advances in our understanding of the biology of genes have given hope that it will be possible to treat inherited genetic disorders by using therapies that either

THE HUMAN GENOME
Chromosomes

A healthy human genome contains 46 individual **chromosomes** arranged in 23 pairs and housed in the nucleus of each cell (Fig. 2.3).[4] Of these 23 pairs of

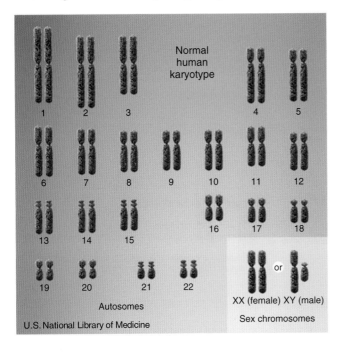

FIGURE 2.3 **Human chromosomes.** Human cells normally contain 23 pairs of chromosomes, with the 23rd pair being the sex chromosomes. (*Source:* https://ghr.nlm.nih.gov/primer/mutationsanddisorders/chromosomalconditions.)

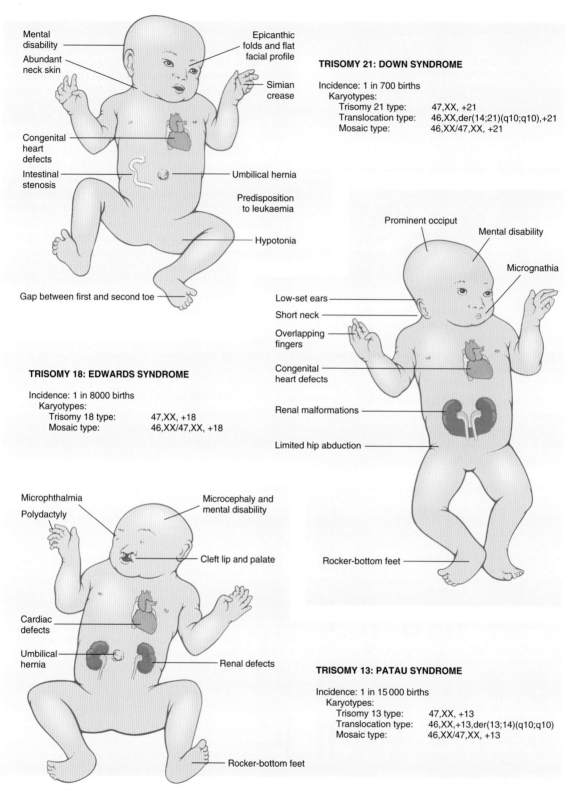

TRISOMY 21: DOWN SYNDROME

Incidence: 1 in 700 births
  Karyotypes:
    Trisomy 21 type: 47,XX, +21
    Translocation type: 46,XX,der(14;21)(q10;q10),+21
    Mosaic type: 46,XX/47,XX, +21

TRISOMY 18: EDWARDS SYNDROME

Incidence: 1 in 8000 births
  Karyotypes:
    Trisomy 18 type: 47,XX, +18
    Mosaic type: 46,XX/47,XX, +18

TRISOMY 13: PATAU SYNDROME

Incidence: 1 in 15 000 births
  Karyotypes:
    Trisomy 13 type: 47,XX, +13
    Translocation type: 46,XX,+13,der(13;14)(q10;q10)
    Mosaic type: 46,XX/47,XX, +13

FIGURE 2.4 **Clinical features and karyotypes of selected autosomal trisomies.** (*Source:* Kumar V, Abbas A, Aster JC. Robbins and Cotran pathologic basis of disease, 9 ed. St Louis: Elsevier; 2015.)

chromosomes, one pair is the **sex chromosomes**: a female will have two X chromosomes (XX) and a male will have one X chromosome and one Y (XY). The remaining chromosomes are called **autosomes**. You inherit one chromosome of each pair from your mother and one from your father. Once united in a new cell, these chromosomes have corresponding sequences of DNA and are termed **homologous chromosomes**. Each chromosome contains many genes. When cells divide, the individual chromosomes split into two thread-like strands, called **chromatids**. Each chromatid is made of double-stranded DNA. A change in the number of chromosomes will lead to issues with development, growth and function.[4] Any increase or decrease in the number of chromosomes is known as **aneuploidy**. An example of this is Down syndrome (trisomy 21): a child born with this condition will have three copies (known as trisomy) of chromosome 21 in each cell, to total 47 chromosomes per cell. Children born with Down syndrome and other trisomies such as Edwards syndrome (trisomy 18) and Patau syndrome (trisomy 13) are born with specific physical features and mental/intellectual disabilities (Fig. 2.4). Many cancer cells contain an abnormal number of chromosomes in their nuclei. Changes in the structure of a chromosome can also lead to diseases affecting development, growth and function. The effect of these changes is predominantly related to size and location of the gene affected and whether genetic material is lost or gained.

Genes

A **gene** is the basic physical and functional unit of heredity.[5] The term **human genome** refers to the complete set of genetic information needed to build and maintain the human organism. This information consists of DNA packaged in genes. Each gene occupies a specific location on a chromosome, known as **locus**. Genes come in slightly different forms in each person. These are known as **alleles** and are characterised by small differences in their sequence of DNA bases.[4] Alleles are always found on the same loci on homologous chromosomes.

Genes contain both coding and non-coding regions of DNA (Fig. 2.5). **Coding DNA** (a sequence of DNA that specifies the amino acid sequence needed to build protein) is found in portions of DNA called **exons**. **Non-coding DNA** (a sequence of DNA that does not encode protein sequence) is stored in sections called **introns**. Genes are inherited or transmitted from parent to offspring and become visible in the offspring's traits. While people have two copies of most genes, one copy inherited from each parent, some people are born with three or more copies of a particular gene or, conversely, one or more genes may be missing. This is known as **copy number variation** and while it impacts gene activity, it mostly causes no harm.[6] The Human Genome Project has determined that the chromosomes constituting the human genome contain approximately 19 000 genes.[4,7] The study of the human genome is known as **human genomics**. Using an individual's own genetic composition

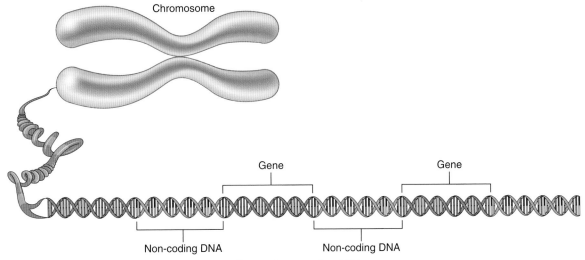

FIGURE 2.5 **Genes contain both coding and non-coding DNA.**

to diagnose a condition and prescribe treatment specific to that composition and person is known as **personalised medicine**.[8]

DNA

DNA is a code that contains a sequence of smaller molecules called **nucleotides**, which are connected by chemical bonds (Fig. 2.6). Each nucleotide has three parts: a sugar group called **deoxyribose**; a **nitrogen base**; and a **phosphate group**. There are four types of nitrogen bases: adenine (A), guanine (G), thymine (T) and cytosine (C).[7] These bases are connected in a specific arrangement, where adenine specifically links to thymine and guanine links only to cytosine. To remember this, the mnemonic <u>A</u>t <u>T</u>he <u>C</u>ricket <u>G</u>round might help (Fig. 2.6).

DNA is a double-stranded molecule, meaning that it is composed of two chains. These chains coil around each other to form a **double helix**, which resembles a spiral shape (Fig. 2.6).[1,7] The capacity to coil is what helps DNA to tightly pack into chromosomes. DNA is housed in the cell nucleus, with smaller amounts also found in mitochondria. Until recently, it was thought that mitochondrial DNA contained only the DNA inherited from the mother. However, there is a suggestion that in some offspring, the DNA may also be inherited from the father.[9] This is a significant discovery that impacts on the inheritance of mitochondrial genetic diseases that impair mitochondria's capacity to produce cell energy.

Another significance of being a double helix is that each strand can act as a template for developing new

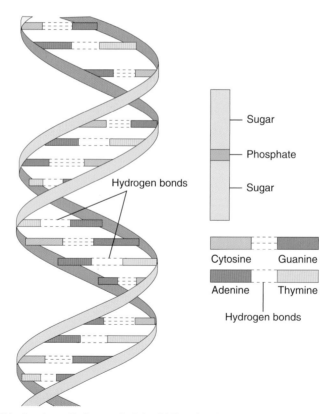

FIGURE 2.6 DNA structure. Each strand of the DNA molecule contains alternating sugar and phosphate groups, with each sugar group joined to the sugar group on the opposite site by a pair of nitrogenous bases. Adenine binds to thymine and cytosine binds to guanine.

copies of DNA, through DNA **replication**.[4,7] In this very complex process that is tightly regulated, DNA makes a copy of itself. The result is the exact number of DNA copies needed for two daughter cells, which are correctly separated during cell division and inherited by the daughter cells. You share 99% of your genome with the rest of the population, while the remaining 1% of your genetic code—that is, the order of the nitrogen bases in your DNA—is what makes you unique.[1] DNA codes for ribonucleic acid (RNA) called messenger RNA.

RNA

Ribonucleic acid (RNA) is also a code that contains a sequence of nucleotides connected by chemical bonds (Fig. 2.7). It is this code that will be translated into protein. Like DNA, each nucleotide that makes up RNA is composed of three parts: a sugar group called **deoxyribose**; a **nitrogen base**; and a **phosphate group**. There are four types of nitrogen bases: adenine (A), guanine (G), uracil (U) and cytosine (C).[4,7] Note that in RNA uracil (U) replaces the thymine (T) in DNA.

RNA is a single-stranded molecule and can be divided into three types: **messenger RNA** (mRNA); **transfer RNA** (tRNA); and **ribosomal RNA** (rRNA). tRNA and rRNA are coded by the non-coding DNA sequence and are examples of non-coding RNA as they do not code for protein structure. The role of tRNA is to read mRNA and translate that code into an amino acid sequence, which will later build a protein. rRNA is a major structural component of **ribosomes**—organelles that are assembled in the nucleus and either float free in the cytoplasm or are bound to rough endoplasmic reticulum.[4] Ribosomes bind mRNA and tRNA together to enable translation of mRNA by tRNA into an amino acid sequence.

Other types of RNA include **heterogeneous nuclear RNA** (hnRNA), **small nucleolar** RNA (snoRNA), **small nuclear RNA** (snRNA) and **small cytoplasmic RNA** (scRNA). For the purposes of this chapter and to understand the function of genes in synthesising protein, you need to understand the link between DNA and three different subtypes of RNA: mRNA, tRNA and rRNA.

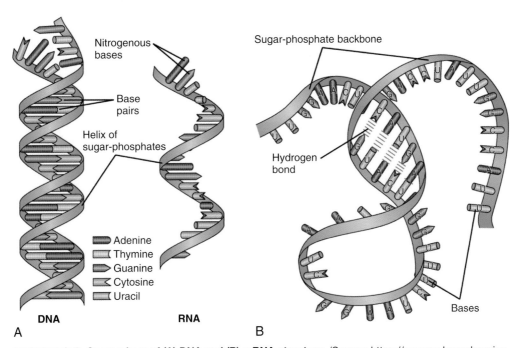

FIGURE 2.7 Comparison of (A) DNA and (B) mRNA structure. (Source: https://courses.lumenlearning.com/microbiology/chapter/structure-and-function-of-rna.)

Protein synthesis

Genes encoded by DNA are copied to mRNA molecules, which use that code to make cell proteins (Fig. 2.8).[10] Prior to being translated into protein, mRNA itself may be edited, at which point changes are made to the RNA nucleotide sequence, such as **insertion, deletion** or **substitution** of the nucleotide.[4,5,10] **Proteins** are one of the main building blocks of cells and their synthesis (formation) is one of the best conserved processes across all animal species. They form cellular structures as well as individual components needed for biochemical reactions occurring in the cells. These components are called **enzymes**. Enzymes regulate the rate (speed) at which biochemical reactions proceed in the cell (Fig. 2.9).[7] To understand the link between DNA and protein, remember that the instructions for synthesising protein are contained in DNA.

You also need to understand that cells synthesise new proteins only when needed rather than continuously. Imagine that your body needs more myosin, a protein molecule needed for muscle structure and function, as part of the repair of an injured muscle. The injury would generate specific cell signals that are sent to the cell nucleus. These signals instruct the nucleus cell machinery to express the gene for myosin. This expression starts with a process called **transcription** and occurs in the

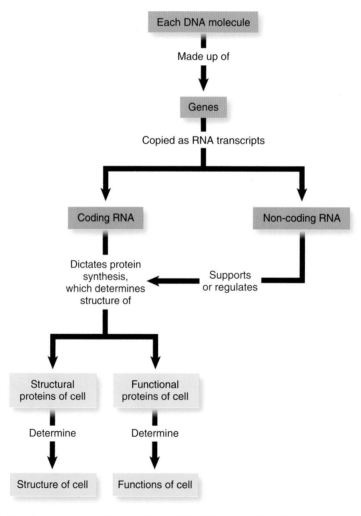

FIGURE 2.8 **Function of genes.** (*Source:* Patton KT, Thibodeau GA, editors. Anatomy and physiology, 10 ed. London: Elsevier Health Sciences; 2017.)

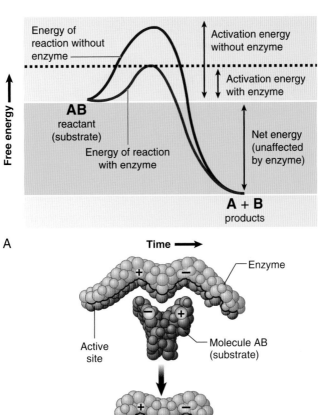

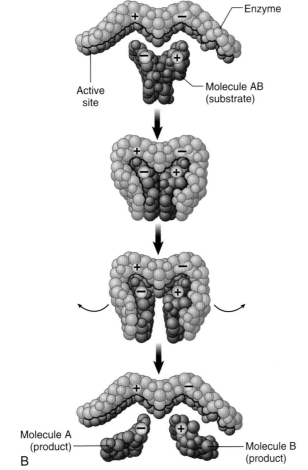

FIGURE 2.9 **Enzymes. A** Enzymes as catalysts. A catalyst is a chemical that reduces the amount of energy required to start a chemical reaction, thus allowing the reaction to occur at normal body temperature. **B** Enzymes have a specific molecular shape that allows them to catalyse chemical reactions. For example, a digestive enzyme acts on substrate molecules AB through a lock-and-key mechanism to produce simpler molecules A and B. (*Source:* Patton KT, Thibodeau GA, editors. Anatomy and physiology, 10 ed. London: Elsevier Health Sciences; 2017.)

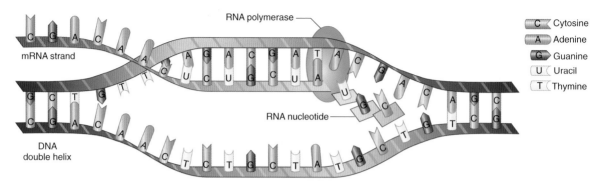

FIGURE 2.10 **Transcription of mRNA.** A DNA molecule unwinds in the region of the gene to be transcribed. RNA nucleotides circulating in the cell nucleus are aligned in a complementary manner (adenine–thymine and cytosine–guanine) and temporarily attach to exposed DNA bases of one of the single strands visible after the DNA was unwound. At this time RNA nucleotides also chemically bond to each other to form a chain of mRNA. The resulting mRNA strand is a copy of the opposite side of the DNA molecule. This reaction is controlled by the enzyme RNA polymerase. (*Source:* Patton KT, Thibodeau GA, editors. Anatomy and physiology, 10 ed. London: Elsevier Health Sciences; 2017.)

cell nucleus (Fig. 2.10).[7] Transcription occurs in three stages: **initiation**, **elongation** and **termination** (Fig. 2.11).[4,7] You can think of this process as simply rewriting information from one source to another, in this case rewriting DNA into RNA.

During transcription, a myosin-coding region of DNA is unwound and separated into single strands, with a small portion of the coding DNA split apart at a time. This initiation stage commences with the binding of RNA polymerase enzyme and one or more transcription

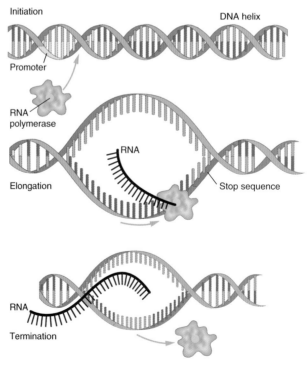

FIGURE 2.11 **Transcription of DNA occurs in three stages: initiation, elongation and termination.**

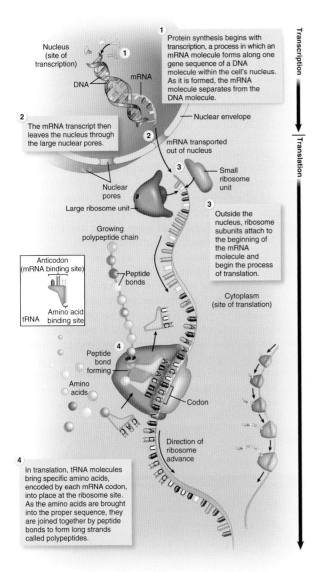

Transcription →

← Translation

1
Protein synthesis begins with transcription, a process in which an mRNA molecule forms along one gene sequence of a DNA molecule within the cell's nucleus. As it is formed, the mRNA molecule separates from the DNA molecule.

Nucleus (site of transcription)

DNA

mRNA

Nuclear envelope

2
The mRNA transcript then leaves the nucleus through the large nuclear pores.

mRNA transported out of nucleus

Nuclear pores

Large ribosome unit

3
Small ribosome unit

3
Outside the nucleus, ribosome subunits attach to the beginning of the mRNA molecule and begin the process of translation.

Growing polypeptide chain

Anticodon (mRNA binding site)

Peptide bonds

tRNA   Amino acid binding site

Cytoplasm (site of translation)

Peptide bond forming

Amino acids

4
Peptide bond

Codon

Direction of ribosome advance

4
In translation, tRNA molecules bring specific amino acids, encoded by each mRNA codon, into place at the ribosome site. As the amino acids are brought into the proper sequence, they are joined together by peptide bonds to form long strands called polypeptides.

FIGURE 2.12 Protein synthesis. Protein synthesis starts with transcription in the cell nucleus, when a mRNA molecule is formed along one gene sequence of a single stranded DNA molecule (1). The newly formed mRNA detaches from the DNA strand, it is proofread and edited for errors. mRNA leaves the nucleus via nuclear pores (2) into the cell cytoplasm. Here ribosome subunits attach to the beginning of the mRNA molecule (recognised through start codon) and commence the process of mRNA translation (3). During translation, tRNA molecules bring specific amino acids, which are encoded by mRNA codons (three base pairs code for one amino acid) to align them at the ribosome site (4). These amino acids are then joined together by peptide bonds (4) as the chain expands to form primary protein structures known as peptides. This process of elongation continues until the complete protein has been formed and a stop codon is reached to signal termination of the process. (*Source:* Patton KT, Thibodeau GA, editors. Anatomy and physiology, 10 ed. London: Elsevier Health Sciences; 2017.)

until the RNA polymerase reaches a specific sequence in the DNA strand known as a **terminator**, which instructs the RNA polymerase to end the **translation process**. The resulting mRNA then carries that information from the nucleus into the cytoplasm for translation into proteins.

Each mRNA encodes the information specific only to that one protein, in this case myosin. Because mRNA molecules are small, they are easily exported from the cell nucleus into the cell cytoplasm where they encounter ribosomes. We covered ribosomes in Chapter 1. Briefly, the ribosomes serve as an assembly point where proteins are made and are composed of two subunits.

mRNA interacts with the larger ribosomal subunit called 60S. This initiates recruitment of tRNA, which carries a specific sequence of three bases, known as **anti-codon**. Each anti-codon codes for a specific amino acid. The human body has 20 amino acids that are combined in numerous ways to make different types of proteins. Each mRNA contains a starting sequence (**start codon**) that is recognised by the tRNA molecule carrying the complementary anti-codon as a site where to bind. That same tRNA also carries an amino acid, a building block of protein. As additional tRNA molecules arrive and find their complementary regions to which they bind, the amino acids are linked by chemical reactions to form an amino acid chain. This process is regulated by ribosomes and uses ATP molecules to form the linking chemical bonds.[7] This process of elongation continues until a **stop codon** (stop sequence) is reached and the **termination** of protein synthesis occurs (Fig. 2.12). The

factors to the region of DNA known as a **promoter**, usually found near the start of a gene. **RNA polymerase**, together with the **transcription factor**, unwinds DNA from a double helix to a single strand. One of these strands is used as a template or code for translation. RNA polymerase reads one nucleotide at a time (adenine, thymine, cytosine, guanine) and adds a complementary nucleotide. For example, if the RNA polymerase reads adenine, it will add uracil; if it reads guanine, it will add cytosine. These additions are chemically linked to produce a chain. This chain (or transcript) is known as the **coding strand**.[7] This process of elongation continues amino acid chain that is formed is referred to as the primary protein structure. This structure can be modified by various cellular processes to yield more complex protein structures that are three-dimensional and have a unique appearance. These proteins are then ferried towards their destination sites and become part of structural or functional aspects of cell machinery.[7,10]

To understand how powerful this process really is, just consider that each time the final product such as myosin protein is synthesised, it must contain the exact sequence of amino acids (the building blocks) to form the same complex shape and integrate into the exact same cell location to be able to perform the exact same function every single time. All this is possible because of the information stored in DNA that regulates the myosin gene and the cellular machinery able to translate that gene.

Cell division

In the human body, cell division occurs by two processes. All body cells, except reproductive cells (sperm and egg), divide through the process of mitosis (Fig. 2.13),[4,7] in which a parent cell gives rise to two daughter cells. The second process, termed meiosis (Fig. 2.14), captures the cell division of male and female reproductive cells or gametes. It is characterised by the birth of four daughter cells from one parent cell. What is common to both processes is that when cells divide, exact copies of chromosomes must be inherited by each daughter cell.

The life cycle of the cell

Before we discuss meiosis and mitosis, you need to understand the events that lead to DNA replication and subsequent cell division, where cytoplasm and organelles are equally divided between daughter cells. In other words, you need to understand the cyclical nature of cell rest, cell growth and cell reproduction, a concept known as the **life cycle of the cell** (Fig. 2.15).[7] When cells are in a resting state—that is, they are not growing or dividing—they are said to be in the G_0 **phase**. In this state, cells simply perform the functions for which they have evolved. For cells that have a very low division rate, like neurons and cardiomyocytes (heart muscle cells), G_0 is a permanent state. If a cell receives a signal from the surrounding environment to divide—for example, to replace tissue lost to injury—the cell will enter a state called **interphase**. Interphase consists of several steps: G_1 phase, S phase and G_2 phase.[7]

During the G_1 **phase**, cells increase in size to accommodate the new copies of organelles they have made and that are needed to build the daughter cells. Cells also synthesise proteins and other biochemical structures that will be used as building blocks for daughter cells. Following this step, cells synthesise a copy of the entire

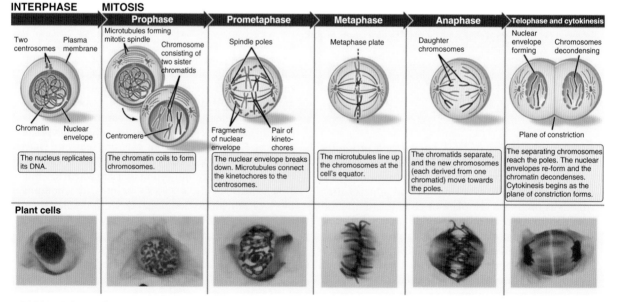

FIGURE 2.13 **The stages of mitosis.** (Source: Discover biology, 3 ed; 2006.)

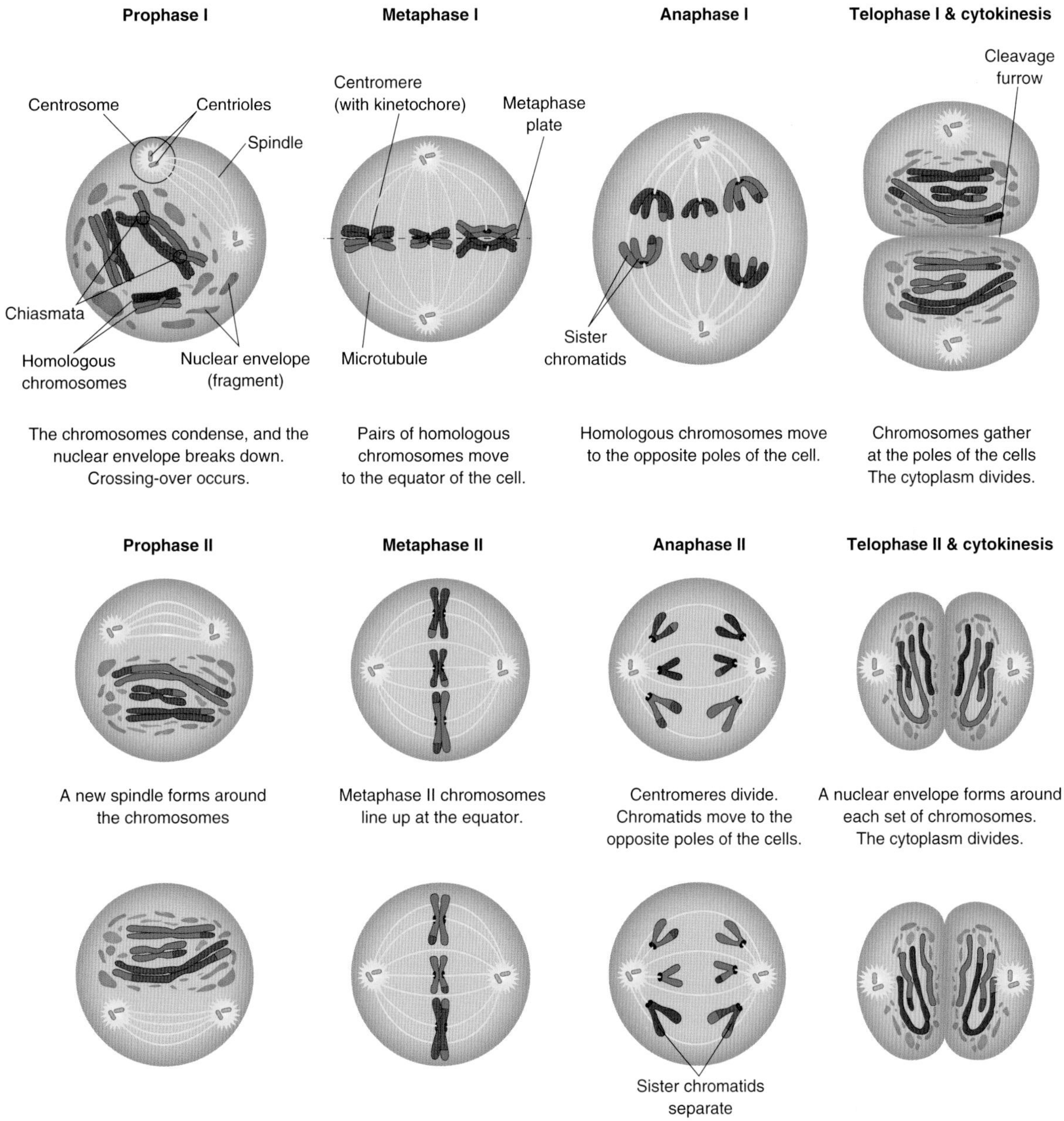

Prophase I

Centrosome   Centrioles

Spindle

Chiasmata

Homologous   Nuclear envelope
chromosomes   (fragment)

The chromosomes condense, and the
nuclear envelope breaks down.
Crossing-over occurs.

Metaphase I

Centromere   Metaphase
(with kinetochore)   plate

Microtubule

Pairs of homologous
chromosomes move
to the equator of the cell.

Anaphase I

Sister
chromatids

Homologous chromosomes move
to the opposite poles of the cell.

Telophase I & cytokinesis

Cleavage
furrow

Chromosomes gather
at the poles of the cells
The cytoplasm divides.

Prophase II

A new spindle forms around
the chromosomes

Metaphase II

Metaphase II chromosomes
line up at the equator.

Anaphase II

Centromeres divide.
Chromatids move to the
opposite poles of the cells.

Telophase II & cytokinesis

A nuclear envelope forms around
each set of chromosomes.
The cytoplasm divides.

Sister chromatids
separate

FIGURE 2.14 **The stages of meiosis.** (Source: Ali Zifan, via Wikimedia Commons.)

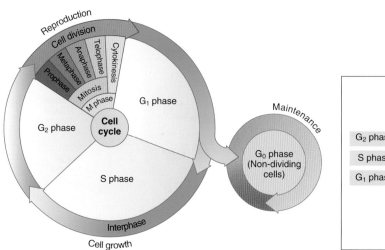

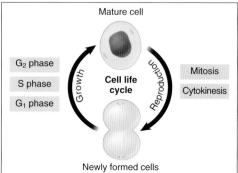

FIGURE 2.15 **Life cycle of the cell.** Cells go through cycles of rest, growth and cell division. Newly formed cells grow to maturity by synthesising new molecules and organelles (G_1 and G_2 phases), including the replication of an extra set of DNA molecules (S phase) in anticipation of reproduction. Mature cells reproduce (M phase) by first distributing the two identical sets of DNA (produced during the S phase) in the orderly process of mitosis, then by splitting the plasma membrane, cytoplasm and organelles of the parent cell into two distinct daughter cells (cytokinesis). Daughter cells that do not go on to reproduce are in a maintenance phase (G_0). (*Source:* Patton KT, Thibodeau GA, editors. Anatomy and physiology, 10 ed. London: Elsevier Health Sciences; 2017.)

DNA that is stored in the cell nucleus and form **centrosomes**, a type of microtubule needed to guide DNA separation in the later stages of cell division. This stage is known as the **S phase**. DNA replication (Fig. 2.16), making copies of the cell's DNA, starts at a specific site, referred to as the **origin of replication**. In this specific DNA sequence the enzyme helicase binds to the origin of replication and unwinds the DNA molecule to expose the base pairs on each DNA strand. Each strand then serves as a **template** to form a complementary strand of new DNA by incorporating the nucleotide present in the cell nucleus into the newly synthesised DNA. Just

to remind you: this is possible because the base pairs always combine in the same way: adenine binds to thymine, and cytosine binds to guanine. This process is referred to as **semi-conservative replication**, meaning that each new double-stranded DNA has one original strand of parent DNA and one new strand of daughter DNA. The enzyme responsible for DNA replication is **DNA polymerase.** Part of this process includes proofreading the new DNA and correcting any errors made during DNA synthesis. However, as we shall see later, the proofreading is not a perfect process.

Cells then enter the **G2 phase**, where they continue to grow as they synthesise additional proteins and cellular structures and start to order those structures for cell division by mitosis.

Mitosis

A hallmark feature of **mitosis**, which is also known as the mitotic phase or **M phase**, is that one mother cell gives rise to two daughter cells. In the M phase the cell nucleus contains chromosome copies, with each chromosome still linked to its sister chromosome. They are known as sister chromatids. The link between sister chromatids occurs via a centromere, a region of DNA where the link is the tightest. A copy of the centrosome is also present.

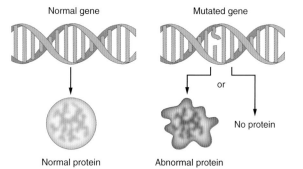

Normal gene   Mutated gene

or

No protein

Normal protein   Abnormal protein

FIGURE 2.16 **DNA replication during cell division.**

During the M phase, two sequential steps occur: cell mitosis and cytokinesis. Mitosis occurs in four consecutive phases: prophase, metaphase, anaphase and telophase.[7] During **prophase** the cell commences changes that alter its structure and prepare it for chromosomal separation. The chromosomes condense and the microtubules assemble to form a mitotic spindle, which captures and organises the chromosomes then acts as a guide for the chromosomes to travel in the right direction in order to later separate into daughter cells. The cell nucleolus, which resides in the cell nucleus, disappears and the nucleus breaks down to release sister chromatids (this stage is also known as prometaphase, the step between prophase and metaphase).

During **metaphase** the sister chromatids line up in a section known as the **metaphase (or equatorial) plate**, which is approximately located in the centre of the dividing cell.[7] The microtubules then pull the chromosomes apart in the opposite direction, which is possible as the centromere holding the sister chromatids together disintegrates. This stage is known as **anaphase**. In telophase, the cell starts to reorganise its internal structures as it forms two nuclei, one for housing each set of chromosomes. Chromosomes also change their appearance and the nucleolus appears. The mitotic spindle is broken down. It is during anaphase and telophase that **cytokinesis** occurs. Here, the contents of the mother cell are equally divided between the two daughter cells and the cytoplasm also divides approximately equally to form two daughter cells. By the time cytokinesis is complete, each daughter cell will have received an identical copy of a set of chromosomes from the mother cell.

Meiosis

The production of gametes—eggs (ova) in females and sperm in males—occurs through **meiosis**.[11] A hallmark of meiosis is that one mother cell gives rise to four daughter cells. Each daughter cell contains only one set of chromosomes rather than the two sets that the mother cell has. When a cell has two sets of chromosomes (46 chromosomes) it is called a **diploid cell**; when it has only one set of chromosomes (23 chromosomes) it is called a **haploid cell**.

Meiosis occurs in two sequential processes, meiosis I and meiosis II,[11] and each process is incredibly complex. **Meiosis I** comprises four consecutive phases: prophase I, metaphase I, anaphase I and telophase I. As in mitosis, parent cells that are meant for division to generate gametes also enter an interphase stage. Again, the cell must grow (G_1 phase), duplicate its chromosomes by duplicating its DNA (S phase) and prepares itself for

cell division and cytokinesis (G_2 phase). During **prophase I** the cell is diploid as it has 46 chromosomes.[7,11] Homologous chromosomes pair with each other and exchange fragments of chromosomes, a process known as **crossing over**. During crossing over, as fragments of chromosomes are exchanged so are the genetic materials responsible for various cell functions or physical or behavioural characteristics. Occasionally this process can go wrong and may generate chromosomes that are defective and therefore likely to give rise to a genetic disorder.[12]

During **metaphase I**, the homologous pairs line up in random orientation at the metaphase plate so that during anaphase I the homologous pairs can separate to opposite sides of the cell, with sister chromatids remaining together. It is the random orientation of the chromosome pairs that dictates which chromosomes will be inherited by the individual gametes. Towards the end of **anaphase I** and during **telophase I**, the cell undergoes cytokinesis and the new cell is haploid with each chromosome containing two sister chromatids, which are not identical to each other.[4,7]

During **meiosis II**, the same stages occur but with a different outcome. Cells that have completed meiosis I and are now haploid enter **prophase II**. Here, the chromosomes condense but the DNA is not copied.[11] The nuclear membrane breaks down and spindle microtubules form. The chromosomes (which are still sister chromatids) line up at the metaphase plate and separate to opposite ends of the cell as part of anaphase II. By this stage each end of the cell will contain chromosomes that have only one chromatid. Cytokinesis commences during telophase I and the newly formed gametes are haploid. The cell nucleus forms again and the spindle is broken down. This process is responsible for the development of very genetically diverse gametes, as each time a process takes place different chromatin cross-overs and different random orientations of the homologous chromosome pairs can take place.[4,7,11]

You may wonder at this stage why you need to learn about the cell cycle and the different types of cell division processes. This knowledge will help you to understand that each time a cell divides, regardless of whether it is a gamete or a somatic cell, the DNA replication process and chromosomal exchange of the chromosome fragments are vulnerable to errors. While the system has evolved so that many of these errors can be detected and corrected, some errors or changes alter the destiny of that section of DNA and with it the gene and the function it encodes. These changes in the DNA sequence are known as mutations.

Mutations

Mutations occur when DNA is copied in preparation for cell division and an error occurs during DNA replication, or when DNA is exposed to injurious agents such as ultraviolet radiation, smoking or chemicals such as benzene and asbestos,[13] all of which are also associated with the development of cancers. Alterations in DNA sequence are unpredictable and permanent. A mutated DNA sequence may either have no effect or result in detrimental outcomes associated with the formation of a defective protein or failure to make that protein. Clinically, this is evident as a spectrum of genetic disorders and some gene mutations can lead to severe consequences so that an embryo cannot develop and miscarriage occurs. At this point it is important to highlight that mutations can occur at both the gene and the chromosomal level.

Gene mutations are classified into hereditary and acquired mutations (Fig. 2.17). **Hereditary mutations** are those inherited from the mother or father, or sometimes both, and are carried by all of the offspring's cells for the duration of the person's life. These mutations are also known as germ-line mutations as the mutation is present in the gametes (egg or sperm) and therefore will be inherited when the affected gamete (e.g. sperm) fertilises an egg to form an embryo. **Acquired (or somatic) mutations** occur in a body (somatic) cell but not in the sperm or egg. These mutations are not inherited and therefore are not passed on to offspring. Although some somatic mutations are caused by exposure to harmful chemicals such as those found in cigarette smoke, many somatic mutations that occur during embryonic development have no known cause.

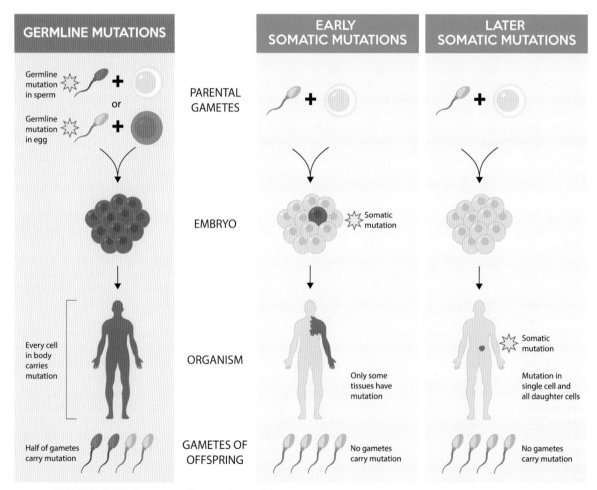

FIGURE 2.17 **Gene mutations and mosaicism.**

The term *de novo genetic mutation*, which is sometimes seen in diagnostic genetic pathology reports, is used to describe a genetic mutation that is identified in a family for the first time. De novo mutations can be hereditary or acquired. **Hereditary mutations** can arise in a single gamete cell (with all other parental gametes not containing that mutation) or in the fertilised egg soon after fertilisation. After the mutation arises, all cells that develop from the parent cell containing the first mutation will subsequently contain that mutation. **Acquired mutations** that develop in a single cell early during embryogenesis will lead to the development of **mosaicism**. This means that the person will have a mixture of cells that contain the mutation and those that don't. An example of such a mutation is overgrowth syndrome, where a mutation in the gene *PIK3CA* results in overgrowth of the affected tissue. If a PIK3CA mutation occurs in the left side of the brain during fetal development, that part of the brain will overgrow, leading to a rare neurological condition known as hemimegalencephaly.[14] The right side of the brain does not contain the mutation and so will develop to normal size. If that same PIK3CA mutation occurs in cells lining the lymphatic vessels (specialised tubes that manage fluid balance in your body and act as channels for immune cells to travel from a site of infection to an immune organ to form the immune response) it will lead to a lymphatic

malformation, which is usually detected during prenatal ultrasound screening or soon after birth.[15] It is likely that the earlier a mutation occurs during embryonic development, the more impact it will have on the function of the organism, including the health and appearance of that organism.

While gene mutations leading to diseases are rare in the general population, genetic changes that do not cause harm are more common. **Polymorphism**, a term that refers to an alternative form of a gene to the one expected to be found, is so common that it is considered to be a part of normal variations in the DNA sequence. Attributes such as hair colour and eye colour are due to polymorphisms.

Gene mutations also vary in size. For example, a mutation can involve a change in a single DNA base pair or affect a large segment of a chromosome that includes many genes. To describe a mutation in a gene, the following terms are used: silent mutation, missense mutation, nonsense mutation, insertion, deletion, duplication, frameshift mutation and repeat expansion (Fig. 2.18).

A **silent mutation** is characterised by the replacement or substitution of a single DNA base pair with another base pair but when that sequence is translated into mRNA and then protein, the same product is made and the protein function is not affected. A **missense mutation** involves a change in a single DNA base pair that leads

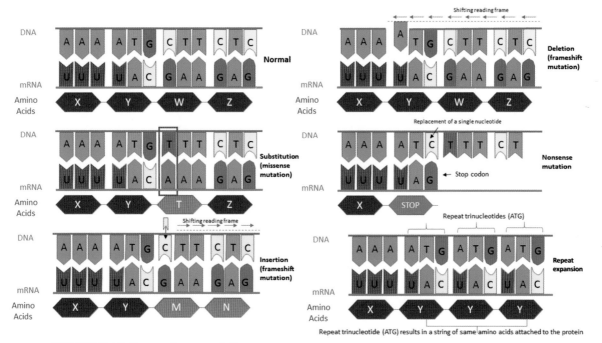

FIGURE 2.18 **Types of gene mutations.**

to substitution of one amino acid for another in the protein that is coded by that gene. A **nonsense mutation** also involves a change in a single DNA base pair, but this change results in premature termination of protein synthesis, thus resulting in the formation of a shorter protein that may fail to function. Silent mutations, missense mutations and nonsense mutations are also known as **point mutations**, as they all involve some form of change to only one DNA nucleotide.

An **insertion** mutation results in the insertion of one or more DNA base pairs, which results in a longer DNA sequence and incorrect code for the protein length. In this case the protein will be longer and is likely to have a defective function. A **deletion** mutation involves the deletion of one or more DNA base pairs; this can range from deleting a fraction to an entire gene, and will lead to synthesis of a defective protein or no protein at all if a whole gene is deleted. A **duplication** mutation involving duplication of a segment of DNA base pairs one or more times also results in defective protein product. A **frameshift mutation** involves the loss or gain of DNA base pairs that alters the reading frame for tRNA to make proteins. A reading frame is a sequence of three DNA base pairs that code for one amino acid. When a frameshift mutation occurs, the reading frame is altered in some way so that it reads differently than

originally intended, and the result is either insertion of a different amino acid in that place or even a premature stop in protein synthesis. Again, the outcome is a protein with altered function. It is important to point out that insertion, deletion and duplication mutations of DNA sequence can all lead to frameshift mutations.

A **repeat expansion** is a mutation that affect a specific region of nucleotide repeats, short DNA sequences that are repeated a certain number of times in that gene. A repeat expansion mutation leads to an increase in the number of times that short DNA sequence of base pairs is repeated in that gene. This type of a mutation also leads to the formation of a dysfunctional protein. When considering dysfunction of the formed protein, scientists usually refer to gain of function, where the protein is more active than would be expected, or loss of function.

With respect to **chromosomal mutations**, the outcome is a change in the number, length or arrangement of the chromosomes. These mutations are classified as duplication, inversion, deletion, insertion and translocation and are summarised in Fig. 2.19.

Patterns of inheritance

We discussed earlier that a child inherits an equal set of genes from the mother and father. What is also important to mention is that in general terms some

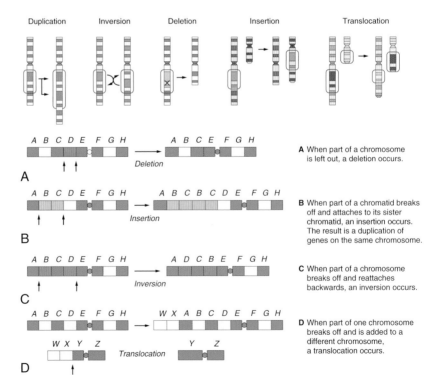

FIGURE 2.19 **Types of chromosome mutations.**

gene alleles can be dominant and some recessive. These terms simply describe how a gene specifies a trait or a characteristic in an organism. Remember that each gene has two alleles. Hence when a gene allele is described as dominant, the characteristic associated with that gene allele would be more obvious to identify. In the case of a dominant allele, only one allele is needed to express this trait. If a gene allele is recessive, that characteristic is harder to observe. For a recessive trait to be seen, you need both alleles of that gene present for the trait to be expressed. In humans, one example is blood group, which is coded by an ABO gene found on chromosome 9. Blood type A is a dominant trait, whereas blood type O is a recessive trait.[16] Let us consider the inheritance of genetic conditions that can be traced to a single gene to understand how this may work in real life.

Assume that a father carries a mutation in a dominant gene and his child inherits one copy of that mutated dominant gene: the child will develop the trait associated with that gene. This type of inheritance is known as **autosomal dominant inheritance**. A parent with an autosomal dominant mutation has a 50% chance of passing that gene trait or disorder onto their child (Fig. 2.20A).

Now imagine that a mother and a father each carry one copy of a mutated gene, but that the gene is recessive. In this case, for their child to inherit the trait (or disease) associated with the recessive gene, the child must inherit a copy of the mutated gene from each parent and therefore have two copies of the recessive alleles of that gene. This is known as **autosomal recessive inheritance**. If two carriers of a recessive gene have a child together, there is a 25% chance that their child will inherit that condition. There is also a 25% chance that the child will not inherit the mutation and a 50% chance that the child will be a carrier of the mutated gene (Fig. 2.20B).

Some genetic diseases are linked to X chromosome only and are known as **X-linked inherited** conditions. Recall that a female has two X chromosomes, whereas a male has one X and one Y chromosome. If we make an assumption that a mother carries a mutation in an X chromosome and the father does not, there is a 25% chance that their daughter will inherit a mutated X chromosome and be a carrier for that condition. However, if the child is male, as he inherits only one X chromosome and it is from his mother, he will be fully affected by that condition. It is common that X-linked genetic conditions affect male children very differently from female children due to the presence of the second non-mutated X chromosome inherited from the father (Fig. 2.20C).

This description of genetic inheritance is a simplistic explanation of what is a very complex process that is also influenced by the person's genetic background (i.e. their other genes) and external factors that influence gene expression and function, which is studied by epigenetics.

Epigenetics

Occasionally, the physical and behavioural characteristics that we inherit from our parents are not a result of DNA sequence or changes in DNA sequence but rather a result of external or environmental factors impacting gene function in terms of gene expression and activity. **Epigenetics** studies how heritable changes in genome that do not involve changes in DNA sequence are caused and how they impact on gene function.[17] Epigenetic changes can occur during fetal development or disease processes as well as cancer. An example of an epigenetic event is the silencing of the second X chromosome in female cells. Female cells apply epigenetic processes to permanently silence one X gene. This is known as X-inactivation and without this process female cells would not survive due to the damaging effects associated with both X chromosomes being active at the same time.[18] Changes in the number and structure of chromosomes and genes as well as the effect of epigenetics on gene function can lead to genetic disorders or diseases. These same changes also underpin the concept of personalised medicine, a medical model of identifying treatments that are most likely to help an individual based on their genetic composition.[8]

Personalised medicine

The philosophy behind **personalised medicine**, also known as precision medicine, is that every individual is different on the genetic and biological levels. Therefore, each of us is likely to respond differently to treatments such as pharmacological agents (medicines). Subsequently, in this transformative approach everyone would receive treatment tailored to their needs and this would lead to the most effective management of a disease. With the advent of technologies that enable scientists to sequence a person's entire genome in a relatively short period of time (about 1 week), it is possible to use this as a diagnostic tool to predict a patient's response to certain medications (a field known as pharmacogenomics) as well as to identify specific therapeutic targets that can be used to tailor the treatment.[19] You may have encountered these concepts already with media coverage of cancer genomics, whereby genetic analysis of a patient's DNA has helped clinicians to find the most effective chemotherapy or other treatment for the patient and impact them positively in terms of increased quality of life and time alive.

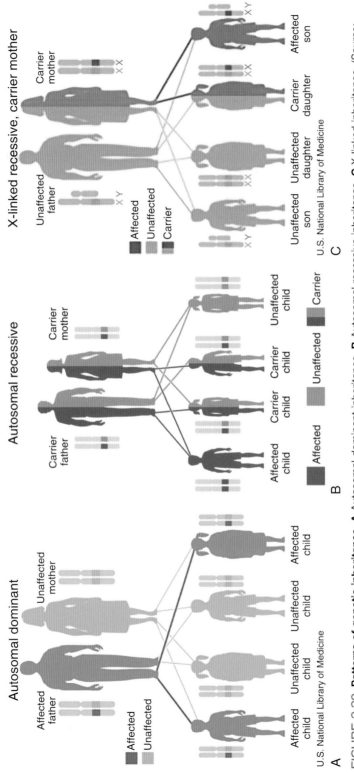

FIGURE 2.20 **Patterns of genetic inheritance. A** Autosomal dominant inheritance. **B** Autosomal recessive inheritance. **C** X-linked inheritance. (*Source:* Modified from http://kintalk.org/genetics-101.)

AGE-RELATED CHANGES

The process of ageing involves many cellular and molecular changes that in time accumulate to form the visible signs of ageing—for example, hair may start to turn grey and wrinkles appear around the eyes. The older person may also feel that they are not as fit as they were in their 20s. It is known that ageing in combination with lifestyle risk factors (such as smoking and drinking heavily) are associated with an increased risk of developing chronic diseases such as heart disease, diabetes and cancer.[20] Despite ageing being part of our natural life span, we understand very little about ageing both from a genetic and cellular process point of view. However, genetic studies comparing people who have lived to 100 years and beyond with people living shorter life spans have identified genetic signatures in terms of polymorphisms that suggest that life span is a polygenic trait. That is, this part of your life is determined by many genes; one study has estimated that as many as 179 genes may be involved in this process.[21] Therefore, you can look to your family's history and combine that with the risks you take (such as smoking, drinking, not exercising) to estimate your biological longevity.[22]

CONCLUSION

Nucleated cells contain genetic code that dictates cell division, migration, responses to external stressors or stimuli and cell death. This genetic code is our DNA. DNA is packaged in our genes, which are ordered in chromosomes. When needed the code is transcribed and translated to generate proteins, which are master regulators of cell structure and function. Errors in DNA codes arising during cell division can lead to hereditary mutations, which affect the development and health of the fetus, or acquired mutations, which can lead to cancers or tissue overgrowth in some settings.

Understanding the sequence of the human genome can be used to develop individualised treatment plans that are expected to improve patient outcomes. This is the basis of personalised medicine. Diagnosis of genetic mutations during pregnancy or within the first few years of life enables parents to effectively prepare for the birth of their child or opt for treatments that will minimise the impact of the genetic disorder. Developments in genetic technologies will continue to improve genetic screening of maternal blood for many fetal abnormalities. The ability to identify babies with rare diseases helps with diagnosis and possible clinical and therapeutic management once the child is born. Knowing this information assists genetic counsellors to better understand the nature of a condition and the associated risks, and to use that knowledge to inform parents of the likely future for their child, enabling them to make evidence-informed decisions regarding their child's care.

CASE STUDY 2.1

Sandra is seven months pregnant. She has just visited her obstetrician and a sonographer for a 28-week ultrasound scan to see if her baby is developing well. The non-invasive prenatal screening test informed Sandra that she is expecting a boy and that no chromosomal abnormalities were detected by the test. During the ultrasound, the sonographer detected that Sandra's baby had a neck mass and as he was not sure what it was, he phoned the radiologist and obstetrician to come to the room. The radiologist suggested that the mass might be a lymphatic malformation, a condition that develops due to a somatic mutation in the *PIK3CA* gene in the cells lining the specialised vessels that regulate fluid balance in the body. Sandra was immediately referred to the children's hospital which has a specialist centre that effectively manages developmental lymphatic malformations.

Q1. During mitosis, the alignment of chromosomes at the metaphase plate occurs prior to:
   a. prophase.
   b. anaphase.
   c. metaphase.
   d. telophase.

Q2. Before a cell can start mitosis, it first must:
   a. undergo cytokines.
   b. undergo metaphase.
   c. replicate its DNA content and duplicate its centrosomes.
   d. develop mitotic spindles.

Q3. What is the division process that regulates the production of gametes called?
   a. Mitosis
   b. Anaphase
   c. Meiosis
   d. M phase

Q4. Suggest why the radiologist might think that Sandra's baby has a condition caused by a somatic mutation.

Q5. Discuss why Sandra's baby's neck mass was seen at the 28-week scan but was not evident at the 12-week scan.

CASE STUDY 2.2

Samantha is a student at a research laboratory. A few weeks ago, she heard that the local clinic was searching for volunteers to donate a blood sample to determine whether a set of four genetic markers linked to heart disease could also be used to identify people at risk of developing heart disease later in life. Knowing that her mother's family had a strong history of heart disease, Samantha contacted the clinic to donate a blood sample. Two weeks later, Samantha received a phone call from the medical officer inviting her to discuss the findings. In Samantha's case, a de novo single point base insertion mutation was discovered in one of the genes that has never been reported in the scientific literature. This de novo mutation has led to a frameshift mutation and the doctors were keen to discuss what impact this might have on Samantha's future health.

Q1. What nucleotide bases make up DNA?

   a. Adenine, guanine, cytosine, uracil
   b. Guanine, adenine, thymine, cytosine
   c. Uracil, adenine, cytosine, guanine
   d. Thymine, uracil, cytosine, guanine

Q2. A single protein product is coded in:

   a. chromosome.
   b. nucleus.
   c. gene.
   d. base pairs.

Q3. In DNA, adenine always pairs up with:

   a. cytosine.
   b. uracil.
   c. thymine.
   d. guanine.

Q4. Explain what a de novo mutation is and how this type of mutation can lead to a frameshift mutation.

Q5. Considering the philosophy behind personalised medicine, discuss how this information could be used to educate Samantha on the likelihood of developing heart disease.

CASE STUDY 2.3

Georgia is a nursing student at the Women's Hospital. As part of her clinical placement, Georgia has been allocated to the maternity ward. Today, together with her nurse educator, she was present at the delivery of an infant diagnosed with Down syndrome during the first trimester (12-week) ultrasound. It is the first time that Georgia has met an infant with Down syndrome and she is keen to understand more about the condition as it may impact on the nursing care that she provides to this infant during the day. Her clinical educator suggests that Georgia review the genetic basis of the condition.

Q1. When the cell nucleus contains an increased or decreased number of chromosomes, the cell is known as:

   a. aneuploid cell.
   b. haploid cell.
   c. diploid cell.
   d. homologous cell.

Q2. Which type of RNA codes for protein?

   a. tRNA
   b. rRNA
   c. mRNA
   d. ssRNA

Q3. Choose the correct statement about mRNA.

   a. It is a double-stranded helix molecule.
   b. It is a single-stranded molecule.
   c. It is attached to an amino acid.
   d. It codes for carbohydrates.

Q4. Down syndrome is classified as trisomy 21. Explain what is meant by this term and discuss how trisomy 21 might have developed in this infant.

Q5. A child born with Down syndrome has specific physical features and varying degrees of intellectual disability. The physical features may include a small chin, slanted eyes, a flat nasal bridge, a single crease of the palm and a protruding tongue. Explain the link between trisomy 21 and the physical and intellectual features associated with this condition.

CASE STUDY 2.4

Tara is 36 years old and is an intensive care nurse who has never smoked or drunk alcohol and exercises regularly. Two weeks ago she gave birth to a baby girl, Zara. The pregnancy was uneventful and the birthing process was without complications. Today, she and her partner, Tom, have taken Zara to see the maternal and child health nurse at the local healthcare centre. During the examination, the maternal and child health nurse noted that Zara's left hand has a single crease extending across the palm. She suggested that Zara should be referred to a genetics specialist at the children's hospital as she might have Down syndrome. Tara disputed this suggestion and informed the maternal and child health nurse that she had a non-invasive prenatal blood test that did not identify trisomy 21 or any other genetic anomaly commonly screened for during pregnancy. Tara also stated that a single transverse palm crease can be found in a small number of healthy people and that Zara was examined by a neonatal paediatrician who declared Zara to be healthy. At home, Tom is concerned that Tara might be wrong and insists on phoning Zara's paediatrician. After phoning the paediatrician, Tom looks relieved as the paediatrician informs him that Zara is a healthy little bub.

Q1. Exposure to environmental stimuli that are harmful to DNA, such as smoking and ultraviolet radiation, may result in:

a. cell breakdown.

b. mutations in DNA sequence.

c. mutations in mitochondrial DNA.

d. no changes to DNA.

Q2. When the DNA sequence of one gene comes in many forms, this is known as:

a. copy number variant.

b. polymorphism.

c. aneuploidy.

d. meiosis.

Q3. Epigenetics is a field of science that studies:

a. how changes in DNA sequence lead to heritable changes.

b. how heritable changes in genome, which do not involve a change in the DNA sequence, occur and impact gene function.

c. how synthesis of mRNA affects heredity.

d. the process of protein synthesis.

Q4. Discuss the non-invasive prenatal genetic screening test that Tara took around the 10th week of her pregnancy to determine whether her baby has chromosomal abnormalities.

Q5. Zara's single transverse palmar crease is thought to be an event driven by genetic polymorphism. Explain what is meant by the term 'polymorphism' and discuss the significance of this in the population.

REFERENCES

1. National Institute of Health, Genetics Home Reference. What is DNA? Available from: https://ghr.nlm.nih.gov/primer/basics/dna.
2. National Institute of Health, Genetics Home Reference. What is noninvasive prenatal testing (NIPT) and what disorders can it screen for? Available from: https://ghr.nlm.nih.gov/primer/testing/nipt.
3. Editorial. The ethics of catching criminals using their family's DNA. Nature 2018;557:5.
4. Patton KT. Genetics and heredity. In: Patton KT, Thibodeau G, editors. Anatomy and physiology. 9th ed. St Louis: Elsevier; 2016. p. 1126–50.
5. National Institute of Health, Genetics Home Reference. What is a gene? Available from: https://ghr.nlm.nih.gov/primer/basics/gene.
6. Clancy S. Copy number variation. Nature Education 2008;1(1):95.
7. Patton KT. Cell growth and development. In: Patton KT, Thibodeau G, editors. Anatomy and physiology. 9th ed. St Louis: Elsevier; 2016. p. 120–36.
8. Blix A. Personalised medicine, genomics and pharmacogenomics. Clin J Oncol Nurs 2014;18(4):437–41.
9. McWilliams TG, Suomalainen A. Mitochondrial DNA can be inherited from fathers, not just mothers. Nature 2019;565:296–7.
10. National Institute of Health, Genetics Home Reference. How do genes direct the production of proteins? Available from: https://ghr.nlm.nih.gov/primer/howgeneswork/makingprotein.
11. Khan Academy. Meiosis. Available from: www.khanacademy.org/science/biology/cellular-molecular-biology/meiosis/a/phases-of-meiosis.
12. National Institute of Health, Genetics Home Reference. Can changes in the structure of chromosomes affect health and development? Available from: https://ghr.nlm.nih.gov/primer/mutationsanddisorders/structuralchanges.
13. Cancer Council Australia. What is a carcinogen? Available from: www.cancer.org.au/about-cancer/causes-of-cancer/environmental-causes/proven-risk.html.
14. Mirzaa G, Conway R, Graham JM Jr, et al. PIK3CA-related segmental overgrowth. In: Adam MP, Ardinger HH, Pagon RA, et al, editors. GeneReviews® [Internet]. Seattle (WA): University of Washington, Seattle; 2013.
15. Lokmic Z, Hallenstein L, Penington AJ. Parental experience of prenatal diagnosis of lymphatic malformation. Lymphology 2017;50(1):16–26.

16. Australian Red Cross Blood Service. Inheritance patterns of blood groups. Available from: https://transfusion.com.au/blood_basics/blood_groups/inheritance_patterns.

17. National Institute of Health, Genetics Home Reference. What is epigenetics? Available from: https://ghr.nlm.nih.gov/primer/howgeneswork/epigenome.

18. Keniry A, Blewitt M. Studying X chromosome inactivation in the single-cell genomic era. Biochem Soc Trans 2018;46(3).

19. Adams J. Pharmacogenomics and personalized medicine. Nature Education 2008;1(1):194.

20. Bauer UE, Briss PA, Goodman RA, et al. Prevention of chronic disease in the 21st century: elimination of the leading preventable causes of premature death and disability in the USA. Lancet 2014;384(9937):45–52.

21. Vinuela A, Brown AA, Buil A, et al. Age-dependent changes in mean and variance of gene expression across tissues in a twin cohort. Hum Mol Genet 2018;27(4):732–41.

22. Passarino G, De Rango F, Montesanto A. Human longevity: genetics or lifestyle? It takes two to tango. Immun Ageing 2016;13:12.

CHAPTER 3

Integumentary system

SUSANNE KAPP, PHD • ZERINA TOMKINS, BAPPSC (MED LAB SCI), BAPPSC (HONS), MNSC (NURS), PHD, GRAD CERT (UNIVERSITY EDUCATION)

KEY POINTS/LEARNING OUTCOMES

1. Describe the structure of the skin.
2. Discuss the function of the skin cells and the cell layers of the epidermis and dermis.
3. Discuss the role of skin wound-healing repair.
4. Explain the significance of the skin's contribution to regulation of body temperature (thermoregulation).
5. Link the function of the skin with other body systems to maintain body homeostasis, such as thermoregulation and wound healing.

KEY DEFINITIONS

- **Dermis:** the layer of the skin located under the epidermis. It is characterised by the presence of blood vessels, hair follicles, sebaceous and sweat glands, and nerves and receptors responsible for the skin's capacity to detect pain, pressure and touch.
- **Epidermis:** the outermost layer of the skin (surface), which lacks blood vessels and nerves. The epidermis acts as a physical barrier to invading microorganisms such as bacteria.
- **Hypodermis (subcutis):** found beneath the dermis, this is an area where a large amount of adipose tissue can be stored.
- **Thermoregulation:** a process that regulates the body's core or baseline temperature in response to changes in environmental temperature or the presence of inflammation or infection.
- **Wound:** an injury that compromises skin or organ integrity.

ONLINE RESOURCES/SUGGESTED READINGS

- **All about the skin** available at www.dermnetnz.org
- **Catalyst: Vitamin D—ABC TV Science** available at www.abc.net.au/catalyst/stories/2514231.htm
- **Clinical Guidelines (Nursing): Wound assessment and management** available at www.rch.org.au/rchcpg/hospital_clinical_guideline_index/Wound_Assessment_and_Management
- **Clinical Practice Guidelines: Burns/management of burns** available at www.rch.org.au/clinicalguide/guideline_index/burns
- **Thermoregulation** available at www.healthline.com/health/thermoregulation

---

INTRODUCTION

The skin, together with the nails, hair and glands, comprises the **integumentary system**. It is a physical barrier that separates the internal structures of the body from the external world. The skin is the most important armour that you will ever wear, as it prevents disease-associated deficits (morbidity) and death (mortality) that would be inevitable were skin unable to respond to a range of insults, such as physical trauma and ultraviolet (UV) radiation.

The skin is responsible for a range of other essential processes that ensure our health and wellbeing. These processes include internal temperature regulation, fluid balance, synthesis of vitamin D and a role in immune responses, which fight infection. The skin can show signs of allergic reactions in the form of rashes. It is rich in sensory receptors that detect pain, differences in environmental temperature, pressure or texture, and it communicates with muscular structures to enable you to move, smile and frown.

The skin has the capacity to heal itself following trauma. Wound healing is an intricate and orchestrated process that typically results in tissue repair. Most wounds are not complex, and many heal without clinical intervention. However, as the skin ages it becomes more susceptible to damage and impaired healing. The presence of other health conditions, such as diabetes, can also impair the skin's capacity to repair. Some wounds, however, are serious; for example, extensive burns and highly virulent skin infections. In these cases, the skin is under significant stress and the outcome can have a detrimental effect on health and even lead to premature death.

This chapter describes the structure and function of the skin and how the skin integrates with other body systems to maintain body homeostasis. It also discusses what occurs when skin integrity is compromised; for example, how the skin responds to environmental changes such as temperature extremes and repairs the damage made to the skin to regain body homeostasis.

STRUCTURE AND FUNCTION OF THE INTEGUMENT

To appreciate the skin's multifaceted functions, it is helpful to consider how the skin differs in some areas of the body. For example, the skin on the palms of the hands and feet is thicker than skin elsewhere on the body and it is also hairless (Fig. 3.1A). This structural difference arises from friction forces associated with the function of the hands and feet as they need to sustain various forms of stress and pressure over a lifetime. Skin on the fingertips has **parallel grooves** that can grip as well as facilitate sensation. This is important given the essential role that the fingers play in everyday activities such as eating, testing the temperate of water and turning the pages of a book. Skin that covers the rest of the body, including the arms, legs and face, is known as 'thin skin' and it contains variable amounts of hair (Fig. 3.1B).

The skin is composed of three structural layers (Fig. 3.2). The layer facing the external environment is the **epidermal layer** or **epidermis**. The layer beneath the epidermis is the **dermal layer** or **dermis**. Underneath the dermis is the **hypodermis** or **subcutaneous layer (subcutis)**, a connective tissue layer that loosely connects the epidermal–dermal layers to underlying structures such as skeletal muscle. The subcutis enables the skin to be pulled in one direction and return to its original position without trauma.[1] This functionality, however, is reduced as the skin ages, and is one of the main causes of bruising, particularly on the back of the hands, in the older person.

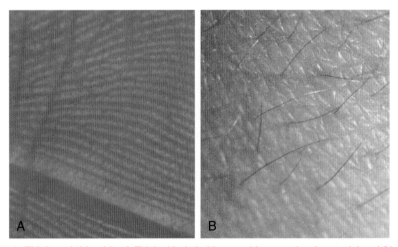

FIGURE 3.1 **Thick and thin skin. A** Thick skin is hairless and has regular deep sulci and friction ridges, which form the 'prints' of the hands and feet. **B** Thin skin has hairs and lacks print-like grooves. (*Source:* Patton KT, Thibodeau GA, editors. Anatomy and physiology, 9 ed. London: Elsevier Health Sciences; 2015.)

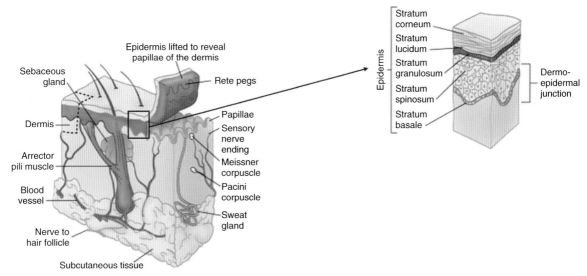

FIGURE 3.2 **The anatomy of the skin and subcutaneous tissue.** Skin is composed of the epidermis, dermis and subcutaneous layer (hypodermis). The epidermis and dermis are separated from each other by a dermal–epidermal junction that contains basement membrane. Note that in contrast to the dermis, the epidermis does not contain blood vessels, glands or nerve endings. The subcutaneous layer is responsible for skin's stretch and movement capacity and it is also a site of adipose tissue storage. (*Source:* Bryant, RA, Nix DP. Acute and chronic wounds: current management concept, 4 ed. St Louis: Mosby; 2012.)

The epidermis and dermis are connected by a **dermal–epidermal junction**. Microscopically, this area resembles finger-like projections known as **dermal papillae** (Fig. 3.2). The dermal–epidermal junction contains a highly specialised structure called the **basal lamina** or basement membrane, which is composed of various connective tissue molecules, such as collagen, predominantly produced by dermal epithelial cells and less so by dermal connective tissue cells (fibroblasts). The basement membrane components modulate cellular activity during tissue development, homeostasis and repair, and it acts as a reservoir for the growth factors that are needed for cell survival and skin repair.[2]

Epidermis

The epidermis is characterised by **stratified squamous keratinised epithelium**, meaning that the epidermal cells (keratinocytes) are organised in layers or strata. From the dermis and moving towards the most external layers, five layers can be distinguished by their appearance (morphology): stratum basale (stratum germinativum), stratum spinosum, stratum granulosum, stratum lucidum and stratum corneum (Fig. 3.3). Each layer represents progressive stages of keratinocyte differentiation and

function. The most undifferentiated (immature) keratinocytes are found in the deeper layers, while more differentiated (mature) keratinocytes are found in the layers closer to the surface of the skin. The most external layer, the stratum corneum, is acellular, meaning that it contains no cells.

The **stratum basale** is comprised of a single layer of cuboidal or columnar epithelial cells. These cells are connected to the basement membrane via stud-like structures called **hemidesmosomes**.[3] Genetic or acquired diseases that affect hemidesmosome structure can lead to skin disorders that present as blisters in the skin and mucous membrane.[2] Epithelial cells in the stratum basale are also connected to each other via localised spot-like cell junctions or **desmosomes**. During a mechanical injury to the skin, such as a knife cut, keratinocytes of the basal layer detach from each other, and from the underlying basement membrane, through dissolution of their intercellular desmosome and hemidesmosome-mediated attachments to the basement membrane.[2,4] These keratinocytes then start to divide with an intent to form a new intact epidermal layer, which occurs typically within 48 hours of injury. This activity is accompanied by deposition of the new basement membrane. Once

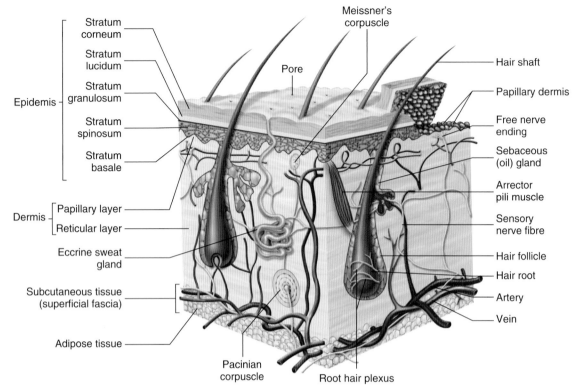

FIGURE 3.3 **Layers of the skin: epidermis, dermis and hypodermis.** (*Source:* Barbara L, Yoost LR. Crawford fundamentals of nursing: active learning for collaborative practice, 2 ed. St Louis: Elsevier; 2020.)

the wound gap has closed, the keratinocytes revert to their normal phenotype and attach to the re-established basement membrane and underlying dermis.[2,4]

The stratum basale **epidermal stem cells** are responsible for skin regeneration. This process occurs through programmed stem cell differentiation to keratinocyte lineage and generation of mature keratinocytes capable of making **keratin**, a key protein that is a structural element of skin, hair and nails. The term 'germinativum' in this case reflects the observation that keratinocyte division occurs in this layer.[1]

The **stratum spinosum**, also known as the spiny or prickle cell layer, is characterised by eight to ten layers of epithelial cells whose microscopic appearance includes cuboidal, polygonal and flattened cells. Characteristic of these cells, the desmosomes connecting keratinocytes pull parts of the plasma membrane of adjoining cells towards one another, giving them a spiky appearance, hence the name prickle cell layer.[1]

It is in the **stratum granulosum** that the epithelial cells of the skin commence the production of keratin.

Keratinocytes are arranged in two to four layers and contain small or oval structures called keratohyaline granules. The keratinocytes that are engaged in programmed cell death (apoptosis) start to break down in this layer.

The **stratum lucidum** is a thin clear layer present in the thick skin. This layer contains flat and closely arranged keratinocytes that mostly lack cells (**anuclear**) and contain eleidin, one of the building blocks of keratin. As keratinocytes break down, residual eleidin and tonofibrils form keratin, the main constituent of the **stratum corneum**. The keratin is further chemically modified, which leads to the formation of a waterproof, tough and durable physical barrier. Any damage to this barrier results in disruption of the protective function of the skin, thus enabling loss of water and entry of microorganisms or environmental debris.[1] **Thick skin** is characterised by a very thick stratum corneum whereas thin skin has a thin epidermal layer, including a thin stratum corneum.

During skin injury, epidermal growth and repair depend on the ability of the keratinocytes in the stratum basale to divide at the same rate as the keratinocytes that are apoptosing and sloughing off at the skin surface. This process is regulated by **epidermal growth factor (EGF)** and a hormone called **insulin-like growth factor (IGF-1)**.[1]

In addition to keratinocytes, the human epidermis contains other cell types. **Melanocytes** are cells that produce melanin, a dark-coloured skin pigment. **Melanin** is transferred to adjacent keratinocytes where it accumulates and protects against exposure to UV radiation by controlling the amount of UV light from the sun that reaches deeper layers of the skin.[1,5] **Epidermal dendritic cells (Langerhans cells)** are antigen-presenting immune cells that continuously check the epidermis for invading bacteria and foreign matter (antigens) so as to process and present them to the immune system for an appropriate response. **Tactile epithelial cells (Merkel cells)** are oval-shaped mechanoreceptors that detect and react to light touch sensations/stimuli and are found predominantly in the stratum basale. These cells are particularly abundant in the fingertips and hair follicles.[1,5]

Dermis

The dermis is comprised of highly vascularised connective tissue linked to the epidermis via dermal–epidermal junctions formed between the hemidesmosomes of the basal keratinocytes and the basement membrane underneath them. Anatomically, the dermis is composed of two sublayers: the thin papillary layer and the reticular layer. The **papillary layer**, which includes the dermal papillae, is composed of strong connective tissue built predominantly by type I and III collagen fibres, and fibroblasts, mast cells, macrophages and antigen-presenting cells.[2,5] The anchoring fibrils of a finer (type VII) collagen fibre connect the dermis to the epidermis by projecting into the basement membrane. The **reticular layer** is a connective tissue layer composed predominantly of bundles of type I collagen and a network of elastic fibres, which are responsible for the elastic properties of the skin, such as stretch and ability to rebound.[2,5]

The dermis contains hair follicles, sweat glands, sebaceous (oil) glands, and smooth and skeletal muscle fibres. This layer also contains an extensive network of blood vessels and lymphatic vessels, nerve fibres and sensory receptors that collectively enable the sensory function of the skin, fluid balance and regulation of body temperature.[1] Evidence of communication between the skin and skeletal muscle (voluntary) fibres is best seen in our facial expressions such as a smile. In the dermis of the testes and nipples, smooth muscle fibres

are responsible for elevation of the testes and erection of the nipples, respectively.

Hypodermis

The hypodermis is the deepest layer of the skin. Composed predominantly of adipose tissue, it contains macrophages, fibroblasts, nerves, blood vessels and lymphatics. The thickness of the hypodermis is associated with the person's weight; for example, in obese individuals this layer can be more than 10 cm thick due to the deposition of adipose tissue in this layer.[1] It is this layer that facilitates skin gliding over the underlying muscles of the body.

Hair, nails and glands of the skin

Hair is a thread-like structure composed of keratin, which grows from a hair follicle that is highly innervated and richly supplied by the vasculature (Fig. 3.4A). The visible part of the hair is called the hair shaft, while the part in the skin is called the **hair root**. The section of the hair follicle where new hair forms has a bulbous appearance and it is called the **hair bulb**. The hair strand is composed of an inner core, the **medulla**, and an outer section, the **cortex**.[1] The medulla and cortex are enclosed by the **cuticle**. The hair follicle is comprised of epithelial cells which are organised into external and internal **dermal root sheaths**. At the bottom of the hair follicle, a specialised cluster of cells (**germinal matrix cells**) undergoes a differentiation process to generate hair. The germinal matrix is in close communication with the **hair papilla**, which houses blood capillaries that supply the germinal matrix cells with nutrients and oxygen.[1,2,5]

The first hair is apparent *in utero* around the sixth month of pregnancy when the baby's hair follicles produce thin, soft downy hair known as **lanugo**. While rarely seen in full-term newborns, lanugo is evident in pre-term babies. It can also reappear in severely malnourished adults such as those affected by anorexia nervosa.[6] Between 33 and 36 weeks of gestation, the lanugo is replaced by **vellus hair**. Following birth, vellus hair is gradually replaced by **terminal hair**. This is evident in infants when a dark-haired newborn grows fair hair or their eyebrows turn from dark to reddish colour. During puberty, coarse pubic and axillary hair develops and is evident in the adult male on the chest, extremities and beard. In the female adult this process is less dramatic, with the more terminal hair confined to the pubic and axillary areas.[1] Hair colour is determined by the amount, type and distribution of melanin. As we age, 'grey' hairs appear; the colour arises from light refraction through a translucent hair shaft. Whether hair is straight or wavy depends on the shape of the hair shaft.[1] A cylindrical hair shaft will produce straight hair, whereas a flat shaft will produce wavy hair.

Associated with the hair follicle are involuntary **arrector pili muscles** (Fig. 3.4A) and skin glands (Fig. 3.4B).[1] Arrector pili muscles are responsible for movement of hair upwards, thus forming the skin 'goose bumps' we can see when we are cold. Through this function, arrector pili muscles also help regulate core body temperature (see the section below on thermoregulation).

Nails (Fig. 3.4C) are found on the distal end of the fingers and toes and their function is to protect the nail bed from trauma.[1] They grow from the matrix at the base of the nail bed with new cells arising from the stratum basale. The **nail bed** itself is highly vascularised,

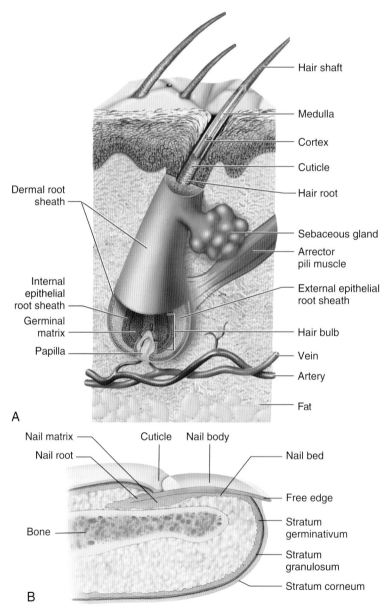

FIGURE 3.4 **A** Structure of the hair follicle and related structures. **B** Skin glands.

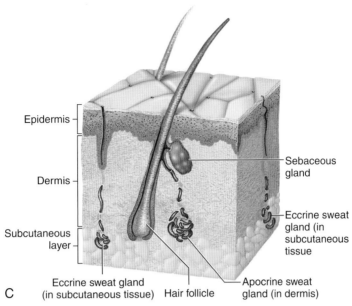

Epidermis

Dermis

Subcutaneous layer

Sebaceous gland

Eccrine sweat gland (in subcutaneous tissue

Apocrine sweat gland (in dermis)

Hair follicle

Eccrine sweat gland (in subcutaneous tissue)

C

FIGURE 3.4, cont'd **C** Sagittal section of a fingernail and associated structures. (*Source:* Patton KT, Thibodeau GA, editors. Anatomy and physiology, 9 ed. London: Elsevier Health Sciences; 2015.)

thus giving nails a pink colour. Patients who have reduced blood oxygen content will have cyanotic (blueish) nail beds, often the first anatomical location where cyanosis is evident. Abnormalities of the nail may reflect cutaneous and systemic disease or exposure to toxic substances.

Sweat glands are also present in the skin and they play a role in sweating (perspiration) (Fig. 3.4B). Sweat is a water-based product containing salts (sodium chloride) and other minor components. Sweat glands are a type of exocrine gland, meaning that they produce and secrete substances by way of a duct. The human body contains two types of sweat glands: eccrine glands and apocrine glands. **Eccrine sweat glands** are found all over the body and their role is to facilitate the evaporation of water (sweat) during the body's attempt to maintain internal body temperature (known as thermoregulation) at homeostatic levels. **Apocrine sweat glands** are confined to the axilla, genital area, face and scalp where they secrete various products but do not participate in thermoregulation. Sebaceous glands, which are found in the vicinity of hair follicles, express oily secretions and sebum onto the skin surface to protect the hair.

Thermoregulation

In humans, the normal body temperature range is 36.2° to 37.7°C. Temperature variations have been observed in different parts of the body; for example, the hands and feet are cooler than the trunk. Slight temperature variations also occur in response to activity, environmental temperature and circadian rhythm (also known as the sleep/wake cycle). The body's temperature is tightly controlled through the process of **thermoregulation** (Fig. 3.5) as it is a critical parameter needed for optimal cell function and survival. The process is a complex mechanism that relies on the integrated responses coordinated between the skin, the cardiovascular system, the respiratory system and the nervous and endocrine systems.

The skin is constantly involved in regulation of body temperature homeostasis via communication with the nervous system, namely the hypothalamus and the sympathetic nervous system, a component of the autonomous nervous system (addressed in Chapter 7). Thermoreceptors located in the skin, abdominal organs and spinal cord inform the hypothalamus on skin surface temperature (which reflects the external or environmental temperature) and core (internal) body temperature. When exposed to temperature extremes, the hypothalamus, in collaboration with the nervous and endocrine systems, responds to input from the thermoreceptors by activating an appropriate response with the aim to maintain the normal body temperature. Specifically, the hypothalamus can activate heat production, heat conservation or heat loss mechanisms.

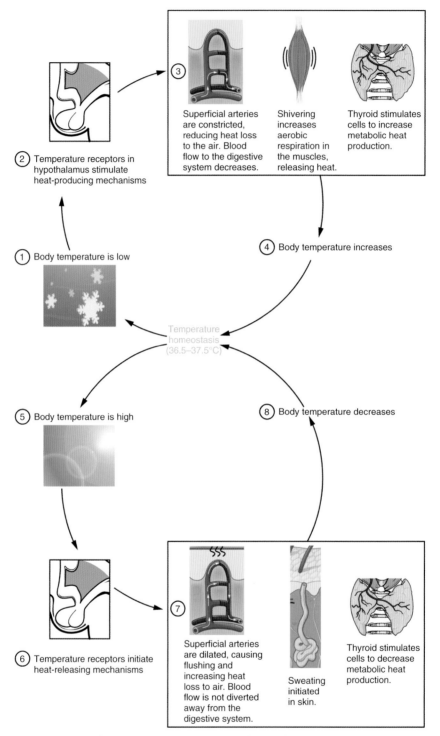

FIGURE 3.5 Thermoregulation is an integrated process that involves communication between the skin and hypothalamus. (*Source:* https://opentextbc.ca/anatomyandphysiology/chapter/24-6-energy-and-heat-balance.)

If you find yourself trapped in a very cold environment, such as being trapped in snow, your hypothalamus will activate mechanisms that will aim to limit heat loss and generate heat through increasing cell metabolism.[2] To produce heat, the hypothalamus synthesises and releases thyroid-stimulating hormone–releasing hormone (TSH-RH). This hormone stimulates the anterior pituitary gland to release thyroid-stimulating hormone (TSH), leading to stimulation of the thyroid gland to release the hormone thyroxine (T4). Thyroxine acts on the adrenal medulla, causing the release of adrenaline (epinephrine) into the bloodstream. Thyroid hormones also stimulate cellular metabolism to increase heat production which is then conducted to the rest of your body via your blood system. Adrenaline (epinephrine) causes vasoconstriction (improves thermal insulation), stimulates glycolysis (breakdown of glucose, the main energy source for cells) and contributes to an increase in the metabolic rate, thus increasing heat production. Sweat production is reduced to avoid loss of heat by evaporation.[1,2]

To conserve heat, the hypothalamus stimulates the sympathetic nervous system, which initiates an increase in skeletal muscle tone and the shivering response, thus increasing aerobic respiration in the muscles and heat release. The skin arteries vasoconstrict, further reducing heat loss. Communication between the hypothalamus and the cerebral cortex results in you becoming conscious of being cold,[2] and leading you to either move around or add more warm clothing. Once you are warm enough, this mechanism is switched off.

If, on the other hand, you find yourself outdoors on a 46 °C day, your hypothalamus will activate heat loss mechanisms by reversing the above processes. Heat loss also occurs through sweating, as heat is lost as sweat evaporates from the surface of your skin. This is known as a negative feedback loop.

Burns

To clinically apply your knowledge of skin structure, consider the damage inflicted by burns to the skin (Fig. 3.6). **Burns** are classified according to severity and depth of injury to skin layers, as follows: superficial burn (first-degree burn), partial-thickness burn (second-degree burn) and full-thickness burn (third-degree burn).[1] A fourth-degree burn is an injury extending deeper than the skin and involving the underlying muscle and bone.

- A **first-degree burn** results in damage that is limited to the superficial layer of epidermis. This type of burn is observed as redness and erythema, and is associated with pain and mild tissue swelling.
- A **second-degree burn** has damage that extends into the epidermis and superficial dermis. Blisters, tissue swelling and pain are typically present; however, hair follicles and glands in the dermis are unaffected.
- A **third-degree burn** involves the entire skin, and all vascular, neuronal and structural elements within the injured area. A third-degree burn presents as dense, white, waxy, leathery and/or hard skin. The skin may also be charred. There is typically accompanying loss of function in the affected area and, if muscle, bone and tendons are involved, the patient is at high risk of

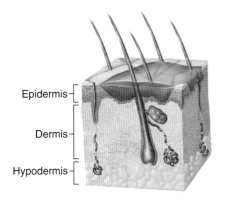
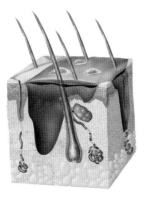
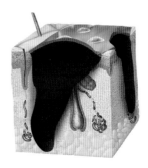

Epidermis

Dermis

Hypodermis

Partial-thickness burns	First-degree burn: damaged epidermis and oedema	Second-degree burn: damaged epidermis and dermis	Full-thickness burns	Third-degree burn: deep-tissue damage

FIGURE 3.6 **Classification of burns by depth of injury.** (*Source:* Patton KT, Thibodeau GA, editors. Anatomy and physiology, 7 ed. London: Elsevier Health Sciences; 2010.)

developing contractures. A contracture is a deformity that arises from loss of elasticity in the skin following a burn and is characterised by tightening of the skin in the region affected by burn scar formation.[1,2]

INTEGRATION WITH OTHER BODY SYSTEMS

To act as a barrier to pathogens, prevent deeper injury associated with physical trauma or exposure to UV radiation, regulate body temperature, maintain fluid balance, synthesise vitamin D and detect pain, the skin communicates with other body systems to perform these functions correctly. Furthermore, skin repair and regeneration are dependent on the person's nutritional status, age and general health. The following section discusses how the skin communicates with other body systems to maintain body homeostasis, such as thermoregulation and wound repair following skin injury.

Cardiovascular system

The link between the cardiovascular system and the integumentary system lies in the rich vascularisation supplying the skin and its appendages. The role of blood vessels is to supply oxygen and nutrients to the cells of the skin via arterial blood that is delivered into tissue capillaries, and to remove metabolic waste products, including carbon dioxide, via capillaries into the venous

system. The circulation of blood in the skin commences in the arteries, which give rise to two plexuses of anastomosing vessels (Fig. 3.7). The first plexus, which is found at the junction of the subcutis and the dermis, is called **cutaneous or deep plexus**.[5] This plexus supplies the adipose tissue of the subcutis, the deeper dermis and the capillaries that supply the hair follicles, deep sebaceous glands and sweat glands. The second plexus is called the **superficial or subpapillary plexus**, and is found at the junction between the papillary and reticular dermis.[5] This plexus supplies the upper dermis and gives rise to a capillary loop in each dermal papilla. The blood from these capillaries then enters the venules of the venous drainage system, which is arranged in plexuses corresponding to arterial supply.[5]

The vessels of the skin participate in regulation of blood flow (haemodynamics) through modulation of **vascular peripheral resistance** (see Chapter 13). Skin **arteriovenous anastomoses** or **shunts**, also known as **glomus bodies**, are unique structures that directly connect arteries to veins, thus bypassing the capillary blood network.[5] As part of the thermoregulatory role, in cold conditions the arteriovenous shunts reduce blood flow through the papillary layer to minimise heat loss. In hot conditions, blood flow is increased to facilitate heat release.

Another fundamental role of the cardiovascular system is evident following injury to the skin (Fig. 3.8). In this

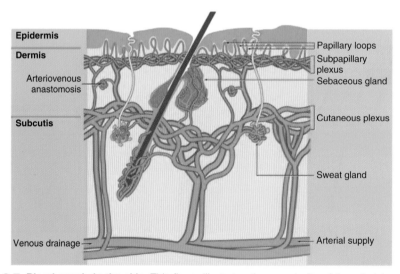

FIGURE 3.7 **Blood supply in the skin.** This figure illustrates the complexity of the arterial, capillary and vein structures that deliver oxygen and nutrients and remove toxic metabolic waste and carbon dioxide while participating in continuous thermoregulation. (*Source:* Wysocki AB. Anatomy and physiology of skin and soft tissue. In: Bryant RA, Nix DP, editors. Acute and chronic wounds: current management concepts, 5 ed: St Louis: Elsevier; 2016.)

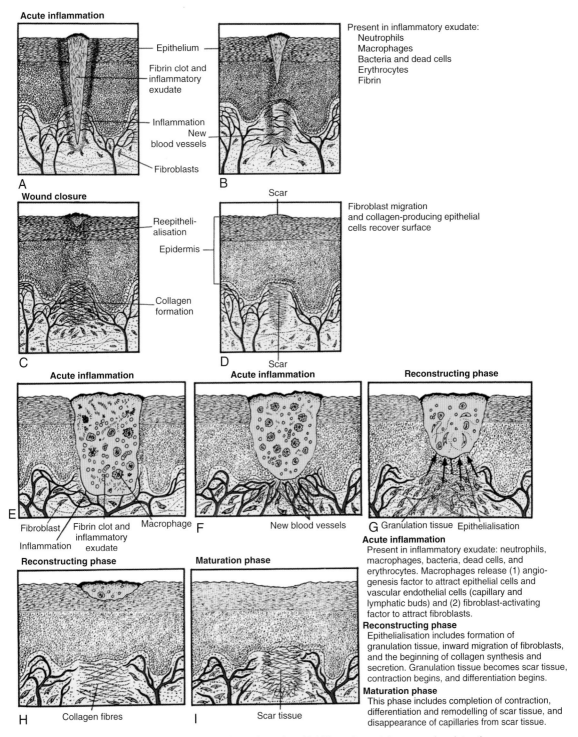

Acute inflammation

Epithelium

Fibrin clot and inflammatory exudate

Inflammation
New blood vessels

Fibroblasts

A

B

Present in inflammatory exudate:
  Neutrophils
  Macrophages
  Bacteria and dead cells
  Erythrocytes
  Fibrin

Wound closure

Reepithelialisation

Epidermis

Collagen formation

Scar

Fibroblast migration and collagen-producing epithelial cells recover surface

C

D

Scar

Acute inflammation

Fibroblast / Fibrin clot and inflammatory exudate   Macrophage
Inflammation

E

Acute inflammation

New blood vessels

F

Reconstructing phase

Granulation tissue   Epithelialisation

G

Acute inflammation
Present in inflammatory exudate: neutrophils, macrophages, bacteria, dead cells, and erythrocytes. Macrophages release (1) angiogenesis factor to attract epithelial cells and vascular endothelial cells (capillary and lymphatic buds) and (2) fibroblast-activating factor to attract fibroblasts.

Reconstructing phase
Epithelialisation includes formation of granulation tissue, inward migration of fibroblasts, and the beginning of collagen synthesis and secretion. Granulation tissue becomes scar tissue, contraction begins, and differentiation begins.

Maturation phase
This phase includes completion of contraction, differentiation and remodelling of scar tissue, and disappearance of capillaries from scar tissue.

Reconstructing phase

H   Collagen fibres

Maturation phase

I   Scar tissue

FIGURE 3.8 **A–D** Wound repair by primary intention. **E–I** Wound repair by secondary intention.
(*Source:* Huether K, McCance S. Pathophysiology: the biologic basis for disease in adults and children. 8 ed. St Louis: Elsevier; 2019.)

case blood vessels facilitate initiation of the inflammatory process, known as the **acute inflammation phase** (discussed in Chapter 16). This response is essential for repair of skin wounds and return of an injured organ to homeostasis. If the tissue injury results in severing of the blood vessel, that vessel will participate in blood coagulation, a process of blood clotting that leads to formation of a gel-like clot composed predominantly of fibrin, platelets and coagulation factors (see Chapter 11). The endothelial cells lining the capillaries in the injured area rapidly proliferate to form a new vascular network, a process known as angiogenesis. This vascular network is very dense and temporary in nature and aims to deliver more oxygen and nutrients to the repair area.[1]

The fibrin-rich clot provides a provisional scaffold for the uninjured connective tissue cells and blood vessels to migrate into the wound gap and synthesise new connective tissue matrix to close the wound gap. Once the gap created by the injury is sealed, a **reconstruction phase** commences. This phase is characterised by extensive remodelling in the connective tissue first deposited in the wound area, whereby the initial collagen fibres are replaced by tougher collagen fibres. As the need for oxygen and nutrients in the repairing tissue eases, some of the vessels start to apoptose, leading to a reduction in the number of vessels in that area.[4,7,8] The **maturation phase** ensues and is characterised by further remodelling of the connective tissue to form an avascular scar, which is characterised by an absence of blood vessels in the scar tissue.[8,9]

Clinically, changes in skin colour can be associated with changes in blood flow to the skin. For example, when you blush, due to endocrine effects the blood vessels dilate to facilitate increased blood flow to the skin. As the oxygenated haemoglobin in red blood cells has red pigment, your skin temporarily changes colour to a deeper red (blushing colour). A similar process occurs during inflammation and when fever is present, as an increase in vessel permeability and blood flow associated with the inflammation gives the skin a brighter red appearance. Similarly, if you look pale when you are cold, your blood vessels have constricted to conserve heat, thus reducing blood flow to your cheeks. If a person has a bluish appearance, this may be due to haemoglobin carrying high levels of carbon dioxide, a condition referred to as cyanosis. Trauma to blood vessels, such as that inflicted by physical injury, results in deposition and trapping of red blood cells in the damaged area. As the trapped red blood cells lose their oxygen they turn a bluish colour and you see this as a bruise.[1] Over time, as tissue macrophages start to repair tissue and digest red blood cells, a breakdown of haemoglobin to haemosiderin iron-free bile pigments will occur. **Haemosiderin** is an orange-brown colour while iron-free bile pigments range from green to yellow in colour. You can see evidence of these changes on your skin as a bruise changes colour from dark blue to purple to green and then yellow until it disappears. This disappearance is associated with recovery of the damaged blood vessels and removal of cellular debris by macrophages.

Lymphatic system

The relationship between the skin and the lymphatic system is most evident in the maintenance of skin fluid homeostasis and the transport of foreign antigens from skin to lymph nodes, where the immune response takes place. As blood flows from arteries to veins through the capillary network, some fluid leaks from the capillaries into the skin layers. This fluid is known as **interstitial fluid**. To prevent accumulation of interstitial fluid in the skin, the lymphatic vessels (see Chapter 14) of the skin, which start as closed-ended unidirectional capillaries in the superficial layers of the dermis, collect the interstitial fluid. Once inside the initial lymphatic capillary, the interstitial fluid is called **lymph**. The lymph is transported to the pre-collecting vessels, which are found in the deeper layers of the dermis. These merge into larger lymphatic ducts, which predominantly reside in the hypodermis. From there the lymphatic vessels join the systemic lymphatic vessel network to return lymph to the central venous circulation via lymphatic ducts. Patients who lack functional lymphatic vessels will experience a build-up of interstitial fluid in the skin, which is evident as **oedema**. Chronic presence of oedema, known as **lymphoedema**, can lead to inflammation and cause disruption of skin integrity, leading to skin infection known as **cellulitis**. Impairment of the skin barrier weakens the skin's capacity to act as a barrier to microorganisms. The skin's resident immune cells immediately respond to any microorganisms that enter the broken area by either activating on-site immune response or transporting captured components of the microorganisms to the lymph nodes, where the systemic immune response can be mounted. This transport of skin immune cells is facilitated by the lymphatic system.

Nervous system

Integration between the nervous system (see Chapter 7) and the skin is evident in many aspects. For example, the effective function of skin blood vessels, skin glands, the base of hair follicles in the dermis and arrector pili muscle fibres is due to them being innervated. The skin's role in transmitting sensations of pain, pressure, vibrations, touch and temperature is also enabled by the presence of specialised peripheral nerves and their communication with the central nervous system. Collectively, these processes protect the human body from events that would otherwise result in harm. For example, an inability to sense that a surface is hot would result in a burn that could compromise skin integrity and predispose the person to infection. Ability to detect different type of sensations is due to the presence of a dense network of free nerve endings in the epidermis. These nerve endings act as sensory receptors and are called **exteroceptors**, meaning they are located very near the surface of the body. Exteroceptors are classified by structure and referred to as either **free nerve endings** or **encapsulated nerve endings**, the distinction being the type of connective tissue capsule that surrounds the nerve terminal end. In the skin, free nerve endings are seen in primary sensory pain receptors (**nociceptors**), tactile discs and root hair plexuses, which control hair movement.

Thermoreceptors, which can be cold receptors or warm receptors, are free nerve endings that are crucial in thermoregulation. Warm receptors are activated above 25°C and increase their nerve impulse firing until 46°C. Thereafter, the sensation of burning pain begins. Cold receptors are activated between 10°C and 40°C, with a gradual decrease in functional capacity below 10°C evident as pins and needles experienced when freezing cold. **Tactile receptors** can be either free nerve endings without encapsulation or with encapsulation at the endings. Free nerve endings are responsible for sensing skin movement, itches and tickles. Discrimination between light and deep touch is possible on account of the structural differences in tactile receptors. Free nerve endings called **Merkel discs** detect light touch, whereas Meissner corpuscles, which are encapsulated mechanoreceptors, detect deep touch. **Meissner corpuscles** have two anatomical variants: a bulboid corpuscle, also known as a Krause end bulb; and a bulbous corpuscle, also known as a Ruffini corpuscle. **Bulboid corpuscles** detect touch and low-frequency vibrations, whereas bulbous corpuscles detect crude, heavy and persistent touch. **Lamellar corpuscles** (Pacini corpuscles), characterised by thick laminated connective tissue, located deep in the dermis, detect sensations of tissue distortion due to deep pressure, high-frequency vibrations and stretch. Extensive injury to these receptors, such as a deep burn, leads to loss of function of these receptors.

Muscular system

The skin is closely integrated to the underlying skeletal muscles through retinacular ligaments, blood vessels, lymphatic vessels and nerves that link the hypodermis and the skeletal muscle.[1] These links enable the skin to glide over muscles as movement or muscle contraction occurs. This can easily be demonstrated by observing what occurs to the skin covering your forearm as you flex your fist and rotate it. Degeneration of these connections results in restrictions of movement in the affected part; for example, as seen during extensive permanent skin scarring (contractures) associated with a full-thickness burn.[1] As discussed in the section on thermoregulation, the arrector pili muscles, which are attached to hair follicles in the dermis and help thermoregulation, are bundles of smooth muscle. These muscles are involuntary and are innervated by the sympathetic neurons derived from the autonomic nervous system.

Immune system

Skin epithelial cells create a keratinised barrier that provides a physical barrier against invading microorganisms. The immune cells residing in the skin include epidermal antigen-presenting Langerhans cells, dermal interstitial dendritic cells, tissue macrophages, histamine-containing mast cells, dendrocytes and T- and B-lymphocytes.[1,2] Such a wide range of cell types, which regularly participate in surveillance of the tissue for microorganisms, provides a broad spectrum of immune responses ranging from combating the invading microorganism on site through to a localised immune response to facilitating the transport of the antigens to lymph nodes and to an immune response at the systemic level. Epidermal **Langerhans cells** and dermal **dendritic cells** have the capacity to recognise and uptake a foreign antigen, which is then processed and presented to sensitised T regulatory lymphocytes.[1,2] **Dermal macrophages**, which are derived from blood-circulating monocytes, act as scavengers as they engulf and digest the microorganism (known as **phagocytosis**) or cellular debris. Mast cells are concentrated in the dermal papilla, near epidermal appendages, blood vessels and nerves. Their role is most prominent in allergic reactions and during inflammation, when they release histamine, which increases vascular permeability and promotes phagocytosis and white blood cell migration into the injured area. Dermal dendrocytes are also phagocytes, which are distributed through the dermis, near vessels in the subpapillary plexus, reticular dermis and subcutaneous fat.[1,5]

Endocrine system

Skin structures respond to various hormones that facilitate skin's capacity to repair and maintain skin integrity. However, the most significant connection between the skin and the endocrine system where skin

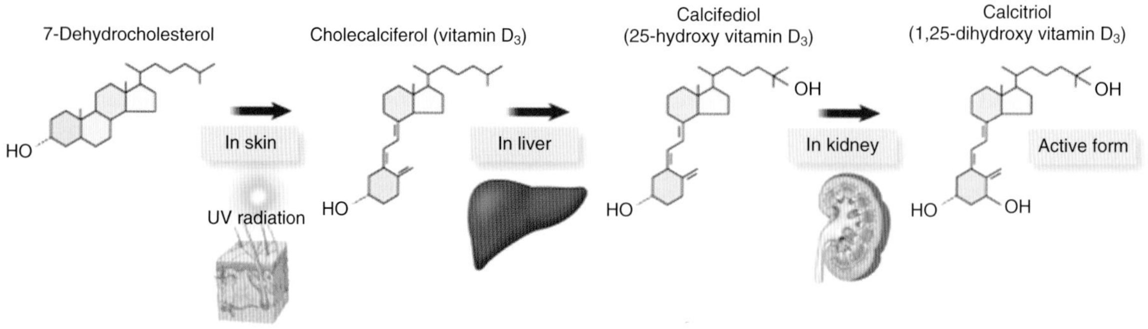

FIGURE 3.9 **The first step in the synthesis of vitamin D is skin exposure to sunlight, which leads to conversion of 7-dehydrocholesterol to cholecalciferol.** Cholecalciferol is then transported to kidneys and liver, where it is converted to calcitriol, an active form of vitamin D. (*Source:* Patton KT, Thibodeau GA, editors. Anatomy and physiology, 9 ed. London: Elsevier Health Sciences; 2015.)

plays a direct role is that of vitamin D synthesis (Fig. 3.9). The synthesis of vitamin D, which is actually a hormone, starts in the skin through skin exposure to sunlight, forming a vitamin D precursor that is then transported to the kidneys and liver for activation. Specifically, the UV rays convert vitamin D precursor (7-dehydrocholesterol, also known as pro-vitamin D3) to pre-vitamin D3 (**cholecalciferol**). So how does this occur? The skin stores a sterol compound called 7-dehydrocholesterol. Upon exposure to sunlight's UV rays, this compound is converted to cholecalciferol or vitamin D. This compound is also present in the vitamin D pills that your doctor will recommend if you are deficient in vitamin D. Cholecalciferol is then transported to the kidneys and liver where it is converted to calcitriol, an active form of vitamin D.[1] Vitamin D is needed for calcium and phosphate metabolism and bone mineralisation.[1,5] Calcium is effectively used to build bones is affected by exposure to sun, which can be low due to high concerns of developing skin cancers. According to Cancer Council Australia: 'Approximately two in three Australians will be diagnosed with skin cancer by the time they are 70, with more than 750,000 people treated for one or more non-melanoma skin cancers in Australia each year.'[10]

Children who are deficient in vitamin D due to low exposure to sun and poor dietary intake experience softening and weakening of bones and can develop fractures and skeletal deformities. Adults experience a similar clinical presentation and the condition is referred to as osteomalacia. Synthesis of vitamin D is higher in lightly pigmented skin and lower in darkly pigmented skin due to the amount of melanin present in the skin.[1] Melanin, a dark pigment responsible for producing skin colour, is transferred to adjacent keratinocytes where it accumulates to protect the skin by absorbing the incoming UV rays and preventing them from reaching deeper skin layers. Other clinical conditions that have also been linked to vitamin D deficiency include childhood allergies, negative mood changes, impaired cognitive status, cardiovascular disease, diabetes and some cancers.[5]

AGE-RELATED CHANGES

The ageing of the skin is the result of internal and external factors that the person is exposed to as a function of time. As we age, the skin starts to look thinner, paler and more translucent. External factors that can often accelerate skin ageing include excessive exposure to sun, cigarette smoking, poor health status and prolonged exposure to environmental toxins. Intrinsic factors include genetically driven processes such as modification of the genes regulating skin function, age-associated loss of connective tissue elasticity needed to maintain the mechanical properties of the skin, and decreased cell division capacity. Thus, imbalances in internal factors affecting skin homeostasis lead to wrinkle formation and hair loss, blisters and rashes, and life-threatening cancers and disorders of immune regulation. For example, while long-term exposure to sunlight results in premature skin ageing, it also blunts immunological responses to invading microorganisms and increases the likelihood of developing a variety of skin cancers.[5] While natural age-related changes in skin characteristics cannot be changed, reducing exposure to harmful extrinsic factors such as excessive exposure to UV and cigarette smoking may delay the appearance of age-related changes.

CONCLUSION

The skin, nails, hair and sweat glands comprise the integumentary system. As an elastic physical barrier that separates the internal structures of the body from the external world, the skin supports changes to body contours without injury. As the body's largest organ, the skin has a protective role against infection, injury, UV exposure and heat, and is responsible for a range of other essential processes that ensure body homeostasis. These include detection of pain, changes in pressure or texture, internal temperature regulation, fluid balance, synthesis of vitamin D, participation in immune responses, excretion of sweat and manifestation of signs of allergic reactions. Furthermore, the skin responds to different types of injury to repair and regenerate the injured area. To perform these functions effectively, the skin communicates with other body systems. Inability to integrate with other body systems results in loss of skin integrity. Age-related changes predominantly affect mechanical properties of the skin with increased decline more obvious as a person gets older. These changes cannot be stopped or reversed; however, decreasing exposure to factors that lead to accelerated age-related changes can be slowed down.

CASE STUDY 3.1

Following his morning shower, 65-year-old wheat farmer Joe dried his skin and proceeded to dress for the day ahead working in the cane fields. After applying his wristwatch, he hastily pushed the watchband up his forearm, causing his skin to tear. Joe placed a clean towel on the wound to stem the bleeding and applied moderate pressure. After 10 minutes the wound stopped bleeding and Joe identified a 3 cm wide, triangular shaped superficial skin tear. The flap of skin that had torn was still attached to one side of the wound. Joe carefully removed his wristwatch and proceeded to rinse the skin tear for 10 minutes under a gentle stream of warm water. While doing so the flap of skin moved back into its original position. Joe applied a sterile, low-adhesive foam dressing carefully over the wound. He then secured the dressing in place with a firm bandage.

Q1. Which skin layer contains blood vessels, nerve structures and sweat glands?

    a. Epidermis

    b. Dermis

    c. Subcutaneous layer

    d. Stratum germinativum

Q2. In which layers of the epidermis does keratin formation start?

    a. Stratum spinosum

    b. Stratum granulosum

    c. Stratum germinativum

    d. Stratum lucidum

Q3. Which of the following roles of the skin was most significantly compromised as a result of Joe's skin tear?

    a. Thermoregulation of body temperature

    b. Protective barrier

    c. Sweat excretion

    d. Production of sebum

Q4. Suggest which skin layers were most likely affected when Joe sustained his skin tear.

Q5. Outline age-related changes that have contributed to Joe's skin tearing.

CASE STUDY 3.2

Dave and Zara went to Mount Kosciuszko for a camping trip. Dave was an experienced camper and he packed the camping gear to suit the cold dry winter conditions. There was no snow yet, but the nights were cold, so Dave packed sleeping bags for subzero temperatures. Zara is not an experienced camper and Dave knows that occasionally she will wake up in the middle of the night feeling cold, so he packed a spare sleeping bag that could be used as a cover. During the night, while Dave slept, Zara struggled to fall asleep as her feet were cold. She unzipped her sleeping bag to put on another pair of socks but she continued to be cold. She started to shiver. Zara then unwrapped the spare sleeping bag, opened it wide and tucked one part of the bag under her own sleeping bag and used the second half to cover herself. Soon she was asleep.

Continued

CASE STUDY 3.2—cont'd

Q1. Adipose tissue can be deposited in which skin layer?
   a. Dermis
   b. Epidermis
   c. Subcutaneous layer
   d. Basement membrane

Q2. When you are cold, goose bumps arise on your skin. These are due to the contraction of the:
   a. biceps.
   b. deltoid muscle.
   c. arrector pili muscle.
   d. gluteal muscles.

Q3. The skin surface is waterproof because:
   a. the superficial layers of the skin contain keratinocytes.
   b. the superficial layers of the skin contain keratin.
   c. skin contains melanin.
   d. skin contains Merkel cells that are waterproof.

Q4. What physiological responses would you expect to be activated to regulate Zara's body temperature?

Q5. Exposed to continuous cold, what has contributed to Zara's shivering?

CASE STUDY 3.3

Toby, a three-year-old boy, was playing in the kitchen when he reached up to the bench and pulled the contents of a cup of tea over his head. Hearing Toby's scream, his mum Erin rushed to pick him up. She saw a red area appear in Toby's left temporal and ear region and grabbed an ice pack, which she wrapped in a wet cloth and strapped around the injured area. She drove him to the nearby medical centre. On arrival, the staff assessed the injury as a superficial burn as there were no blisters and no indication of damage below the epidermis. A soothing gel was applied to the burn and a supply provided to Erin for use over the coming week. Pain relief medication was also provided in a liquid form.

Q1. The epidermis plays an important role in immune defences. Which of the following immune cells are in the epidermis?
   a. Germinal cells
   b. Langerhans cells
   c. Keratinocytes
   d. Endothelial cells

Q2. Pain sensation in the skin is detected by which receptor?
   a. Nociceptors
   b. Chemoreceptors
   c. Photoreceptors
   d. Pacinian corpuscles

Q3. Skin is connected to the underlying muscle by the:
   a. epidermis.
   b. dermis.
   c. subcutaneous layer.
   d. ligaments.

Q4. Toby's burn affected the epidermis. Describe the layers of the epidermis you would expect to be damaged, how this would impact the function of those layers and how this correlated to redness observed in the injured area.

Q5. Superficial skin wounds are often very painful. Why is this so?

CASE STUDY 3.4

Four days ago, Sarah, a 27-year-old barista who spends most of her time indoors, was on her way home from work when she misjudged the roadside kerb, lost her footing and fell onto the ground. During the fall, she braced herself by placing her forearm in front of her face. On contacting the ground, Sara felt immediate pain. Concerned that she might have fractured a bone in her arm, she checked into the local clinic where they did an x-ray. The x-ray showed a fractured radius bone. Four days later, Sarah visited her local GP for a check-up and expressed surprise that the fracture occurred so easily. Concerned that Sarah's lack of sun exposure might have contributed to an increased risk of bone fracture, her GP ordered a blood test to determine Sarah's vitamin D level.

CASE STUDY 3.4—cont'd

Q1. The production of vitamin D commences in the:
  a. liver.
  b. kidneys.
  c. muscles.
  d. skin.

Q2. Exposure to sunlight stimulates the production of melanin. Which cells produce melanin?
  a. Keratinocytes
  b. Endothelial cells
  c. Langerhans cells
  d. Melanocytes

Q3. Vitamin D is created from a substance that is already present in the skin. This substance is:
  a. 7-dehydrocholesterol.
  b. cholecalciferol.
  c. 1,25 dioxyfroxycholecalciferol.
  d. oestrogen.

Q4. Why is lack of sun exposure to the skin associated with vitamin D deficiency?

Q5. Skin is sensitive to UV rays. Which cells protect the skin from UV damage and how is this function performed?

REFERENCES

1. Patton KT, Thibodeau GA. Skin. In: Patton KT, Thibodeau GA, editors. Anatomy and physiology. 9th ed. London: Elsevier Health Sciences; 2015. p. 180–208.
2. Huether SE, Rodway G, DeFriez C. Pain, Temperature regulation, sleep, and sensory function. In: McCance KL, Huether SE, Brachers VL, et al, editors. Pathophysiology: the biologic basis for disease in adults and children. 7th ed. St Louis: Elsevier; 2014. p. 484–526.
3. Hegde S, Raghavan S. A skin-depth analysis of integrins: role of the integrin network in health and disease. Cell Commun Adhes 2013;20(6):155–69.
4. Rousselle P, Braye F, Dayan G. Re-epithelialization of adult skin wounds: cellular mechanisms and therapeutic strategies. Adv Drug Deliv Rev 2018.
5. Wysocki AB. Anatomy and physiology of skin and soft tissue. In: Bryant RA, Nix DP, editors. Acute and chronic wounds: current management concepts. 5th ed. St Louis: Elsevier; 2016. p. 40–62.
6. Williams PM, Goodie J, Motsinger CD. Treating eating disorders in primary care. Am Fam Phys 2008;77(2):187–95.
7. Reinke JM, Sorg H. Wound repair and regeneration. Eur Surg Res 2012;49(1):35–43.
8. Lokmic Z, Darby IA, Thompson EW, et al. Time course analysis of hypoxia, granulation tissue and blood vessel growth, and remodeling in healing rat cutaneous incisional primary intention wounds. Wound Repair Regen 2006;14(3):277–88.
9. Edwards H. Nursing management: inflammation and wound healing. In: Brown D, Edwards H, Seaton L, et al, editors. Lewis's medical-surgical nursing: assessment and management of clinical problems. 4th ed. Chatswood: Elsevier; 2015. p. 144–63.
10. Australia CC. Skin cancer. Available from: www.cancer.org.au/about-cancer/types-of-cancer/skin-cancer.html.

The skeletal system

SONYA MOORE, DHEALTH

INTRODUCTION

The skeletal system encompasses bones and their connective tissues. It is a functionally integrated system comprising all the bones in the body, which are connected by joints, which are in turn lined with cartilage and supported by ligaments. The skeletal system provides a scaffold that is imperatively supported by the muscular system for posture and movement, the neural system for control of movement and the endocrine system for cellular health and adaptation. While a key function of the skeletal system is to give the body shape, and enable movement at joints, it is also important for the production of blood cells and the storage of calcium essential to the function of nearly every cell.

The importance of exposure, responsivity and adaptation to load are increasingly recognised in maintaining a healthy skeletal system. All of the body systems function to prepare for and respond to activities of daily living and to keep the body in balance. Bones adapt to become stronger in response to load demands and will weaken with less use—hence there is truth to the saying 'use it or lose it' in terms of skeletal health. The historical anatomical principle whereby bone continually responds to and adapts to mechanical load and remodels throughout life is referred to as **Wolff's law**.[1] Mechanical load is generated through activities of daily living such as walking, lifting and carrying, and gravitational forces.[2] Mechanical and cellular signalling stimulate a biochemical response in a process called **mechanotransduction**,[1] in turn stimulating **osteogenesis**, the formation of new bone.[2] Muscle contractions are increasingly recognised as the greatest generators of loads and forces on the skeletal system, and therefore significantly stimulate bone adaptation.[2,3] Skeletal system health is therefore strongly correlated with the strength of the muscular system and other systems contributing to the capability to engage in physical activity.

Engaging in physical activity requires several of the body's systems to function together to supply the energy and coordinate the movement requirements for exercise. The gastrointestinal metabolic system drives the availability of energy from the food we eat to the cardiovascular and neuromuscular systems, which are primary determinants of movement and exercise capacity. How efficiently energy is delivered and used by the body determines how long we can exercise for without becoming tired, a concept known as aerobic capacity or endurance. How proficient the muscles are at using energy to generate force is often referred to as strength.

It is important to understand the structure and function of the skeletal system because it plays such a large role in overall health. Promoting physical activity and addressing inactivity are pillars of societal health, for which a healthy functioning skeletal system is integral. Understanding the structure and function helps us to understand why simple activities of normal living can promote this healthy balance. Using the skeleton in a variety of everyday activities enables it to respond and adapt to these demands, which sustains bone health and skeletal system homeostasis.

STRUCTURE AND FUNCTION OF THE SKELETAL SYSTEM

The adult **skeletal system** contains more than 200 bones. It can be divided into the **axial skeleton** (arising from the para-axial mesoderm) comprising the spine and torso; the **appendicular skeleton** (arising from the lateral plate mesoderm) comprising the limb complexes; and the **facial skeleton** (arising from the ectodermal neural crest) (Fig. 4.1).[4] The bone structure of the skeletal system functions to give the body shape and rigidity. Without bones, the human body would be pliable and soft, and unable to bear the required loads of everyday living. Loads of everyday living are synonymous with the forces the body encounters during activities such as walking, getting in and out of a car, climbing stairs or carrying shopping.

The skeletal system is designed for functional load bearing and movement

As the foot strikes the ground with each step (or impact) a proportional and opposite ground reaction force is generated. This ground reaction force is absorbed and transferred from the ground through the feet and lower limbs to the pelvis and spine. The absorption and dissipation of forces acting on the body is a key function of the skeletal system, and one that is supported by neural and muscular control. The more effective the neural and muscular systems are in sustaining optimal alignment of the bones, the more efficiently the skeletal system can function in its load-force-distribution role. The typical pattern of this load transfer and dissipation between the ground and the skeletal system is shown in Fig. 4.2.

The skeleton also serves to provide attachment for muscles. Muscles contract to move the bones at joints, which function like a hinge between two (or more) bony levers. If we did not have bones, the muscle would not have a rigid attachment to pull upon. Joints are not all shaped the same. The shape of joints allows movement in some directions and restricts it in others (see Chapter 5). Ligaments hold joints together and support this directional movement pattern by being thicker and more resistive in some directions and thinner in others to allow movement in desired directions. Fig. 4.3 shows some examples of muscles and their bony attachments to the skeletal system. The muscles pull along the line of their fibre alignment, exerting force on bones at these points. Where muscles cross joints, this allows movement of the bony levers along this line of force.

Bones are shaped according to their specific function

The skull bones serve to provide a protective casing for the brain, and the spinal cord runs through the protective spinal canal, formed between the vertebral bodies and vertebral arch. The spinal canal is a good example of

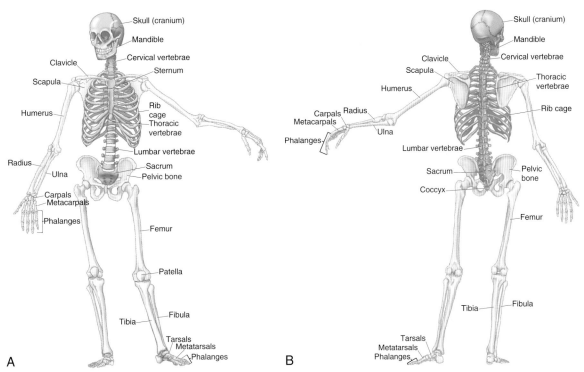

FIGURE 4.1 **Axial and appendicular skeleton. A** Anterior view of the skeleton. **B** Posterior view of the skeleton. Axial skeleton in blue; appendicular skeleton in tan. (*Source:* Muscolino J. Know the body: muscle, bone and palpation essentials. St Louis: Mosby; 2012.)

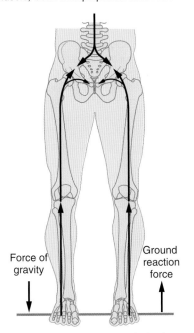

FIGURE 4.2 **Load transfer through the lower limbs and pelvis.**

how the unique shape of the vertebrae supports their key functions, which are to form the vertebral column (a key component of the axial skeleton) and house the spinal cord (Fig. 4.4).

The large pelvic bone complex is shaped effectively for its functional capacity to bear the large body-weight load for standing, walking and other activities. The pelvis is formed by the largely fibrocartilaginous union between the ilia, pubic rami, ischium and sacral bones. This shape and structure enable it to efficiently absorb and dissipate weight-bearing forces from both legs and in the pushing and pulling involved in a variety of physical activities. The large surface area created by the shape of the pelvis provides a large area for muscle attachment, allowing both the bone structure and the attaching muscles to be strong, resilient and capable of managing large, multidirectional forces. The shape of the pelvis also enables it to carry and protect important internal organs and blood vessels. The female pelvis is wider than the male pelvis. This gives it the capacity to completely contain and protect a growing fetus in the first three months of gestation, and further accommodate the developing pregnancy and childbirth (see Chapter 22).

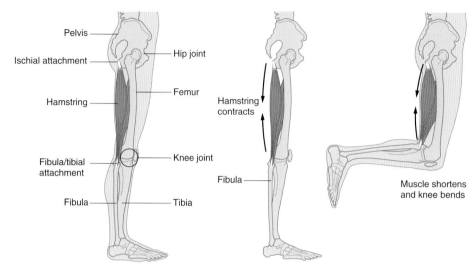

FIGURE 4.3 **Muscle attachments and movement.**

The fibrocartilaginous joints within the pelvis are important in allowing some expansion and flexibility of the pelvic diameter for the baby to grow and for birth.

Ribs are arranged in 'rings' to form a cage that includes a series of small-moving joints with the thoracic spine posteriorly (**synovial joints**) and the sternum anteriorly (**cartilaginous joints**). This arrangement enables the ribs to provide protection and stability for internal organs such as the heart and lungs, while allowing expansion for breathing. While your arms and legs are pumping

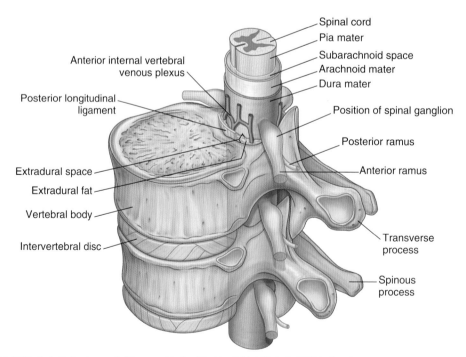

FIGURE 4.4 **Spinal canal.** (*Source:* Drake RL, Vogl W, Mitchell AMW. Gray's anatomy for students. London: Churchill Livingstone; 2005.)

powerfully in a running race, so too are your chest organs. The series of small joints enables the rib cage to expand a small amount at each rib level as lung volume increases with breathing in (inhalation) and decreases with breathing out (exhalation). Meanwhile, because no single joint is moving a lot, the internal organs are protected and trunk stability can be maintained in an upright posture at your maximum running pace. Muscles attaching to the rigid ribs and sternum—particularly the diaphragm—contract to provide the force to expand the rib cage. As the volume inside the chest cavity increases, a negative pressure is created and air is sucked into the lungs. As the muscle relax, the balance of rigidity and elasticity allows the rib cage to recoil to its previous shape and capacity, and air is forced back out of the lungs.

Long bones—typical of the limbs, such as the femur, humerus and tibia—are inherently designed with a hard, compact bone cortex encasing cavity-filled cancellous bone, with a hollow medullary canal to balance rigidity with low weight.[5,6] This facilitates their function as load-bearing bones and levers, which our neuromuscular system can move freely and efficiently in space. While bone strength is crucial, without this less-dense centre it would be very difficult to lift your arms above your head or lift your legs to climb stairs. Because they are shaped like a tube they are particularly resilient to bending and torsion.[6] Fig. 4.5 shows a cross-section of a typical long bone, and the next section discusses the architecture of bone in more detail.

Bone architecture

As well as being essential for structure and movement, the skeletal system provides an essential and specific internal mineralised framework that is home to essential metabolic and endocrine functions. The skeletal system stores 99% of the body's calcium and is also dense in phosphate.[5] Bones are made up of layers: the outside is **cortical bone**, which is harder and stiffer than the inner **cancellous bone**, which is structured by trabeculae and cavities[2] containing yellow or red **bone marrow**.[5] Yellow bone marrow supports blood vessels within its fatty connective tissue matrix. Red bone marrow is where red and most white blood cells are made. Bone surfaces are covered by a dense, fibrous membrane called periosteum, which has a nerve and blood vessel-dense outer layer, an osteogenic inner layer called endosteum, and is attached to the cortical bone by collagenous Sharpey's fibres.[5] Fig. 4.5 shows how periosteum, cortical bone, cancellous bone and bone marrow are structured and organised to form a typical long bone, which is shown in cross-section.

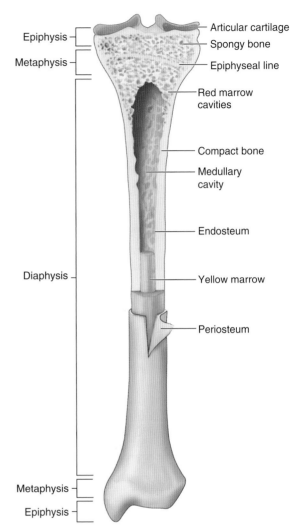

Epiphysis
Metaphysis
Diaphysis
Metaphysis
Epiphysis

Articular cartilage
Spongy bone
Epiphyseal line
Red marrow cavities
Compact bone
Medullary cavity
Endosteum
Yellow marrow
Periosteum

FIGURE 4.5 Cross-section of bone. Longitudinal section of long bone (tibia) showing spongy (cancellous) and compact bone. (*Source:* Huether K, McCance S. Pathophysiology: the biologic basis for disease in adults and children, 8 ed. St Louis: Elsevier; 2019.)

In contrast to the adult skeleton, when we are born, the skeletal system has around 300 bones. As we grow some of these bones fuse and our skeletal system reaches its mature height in adolescence or early adulthood. An x-ray of a growing long bone, for example a femur, shows that the ends of the bone—called epiphyses—are not yet fused to the shaft or diaphysis. The section between the epiphysis and the diaphysis is called the metaphysis, forming a 'growth zone' for new bone. Anatomically, the metaphysis is the hard bony region adjacent to

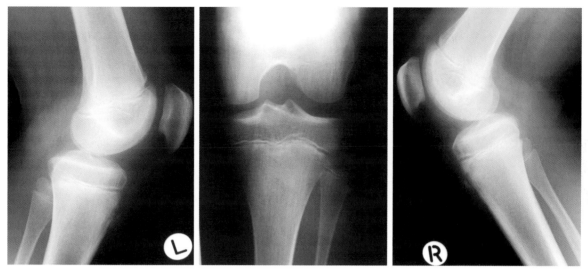

FIGURE 4.6 **X-ray of growing bones.** Open epiphyses of the distal femur, proximal tibia, proximal fibula and tibial apophysis can be seen in this knee x-ray series.

the cartilaginous epiphyseal plate. The epiphyseal plate cannot be visualised as dense bone on an x-ray as it is cartilaginous and has not yet been mineralised (Fig. 4.6). There are points where muscles attach to children's bones that are not fused to the main bone until maturity, known as apophysis.

Overview of bone microarchitecture and remodelling

Bone is made up of a variety of function-specific cells, including osteoblasts, osteocytes and osteoclasts, which are organised within an extracellular mineralised matrix, often termed ground substance. This ground substance is made up of calcium, phosphates and hydroxyapatite (60–70% in a combination that naturally varies within the process of mineralisation), collagen (30–40%) and glycoproteins (5%).[5]

Bone cell turnover and osteogenesis are constant, with new bone cells replacing old ones, and new bone being formed and mineralised in response to load.[2] Therefore, within each bone at any point in time, at a cellular level there will be regions of new bone forming. **Osteoid** is newly deposited or immature bone that has not yet been mineralised and the higher proportion of collagen renders it relatively flexible.[5] Osteoid contains bone-forming cells called **osteoblasts** that synthesise a collagen (mostly type I and some type V) and calcium-rich matrix, which can then be mineralised with calcium, phosphates and hydroxyapatite.[5] Osteoblasts mature

into **osteocytes**, which are interconnected by dendritic processes and maintain the extracellular matrix.[5]

Initially, osteocytes are irregularly arranged with variable diameter collagen to form woven or bundle bone.[5] As bone matures, osteocytes communicate and typically organise into circumferential lamellae around neurovascular bundles to form Haversian systems or osteons.[5] Furthermore, the orientation of osteons and the collagen fibres within them align according to the load and forces on the skeletal system, such that they are arranged longitudinally, obliquely and transversely in areas of tension, compression and the diaphysis periphery, respectively.[5] Strong, mineralised, organised cellular matrix is referred to as mature bone, forming a hard skeletal structure that stores calcium and can withstand force and load-bearing. Picture yourself kicking a soccer ball forwards down the pitch, sideways to a team mate or in a twisting-turning motion to take control of the ball from your opponent—these are examples of the importance of organised cellular matrix providing bone strength in multiple directions.

The bone matrix is constantly being dissolved and reabsorbed by **osteoclasts**, releasing calcium into the bloodstream which is then available for other body systems including cardiac, neural and muscular function. Skeletal system homeostasis therefore involves maintenance of a resilient mature bone structure, balanced by constant processes of bone reabsorption and reformation. This is called **bone remodelling**.

Functional osteogenesis

Osteogenesis is the formation of new bone. Bones grow in distinct patterns: endochondral ossification results in bones growing longer; and periosteal apposition results in circumferential expansion and thickening of the cortex.[2] Normal healing of most fractures involves a combination of periosteal apposition,[5] and endochondral and intramembranous bone formation, including angiogenesis.[7]

Endochondral ossification

The process of osteogenesis, which begins with a cartilaginous scaffold, is called endochondral bone formation[3] and is typical of bone formation in the axial and appendicular skeleton.[4] Bone tissue contains chondrocytes in various stages of a life cycle which transitions through a proliferative state to terminal differentiation and **apoptosis** (cell death).[7] In the epiphyseal plate, chondrocytes in an undifferentiated and non-proliferative state await endocrine signalling to proliferate and form a cartilaginous scaffold or mould, which is then mineralised to form bone and bone marrow.[4,7] Activated and hypertrophic chondrocytes synthesise and mineralise a cartilaginous matrix (including type II collagen, type IX collagen, type XI collagen, aggrecan, chondromodulin 1 and matrilin-3), before undergoing apoptosis.[4] This mineralised cartilaginous matrix is further vascularised and degraded by chondroclasts, and adjacent perichondrial cells differentiate into osteoblasts, which lay down bone matrix onto the cartilaginous scaffold.[4] Osteogenesis occurs within the metaphysis growth zone, and gradually mineralises and matures. Children's bones become gradually longer, and they grow gradually taller. This happens until growth is complete and the epiphyseal plate fuses. Different bones fuse at different ages; for example, epiphyses of long bones typically fuse at the end of adolescence, while epiphyses of the pelvis are later at age 20–25.[5] When all bones have fused, the size and structure of the adult skeleton is reached. Although the blueprint of the human skeleton is genetically determined, individual variation will influence its final and specific form, such as peak bone mass and adult height.[8]

Intramembranous bone formation

Typical of the skull and facial bones is intramembranous bone formation, where mesenchymal cells differentiate directly into osteoblasts which lay down bone matrix, without the cartilaginous scaffold.[4]

Periosteal apposition

Periosteal apposition involves the formation of new woven bone between the outer fibrous layer of periosteum and cortical bone.[5] Fractures involving regions of bone where there is no periosteum can therefore be vulnerable to delayed healing, such as inside joint capsules and articular surfaces and at tendon and muscle attachments.[5] Fractures involving the intra-articular femoral head and neck sites are typically slower to heal or can be problematic.

Children's bones

Children's bones are more flexible than those of adults as a higher proportion of the matrix is not yet organised and the collagen has an irregular, woven or bundle arrangement.[5] The properties of collagen are responsible for many characteristics of bone, including mechanical strength—tolerance to tensile, compressive and shearing loads—and a degree of elasticity. A growing skeleton that has not been fully mineralised and therefore has not reached peak bone mass is more vulnerable to fracture.[8] If a child falls from their bike, they may be particularly susceptible to breaking an arm as children's bones are softer. Furthermore, as children's bones are more elastic, they are less likely to 'snap' in a pattern you might see in a harder adult bone—like breaking a mature wooden stick. Instead, they bend or bow on one side—like if you tried to snap a smaller, softer green branch. This is where the term 'greenstick fracture' comes from, generally occurring in children under 10 years old. It is still considered a break as the bone structure has been disrupted. Fig. 4.7 shows the characteristic greenstick fracture pattern.

Bone density and the life span

Bone density refers to the amount and strength of bone cellular matrix. This cellular matrix provides the scaffolding and gives bone its resilience. In a homeostatic state, the strength of this scaffolding will be maintained

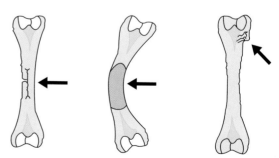

FIGURE 4.7 **Greenstick fracture pattern.** (*Source:* Carson S, Woolridge D, Colletti J, Kilgore K. Pediatric upper extremity injuries. Pediatr Clin North Am 2006 Feb;53(1):41–67.)

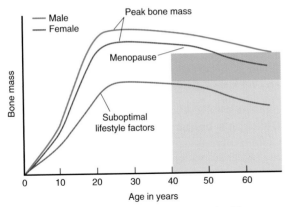

FIGURE 4.8 **Normal bone density over the life span.**

jumping. During youth and the adolescent years, bone density increases with normal growth and development[2,8] as osteogenesis is greater than reabsorption.[6] This reaches a peak around age 30–40, when the adult skeletal system is at its strongest in terms of withstanding and absorbing forces.[2,8] If our same child fell from their bike as an adult, their bones would be better able to withstand the force of the fall. This is then maintained through the middle stages of life before declining in older age.[2,8] This bone loss is referred to as **osteopenia** and parallels age-related skeletal muscle loss, or **sarcopenia** (see Fig. 4.8).[3] Specifically, physical activity, and adequate overall availability of energy, calcium and vitamin D are essential for promoting normal peak bone density.[8] There is evidence that physical activity and the mechanical loading of bone are positively related to bone density (and bone health) throughout the life span and that declining bone density with age is in part attributable to reduced mechanosensitivity and a reduced capacity for adaptation.[6]

Endocrine signalling and osteogenesis

Healthy functioning endocrine and metabolic systems are part of the signalling cascade of physiological processes for osteoblastic activity and energy availability to generate new tissue. This is represented in Fig. 4.9, a

at an adequate level to provide rigidity yet have the capacity to absorb bending and compressive forces. For example, this is like jumping on a trampoline, where the mat and springs must be firm enough to withstand the forces of jumping without breaking, but with enough 'give' to absorb and dissipate components of the force in different directions for smooth body movement.

Healthy bone density changes over the life span[2,8] but needs to be maintained at a level high enough to meet the load demands of everyday living, running and

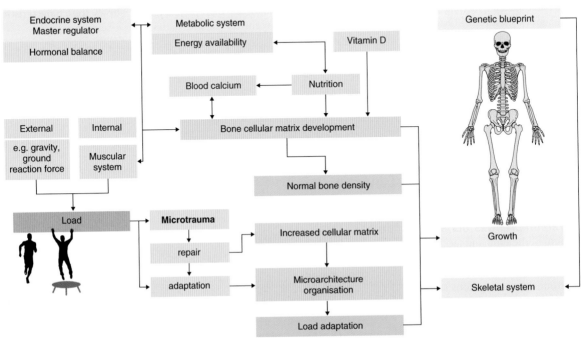

FIGURE 4.9 **System integration in the formation of bone and remodelling concept map.**

concept map of system integration in the formation of bone. The endocrine system (see Chapter 10) and hormonal balance provide essential signalling for osteogenic reabsorption and deposition. The metabolic system (see Chapter 19) provides the energy to form and build the matrix. The vascular system delivers blood to the epiphyseal plate, with glucose and oxygen being metabolised locally to produce the energy needs for new bone formation.[9]

Bone homeostasis and remodelling in response to load

The endocrine system provides the overarching signalling and mediation to maintain bone homeostasis, which is further moderated by mechanical loading and muscle activity.[2,3] Each time we take a step, the equal and opposite reactive force from our foot-strike that is returned to the skeletal system is called the ground reaction force (GRF). This force is transferred to and dissipated throughout the skeletal system. For example, imagine a group of schoolchildren jumping on a trampoline. As they jump, there are several forces at play. As the children land on the trampoline, a reactive force propels them back up in the opposite direction. Meanwhile, some of the landing force is absorbed by the flexible mat with springs, which does not collapse. These same forces are at play on the skeletal system. Just like the trampoline, the skeletal system needs to absorb and redirect components of this force to keep the body in balance. The skeletal system needs to be strong enough to withstand and absorb the forces of running and jumping on all kinds of surfaces such as grass, footpaths and sports courts.

The skeletal system is highly responsive to the loads and forces to which it is subjected. Formation of new bone mass is stimulated in response to loading and muscle activity.[2] So the more the group of schoolchildren run or jump, the greater the stimulus for new bone formation and increased bone density to withstand this load. When they challenge themselves and jump higher or harder than previously, this provides the stimulus for osteogenesis and adaptation to meet the demands. Correspondingly, if the children consistently replace this osteogenesis-stimulating activity with inactive computer games, loads on the skeletal system are less and bone may instead be reabsorbed. The **mechanostat theory** refers to the dose-response of load applied to the skeletal system, whereby bone will be reabsorbed if the stimulus is too low, will adapt with optimal loading above the threshold, or will structurally fail if the load is too high.[2] If you were to set a goal of training for a marathon, it would be unwise to try to run the whole distance in your first attempt. Rather, running volume should be gradually built up over time to allow the skeletal system to repair microtrauma and gradually adapt to the increasing load with a stronger matrix. As familiarity with running improves, the skeletal system will be more resilient to these familiar forces and the risk of bone stress injury is less.

The role of muscle in osteogenesis

Muscle is a major stimulus for bone adaptation in its capacity to provide bone-stimulating mechanical loading[2,3] and deliver blood and trophic factors via their attachments.[2] Furthermore, emerging evidence explores and supports the concept of site-specific loading and osteogenesis, which is an important consideration in advocating engagement in a variety of physical activities and designing specific rather than general exercise interventions to optimise bone health.[2,10] Rarely do our bodies move only in straight, controlled lines. Muscles therefore exert pulling, shear and compression forces in different directions on the bones they attach to. This creates macroscopic stress or load (external force) and strain (structural deformation) on bone tissue that is specific to each region of each bone, and in turn allows the skeletal system to adapt very specifically to typical movement demands.[2] Inversely, compromised muscle function and fatigue can result in suboptimal movement mechanics and consequently undesirable or changed bone loading patterns; for example, when a runner is tired and loses form. This can contribute to bone stress injury as the bone has not accommodated to the irregular pattern of stress loading.[2] A strong versatile skeletal system that has adapted to the variable demands placed on it as part of daily life enables healthy and continued participation in physical activity.

Haemopoiesis

Bone marrow is the primary site of blood cell formation, which primarily occurs in the red bone marrow–rich bones of the sternum, ribs and hips. This process is called **haemopoiesis**. Haematopoietic stem cells differentiate and mature into oxygen-carrying **erythrocytes** (red blood cells) and immune system responsive **leucocytes** and **lymphocytes** (white blood cells). These cells are released into the bloodstream, circulating throughout the body and into the tissues and lymph system to perform their functions.

Some blood cells fulfil their function within the bloodstream, such as erythrocytes and clot-regulating platelets. Different types of leucocytes travel via the circulatory system to where they are needed in response to injury, invasion or infection, and will transit through

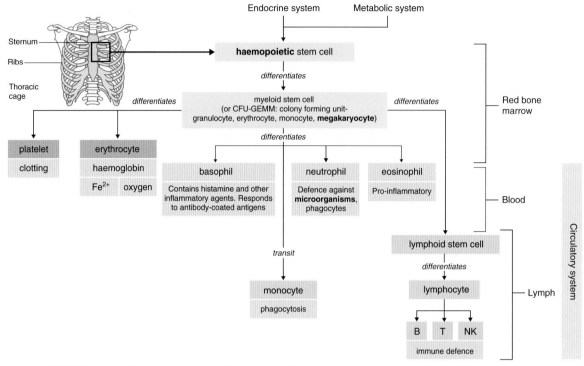

FIGURE 4.10 **Skeletal system and haemopoiesis concept map.** The process of haemopoiesis is demonstrated as a concept map, including the integration with several body systems.

the bloodstream to the lymphatic system, immune system and interstitial spaces, where they can participate in specific immune responses. Bone marrow-produced basophils contain histamine and other inflammatory agents and respond to antibody-coated antigens. Bone marrow-produced monocytes and neutrophils defend the body against microorganisms and engulf the bacteria through phagocytosis. Bone marrow-produced lymphoid stem cells differentiate into lymphocytes with specific functions in immune defence. Fig. 4.10 demonstrates the process of haemopoiesis as a concept map, including the integration with several body systems.

INTEGRATION OF THE SKELETAL SYSTEM WITH OTHER BODY SYSTEMS
Endocrine system, skeletal system and calcium balance
The endocrine system is the master regulator of the body's response to stimuli and environmental changes to maintain homeostasis, including calcium homeostasis. Calcium availability is crucial to many functions including normal heart rhythm, nerve conduction, muscle contraction, blood clotting and enzyme action. While

the skeletal system requires a calcium-dense matrix for its resilient structure, this also serves as the body's calcium stores. Bone remodelling and the balance between building bone density and releasing stored calcium into the bloodstream for the rest of the body is regulated by the endocrine system. This requires intricate communication between the two systems.

Take, for example, a runner, who needs calcium to maintain a steady heart rhythm while she runs. At the same time, she needs calcium for nerve signalling to the muscles, which in turn need calcium to contract. To regulate blood calcium levels for these requirements, the endocrine system signals the release of parathyroid hormone from the parathyroid glands. This stimulates osteoblasts and promotes calcium release into the bloodstream from the skeletal system, keeping blood calcium levels within the normal range and meeting the ongoing needs for running. When she has finished running, this osteoblast activation continues, triggering bone remodelling. Along with the mechanical loading of the skeletal system, bone formation and adaptation to the demands of running are promoted. Dietary calcium intake and absorption need to be adequate to meet her overall requirements during running and to replenish skeletal system stores used during running. Over and above this, dietary calcium and energy intake needs to meet the additional demands of bone adaptation, as the skeletal system responds and adapts to the forces of running by increasing calcium and bone matrix density.

Neural system, muscular system, skeletal system and bone remodelling

The shape and structure of bones within the skeletal system are especially designed to meet functional demand. Some bones are designed for weight-bearing, while others are designed for muscle attachment and transfer of force. Some bones are designed to protectively house structures such as the brain, ribs, heart/lungs, vertebrae/spinal cord, pelvis great vessels and internal organs when running at pace, for instance. Fig. 4.11 shows examples of the different structures of bones and the relationship to their unique functions. These functions are possible because the skeletal system is integrated with the neural and muscular systems to produce coordinated body movement. Nerves control muscle activation patterns, which in turn act upon the skeleton to move or stabilise it. When a gardener digs a shovel into the ground, the brain sends signals along nerves to the muscles about where he needs to position his arms—first to raise the shovel, then to drive to it into the ground. The nervous system provides the information about the coordination of these movements and how much force is needed to complete the task. This neural signalling tells the muscles to grip the shovel strongly, contract quickly to power the dig, and to brace the body to resist and control the ground reaction force that will return up the shovel as it hits the ground. These forces from the ground and contracting muscles are transferred to, absorbed and dissipated by the skeletal system. Bone remodelling occurs in response to the forces exerted upon it by the muscular system,[2,3,10] enabling the skeletal system to meet the demand to provide a rigid and resilient scaffold.

Immune system, cardiovascular system and lymph system

The skeletal system houses bone marrow for production of blood cells in a healthy functioning immune system and is therefore part of the integrated system cascade response when the immune system is activated. For example, when a splinter is embedded under the skin, locally circulating mast cells that have been synthesised in the bone marrow recognise the invasion of a foreign body and release histamine. This initiates the further immune signal cascade. More bone marrow-produced leucocytes (white blood cells) are released from the skeletal system into the bloodstream, where they are circulated throughout the body. They engulf foreign cells and bacteria in a process called **phagocytosis** and activate further immune responses. Blood flow, vessel dilation and cellular influx to the area cause local redness, oedema and fluid around the splinter. These are signs that the immune cells are actively fending off bacteria and germs associated with the foreign body. When the splinter is removed, the lymphatic system from the neighbouring muscles balances this circulatory influx and immune response by reabsorbing and returning inflammatory by-products, debris and oedema to the central circulation. Normal balance is restored.

Energy requirements of the skeletal system: nutrition and metabolism, cardiac system and blood

So how does the skeletal system resource the energy required for bone growth, constant bone remodelling and haemopoiesis? The cardiovascular system transports nutrients and glucose-rich blood for local oxidation to meet the energy requirements for chondrocyte activity, cell division, synthesis of extracellular matrix and bone.[9] Adequate overall availability of energy, calcium and vitamin D is essential for promoting normal peak bone density and bone health.[8]

AGE-RELATED CHANGES

Perhaps the best-known age-related change in the human body is that of loss of calcium in bones, which leads to diminished bone density in women and men. This loss of density in turn leads to bone fragility and increased risk of bone fracture even if small force is exerted on the ageing bone. During their reproductive years, women are in part protected by oestrogen. However, once menopause starts, the loss of calcium is rapid and more severe.[12] An ageing body also produces fewer proteins like collagens and fibres that provide bone strength and flexibility. Collagen-depleted bone becomes more brittle, again making the person more susceptible to fractures. Bone reabsorption occurs in the absence of continuous formation of new bone, resulting in the formation of larger centrally located medullary cavities of the long bone and loss of wall thickness of the compact bone.[11]

CONCLUSION

The skeletal system is structured to give the body shape and rigidity; enable movement and bear load; store and release the body's calcium; and house bone

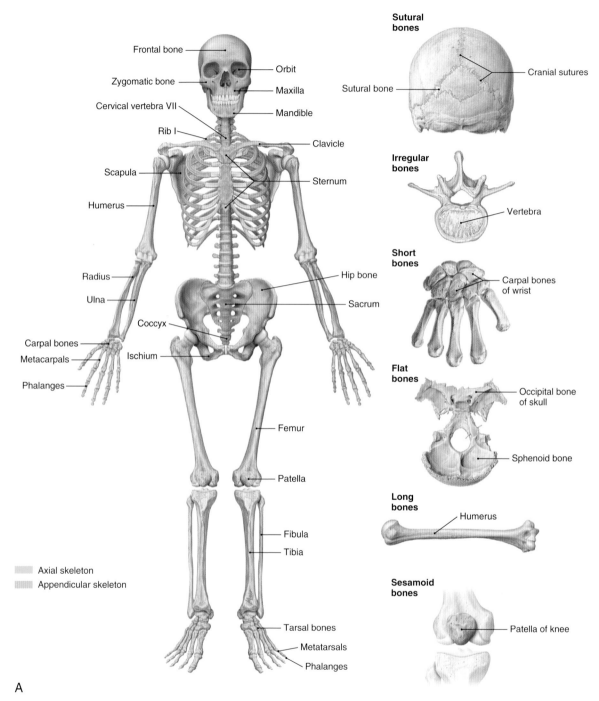

FIGURE 4.11 **Structure of bones and their function. A** Types of bones.

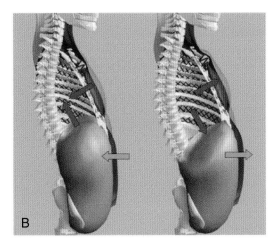

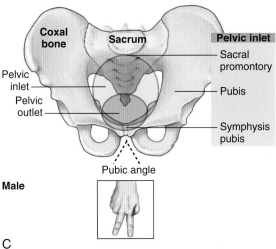

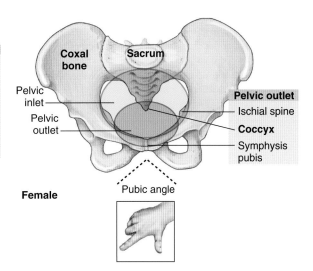

FIGURE 4.11, cont'd **B** Bucket-handle action of ribs. Rib movement is produced by the action of the diaphragm and other inspiratory muscles, which expand the rib cage diameter with inhalation. **C** Male vs female pelvis. (*Source:* A, Hombach-Klonisch S, Klonisch T, Peeler J. Sobotta clinical atlas of human anatomy. Elsevier; 2019. B, Zordan V, Celly B, Chiu B, DiLorenzo P. Model and control of human respiration for computer animation. Elsevier; 2006. C, Niedzwiecki B, Pepper J, Weaver A. Kinn's medical assisting fundamentals: administrative and clinical competencies with anatomy and physiology. Elsevier; 2019.)

marrow where haemopoiesis occurs. These processes are meticulously integrated with all other body systems to maintain whole body homeostasis and optimal function.

The skeletal system is responsive and adaptable to meet the dynamic environmental demands of everyday living. In a process of bone remodelling, the skeletal system lays down calcium-rich cellular matrix in response to the loads it encounters so that it can withstand the demands of daily life. The neuromuscular system is a key driver of these load responses, including generating a mechanical stimulus for osteogenesis and moderating forces encountered in day-to-day activities such as running and jumping. The endocrine and metabolic systems are integral to the cellular signalling and cascade of events that support bone growth and remodelling.

Although the structure and function of the human skeleton is predetermined by a genetic blueprint, integration across several systems strongly influences homeostasis and the capacity for optimal function.

CASE STUDY 4.1

When walking your dog, instead of sticking to the usual footpath you head through a different park that has small hills and large rocks to add variety to the routine. Your dog escapes its lead and you give chase for some time as you both leap and bound to navigate the terrain. The next day you discuss your adventure with a friend, who laughs at your account and sympathises with your aching legs. You wonder whether you should do more of that kind of activity or stick to the footpath to avoid the feeling of aching legs in the future.

Q1. Skeletal structure and function refers to which characteristics?

    a. Bone shape

    b. Bone function

    c. Bony architecture

    d. All of the above

Q2. Normal structure and function of particular regions of the skeletal system is determined by:

    a. fit-for-purpose bone shape, joint characteristics and the attaching muscles.

    b. bone height, joints, immune function.

    c. the skeletal system alone.

    d. blood calcium balance and the endocrine system.

Q3. The skeletal system manages ground reaction force and weight-bearing load by:

    a. resisting forces through rigid bony structure.

    b. absorbing forces through 'give' in bones and joints.

    c. having a balanced pattern of force absorption, transfer and dissipation through the skeletal system, supported by the muscular system.

    d. muscles contracting to resist the forces applied to the skeletal system.

Q4. How are the ribs especially designed to ensure that you can breathe deeply while chasing your dog?

Q5. In terms of skeletal adaptation, why would you decide to walk your dog on a flatter more predictable landscape tomorrow?

CASE STUDY 4.2

Two small children are kicking a ball around at the park, until a wayward pass lands the ball in a nearby tree. One of the children climbs the tree but falls and sustains a forearm growth plate and greenstick fracture.

Q1. Why are immature bones more flexible than mature (adult) bones?

    a. Because they are not fully grown

    b. Because they have less rigid cells

    c. Because the microarchitecture of immature bone is not yet organised, and it is the organisation of the cellular and extracellular matrix that gives bone its mechanical strength and resilience

    d. Because children are generally more flexible than adults and we become stiffer as we get older

Q2. What is the main structure and related function of the epiphyseal plate?

    a. Cartilaginous, to give immature bones some flexibility as children fall over a lot

    b. Cartilaginous, as it is the growth zone of bone that has not yet mineralised and hardened

    c. Cancellous bone, as growing bones need strength

    d. Red marrow, as it contains cavities that are not visible on x-ray

Q3. How do bones fuse to form a certain size and shape in adulthood?

    a. Genetics: this is predetermined by our genetic makeup

    b. The stronger the muscles and the more energy available, the larger bones will grow

    c. The more weight-bearing load, the faster they fuse in response to force

    d. A combination of genetics, signals from the endocrine system, energy availability, inherent skeletal system structure and supporting muscle function

Q4. Why does this child sustain two types of bone fracture that are not seen in adults?

Q5. How do other body systems influence the healing of a greenstick fracture?

CASE STUDY 4.3

Several schoolchildren are jumping on a trampoline. As they jump, there are several forces at play. As the children land on the trampoline, a reactive force propels them back up in the opposite direction. Meanwhile, some of the landing force is absorbed by the flexible mat and springs. These same forces are at play on the skeletal system. The equal and opposite reactive force from a foot strike or jump landing is called the ground reaction force (GRF). Just like the trampoline, the skeletal system needs to absorb and redirect components of this force to keep the body in balance.

Q1. What is bone remodelling and why is it important?
   a. Bone reabsorption, which is important for releasing calcium into the bloodstream, which is then available for other body systems
   b. Bone reformation, which is important in the maintenance of a resilient mature bone structure
   c. Bone matrix adaptation in response to load
   d. All of the above

Q2. The more you run and jump:
   a. the weaker bones become as they are subject to large forces.
   b. the greater the stimulus for bone remodelling in response to load.
   c. the more dense the bone microarchitecture becomes with adaptation over time.
   d. both b and c.

Q3. Which systems need to be functioning in balance to maintain healthy bone density?
   a. Skeletal system
   b. Muscular system
   c. Endocrine system
   d. All of the above

Q4. How does the microarchitecture of bone contribute to withstanding the forces of jumping?

Q5. How is bone density homeostasis supported by other body systems?

CASE STUDY 4.4

Some middle-aged friends gather to watch a younger generation of men and women play football at their local football ground. They observe the typical similarities and differences between male and female styles of play, and discuss the decline in their own athletic capacity compared with their playing days. One of the members, a 50-year-old female, mentions that she noticed some hip and pelvic unsteadiness when coming down stairs, which was accompanied by feeling tired and puffed. Her doctor has organised bone density tests and blood tests to check for iron deficiency anaemia.

Q1. What is haemopoiesis?
   a. The production of blood cells in red bone marrow
   b. The process of phagocytosis of microorganisms in the bone marrow
   c. Another name for haematopoietic stem cells
   d. When haemoglobin binds to erythrocytes in the bloodstream

Q2. Red bone marrow is primarily found in which bones?
   a. Femur and tibia
   b. Sternum, ribs and hips
   c. Skull
   d. All bones

Q3. Blood cells formed in skeletal system bone marrow fulfil their functions within which other systems?
   a. Endocrine system
   b. Bone marrow and the skeletal system
   c. Immune system
   d. Blood, circulatory, lymph and immune systems as part of a coordinated system response to injury, invasion and infection

Q4. What are the key design components that relate to the function of the pelvis?

Q5. Particularly in older age, why would it be important to maintain strong muscles around the pelvis?

REFERENCES

1. Teichtahl AJ, Wluka AE, Wijethilake P, et al. Wolff's law in action: a mechanism for early knee osteoarthritis. Arthritis Res Ther 2015;17(1):207. doi:10.1186/s13075-015-0738-7.
2. Hart N, Nimphius S, Rantalainen T, et al. Mechanical basis of bone strength: influence of bone material, bone structure and muscle action. J Musculoskelet Neuronal Interact 2017;17(3):114–39.
3. DiGirolamo DJ, Kiel DP, Esser KA. Bone and skeletal muscle: neighbors with close ties. J Bone Min Res 2013; 28(7):1509–18.
4. Hojo H, Ohba S, Yano F. Coordination of chondrogenesis and osteogenesis by hypertrophic chondrocytes in

endochondral bone development. J Bone Miner Metab 2010;28:489.

5. Standring S, editor. Grey's anatomy. 39th ed. Edinburgh: Elsevier; 2005.

6. Birkhold AI, Razi H, Duda GN, et al. The periosteal bone surface is less mechano-responsive than the endocortical. Sci Rep 2016;6:23480. doi:10.1038/srep23480.

7. Kostenuik P, Mirza FM. Fracture healing physiology and the quest for therapies for delayed healing and nonunion. J Ortho Res 2016;35(2):213–23.

8. Weaver C, Gordon C, Janz K, et al. The National Osteoporosis Foundation's position statement on peak bone mass development and lifestyle factors: a systematic review and implementation recommendations. Osteoporos Int 2016; 27:1281–386. doi:10.1007/s00198-015-3440-3.

9. Shapiro IM, Srinivas V. Metabolic consideration of epiphyseal growth: survival responses in a taxing environment. Bone 2006;40(3):561–7.

10. Fuchs RK, Kersh ME, Carballido-Gamio J, et al. Physical Activity for Strengthening Fracture Prone Regions of the Proximal Femur. Curr Osteoporos Rep 2017;15(1):43–52.

11. Aging changes in the bones—muscles—joints. Medline Plus; May 2019. Available at: https://medlineplus.gov/ency/article/004015.htm.

12. Schneidmüller D, Röder C, Kraus R, et al. Development and validation of a paediatric long-bone fracture classification. A prospective multicentre study in 13 European paediatric trauma centres. BMC Musculoskelet Disord 2011;12:89. doi:10.1186/1471-2474-12-89.

CHAPTER 5

Joints

KIM ALLISON, PHD

KEY POINTS/LEARNING OUTCOMES

1. Describe the type and structure of joints within the skeletal system.
2. Explain the basic function of the different types of joints and the distinct components of joints within the skeletal system.
3. Understand how joint structure impacts on joint function.
4. Discuss how homeostasis of joint structure is maintained.
5. Explain how joints contribute to the maintenance of general body homeostasis.

KEY DEFINITIONS

- **Cartilage:** connective tissue covering joint surfaces.
- **Fibrous joint:** joint that permits little movement, characterised by bony components being united by fibrous tissue.
- **Joint:** an articulation between two or more bones of the skeleton.
- **Proprioception:** a neurological function that provides the sense of where a part of the body is in space; with respect to joints, an awareness of joint position.
- **Synovial joint:** joint designed for human mobility, characterised by bony components covered in hyaline cartilage and enclosed in a synovial sheath (joint capsule).

ONLINE RESOURCES/SUGGESTED READINGS

- Levangie PK, Norkin CC. Joint structure and function: a comprehensive analysis. Philadelphia, PA: FA Davis; 2011
- **Bones, Joints & Muscles: Human Anatomy Facts 360** app, available for iOS devices from App Store
- **How different joints work in human?** 3D animation, available at www.youtube.com/watch?v=Un_iG74R_TI
- **International Cartilage Repair Society** videos and 3D animations, available at https://cartilage.org/patient/video
- **Ligaments, tendons and joints** available at www.khanacademy.org/science/high-school-biology/hs-human-body-systems/hs-the-musculoskeletal-system/v/ligaments-tendons-and-joints

INTRODUCTION

The human skeletal system is designed for movement, to facilitate locomotion and to enable positioning of the limbs in space for function. It is the joints of the skeletal system, together with the neuromuscular system, that enable this movement. Joints exist to join the bony segments of the body; that is, when the end of a bone articulates (joins) with another bone, a joint is formed. This joint is often referred to as an **articulation** or **arthrosis**.

More simply, the long bones of the body can be considered as levers that can transmit, accept and modify force and motion, whereas it is around the axis of the joints that join these levers that movement occurs. Joints in series have a relationship whereby movement around one joint influences movement at another joint (Fig. 5.1). Depending on the type of joint, movement can be extreme across large ranges or very minimal.

There are several types of joints in the human body, the structure of which dictates the movement and function permitted at each joint. Generally, joints are classified as **non-synovial joints** (synarthrosis) and **synovial joints** (diarthrosis) based on the material that comprises the

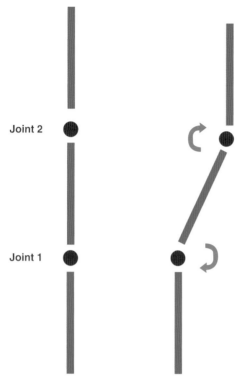

FIGURE 5.1 **Joints act as an axis for movement between bones of the skeletal system.** Joints may be connected in series such that movement at one joint (joint 1) influences movement at the joint above or below (joint 2).

joint. Non-synovial joints are categorised as either **fibrous** or **cartilaginous**. Synovial joints are the most common joints in the body and enable movement of the limbs. Joints of the upper limbs have an innately different function than those of the lower limbs, given that humans use the upper limbs for tasks involving reaching and grasping, while the lower limbs are used in locomotion. It can be helpful to consider the functional demands on the joints—for example, a weight-bearing joint such as the knee—when attempting to understand the structural components of a joint, as there is a bilateral relationship between structure and function which changes across the life span. In this chapter we explore the basic structure and function of the joints of the skeletal system and how these are maintained by relationships with other systems in the body.

STRUCTURE AND FUNCTION OF THE JOINTS
Fibrous joints

A **fibrous joint** is an articulation between two bones that is joined by fibrous tissue. Fibrous tissue is comprised predominantly of collagen produced by resident fibrocytes and organised in a dense network. This key structural feature means that very little movement can occur at a fibrous joint. There are three types of fibrous joints: suture, gomphose and syndesmosis.

Suture

Sutures are bony articulations shaped so they interlock or overlap on one another and are united by a fibrous membrane. They are found only in the skull and they permit very little movement to occur (Fig. 5.2). At birth,

FIGURE 5.2 **The suture is a strong fibrous joint uniting the flat bones of the skull.**

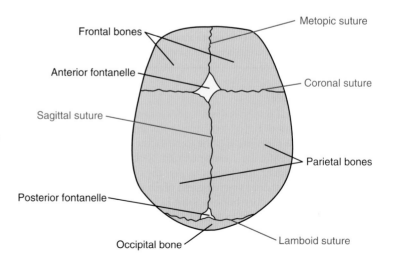

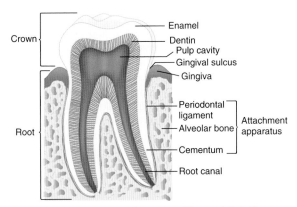

FIGURE 5.3 **The gomphose is a fibrous joint: the peg-shaped tooth is held in the mandible or the maxilla with fibrous tissue.** (*Source:* Buttaravoli P, Leffler SM. Minor emergencies, 3 ed. Elsevier Saunders, 2012.)

some movement is permitted at these joints to facilitate compliance and elasticity of the skull during the birthing process. In early development it supports the growing brain. During the first two years of life, sutures become more rigid and fixed for adulthood.

Gomphose

A **gomphose** is a unique fibrous joint in which a bone fits into another bone like a peg in a socket. The only place that gomphoses occur is in the mandible and maxilla (jaw) (Fig. 5.3), where the peg-like root of a tooth fits into a tooth socket. Structurally, very little movement occurs at this joint in an adult.

Syndesmosis

A **syndesmosis** occurs when two bones that do not have good bony congruence or fit are held together by a fibrous ligament or aponeurosis, often reinforced by ligaments. The most common example of a syndesmosis is the radioulnar joint, where the radius and ulna bones of the forearm are held together by a long sheet of connective tissue (Fig. 5.4). A small amount of movement occurs

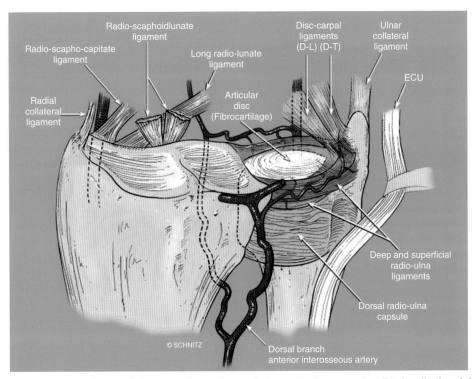

FIGURE 5.4 **A syndesmosis between the radius and ulna of the forearm: the distal radioulnar joint.** The connective tissue between the two bones also serves as an attachment site for muscle tissue. (*Source:* Kleinman WB. Stability of the distal radioulnar joint: biomechanics, pathophysiology, physical diagnosis and restoration of function what we have learned in 25 years. J Hand Surg Am 2007;32(7):1086–106.)

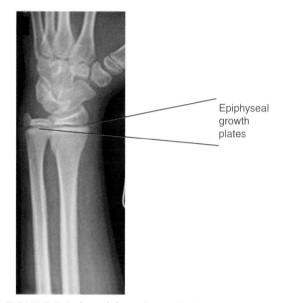

FIGURE 5.5 An epiphyseal growth plate is a primary cartilaginous joint. The epiphyseal plate is a region of cartilage in the long bones that has not ossified and exists to facilitate the increase in length of the long bones with growth and development.

at this joint to enable pronation and supination for positioning the hand in space. What is interesting about this joint is that bony articulations are not necessarily shaped to fit to one another (lack of congruence).

Cartilaginous joints

Cartilaginous joints are distinct from fibrous joints due to the nature of the material that binds the joint surfaces together at the bone-on-bone interface, namely fibrocartilage or hyaline cartilage. Hyaline cartilage is comprised of chondrocyte cells and the extracellular matrix of predominantly collagen and proteoglycans, which they produce. In contrast, the cellular composition of fibrocartilage includes both fibrocytes and chondrocytes. **Fibrocartilage** is considered a transitional tissue, with varying amounts of type I and type II collagen,[1] the cross-links between which make it a very strong tissue. Cartilaginous joints are categorised into primary cartilaginous joints and secondary cartilaginous joints.

Primary cartilaginous joints

Primary cartilaginous joints exist as cartilage regions of bones that articulate the ossifying regions of a bone together (Fig. 5.5). Their function is to enable slight bending of the long bones during early life and to permit the bones to grow in length. These primary cartilaginous joint regions convert to bone once bone growth and maturity are achieved; hence they are considered temporary joints. Thus, primary cartilaginous joints are not joints that function in the standard sense of allowing significant amounts of movement to occur. Instead, they exist to facilitate the increase in length of long bones during development.

Secondary cartilaginous joints

Secondary cartilaginous joints are also known as '**symphysis**' joints. They comprise two bony articulations covered with hyaline cartilage. These joints are considered very stable due to the tight fibrocartilage that spans between the articulating surfaces. However, these joints still permit small amounts of movement due to the ability of the collagen fibres to undergo stretch or deformation. The simplest examples of secondary cartilaginous or symphysis joints are the pubic symphysis in the midline of the pelvis (Fig. 5.6) and the intervertebral joints between the vertebral bodies in the spinal column.

FIGURE 5.6 The pubic symphysis joint. The pubic symphysis joint is a secondary cartilaginous joint found in the midline of the body; it permits very little movement.

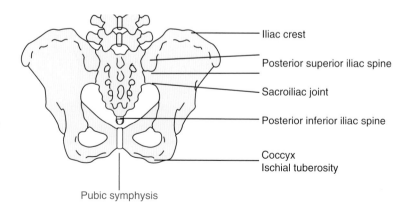

Synovial joints

Synovial joints are the most common joint in the human body. They allow the greatest degree of movement due to the shape of the articulating surfaces and loose joint capsules and are typically the easiest for clinicians to conceptualise. They are comprised of two bony components whose articulating surfaces are covered with hyaline cartilage. These articulating surfaces are only indirectly connected to one another by a joint capsule and associated ligaments. Synovial joints also have a joint cavity, which is enclosed by a joint capsule, and have a synovial lining on the inside of the joint capsule. This synovial lining produces a synovial fluid that covers the joint surfaces. Synovial joints have associated ligaments to support the joint in addition to other accessory structures to augment stability and mobility including fibrocartilaginous discs, menisci, labrums, fat pads and tendons.

Structurally, synovial joints can be categorised by the shape of their articular surfaces. The orientation, size and shape of the articular surfaces of a synovial joint dictate the movements that can occur at each joint (Table 5.1). Regardless of the shape of the articular surfaces of a synovial joint and its subsequent categorisation, the features of synovial joints are homogeneous.

Hyaline cartilage

Hyaline cartilage is a smooth, translucent form of cartilage that lines the articulating surfaces of a synovial joint. The role of hyaline cartilage is to enable the joint surfaces to move smoothly on one another, reduce friction between the joint surfaces and, in a weight-bearing synovial joint, provide some shock absorption.[2] Hyaline cartilage is comprised of chondrocyte cells and the extracellular matrix of predominantly collagen and proteoglycans, which they produce and maintain.[2] The cartilage extracellular matrix is comprised predominantly of:

- proteoglycans (core proteins with glycosaminoglycan chains comprised of negatively charged carbohydrate polymers, mainly aggrecan in hyaline cartilage) and water they attract
- collagen network (white fibres of connective tissue, predominantly type II) in which the proteoglycans are embedded
- other non-collagen proteins (non-proteoglycan polysaccharide proteins).

Proteoglycans interact with one another to attract water to provide swelling pressure, which is resisted by tension within the collagen network, to enable the cartilage tissue to distribute and withstand load in the synovial joint.[3] When a compressive load is applied,

TABLE 5.1		
Categorisation of synovial joints		
Type of joint	**Description**	**Example**
Ball and socket	A rounded joint surface (ball or head) articulates with a concave surface (socket). This articulation configuration of spherical surfaces enables movement on several axes (flexion/extension; rotation; abduction/adduction)	Glenohumeral (shoulder) joint
Hinge joint	A hinge joint is comprised of two joint surfaces that permit movement in one plane (uniaxial), allowing flexion and extension only	Elbow joint
Plane joint	Two planar, or relatively flat, surfaces articulate with one another enabling only sliding or gliding of the surfaces on one another; plane joints are typical uniaxial (permit movement in one plane only)	Acromioclavicular joint
Saddle joint	A saddle joint is comprised of two articulating surfaces shaped like a saddle that fit with one another (where they articulate, one surface is concave and the other is convex); this bony orientation allows for movement in two different planes	First carpometacarpal joint (thumb)
Condyloid joint	A condyloid joint is comprised of two spherical joint surfaces which enable movement in two planes, including combined movements	Metacarpophalangeal joints
Pivot joint	Pivot joints are rare in the human body and are comprised of a round projection from a bone fitting into a round socket made from a ligamentous structure, rather than a bony structure	Atlantoaxial joint

some of the water content of the cartilage is released; when the compressive load is removed, this fluid moves back into the cartilage. **Collagen** makes up the bulk of the tissue volume and gives cartilage the ability to resist load as well as a smooth surface for the articulating surfaces. The strength of the collagen matrix is dependent on the nature and extent of the cross-links that exist between the collagen fibrils and the orientation of the fibrils (vertical in the deepest layers, becoming more horizontal in the superficial layers).[2]

There are four distinct regions or layers within hyaline cartilage, the structure of which reflects their function (Fig. 5.7). In **layer 1** (outermost layer), collagen fibres are aligned horizontally, parallel to the surface to create a smooth outermost layer. In **layer 2** (mid zone), collagen fibres are aligned in a loose framework or latticework,

enabling deformation and shock absorption. In **layer 3** (deep zone, also known as the radiate stratum), collagen fibres are aligned vertically extending into the calcified regions of cartilage above the subchondral bone to integrate the superficial to the deep layers. **Layer 4** (calcified zone deepest layer adjacent to bone) is a calcified region of cartilage adjacent to the subchondral bone, anchoring the hyaline cartilage to the bone.

Two additional characteristic structural features of hyaline cartilage are that it lacks neurons (it is aneural) and vascular structures (it is avascular). The absence of a blood and nerve supply enables large forces to be transmitted through the articulating joint surfaces such as those that are absorbed through the knees during running, without pain. Being avascular in nature means hyaline cartilage needs to receive nutrition from the

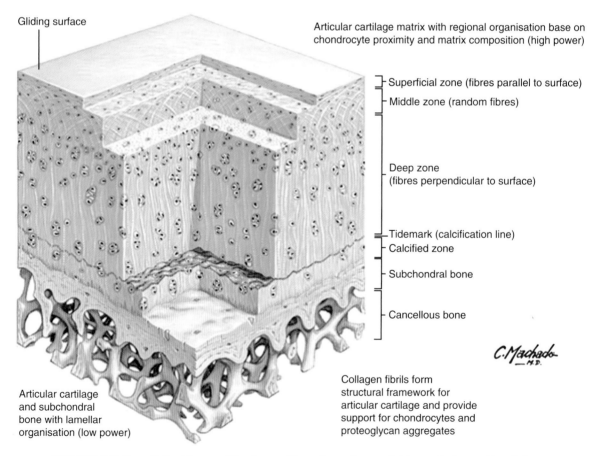

Gliding surface

Articular cartilage matrix with regional organisation base on chondrocyte proximity and matrix composition (high power)

Superficial zone (fibres parallel to surface)

Middle zone (random fibres)

Deep zone (fibres perpendicular to surface)

Tidemark (calcification line)

Calcified zone

Subchondral bone

Cancellous bone

Articular cartilage and subchondral bone with lamellar organisation (low power)

Collagen fibrils form structural framework for articular cartilage and provide support for chondrocytes and proteoglycan aggregates

C. Machado
— M.D.

FIGURE 5.7 Four distinct layers of hyaline cartilage. Layer 1, superficial zone (outermost layer); layer 2, the mid zone; layer 3, the deep zone; layer 4, calcified layer adjacent to bone. (*Source:* Green WB. Netter's orthopaedics. Philadelphia, Elsevier, 2006.)

subchondral surface below and the synovial fluid above. Importantly, for homeostasis and nutrition of the cartilage, the flow of synovial fluid that occurs within a joint with movement is integral for cartilage health. Thus, joint movement and physical activity are integral to joint homeostasis.

Joint capsule

The **joint capsule** is a loose sleeve, similar to a balloon, that forms a sealed enclosure around the articulating bones to which it attaches. The capsule itself is comprised of thick, dense collagenous and fibrous tissue, giving it significant strength.[4] As with cartilage, the orientation of the fibres that make up the capsule varies regionally depending on the stresses the tissue must withstand. The joint capsule is reinforced regionally by ligaments that span the width of the articulation to resist stresses that stretch or strain the joint through the extremes of range of movement. For example, in the hip joint, there are four large ligaments that reinforce the joint capsule, all running in different directions (Fig. 5.8); they are ultimately indistinguishable from the capsule due to the degree to which they blend into the joint capsule itself. The ligaments anterior to the joint provide resistance and limit hip extension as they are stretched as the hip moves into extension.

Unlike cartilage, the joint capsule has a nerve supply and a blood supply, albeit a small one. Both proprioceptive and pain nerve endings have been identified in the capsule, which indicate that capsular innervation has a role in proprioception and protecting the joint from extremes of movement. Proprioceptive receptors in the joint capsule include both Ruffini (stretch) receptors and Pacinian receptors (responsive to compression and changes in hydrostatic pressure in the joint).[5]

Ligaments

Ligaments are dense bands of collagen fibres that provide passive stability and reinforcement to joints in the human body.[6] To this end, and distinct from tendons that attach muscles to bone, ligaments run between and connect two articulating bony surfaces. With respect to synovial joints, ligaments can be classified as **extra-capsular ligaments** that run outside the joint capsule (e.g. lateral collateral ligament of the knee) and **intra-capsular ligaments** (e.g. anterior and posterior cruciate ligaments of the knee) that span between two articulating surfaces but inside the capsule of the joint. The function of both intra- and extra-articular ligaments is to enhance the stability of the synovial joint. This is enabled by their inherent relatively stiff, strong collagenous structure and via their proprioceptive innervation.[6]

Depending on the orientation of the ligament, the direction in which the ligament runs will dictate what

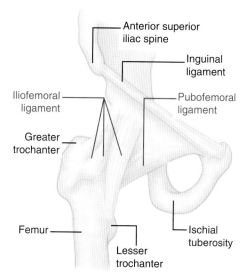

FIGURE 5.8 The hip joint ligaments reinforce the joint capsule, blending with this tissue so the two are indistinguishable. They are named after the bone they originate from and attach to. The ischiofemoral ligament runs posterior to the joint.

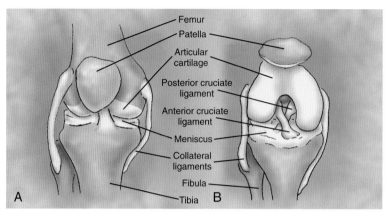

FIGURE 5.9 **The extra- and intra-articular ligaments of the knee shown with the joint in extension A and flexion B.** Extra-articular ligaments: the medial collateral ligament blends with the joint capsule, whereas the lateral collateral ligament is more pronounced. These ligaments resist forces of the joint in the frontal plane. Intra-articular ligaments: the anterior and posterior cruciate ligaments, named by their relative origin on the tibial plateau, resist anterior and posterior translation of the tibia on the femur. (*Source:* Madick S. Anterior cruciate ligament reconstruction of the knee, AORN J 2011;93(2):210–25.)

forces or direction of movement the ligament will pursue. For example, at the knee the two extracapsular ligaments are the medial collateral ligament, spanning between the medial femoral condyle and the medial aspect of the tibia, and the lateral collateral ligament, running between the lateral femoral condyle and the head of fibula (Fig. 5.9). These two ligaments run in parallel on either side of the knee joint in the frontal plane and will resist opposite forces and movements to one another (Fig. 5.10). The medial collateral ligament

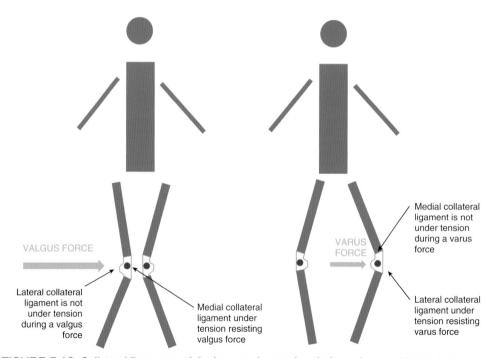

FIGURE 5.10 **Collateral ligaments of the knee under tension during valgus and varus forces.**

will resist a valgus force to the knee, or a knock-knee position, where the medial femoral condyle is forced away from the medial aspect of the tibia. In contrast, the lateral collateral ligament will resist a varus force to the knee, or a bow-knee position, where the lateral femoral condyle is stretched away from the head of the fibula. However, ligaments are a little more complex than this simplistic model.

A ligament itself is comprised of many bundles of predominantly (~85%) type 1 collagen aligned along the length or axis of the ligament.[6] Ligament structure is very similar to that of muscle tendon: a hierarchical organisation of bundles of type 1 collagen aligned in the direction of regional stress that are produced by resident fibroblasts that respond to load. However, fibroblasts in ligament are more rounded in shape and produce slightly less organised collagen fibres. These collagen fibres sit in a ground substance of other proteoglycans and water, with crosslinks developed between the individual fibres for strength.

When the synovial joint is in a neutral position—so the ligaments that reinforce the joint are not under stretch or strain—there is a 'crimping' of the collagen. That is, the length of the collagen fibre is wavy at rest, so that the ligament has capacity to lengthen and resist tensile load or stretching of the joint and ligament. As a ligament is stretched or exposed to tensile load, also known as strain, it will deform ('creep') in a non-linear manner (Fig. 5.11). However, like all visco-elastic materials, ligament will return to its resting length once the load is removed, unless the load applied exceeds the capacity of the ligament to withstand tensile load, as occurs in a joint sprain, where a region of the ligament will tear. Under normal conditions, once a submaximal load is removed, depending on the time and magnitude of force applied, the time the collagen fibres take to return to their resting length will vary. This creep phenomenon happens at a microscopic level—and at the macroscopic level of a ligament no changes in length are physiologically perceivable under normal conditions.[7]

The nature of ligament insertion into the bones from which it originates is complex. Simply, ligaments have either a direct (fibrocartilaginous) insertion or an indirect (fibrous) insertion defined by the predominant connective tissue of the insertion. Direct insertion comprises four zones of the connective tissue: ligament, fibrocartilage, mineral fibrocartilage becoming bone/periosteum. Indirect insertion has both superficial components that insert into the periosteum and deep components (Sharpey fibres) and collagen fibres that anchor directly into the bone. Under normal healthy conditions, ligament insertions are very strong and robust.

Ligaments, and the synovial joints they reinforce, are protected from excessive forces by the proprioceptive innervation of the ligaments themselves. Proprioceptive nerves are characterised by **mechanoreceptors** (sensory transducers at the end of afferent nerves including Ruffini, Pacini corpuscles and Golgi-type nerve endings)[8] that are responsive to stretch and send signals to the central nervous system about the position of a joint in space. It is by this nature of innervation of ligaments that they can play a vital role in joint stability.

Synovial lining (stratum synovium)
Lining the interior aspect of the joint capsule is the **synovial lining**, a layer of connective tissue that produces synovial fluid. In addition, the synovial lining contains proprioceptive Golgi receptors that respond to pressure changes within the joint at extreme ranges of movement.[4] The synovial lining can be considered to have two layers: the intima and the subsynovial tissue.

Intima. The intima is comprised of specialised fibroblasts called synoviocytes that sit within an extracellular matrix of proteins and of which there are two types. **Type A synoviocytes** are responsible for synthesis of phagocytotic enzymes whose role is to clear debris from the joint space. This role is balanced by **type B synoviocytes**, which secrete enzymes that inhibit excessive destructive action of type A synoviocytes. In normal synovium, there is a greater prevalence of type B synoviocytes than type A synoviocytes, to ensure that there is not excessive degradative enzymatic activity that could be destructive to the joint structure. Both type A and B synoviocytes synthesise products that constitute the synovial fluid and the extracellular matrix in which the cells sit, as

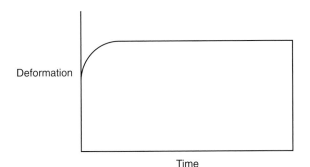

FIGURE 5.11 Collagen fibres in ligament exhibit creep when a constant load is applied. As a constant tensile load is applied, the collagen fibres will initially rapidly deform, as evidenced by the initial steep curve of the graph, and then more gradually deform over time.

well as cytokines and growth factors.[9] Type B also secrete antigens and thus have a key role in the immune response. The balanced interaction of local cytokines either stimulating or inhibiting activity of type A or B synoviocytes enables repair of synovium, response to immune threats and destruction of tissue or loose bodies in the joint. The intima is richly innervated and dense with small blood vessels (capillaries) and the accompanying lymphatics, all of which interact to support the synoviocyte cell function.

Subsynovial tissue. The subsynovial tissue lies between the intima and the joint capsule and inserts into the bony surfaces. Essentially the role of this layer of synovium is to form the attachment to the capsule and to support the cells of the intima above through the rich blood supply that originates in this region. The subsynovial tissue also has a rich sympathetic nerve supply that supports the blood supply to the synovium.

Synovial fluid

Synovial fluid is a clear, lubricating fluid that is a distinguishing feature of all synovial joints. The nature of synovial fluid has been described as analogous to blood plasma;[7] however, it also contains hyaluronic acid and a glycoprotein, lubricin. The role of **lubricin** is to provide lubrication to the cartilage surfaces, while hyaluronic acid acts to reduce the friction between the folds of the capsule and the articular surfaces. The synovial fluid reduces friction between the components of the joint and keeps the joint lubricated. As discussed, the synovial fluid also has a role in providing nutrition to the chondrocyte cells of the hyaluronic cartilage to ensure

that they maintain optimal function and integrity of the cartilage of the joint.[9]

Menisci, labrums, fat pads and bursae associated with synovial joints

The key features of synovial joints are hyaline cartilage covering the articular surfaces, a joint capsule lined by a synovial membrane supported by intra- and extra-articular ligaments and lubricating synovial fluid (Fig. 5.12). There are other components that are associated with some synovial joints throughout the body that have a function specific to their associated joint and are important to appreciate, specifically the menisci in the tibiofemoral (knee joint), labrums (which line the socket of a ball-and-socket joint), fat pads (associated with the patellofemoral joint and the subtalar joint) and bursae (located throughout the body). These accessories to a joint act to increase stability, redistribute load and minimise friction between any two surfaces.

Menisci are found in knee joints of all weight-bearing mammals. They are moon-shaped shock-absorbing discs that protect the joint surfaces by redistributing load and, in humans, by increasing congruence between the large femoral condyles and shallow tibial plateau (Fig. 5.10). Menisci are attached to the tibial plateau around their border by a mixture of calcified and uncalcified fibro-cartilage. The knee joint undergoes significant loads during weight-bearing activities. The role of menisci is to redistribute load across the joint surfaces, essentially acting as shock absorbers. Like hyaline cartilage, menisci are relatively hypocellular but dense in collagen, organised in line with the circumference in a crescent shape. The outer third of the menisci receives a blood and

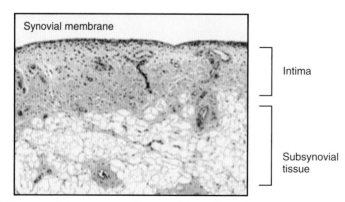

FIGURE 5.12 **The synovial membrane.** The synovial membrane has two layers: the intima, which is rich in synoviocyte cells; and the sub-synovial tissue layer, which attaches to the capsule. (*Source:* Modified from Block J, Scanzello C. Osteoarthritis. In: Goldman L, Goldman-Cecil medicine, 25 ed. Philadelphia, PA: Elsevier; 2016.)

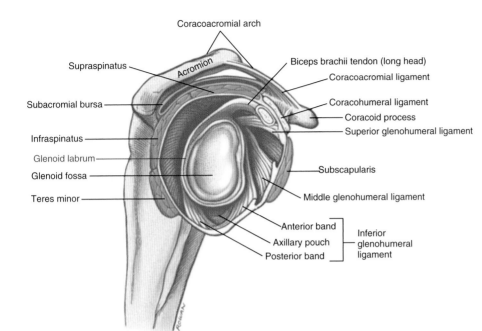

FIGURE 5.13 **The glenoid labrum extends the articular surface of the glenoid fossa, increasing the articulation congruence between the large ball (humeral head) and the shallow socket (glenoid fossa).** (*Source:* Modified from Magee D. Shoulder. In: Kinesiology of the musculoskeletal system: foundations for rehabilitation. St Louis: Mosby; 2014.)

nerve supply, whereas the inner portion does not, with implications for healing and regenerative capacity. Given the role of menisci in absorbing and redistributing load through the knee, any changes to meniscus integrity and health will have an impact on cartilage loading and health.

A **labrum** is a fibrocartilage ring or rim that lines the socket of a ball-and-socket joint, such as the glenohumeral joint (shoulder) (Fig. 5.13)[10] and femoroacetabular joints (hip),[11] with the primary purpose to deepen the socket and increase the stability of the joint. Other functions include acting as the insertion and attachment site for the joint capsule, ligaments and tendons. A labrum typically can be considered to have three surfaces: a base that attaches to the bony rim of the socket; an external surface that contacts the joint capsule; and an internal surface that acts as an articulating surface for the 'ball' of the ball-and-socket joint. Similar to the meniscus, the blood supply to the labrum is restricted to the periphery, with consequent relevance for healing.

Fat pads can be intra- or extra-articular associated with a synovial joint (Fig. 5.14). That is, they can occupy space within a joint, themselves covered by synovial membrane such as the infra-patella fat pad which sits in the patellofemoral joint space,[12] or they can be external to the joint space and joint, such as the fat pad under the calcaneus that assists shock absorption through the subtalar and talocrural (ankle) joints. As the name suggests, fat pads are comprised of a mass of closely

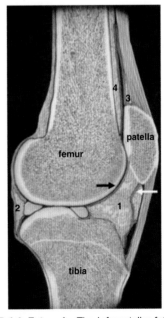

FIGURE 5.14 **Fat pads.** The infrapatellar fat pad (1) is the largest fat pad in the knee and is thought to act as a biomechanical cushion between the patella and the tibia. The posterior fat pad (2), anterior suprapatellar fat pad (3) and suprapatellar fat pad (4) are smaller fat pads associated with the knee joint. (*Source:* Clockaerts S et al. The infrapatellar fat pad should be considered as an active osteoarthritic joint tissue: a narrative review. Osteoarthritis Cartilage 2010;18(7):876–82.)

packed fat cells within honeycomb-like septa of fibrous tissue.[13] Unlike other accessory features of a synovial joint, fat pads receive a rich blood and nerve supply, and thus can become inflamed or painful when irritated.

Fat pads are unique in that although they are similar to subcutaneous fat cells, they are not metabolised, nor do they increase in size or volume depending on energy intake and body mass index. Fat pads are thought to play mainly a biomechanical role. At the knee, the infrapatellar fat pad occupies dead space within a joint. Together with its synovial membrane covering, it is thought to increase surface area for the synovial membrane and thus synovial fluid production for lubrication, and change the flow of synovial fluid within the joint to facilitate greater lubrication.[14] Fat pads also act as biomechanical 'cushions' or shock absorbers. For example, the infrapatellar fat pad, which lies between the tibia and the patella tendon, and the posterior fat pad of the elbow, which lies between the triceps tendon and olecranon, provide protection for these tendons. There are suggestions that fat pads may also have a non-biomechanical role, as adipose tissue is considered an endocrine organ capable of producing cytokines, interleukins and growth factors.[14] In the context of the synovial joint, these mediators have been found in synovial fluid and are able to influence cartilage and synovium metabolism.[14]

Bursae are extra-articular fluid-filled sacs that act to minimise friction between bone and overlying connective or soft-tissue structures, such as the subacromial bursae which lie between the acromium and the supraspinatus tendon to provide protection in the subacromial space (Fig. 5.15). Bursae are similarly lined with a synovial membrane that produces synovial fluid that fills the bursae.

INTEGRATION OF THE SKELETAL JOINTS WITH OTHER BODY SYSTEMS

Muscular system

The joints of the skeletal system provide the system with flexibility and the opportunity to position the limbs and levers of the skeletal system in space for function. The muscular system (Chapter 6), specifically the individual muscles that cross a joint, driven by the central nervous system, is responsible for creating movement around a joint and providing active stability to support the passive stability structures (such as ligaments). The proprioceptive fibres within the joint capsule and associated ligaments in a synovial joint provide feedback to the range and speed of movement occurring at the joint

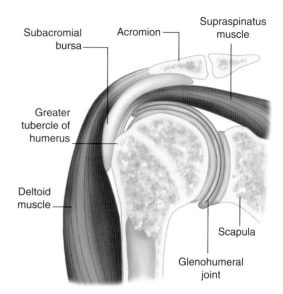

FIGURE 5.15 Subacromial bursa of the glenohumeral joint of the shoulder. The bursa is a fluid-filled sac that lies between the supraspinatus tendon and the bony acromium above. (*Source:* Biundo JJ. Bursitis, tendinitis, and other periarticular disorders and sports medicine. In: Goldman L, Andrew I. Goldman-Cecil medicine, vol 2, 24 ed. Philadelphia, PA: Elsevier; 2012, p. 1676–81.)

to regulate the amount of muscle activity required to maintain joint stability and the forces acting across the joint within a safe range. In addition to facilitating movement at a joint, the stabilising and prime mover muscles, which cross an articulation, also actively absorb force in weight-bearing activities and help reduce the load through the articular surfaces. Being physically active is crucial for homeostasis of muscle, bone and joint tissue as these tissues are metabolically active in response to load. Thus, muscle health and fitness are equally important for joint health. For example, sustained suboptimal postures, such as prolonged sitting in thoracic kyphosis over an ill-positioned laptop for prolonged and repeated bouts of time where the thoracic extensor muscles are on stretch rather than being active, deprives the joint tissues from any stretch or movement stimulus and can result in stiffness of the costovertebral and intervertebral joints in this region.

Immune system

Homeostasis of the immune system is a complex phenomenon (Chapter 15). When considering the most common joints in the human body, the synovial joints, there are several resident specialised cells that can be considered immune cells and that play a role in regulating an inflammatory response within the joint and communicate with the broader immune system, similar to those in other body systems. Type A synoviocytes, which sit in the intimal layer of the synovial lining, are macrophage-type cells derived from blood-borne mononuclear cells. In addition to the ability to phagocytose debris in the joint, type A synoviocytes are immunoreactive to several antibodies and can express antigens as part of an early immune response.[15] As explored in this chapter, under normal conditions type A synoviocytes secrete lysosomal enzymes to phagocytose debris in a joint, but they can also be involved in inappropriate immune responses (e.g. excessive degradation, formation of reactive oxygen species). The presence and nature of type A synoviocytes can result in synovial joints being involved in a more systemic, widespread immune response in the body and this is related to the presentation of autoimmune disease such as rheumatoid arthritis.

Endocrine system

In addition to its other functions, oestrogen is known as a regulatory hormone in the metabolism of connective tissue, including ligaments and cartilage. Oestrogen receptors have been identified within ligament tissue, and there is a building body of evidence that collagen synthesis decreases with lower oestrogen levels.[16] This has relevance for ligament strength and stiffness. For example, anterior cruciate ligament (ACL) injury is three to five times more common in women than men[17] and on this basis, extensive research has explored the relationship between the hormonal cycle and ligament laxity. A reduction in oestradiol (a form of oestrogen) has been shown to be associated with a reduction in collagen synthesis, and during the phase of the menstrual cycle when oestradiol is at its lowest, there is some evidence that ACL ligament laxity, measured by clinical tests, increases.[16] During pregnancy, the laxity of the typically relatively immobile sacroiliac joints increases, thought historically to be due to increased levels of the hormone relaxin circulating in the system.

AGE-RELATED CHANGES

Throughout life the skeletal joints change as part of the ageing process. This process is unique and depends on the type of joint (e.g. fibrous versus cartilaginous), the location of the joint in the body (i.e. weight-bearing or non-weight-bearing) and the loads placed on the joint throughout the life span.

For joints that permit movement and growth (fibrous sutures of the skull and the primary cartilaginous joints [growth plates of the long bones]), these changes happen rapidly in early life. The fibrous sutures of the skull become more rigid and fixed within the first two years of life as the skull becomes fixed for adulthood. The primary cartilaginous joints (growth plates) are ossified (converted to bone) between the ages of 11 and 19 years,[18] with growth plate closure typically happening later in males than in females (which is why adolescent males tend to have later 'growth spurts' than females).

Secondary cartilaginous joints (those that are located in the midline and permit little movement because of the tight fibrocartilage connecting the two bones) undergo load and age-related changes as we age. For example, it is very common for the fibrocartilage discs in the spine between the vertebral bodies to reduce in height due to a reduction in water content, resulting in a loss of height, and for the zygapophyseal joints between the lamina of the vertebral bodies to come closer together, stimulating bone growth (osteophytes).[7]

With respect to synovial joints, there are some frequently seen age-related changes, particularly in the hip, knee and first toe (joints that undergo significant load during gait and activities of daily living). Chondrocytes (the metabolically active cells of cartilage) become less active and produce smaller and fewer proteoglycans, which can lead to reduced water content and shock absorption capacity, thus increasing loads on the subchondral bone and subsequent thickening of bone in this region.[19] As cartilage narrows, this brings the joint surfaces closer together, reducing the joint space and resulting in a shortening of the supporting ligaments, both of which can contribute to joint stiffness.[20] It is thought that age-related changes to joints can be mitigated by staying physically active and maintaining muscle mass to improve function and the shock-absorbing capacity of the musculoskeletal system.

CONCLUSION

The joints of the skeletal system, together with the muscular system, are integral for skeletal movement generated by the muscular system. The function of a joint is directly related to its structure and conversely structure to function, including the shape of the articulating bony surfaces, the type of connective tissue lining the articulating surfaces and the resident cells within a joint (e.g. synoviocytes). Movement and loading are fundamental to joint and body homeostasis.

CASE STUDY 5.1

Alice has just had her first child and at her maternal nurse education session, the nurse spends some time on the importance of variability in resting positions for the baby for development. It is not uncommon for newborn children to have an asymmetrical or partially flattened head shape.

Q1. Synarthrosis joints include:
  a. fibrous and cartilaginous joints.
  b. fibrous and synovial joints.
  c. cartilaginous and synovial joints.
  d. synovial joints.

Q2. The features of fibrous joints include:
  a. a joint that is found only in the skull.
  b. a bony articulation that directly unites bone to bone via fibrous tissue.
  c. a bony articulation that unites bone to bone via a capsule.
  d. a joint that is found only in the midline.

Q3. Mobility of the fibrous joints of the skull (sutures) is designed to:
  a. provide flexibility of the skull to control intracranial blood pressure.
  b. provide flexibility of the skull to enable brain growth during childhood.
  c. provide flexibility of the skull to enable brain growth during childhood and for deformation for passage through the birth canal.
  d. do nothing as there is no mobility of the fibrous joints of the skull.

Q4. What type of joints are present in the skull and what is the structure and function of these joints that has relevance for head shape in a child?

Q5. Suggest what might be a consequence for the development of a child's brain if the joints that are present in the skull fuse too early.

CASE STUDY 5.2

Jenny is in her early 20s and recently started working at a law company in the central business district. She was wearing high heels every day, which forced her to walk more on the lateral aspect of her foot. She also sat at her desk with her right foot crossed over her left all day, such that the outside of her ankle was constantly under stretch. When she walked on the uneven surface of her driveway, she noticed than her right ankle felt a little 'looser' and had a little more movement than her left ankle. Subsequently, she started wearing flats and making a conscious effort to sit with good posture, her feet flat upon the floor. After doing so, she no longer has the same perception of joint laxity.

Q1. Which of the following are passive stabilisers of a synovial joint?
  a. Joint capsule, hyaline cartilage, intra-articular ligaments
  b. Joint capsule, intra-articular ligaments, synovial fluid
  c. Joint capsule, intra-articular ligaments, extra-articular ligaments, labrum
  d. Intra-articular ligaments, extra-articular ligaments, synovial fluid, labrum

Q2. Which of the following statements is true?
  a. Ligaments are comprised predominantly of type 1 collagen and deform under stretch in a non-linear manner. Once a load is removed, collagen has the capacity to return to its pre-stretch length.
  b. Ligaments are comprised predominantly of proteoglycans and deform under stretch in a non-linear manner. Once a load is removed, collagen has the capacity to return to its pre-stretch length.
  c. Ligaments are comprised predominantly of proteoglycans and deform under stretch in a linear manner. Once a load is removed, a ligament will stay at its stretched length.
  d. Ligaments are comprised of predominantly type 1 collagen and deform under stretch in a linear manner. Once a load is removed, a ligament will stay at its stretched length.

Q3. Which of the following is true?
  a. Ligaments are highly innervated by proprioceptive nerve fibres which are involved in the perception of pain.
  b. Ligaments have sparse nerve supply and are purely passive collagenous structures to provide rigid support to a joint.
  c. Ligaments are richly innervated by proprioceptive nerve fibres which are responsive to stretch and signal to the central nervous system about the rate of stretch to provide information about joint position sense and the position of the joint in space.
  d. Ligaments have a rich blood and nerve supply.

Q4. What elements are responsible for the stability of a synovial joint? What is the structure of the key passive stability structures? Consider your answer with respect to the talocrural joint, which is a hinge joint.

Q5. What other systems would be influenced in this scenario?

CASE STUDY 5.3

David has just had his 67th birthday. He has been a recreational runner all his life, running 5–6 km two to three times per week. Since he turned 50 he has gradually become more aware of the impact forces through his knees during running and prefers to run on grass rather than asphalt paths, and rather than running on consecutive days he requires a day off between sessions. He mentions this to the members of his mature-aged running club and finds that everyone has similar experiences but they are still able to enjoy running.

Q1. Hyaline cartilage is a unique tissue that lines the articulating surfaces of a joint to reduce friction and provide shock absorption. Chondrocytes are responsible for the maintenance of cartilage structure and receive their nutrition from:

   a. the blood vessels that run within the hyaline cartilage matrix.

   b. the blood vessels that run within the hyaline cartilage matrix and the subchondral bone below.

   c. the blood vessels that run within the hyaline cartilage matrix and the circulating synovial fluid.

   d. the circulating synovial fluid and subchondral bone.

Q2. Which of the following is true of chondrocyte cells?

   a. Chondrocyte cells are rounded, specialised fibroblasts that respond to load to produce type 1 collagen and proteoglycans to maintain the extracellular matrix.

   b. Chondrocyte cells respond to substances in the synovial fluid to produce type 1 collagen and proteoglycans to maintain the cellular matrix.

   c. Chondrocyte cells are categorised as type A or type B cells depending on their metabolic function.

   d. Chondrocyte cells are organised alongside blood vessels in line with the orientation of the collagen fibres.

Q3. What other features specific to the knee joint can contribute to shock absorption and load distribution?

   a. Fat pads

   b. Menisci

   c. Labrum

   d. Bursae

Q4. What structures of the knee joint are responsible for shock absorption and what is the normal influence of ageing on this structure?

Q5. What other systems could influence the perception of shock absorption?

CASE STUDY 5.4

Scott is 10 years old and at his school fete he sees that one of the stalls is creating fake plaster casts for students to wear. Scott has a plaster cast made that fits over his left wrist and thumb but is open to allow him to take it on and off. He loves the cast and wears it for a week, getting signatures from all his friends and family on the cast. After a week, his mum makes him take it off. Scott finds that his left thumb feels stiff and is not moving as freely as his right thumb. This feeling resolves after a day or two.

Q1. Which of the following is needed as a stimulus for maintenance of homeostasis in a synovial joint?

   a. Movement

   b. Heat

   c. Cold

   d. Training overload

Q2. Which of the following is true about synovial fluid?

   a. It is comprised of lubricin and hyaluronic acid secreted by type A synovial cells in isolation in the intimal lining of the synovial membrane and is rich in immune cells.

   b. It is a feature of all joints and is comprised of lubricin and hyaluronic acid secreted by both type A and type B synovial cells and acts as a lubricant for the joint.

   c. It is a feature of all joints of the body and is comprised of lubricin and relaxin secreted by type A synovial cells in isolation.

   d. It is comprised of lubricin and hyaluronic acid secreted by type A and B synovial cells and acts as a lubricating fluid for the joint, the movement of which provides nutrients to the chondrocyte cells of hyaline cartilage.

Continued

CASE STUDY 5.4—cont'd

Q3. Which of the following is true about immobilisation?

    a. Immobilisation has a negative effect on homeostasis of a joint, the effects of which are irreversible.

    b. Immobilisation does not affect the homeostasis of a joint because no metabolically active cells in the joint structures rely on load for normal function.

    c. Immobilisation has a negative effect on normal metabolism of the cells within ligament, cartilage and the synovium, the effects of which can be reversed with mobilisation.

    d. Immobilisation has a negative effect on the metabolically active cells within the cartilage only.

Q4. Why does Scott experience stiffness and decreased movement in his left thumb? When answering the question, consider the consequences of immobilisation on the structures in a synovial joint.

Q5. What effect does immobilisation have on the venous and lymphatic systems in this case? You may want to look at Chapter 13 on the cardiovascular system and Chapter 14 on the lymphatic system in considering your answer.

REFERENCES

1. Benjamin M, Ralphs JR. Biology of fibrocartilage cells. Int Rev Cytol 2004;233:1–45.
2. Cohen NP, Foster RJ, Mow VC. Composition and dynamics of articular cartilage: structure, function, and maintaining healthy state. J Orthop Sports Phys Ther 1998;28(4):203–15.
3. Franz T, Hasler EM, Hagg R, et al. In situ compressive stiffness, biochemical composition, and structural integrity of articular cartilage of the human knee joint. Osteoarthritis Cartilage 2001;9(6):582–92.
4. Ralphs J, Benjamin M. The joint capsule: structure, composition, ageing and disease. J Anat 1994;184(3):503–9.
5. Hogervorst T, Brand R. Mechanoreceptors in joint function. J Bone Joint Surg 1998;80(9):1365–78.
6. Frank C. Ligament structure, physiology and function. J Musculoskelet Neuronal Interact 2004;4(2):199–201.
7. Levangie P, Norkin C. Joint structure and function: a comprehensive analysis. 3rd ed. Canada: FA Davis; 2001.
8. Halata Z, Rettig T, Schulze W. The ultrastructure of sensory nerve endings in the human knee joint capsule. Anat Embryol (Berl) 1985;172(3):265–75.
9. Smith MD. The normal synovium. Open Rheumatol J 2011;5:100.
10. Hill AM, Hoerning EJ, Brook K, et al. Collagenous microstructure of the glenoid labrum and biceps anchor. J Anat 2008;212(6):853–62.
11. Grant AD, Sala DA, Davidovitch RI. The labrum: structure, function, and injury with femoro-acetabular impingement. J Child Orthop 2012;6(5):357–72.
12. Labusca L, Zugun-Eloae F. The unexplored role of intra-articular adipose tissue in the homeostasis and pathology of articular joints. Front Vet Sci 2018;5:35.
13. Vahlensieck M, Linneborn G, Schild H, et al. Hoffa's recess: incidence, morphology and differential diagnosis of the globular-shaped cleft in the infrapatellar fat pad of the knee on MRI and cadaver dissections. Eur Radiol 2002;12(1):90–3.
14. Clockaerts S, Bastiaansen-Jenniskens YM, Runhaar J, et al. The infrapatellar fat pad should be considered as an active osteoarthritic joint tissue: a narrative review. Osteoarthritis Cartilage 2010;18(7):876–82.
15. Toshihiko I, Mitsumori S, Hiroko K, et al. Morphology and functional roles of synoviocytes in the joint. Arch Histol Cytol 2000;63(1):17–31.
16. Herzberg SD, Motu'apuaka ML, Lambert W, et al. The effect of menstrual cycle and contraceptives on ACL injuries and laxity: a systematic review and meta-analysis. Orthop J Sports Med 2017;5(7).
17. Angel J, Arendt EA, Bershadsky B. Anterior cruciate ligament injury in national collegiate athletic association basketball and soccer: a 13-year review. Am J Sports Med 2005;33(4):524–31.
18. Crowder C, Austin D. Age ranges of epiphyseal fusion in the distal tibia and fibula of contemporary males and females. J Forensic Sci 2005;50(5):JFS2004542-7.
19. Vo N, Niedernhofer LJ, Nasto LA, et al. An overview of underlying causes and animal models for the study of age-related degenerative disorders of the spine and synovial joints. J Orthop Res 2013;31(6):831–7.
20. Hughes VA, Frontera WR, Roubenoff R, et al. Longitudinal changes in body composition in older men and women: role of body weight change and physical activity. Am J Clin Nutr 2002;76(2):473–81.

CHAPTER 6

Muscular system

MICHAEL LEE, BSC, MPHTY, MCHIRO, PHD

KEY POINTS/LEARNING OUTCOMES

1. Provide an overview of the structure and function of skeletal muscle.
2. Describe the microscopic anatomy of skeletal muscle fibre.
3. Describe the different types of muscle fibres.
4. Discuss the physiological processes of muscle contraction and relaxation.
5. Describe the structure and function of a motor unit.
6. Describe different types of muscle actions.

KEY DEFINITIONS

- **Acetylcholine (ACh):** a neurotransmitter released by many somatic and peripheral nervous system neurons. It acts at the neuromuscular junction and functions as a neuromodulator.
- **Adenosine triphosphate (ATP):** an organic compound composed of adenosine and three phosphate groups. It is the main energy currency for many metabolic processes.
- **Contractility:** the ability of muscle tissue to contract.
- **Extensibility:** the ability of muscle tissue to stretch without being damaged.
- **Hypertrophy:** an enlargement of existing muscle fibres.
- **Motor unit:** a motor neuron and the muscle fibres it innervates.

ONLINE RESOURCES/SUGGESTED READINGS

- **Function & anatomy of the muscles of the face, neck & back** available at https://study.com/academy/lesson/function-anatomy-of-the-muscles-of-the-face-neck-back.html
- **Muscular system** available at www.innerbody.com/image/musfov.html
- **Skeletal structure and function** available at www.khanacademy.org/science/high-school-biology/hs-human-body-systems/hs-the-musculoskeletal-system/v/skeletal-structure-and-function
- **Types of muscle tissue: skeletal, cardiac & smooth** available at https://study.com/academy/lesson/types-of-muscle-tissue-skeletal-cardiac-smooth.html

INTRODUCTION

Muscle tissue is highly specialised owing to its unique ability to contract. The human body is comprised of three types of muscle tissue: cardiac muscle, smooth muscle and skeletal muscle. **Cardiac muscle** is found only in the heart and forms most of the heart wall. Individual heart muscle cells (cardiomyocytes) are connected by intercalated discs, which allow groups of heart muscles to contract and relax together. Contraction and relaxation of the heart are not under conscious control (i.e. these actions are involuntary). The primary function of cardiac muscles is to 'pump' blood through the circulatory system. The structure and function of cardiac muscle is discussed in Chapter 13.

Smooth muscle is the primary muscle found in the walls of hollow internal organs, airways and blood vessels. Smooth muscle produces a rhythmic contraction (peristalsis) that pushes materials/substances into and out of the body. This action is generally involuntary. Both smooth muscle and cardiac muscle are controlled by neurons governed by the autonomic nervous system. The structure and function of smooth muscle is discussed in Chapter 20.

Skeletal muscle is the most abundant of the three types of muscle in the human body and constitutes approximately 40% of the total body weight in an adult human.[1] There is a gender difference for total body muscle mass, approximately 38% in males and 31% in females.[2] Given that skeletal muscle mass has a large influence on bone mineral density,[3] the higher prevalence of osteoporosis in women may be associated with their lower total body muscle mass.[2] Similar to cardiac muscle, skeletal muscle is striated (because of its light and dark banded patterns when viewed under a microscope) but is under voluntary control of the somatic nervous system. Skeletal muscles contract only in response to signals from a motor neuron (a specialised nerve cell that sends electrical output signals to muscles). This chapter focuses on the function and structure of skeletal muscle, which comprises the **muscular system** of the body.

FUNCTION AND STRUCTURE OF SKELETAL MUSCLE

Function of skeletal muscle

Skeletal muscle has five key functions in the human body:
1. production of body movements
2. maintenance of body position and posture
3. stabilisation of joints
4. generation of heat
5. storage of water.

Production of body movements

Most skeletal muscles are attached to bones via tendons; when skeletal muscles contract, they pull on the tendons, which in turn move the bones of the skeleton and thereby produce body movements. These movements are dependent on what the muscles are attached to. Generally speaking, an **origin** is a muscle attachment site on a bone that is either fixed or less movable (i.e. more stationary) during contraction, while an **insertion** is the more movable part of the bone during contraction. Most body movements are produced by a group of muscles rather than one muscle. However, one muscle may be responsible for most of the movement, and this muscle is called the **prime mover**. Other muscles that assist the prime mover to produce the movement are called **synergists**, while muscles that oppose the prime mover are called **antagonists**.

To produce a purposeful voluntary movement, coordination between the prime mover, synergists and antagonists are crucial and are precisely controlled by the central nervous system. For example, when you try to take a sip of coffee from a cup, your finger flexors contract to hold the cup while your wrist flexors and extensors co-contract to provide stability at the wrist joint. You then bend your arm at the elbow joint using the biceps brachii as the prime mover (Fig. 6.1A). This action is assisted by the synergist muscles (brachialis and brachioradialis), while the antagonist (triceps brachii) relaxes to allow the elbow to bend so that you can bring the cup to your mouth. Similarly, to straighten your elbow, the prime mover of elbow extension (triceps brachii) contracts while the biceps brachii and other flexors of the elbow (antagonists to elbow extension) relax (Fig. 6.1B). Generally speaking, purposeful movements such as these are under voluntary control (i.e. under conscious control); however, involuntary spinal reflex pathways (e.g. reciprocal inhibition) also play a

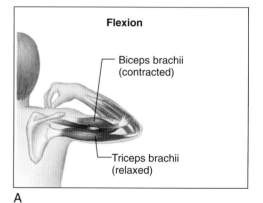

A

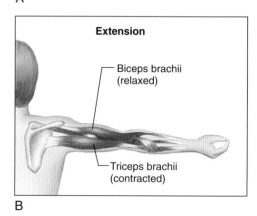

B

FIGURE 6.1 **Production and control of body movement. A** Contraction of the biceps brachii to flex the elbow. **B** Contraction of the triceps brachii to extend the elbow. (*Source:* Patton KT, Thibodeau. The human body in health and disease, 6 ed. St Louis: Mosby; 2014.)

critical role in the control of movement. This is discussed in more detail in Chapter 7.

Maintenance of body position and posture

Skeletal muscle plays a critical role in maintaining body position and posture (e.g. standing or sitting). This is achieved via sustained and coordinated contractions of muscles that span the axial skeleton. For example, sustained contraction of the neck muscles supports the head in an upright position.

Stabilisation of joints

Skeletal muscles provide joint stability during dynamic movements. Simultaneous contraction (co-contraction) of the agonist and antagonist muscles acting about a joint produces a compressive force, which increases stiffness of the joint and allows it to become more stable (or less influenced by external perturbation). This stabilisation mechanism is important when unexpected load is imposed on the body during voluntary movements.

Generation of heat

Skeletal muscle plays an important role in regulating and maintaining normal body temperature. During skeletal muscle contraction, **adenosine triphosphate (ATP)** is used as an energy source. Nearly three-quarters of this energy is released as heat, a process known as **thermogenesis**.[4] Involuntary contractions of skeletal muscles (shivering when we are cold) help increase the rate of heat production to regulate optimal body temperature.

Storage of water

Skeletal muscle is a reservoir for water, storing approximately 75% of the body's water. In addition, skeletal muscle contractions help facilitate flow of lymphatic fluid and blood to the heart.[4]

Structure of skeletal muscle

Skeletal muscles are the primary tissues that make up the muscular system. Each skeletal muscle is comprised of muscle fibres (specialised muscle cells), connective tissue, blood vessels and nerves.[4] A dense layer of connective tissue known as **fascia** surrounds the muscle, enabling freedom of movement as well as providing a passage for nerves, lymphatics and blood vessels to enter and exit the muscle. Three layers of connective tissue extend from the fascia to provide additional support and protect the skeletal muscle (Fig. 6.2): the endomysium, perimysium and epimysium. The **endomysium** is a delicate, thin layer of connective tissue that encloses each individual muscle

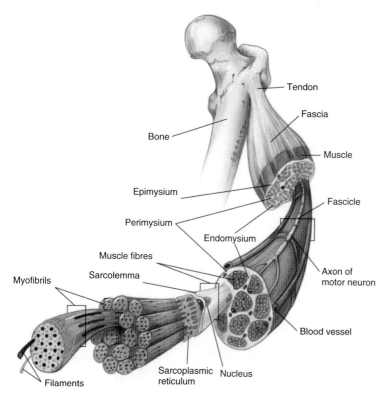

FIGURE 6.2 **Connective tissue surrounding skeletal muscle.** (*Source:* Caballero B, Finglas PM, Toldrá F. Encyclopedia of food and health. Elsevier; 2016.)

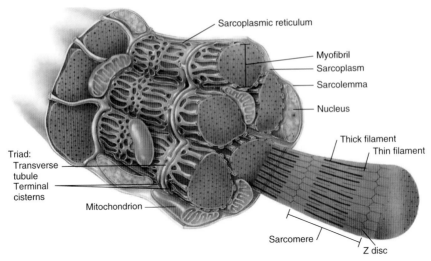

FIGURE 6.3 **Microscopic anatomy of skeletal muscle fibre.** (*Source:* Tortora GJ, Derrickson BH. Principles of anatomy and physiology, vol 1, 12 ed. Hoboken, NJ: John Wiley & Sons; 2009.)

fibre. The **perimysium** is a layer of dense connective tissue that surrounds bundles of muscle fibres known as fascicles. Many fascicles are bound together by a dense and tough layer of connective tissue called the **epimysium**. The epimysium surrounds the entire muscle.[4,5] The epimysium is continuous with the connective tissue that attaches skeletal muscles to bones. It blends to form either a cord-like tendon (e.g. the Achilles tendon, which connects the gastrocnemius muscle to the calcaneus) or a broad sheet-like **aponeurosis** which attaches muscle to other muscles (e.g. the linea alba, which connects the transversus abdominis and the oblique muscles).

Anatomy of skeletal muscle fibre

Skeletal muscles are composed of a collection of specialised muscle cells known as **muscle fibres**. Each muscle fibre is a long cylindrical cell with multiple nuclei (up to several hundred) located just beneath the plasma membrane of the muscle cell (the sarcolemma).[1] Skeletal muscle fibres are among the largest cells in the human body and are formed by fusion of various embryonic mesodermal cells, also known as **myoblasts**. The number of muscle fibres an individual has is genetically determined and remains fairly constant throughout life; it does not seem to increase with exercise or training.[6]

Microscopically, skeletal muscle fibre has several cellular components (Figs 6.3 and 6.4):

- **Sarcolemma** is the cell membrane of muscle fibre.
- **Sarcoplasm** is the cytoplasm of the muscle fibre. The sarcoplasm is rich in mitochondria and contains large amounts of glycogen, which is used to

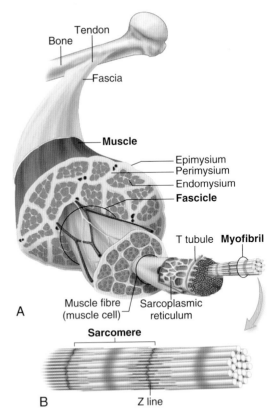

FIGURE 6.4 **A** Anatomy of myofibril. **B** Anatomy of sarcomere. (*Source:* Modified from Patton KT, Thibodeau GA. Anatomy and physiology, 9 ed. St Louis: Mosby; 2016.)

produce ATP during muscle contractions.[4] Myoglobin (red-coloured protein) is found in abundance in the sarcoplasm, which binds to oxygen. Oxygen is released from the myoglobin by the mitochondria to generate ATP.[4]

- **Transverse T-tubules** are a network of narrow tubules with openings to the outside of the muscle fibre; they are filled with extracellular fluid.[7]
- **Myofibrils** are contractile structures of muscle fibre. They are long thread-like structures that extend the entire length of the muscle and are made up of bundles of myofilaments.
- **Myofilaments** are small protein structures found within the myofibrils. There are two types of myofilaments, thin and thick, and both are involved in the contractile process. **Thin filaments** are primarily composed of a protein called actin, and **thick filaments** are mainly made up of a protein called myosin. Thin filaments also contain two other proteins, tropomyosin and troponin, which prevent actin from binding to myosin and hence prevent muscle contractions.
- **Sarcoplasmic reticulum** is a fluid-filled sac that wraps around the myofibril. Sarcoplasmic reticulum stores calcium ions.
- **Sarcomeres** are the basic functional units of the myofibril. Each sarcomere is delineated by **Z discs** and consists of several distinct bands and zones. Under a light microscope, the I band is the lightest colour band and is a region occupied only by the thin filaments, while the A band is the darkest band and extends the entire length of the thick filaments. The middle section of the A band (also known as the H zone) is exclusively occupied by thick filaments. The thick and thin filaments overlap at the periphery of the A band. The centre of the H zone is known as the M line, and is formed by proteins that bond the thick filaments together.

Skeletal muscle contraction and relaxation

Contraction of muscle fibres produces force. This remarkable process enables us to move or to resist an external load. For muscle contraction to occur, skeletal muscle fibres must be stimulated by nerve impulses. Each muscle fibre is controlled by a **motor neuron** (a specialised nerve cell). Each motor neuron innervates a few to several hundred muscle fibres.[5] A motor neuron and the muscle fibres it innervates are known as a **motor unit** (Fig. 6.5).

Skeletal muscle contracts in response to activation of the respective motor neuron. Nerve impulses initiated in the brain are transmitted by action potentials along motor axons, which are long, threadlike extensions of neurons.

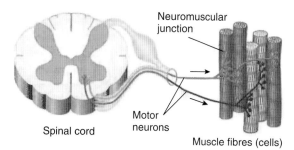

FIGURE 6.5 **Motor unit.** (*Source:* Tortora GJ, Derrickson BH. Principles of anatomy and physiology, vol 1, 12 ed. Hoboken, NJ: John Wiley & Sons; 2009.)

When the action potential reaches the axon terminal (the end of the motor neuron), a neurotransmitter called **acetylcholine (ACh)** is released into the synaptic cleft between the motor neuron and the motor endplate. This junction or synapse between the motor neuron and skeletal muscle fibre is known as the neuromuscular junction (refer to Chapter 7).

ACh molecules bind to ACh receptors on the motor endplate and cause a change in the permeability of the sarcolemma to allow influx of sodium (Na^+) into the sarcoplasm and potassium (K^+) out of the muscle fibre. However, more Na^+ ions enter than K^+ ions leave, and this leads to an increase in the positive charge ions inside the cell and produces a local change in the electrical condition of the membrane (depolarisation). This movement of ions generates an electrical current known as an **action potential**, which spreads across the entire surface of the sarcolemma, conducting electrical impulses from one end of the cell to the other, continues down the T-tubules and initiates the release of calcium ions (Ca^{2+}) from the sarcoplasmic reticulum into the sarcoplasm, which leads to contraction of muscle fibre. As such, the concentration of calcium ions is critical in muscle contraction. An increase in the concentration of calcium ions will initiate muscle contraction, whereas a decrease in calcium ion concentration will prevent or cease muscle contraction. A single nerve impulse can only produce one contraction; the reason for this is that the effects of ACh binding last only momentarily. ACh is rapidly broken down into acetyl and choline by an enzyme called acetylcholinesterase (AChE), which is present in the extracellular matrix of the synaptic cleft and on the sarcolemma. With the depletion of ACh, the muscle fibre relaxes and will only contract if another nerve impulse triggers more release of ACh.

While contraction creates tension in the muscle and is an active process that requires ATP, **relaxation** is the release of tension produced by a contraction. Proposed by Huxley and Niedergerke in 1954, the **sliding filament mechanism** remains the most well-accepted theory of muscle contraction.[8] It is hypothesised that in the resting state, there is a small overlap between the thin and thick filaments at both ends of a sarcomere (Fig. 6.6). During muscle contraction (when a nerve impulse activates muscle fibres as described above), the myosin heads attach to the binding sites on the thin (actin) filaments to form 'cross bridges', a process that requires calcium ions and ATP. ATP 'energises' the myosin heads, which in turn generates tension that helps pull the thin filaments towards the centre of the sarcomere. As a consequence, the thin and thick filaments slide past each other and bring the Z discs of the sarcomere closer together. This results in shortening of the sarcomere. Despite the shortening of the sarcomere, the length of

the A band remains unchanged. These observations are consistent with the sliding of the thin (actin) filaments along the thick (myosin) filaments, which draws the thin filaments towards the centre of the H zone (i.e. the M line). The sliding filament theory provides an explanation for why muscle contraction can create force without necessarily producing movement.[1] The contraction cycle continues as long as there are sufficient ATP and calcium ions.

Types of skeletal muscle fibre

There are three types of muscle fibres found in skeletal muscles:

1. slow oxidative fibres
2. fast oxidative-glycolytic fibres
3. fast glycolytic fibres.

Slow oxidative fibres are small-diameter fibres containing a large amount of myoglobin (and hence are dark-red in appearance) and a high concentration of mitochondria. These fibres produce ATP by aerobic respiration.[1,4] This process involves metabolism of oxygen (from haemoglobin or myoglobin) and glucose to form ATP. During contractions, slow oxidative fibres use ATP relatively slowly with a slower contraction cycle (compared with fast oxidative-glycolytic and fast glycolytic fibres). Slow oxidative fibres are the least powerful type of muscle fibre but are capable of prolonged, sustained contractions and are less susceptible to fatigue.[1,4] As such, they are also known as 'slow-twitch' fibres (or type I fibres) and are associated primarily with long duration/endurance activities such as running a marathon and maintenance of body posture (e.g. standing or sitting).[1,4,6]

Fast oxidative-glycolytic fibres and **fast glycolytic fibres** are classified as 'fast-twitch' fibres. Fast oxidative-glycolytic fibres (also known as type IIa fibres) are intermediate in diameter and are capable of producing ATP via both aerobic respiration and anaerobic glycolysis.[1,4] The rate at which ATP is used is much faster than with slow oxidative fibres. Fast oxidative-glycolytic fibres contract and relax more quickly than slow oxidative fibres and are used during activities such as walking and sprinting.[1,4,6]

Fast glycolytic fibres (also known as type IIb fibres) are large-diameter fibres (the largest of the three) with the lowest myoglobin content and relatively few mitochondria. Fast glycolytic fibres contain the largest number of myofibrils. They produce ATP primarily by anaerobic glycolysis and are capable of generating quick and forceful contractions but have the tendency to fatigue more quickly and easily than fast oxidative-glycolytic and slow oxidative fibres.[1,4,6] Fast glycolytic fibres respond favourably to resistance training; that is, they increase in size (i.e. leading to muscle hypertrophy; see below) and

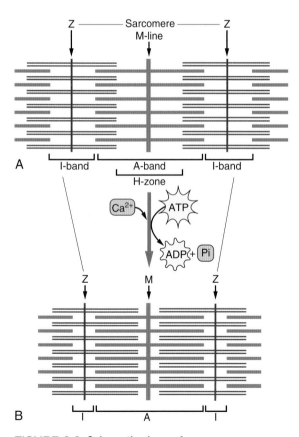

FIGURE 6.6 Schematic views of a sarcomere.
A Relaxed state. **B** Contracted state. (*Source:* Baynes JW, Dominiczak MH. Medical biochemistry, 5 ed. Elsevier; 2019.)

glycogen content when an individual participates in regular resistance training.[1,4]

Ratio of slow-twitch to fast-twitch fibres in skeletal muscle.

Both slow-twitch and fast-twitch fibres are found in all skeletal muscles but in different proportions and this varies between individuals.[9] Muscles whose primary function is to maintain posture have a higher percentage of slow-twitch fibres, whereas muscles that are used to produce ballistic, forceful contractions have higher percentage of fast-twitch fibres.[6] A person's ratio of slow-twitch to fast-twitch fibres is genetically determined.[1,4] Those with a high percentage of slow-twitch fibres are better at endurance activities such as marathon running[1,4] while those with a high proportion of fast-twitch fibres are better in sports that require explosive movements such as weight-lifting and sprinting.[4,10] It is well-accepted that the number of fibres remains fairly constant throughout life and does not change with exercise,[4,6,11] although the characteristics of existing fibres may change to some extent if muscles are repeatedly exposed to certain types of aerobic or anaerobic training.[4,12]

Muscle hypertrophy and atrophy

Repeated, forceful voluntary muscular activity (e.g. resistance training) can lead to **muscle hypertrophy**, which is an increase in the size/diameter of muscle fibres secondary to an increase in the production of myofibrils, mitochondria, sarcoplasmic reticulum and other organelles. Because the hypertrophied muscles contain more myofibrils, they can generate more forceful contractions. In contrast, **muscle atrophy** is a decrease in the size of muscle fibres due to progressive loss of myofibrils. Muscle atrophy is a common consequence of lack of use (or 'disuse'). *Disuse atrophy* can occur in individuals who are bedridden due to chronic illness or forced immobilisation (e.g. post fracture immobilisation). Furthermore, if the nerve supply to a muscle is disrupted (e.g. peripheral nerve injury or a severed nerve), the muscle can undergo *denervation atrophy*. Similarly, degeneration of motor neurons can result in progressive muscle atrophy because the muscles have lost their nerve supply (e.g. in motor neuron disease or amyotrophic lateral sclerosis). The atrophied muscles contain fewer myofibrils, so their force-generating capacity is compromised (i.e. weaker contractions) and is more susceptible to fatigue.

Muscle injury/damage

Injury to muscles or 'muscle strain' may occur when the musculotendinous unit is forced to contract against too much load or resistance exceeding its tensile capability. Injury can also occur when the muscle is overstretched (i.e. exceeding its extensibility limit). In the acute stage, muscle strain is associated with inflammation and development of swelling and oedema, which contributes to muscle pain. Damage may occur to the muscle fibres, at the musculotendinous junction, in the tendon or the tendinous attachment to the bone.

The extent of muscle strain can be graded using a simple classification system:
- **Grade 1 strain:** some muscle fibres have been stretched and may be torn. Active movement involving the muscle causes pain locally but there is usually no loss of range of movement.
- **Grade 2 strain:** some muscle fibres have been torn and voluntary (active) contraction of the muscle is extremely painful. There is usually a palpable divot in the belly of the muscle at the spot where the muscle fibres have been torn. This is often associated with increased swelling due to bleeding of the capillaries.
- **Grade 3 strain:** there is a complete rupture of muscle fibres and this can occur in the belly of the muscle, in the musculotendinous junction or near the insertion of the tendon to bone.

Types of muscle action

As described above, one of the main functions of skeletal muscle is the production of body movements. It was noted that muscle contraction produces force to generate movement. However, muscles can also produce force without generating movement. The actions produced by muscle may be classified as either isotonic or isometric. Traditionally, in **isotonic contractions** the length of the muscle changes while the tension produced remains equal or constant. There are two types of isotonic contractions: concentric and eccentric. During *concentric contractions*, the force generated by the muscle overcomes the load/resistance imposed on it while the length of the muscle *shortens*. An example is lifting a box from the ground to your chest. During this action, the biceps brachii muscle shortens to bend or flex the elbow joint. Now imagine lowering the box back down to the ground: the biceps brachii is still contracting, but its length is *increasing*. This action is an example of an *eccentric contraction*. Eccentric contractions are thought to produce more tension than concentric contractions and contribute more to cellular damage as well as the development of **delayed-onset muscle soreness**, which typically peaks one to three days after unaccustomed eccentric exercise.[13,14] In **isometric contractions**, the force produced does not exceed the load or resistance imposed on the muscle and, as such, there is no change in muscle length and hence no movement. Isometric contractions are essential for the maintenance of body posture and stabilisation of joints.

INTEGRATION OF THE MUSCULAR SYSTEM WITH OTHER BODY SYSTEMS
Skeletal system, nervous system and joints

As most skeletal muscles are attached to bones of the skeleton, contraction of skeletal muscles will in turn move the bones to produce body movement. Some skeletal muscles, especially those spanning a joint, provide additional dynamic support to the passive stability structures such as ligaments and joint capsules. The active dynamic stabilisation provided by skeletal muscles is especially important for joints that are innately mobile (e.g. the glenohumeral joint). Coordinated and purposeful body movements are the result of integration of the muscular system, the nervous system and the skeletal system. Voluntary movements begin with 'motor planning' in the brain, which involves a set of processes related to the preparation of motor activity with appropriate sequencing and timing of various body segments. Neural impulses from the brain then send signals to the relevant muscles to contract. During performance of a motor task, the nervous system continuously provides feedback to the agonist, antagonist and synergist muscles to provide and maintain the appropriate level of force and trajectory required to complete the intended motor task.

AGE-RELATED CHANGES

As we age, there is a gradual decline in both the size of the muscle fibres and the number of myofibrils.[1,7] Muscles that contain fewer myofibrils have less force-generating capacity and are prone to early fatigue and may contribute to a lower tolerance for exercise.[15] The loss of muscle strength is also related to an individual's level of physical activity.[1] Those who are more active or perform more regular exercises have a slower decline in muscle strength with age.[1] More specifically, regular resistance training is particularly effective at slowing age-related decline in skeletal muscle strength and function. Furthermore, as we age, skeletal muscles lose their elasticity/extensibility due to an increase in the concentration of connective tissue in the endomysium and perimysium, a process known as fibrosis.[7] This increase in connective tissue is associated with an increase in muscle stiffness with ageing.[16]

CONCLUSION

There are three different types of muscle tissue: skeletal, cardiac and smooth. The primary function of skeletal muscle is to contract, which in turn generates tension. Through contraction and relaxation, skeletal muscle performs a range of important functions: producing body movements, maintaining body position and posture, stabilising joints, generating heat and serving as a reservoir for water.

CASE STUDY 6.1

Jessica is a 27-year-old marathon runner who has been participating in long-distance running for more than 10 years. She now wants to start training for a 100-metre sprint event.

Q1. Specialised muscle cells are also known as:
  a. muscle fibres.
  b. muscle spindles.
  c. microfilaments.
  d. motor neurons.

Q2. Which type of muscle tissue is the most abundant in the human body?
  a. Cardiac
  b. Smooth
  c. Skeletal
  d. Endothelial

Q3. Which muscle fibre increases in size when a person undertakes a regular resistance training program?
  a. Fast glycolytic
  b. Slow oxidative
  c. Fast oxidative
  d. Fast oxidative-glycolytic

Q4. The number of muscle fibres an individual has is predetermined before birth. Which muscle fibres do you think Jessica has a larger proportion of?

Q5. Based on your knowledge of muscle physiology, why do you think training for a 100-metre sprint event may be a difficult task for Jessica?

CASE STUDY 6.2

Jason is a 21-year-old university student presenting with pain in the back of his right thigh. The pain started yesterday during a soccer game. Jason went to kick the ball and felt an immediate 'pull' in the back of his right upper thigh. He had to limp off the field and reported mild pain in his right hamstring muscles with most active movements involving knee flexion and extension. Jason can still walk around without too much discomfort.

Q1. A type of muscle contraction in which the muscle lengthens as it contracts is known as:

    a. a concentric contraction.

    b. an isometric contraction.

    c. an isotonic contraction.

    d. an eccentric contraction.

Q2. Muscle soreness that develops 24–72 hours after unaccustomed activity or exercise is known as:

    a. accelerated muscle soreness.

    b. delayed-onset muscle soreness.

    c. advanced-onset muscle soreness.

    d. chronic compartment syndrome.

Q3. A muscle is strained or torn when excessive tension or tensile forces within the muscle cause muscle fibres and their surrounding connective tissues to fail. Which type of muscle contraction is known to produce the most tension and contribute more to cellular damage?

    a. Isometric

    b. Concentric

    c. Eccentric

    d. None of the above

Q4. What is the most likely cause of Jason's pain?

Q5. Suggest what type of injury Jason has sustained and discuss what structures are typically damaged in muscle strain.

CASE STUDY 6.3

Bob is 60 years old and recently had surgery to repair a grade 3 rotator cuff tear in his right shoulder. His shoulder was immobilised in a sling (with the elbow bent at 90° and the forearm resting in front of his stomach) for six weeks. Today he was advised by his surgeon to begin exercise rehabilitation with his local physiotherapist. Bob reports that his right shoulder feels 'weak' and 'stiff' when he tries to lift his arm above his head and the girth of his shoulder muscles 'feel smaller'.

Q1. Which types of muscle tissue are striated?

    a. Smooth and cardiac

    b. Cardiac and skeletal

    c. Skeletal and smooth

    d. Skeletal muscle only

Q2. Atrophy of skeletal muscle secondary to peripheral nerve injury is known as:

    a. disuse atrophy.

    b. denervation atrophy.

    c. discontinue atrophy.

    d. degenerative atrophy.

Q3. The wasting away of muscle due to lack of use or restricted use is known as:

    a. muscular dystrophy.

    b. muscle hypertrophy.

    c. disuse atrophy.

    d. myopathy.

Q4. Why does Bob's shoulder feel weak and stiff after six weeks of immobilisation in an arm sling?

Q5. What structures are responsible for the banding pattern of skeletal muscle fibre?

CASE STUDY 6.4

A 67-year-old retired accountant has expressed his concerns that he is 'not as strong' as he used to be. He does not partake in any form of regular exercise and he feels that his body is getting progressively 'stiffer' and 'tighter' every year.

Q1. Which of the following statements regarding skeletal muscle fibre is true?

    a. The number of muscle fibres remains fairly constant throughout life.

    b. The number of muscle fibres can increase with regular exercise.

    c. The number of muscle fibres reduces with age.

    d. Atrophied muscles contain more myofibrils.

Q2. Which neurotransmitter is released by motor neurons?

    a. Glutamate

    b. Dopamine

    c. Noradrenaline (norepinephrine)

    d. Acetylcholine

Q3. During muscle contraction, which of the following does *not* occur?

    a. The Z discs of the sarcomeres are drawn towards each other.

    b. The concentration of calcium in the sarcoplasm increases.

    c. ACh is released into the neuromuscular junction.

    d. The thick filaments slide inwards towards the M line.

Q4. What are the effects of ageing on skeletal muscle?

Q5. What is the direct source of energy used by muscle fibres for contraction?

REFERENCES

1. Silverthorn DU, editor. Human physiology: an integrated approach. 5th ed. Upper Saddle River, NJ: Pearson Education; 2010.
2. Janssen I, Heymsfield SB, Wang ZM, et al. Skeletal muscle mass and distribution in 468 men and women aged 18–88 yr. J Appl Physiol 2000;89(1):81–8.
3. Snow-Harter C, Bouxsein M, Lewis B, et al. Muscle strength as a predictor of bone mineral density in young women. J Bone Miner Res 1990;5(6):589–95.
4. Tortora GJ, Derrickson B, editors. Principles of anatomy and physiology. 14th ed. New York: Wiley; 2014.
5. Marieb E, Keller SM, editors. Essentials of human anatomy and physiology. 12th ed. San Francisco: Pearson; 2018.
6. Prentice W, editor. Rehabilitation techniques for sports medicine and athletic training. 6th ed. Thorofare, NJ: SLACK Incorporated; 2015.
7. Martini F, Bartholomew E, editors. Essentials of anatomy & physiology. 7th ed. Upper Saddle River, NJ: Pearson Education; 2017.
8. Huxley AF, Niedergerke R. Structural changes in muscle during contraction; interference microscopy of living muscle fibres. Nature 1954;173(4412):971–3.
9. Hickson RC, Hidaka K, Foster C. Skeletal muscle fiber type, resistance training, and strength-related performance. Med Sci Sports Exerc 1994;26(5):593–8.
10. Costill DL, Daniels J, Evans W, et al. Skeletal muscle enzymes and fiber composition in male and female track athletes. J Appl Physiol 1976;40(2):149–54.
11. Booth FW, Thomason DB. Molecular and cellular adaptation of muscle in response to exercise: perspectives of various models. Physiol Rev 1991;71(2):541–85.
12. Bandy WD, Lovelace-Chandler V, McKitrick-Bandy B. Adaptation of skeletal muscle to resistance training. J Orthop Sports Phys Ther 1990;12(6):248–55.
13. Sargeant AJ, Dolan P. Human muscle function following prolonged eccentric exercise. Eur J Appl Physiol Occup Physiol 1987;56(6):704–11.
14. Stauber WT. Eccentric action of muscles: physiology, injury, and adaptation. Exerc Sport Sci Rev 1989;17:157–85.
15. van Soest AJ, Bobbert MF. The contribution of muscle properties in the control of explosive movements. Biol Cybern 1993;69(3):195–204.
16. Williams PE, Goldspink G. Changes in sarcomere length and physiological properties in immobilized muscle. J Anat 1978;127(Pt 3):459–68.

CHAPTER 7

Nervous system

KIRYU YAP, BMEDSC, MBBS

KEY POINTS/LEARNING OUTCOMES

1. Outline the anatomical and functional divisions of the nervous system.
2. Describe the structure and function of the central nervous system.
3. Describe the structure and function of the peripheral nervous system.
4. Describe the components and function of the autonomic nervous system.
5. Link the integration of the central, peripheral, somatic and autonomic nervous systems to cognition, sensorimotor function and autonomic control of the body.
6. Outline the nervous system's relationship with other systems in the body.

KEY DEFINITIONS

- **Autonomic nervous system:** the portion of the peripheral nervous system that controls involuntary regulation of essential visceral functions.
- **Central nervous system (CNS):** the main command centre of the nervous system and body consisting of the brain, brain stem and spinal cord, which are in continuity with each other.
- **Cognition:** the process of acquiring and processing input signals to derive awareness, thought and learning, which may result in a perception, emotion or decision which results in a command or action.
- **Nerves:** the 'wiring' of the nervous system that transmits sensory information to the brain and spinal cord, as well as commands from the brain and spinal cord to target tissues and organs such as skeletal muscles or glands.
- **Peripheral nervous system (PNS):** components of the nervous system that lie outside of the central nervous system and communicate with target tissues and organs. This consists of ganglia (aggregates of nerve cell bodies) and nerves (fibres that contain neurons).
- **Reflex arc:** a neural pathway where sensory neurons synapse in the spinal cord with motor neurons to compute sensory input into a motor command without involving the brain; therefore, there is no voluntary control.
- **Somatic nervous system:** associated with body movement through voluntary control of skeletal muscles or involuntary reflex arcs.
- **Synapse:** the connection point between two neurons (nerve cells).

ONLINE RESOURCES/SUGGESTED READINGS

- **Nervous system** available at www.nature.com/subjects/nervous-system
- **Overview of neuron structure** available at www.khanacademy.org/science/health-and-medicine/human-anatomy-and-physiology/nervous-system-introduction/v/overview-of-neuron-structure
- **Structure of the nervous system** available at www.khanacademy.org/science/high-school-biology/hs-human-body-systems/hs-the-nervous-and-endocrine-systems/v/structure-of-the-nervous-system
- **Types of neurotransmitters** available at www.khanacademy.org/science/health-and-medicine/human-anatomy-and-physiology/nervous-system-introduction/v/types-of-neurotransmitters

INTRODUCTION

The nervous system is the control system for the body, providing all of its wiring (peripheral nerves), which relays signals to and from tissues and organs to the body's central command centres, the brain and spinal cord. The nervous system regulates organ function during normal homeostasis and facilitates the body's response to emergency situations. Anatomically, it can be divided into two major regions: the **central nervous system (CNS)**, which consists of the brain and spinal cord; and the **peripheral nervous system (PNS)**, which consists of nerves and ganglia (clusters of nerve cells). Functionally, the CNS and PNS work together to obtain sensory inputs from the body, integrate incoming information and make decisions, and provide feedback to other body tissues and organs to create a response.[1]

The PNS consists of the **somatic nervous system** (associated with body movement through either voluntary control of skeletal muscles or involuntary reflex arcs) and the **autonomic nervous system** (associated with the involuntary control of visceral functions). The somatic nervous system contains all the spinal nerves and plexuses (nerve networks) exiting the spinal cord, as well as the peripheral nerves that innervate distal tissues and organs. This provides sensory motor information to and from the body. In the head and neck, the somatic nervous system also encompasses the cranial nerves, which exit the brain and brain stem but are not considered part of the CNS (except for the optic nerve, which is derived from an outpouching of the brain during embryonic development and is therefore considered part of the CNS). The autonomic nervous system innervates smooth muscles and glands, and control is exerted via its three divisions—namely, the parasympathetic, sympathetic and enteric nervous systems. Divisions of the nervous system are covered in Fig. 7.1.

CELL ANATOMY AND PHYSIOLOGY

Nervous tissue, regardless of location, is made of two types of cell: neurons, which are the cells responsible for communication (and therefore the main cells in the nervous system); and glial cells, which are support cells. Electrophysiological (electric) impulses enter neurons via structures called dendrites (Fig. 7.2). From the cell body (also called the soma), impulses travel out of the neuron via long channels called axons, and these connect onto the next neuron or target tissue via specialised connection points called synapses. Axons can travel a long distance, and the conductivity of impulses is enhanced by encasing axons with myelin, a lipid-rich insulating material produced by glial cells which wrap around the axon. Myelin-producing glial cells in peripheral nerves are called Schwann cells, and in the CNS they are called oligodendrocytes. Cell bodies are organised into localised structures referred to as a nucleus in the CNS and a ganglion in the PNS. Axons arising from such clusters are bundled together to form fibres referred to as a tract in the CNS and a nerve in the PNS. A network of ganglia and nerves in the PNS is also referred to as a plexus (e.g. brachial plexus).[1]

Synapses allow neurons to transmit their nerve impulses, called action potentials. Action potential refers to the change in the electrical state of the nerve cell's membrane (membrane potential), which is regulated by ions such as potassium, sodium and calcium moving in and out of the cell via ion channels. The membrane potential is effectively the difference between the electrical charge within the cell and in the external

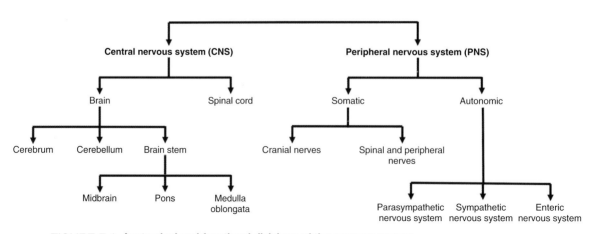

FIGURE 7.1 **Anatomical and functional divisions of the nervous system.**

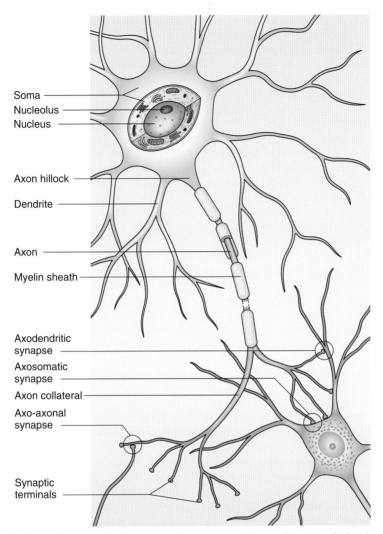

FIGURE 7.2 **Basic structure of interconnected neurons.** (*Source:* Standring S. Gray's anatomy, 41 ed. New York: Elsevier; 2016.)

Soma
Nucleolus
Nucleus
Axon hillock
Dendrite
Axon
Myelin sheath
Axodendritic synapse
Axosomatic synapse
Axon collateral
Axo-axonal synapse
Synaptic terminals

micro-environment. At a resting state where a cell is not transmitting an electrical signal, the resting membrane potential is approximately −70 mV (the exact voltage depends on the cell and location) and is carefully maintained by regulating the intracellular concentration of ions. In this state, the concentration of potassium (K^+) in the cells is much higher than in the external environment, whereas the concentration of sodium (Na^+) is 10 times greater outside of the cell.

A nerve cell can be stimulated to open its Na^+ channels and allow Na^+ to enter the cell through a variety of mechanisms. This may include a mechanical stimulus that distorts the cell membrane and opens a mechanically

gated ion channel, or the binding of a chemical signal to open a ligand-gated Na^+ channel. These events start to depolarise the membrane (so there is less of a difference between the Na^+ concentration internal and external to the cell as Na^+ is allowed into the cells). Depolarisation of up to −55 mV does not lead to the transmission of an electrical signal from one area of the cell membrane to another via an action potential. However, once the membrane potential reaches −55 mV or higher, a special channel called the voltage-gated Na^+ channel opens, which leads to a large influx of Na^+ into the cell and a rapid change in the membrane potential, which continues up to +30 mV. This is an action potential and its activity spreads further by depolarising the voltage-gated Na$^+$ channels of the adjacent area, resulting in the transmission of signals from one area to another. Following depolarisation and an action potential, the exchange of Na$^+$ and K$^+$ returns that part of the membrane to its resting potential. In this manner, action potentials can be transmitted along the neuron's axon via continuous conduction.

Axons that are myelinated are wrapped by Schwann cells or oligodendrocytes, which produce lipid-rich myelin to act as an electrical insulator to promote transmission of action potentials. Ionic exchange occurs only in specific areas interspersed along the axon that are non-myelinated and are called nodes of Ranvier. Once an action potential occurs at one node, it travels rapidly along a myelinated region of the axon without the need for further voltage-gated Na$^+$ channel depolarisation until it reaches the next node. Action potentials travel along this myelinated corridor much more quickly than in continuous conduction; this mode of perpetuating action potentials is referred to as saltatory conduction (from the Latin word *saltare*, meaning to leap).[2]

At the end of an axon, transmission of signals from one neuron to another occurs via either a chemical synapse or an electrical synapse (the junction between one neuron and another neuron or target structure). In a chemical synapse, chemical signalling in the form of neurotransmitters released from the pre-synaptic neuron bind to receptors on the post-synaptic cell and modulate their ability to fire an action potential. Examples of neurotransmitters include acetylcholine, adrenaline (epinephrine), noradrenaline (norepinephrine), serotonin, histamine and dopamine. The neuromuscular junction (connection between a neuron and a muscle fibre, described in Chapter 6) is an example of a chemical synapse. Once an action potential reaches a neuromuscular junction, it causes the neurotransmitter acetylcholine to be released from the neuron into the space between the nerve and muscle fibre within the neuromuscular junction (called the synaptic cleft). Binding of acetylcholine to specific nicotinic receptors on the cell membrane of a muscle fibre leads to its depolarisation and a sequence of events leading to muscular contraction. In an electrical synapse, ions flow between the pre-synaptic and post-synaptic cells through a direct connection in the form of gap junctions.

STRUCTURE AND FUNCTION OF THE CENTRAL NERVOUS SYSTEM

The brain and spinal cord are continuous structures (Fig. 7.3) and within them are regions referred to as grey and white matter. Grey matter is a region densely populated with cell bodies and dendrites, while white matter is the region where lipid-rich (fatty) white axons travel through.

Apart from oligodendrocytes that produce myelin to ensheath axons in the CNS, there are several other types of glial cells. Astrocytes are the most common glial cells, and in fact are the most common cell type found in the brain. These star-shaped cells play several important roles, including supporting the endothelial cells of the blood–brain barrier, providing metabolic support to neurons, modulating synaptic transmission, promoting nerve myelination by oligodendrocytes and facilitating nervous system repair. Microglia are resident macrophage cells in the CNS and act as scavenger cells to remove dead cells, waste and debris. Ependymal cells line spaces in the CNS that contain **cerebrospinal fluid (CSF)** and have beating hair-like cilia to promote CSF movement. The delicate brain and spinal cord have several protective layers (Fig. 7.4). The bony coverings are the cranial bones encasing the brain and the vertebral column covering the spinal cord. Within the bony covering lie three membrane layers that are collectively referred to as the meninges: the thick **dura mater** (external), the **arachnoid mater** and the innermost **pia mater**, which contains blood vessels. In the skull, the periosteum covers the external surface of the cranial bones, and the internal surface is covered by the dura mater, which is continuous with the periosteum.

The meninges are associated with three spaces. The **epidural space** lies between the dura mater and bony covering. In the spine this contains fat and connective tissue, but in the head because the dura mater serves as the inner periosteum there is usually no potential space. The **subdural space** lies between the dura mater and the underlying arachnoid mater and contains lubricating serous fluid. The **subarachnoid space** lies between the arachnoid mater and pia mater and contains CSF.

CSF flows through specific spaces within the CNS and functions to provide a fluid-filled protective cushion. Regulation of CSF flow and volume can regulate intracranial pressure, and CSF also has essential functions in homeostasis as it is closely monitored by receptors that are involved in respiratory control and pH regulation. Cellular metabolic waste is also excreted into CSF and absorbed into blood. About 125–150 mL of CSF is present, although a total of approximately 500 mL of CSF is produced daily at a rate of about 25 mL/hour. CSF is produced via filtration of blood plasma through the choroid plexus, specialised capillary networks present within large CSF spaces within the brain called the

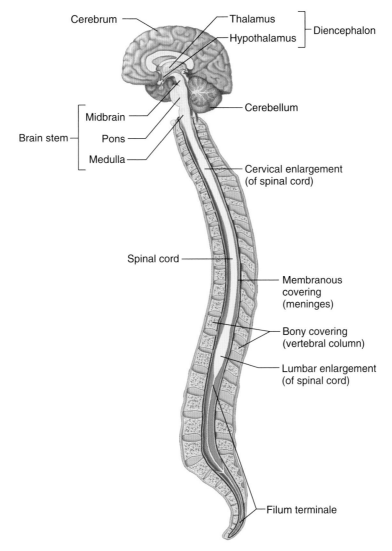

Cerebrum

Thalamus ⎤
Hypothalamus ⎦ Diencephalon

Cerebellum

Brain stem ⎡ Midbrain
⎢ Pons
⎣ Medulla

Cervical enlargement
(of spinal cord)

Spinal cord

Membranous
covering
(meninges)

Bony covering
(vertebral column)

Lumbar enlargement
(of spinal cord)

Filum terminale

FIGURE 7.3 **General structure of the CNS.** (*Source:* Patton KT, Thibodeau GA, editors. Anatomy and physiology, 9 ed. London: Elsevier Health Sciences; 2015.)

ventricles. CSF drains throughout the CSF spaces within the CNS as well as the lymphatic system, then recirculates back into the blood by passing through the arachnoid mater via arachnoid granulations—finger-like projections into the brain's large veins (dural venous sinuses) that contain valves to ensure one-way circulation.

The microvasculature of the CNS tightly regulates the movement of cells and molecules from the systemic blood supply into the CNS. The physiological barrier, the **blood–brain barrier**, is maintained by specialised endothelial cells that line the CNS microvasculature and interact with supporting pericytes and

vascular smooth muscle cells, as well as glial cells and neurons.

Brain

The brain is a large organ of about 1.4 kg in most adults,[3] with a soft paste-like consistency. It is divided into two hemispheres, and contains the cerebrum, diencephalon and cerebellum. These structures are in close proximity and are continuous with the brain stem, which leads onto the spinal cord. The **cerebrum** contains the large dome-shaped hemispheres at the cranial end of the CNS, and the smaller **diencephalon** lies underneath the

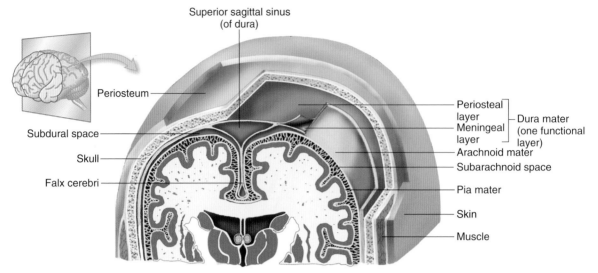

FIGURE 7.4 Coronal section of the head demonstrating the skull and meninges covering the brain. (*Source:* Patton KT, Thibodeau GA, editors. Anatomy and physiology, 9 ed. London: Elsevier Health Sciences; 2015.)

cerebrum, over the brain stem. The **cerebellum** lies on the posterior aspect of the brain underneath the cerebrum, wrapping around the back of the brain stem.

The surface of the cerebrum (the cerebral cortex) contains six layers of interconnecting neurons, with the dense cell bodies resulting in the cortex being the grey matter. The cortex is a very wrinkled layer that contains prominent grooves called sulci interspersed between raised folded tissues called gyri. Clusters of gyri and sulci are divided into functional regions within the cortex called lobes, demarcated by deep sulci called fissures (Fig. 7.5).

The functions of the cerebral cortex are complex, and the plasticity of the cells in each lobe to take on the function of another lobe is still not completely understood. However, the major lobes (demarcated by fissures and the name of the cranial bones that overlie them) and their main functions have been well described. These five paired (left and right) lobes are the frontal lobe, parietal lobe, temporal lobe, occipital lobe and insula (Fig. 7.5). An overall description of the brain's various functions can be found in Table 7.1.

The **frontal lobe** lies behind the forehead and plays a role in motivation, memory, problem solving, impulse control, judgement and control of social and sexual behaviour. It is separated from the parietal lobe by the central sulcus. The pre-central gyrus is the last gyrus of the frontal lobe that lies anterior to the central sulcus and is responsible for motor control. It contains specific clusters of neurons that control different parts of the body, and this neurological map of the body on the motor strip is called the motor homunculus (Fig. 7.6). The frontal lobe also contains an area responsible for controlling our ability to speak (motor speech). This specific region, called Broca's area, is present in only one cerebral hemisphere, more frequently in the left frontal lobe.

The **parietal lobe** lies behind the central sulcus, and the first gyrus (the post-central gyrus) is responsible for sensory input. Again, regions of the body are mapped onto specific areas of the post-central gyrus and this is called the sensory homunculus. The parietal lobe is involved in the processing and integration of sensory input. It also facilitates spatial awareness of our environment, which enables coordination of our behaviour and movements.

The **temporal lobe** is also involved in the processing of sensory input, including visual and auditory information. It is involved in visual and verbal memory, object recognition, language recognition and emotional association. It contains the primary auditory cortex, which receives auditory information and computes this into meaningful sounds and speech. In one cerebral hemisphere (often the left) it contains Wernicke's area, which is responsible for language development and the understanding of speech (receptive speech). The temporal lobe also contains the amygdala, an almond-shaped structure involved in the processing of emotions, as well

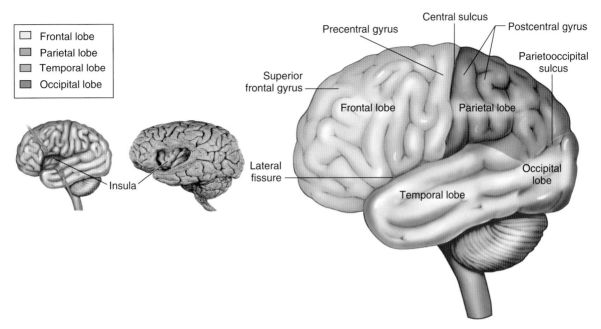

- ☐ Frontal lobe
- ▨ Parietal lobe
- ▨ Temporal lobe
- ▨ Occipital lobe

Central sulcus
Precentral gyrus
Postcentral gyrus
Parietooccipital sulcus
Superior frontal gyrus
Frontal lobe
Parietal lobe
Occipital lobe
Lateral fissure
Temporal lobe
Insula

FIGURE 7.5 **Lobes of the cerebral cortex.** (*Source:* Patton KT, Thibodeau GA, editors. Anatomy and physiology, 9 ed. London: Elsevier Health Sciences; 2015.)

TABLE 7.1
Summary of functions of the major regions in the brain

Area of brain	Function
Frontal cortex	Motivation, memory, problem solving, impulse control, judgement and the control of social and sexual behaviour
	Motor homunculus
	Contains Broca's area (motor speech)
Parietal cortex	Sensory homunculus
	Processing/integration of sensory input and spatial awareness
Temporal cortex	Processing sensory input
	Visual and verbal memory, objection recognition, language recognition
	Contains Wernicke's area (receptive speech)
	Includes hippocampus (controls memory) and amygdala (emotional processing)
Occipital cortex	Vision
Insular cortex	Language, decision making, self and emotional awareness, pain perception
Thalamus	Transmits sensory input to cerebral cortex, regulates sleep and consciousness
Hypothalamus	Automatic control of key survival processes such as heart rate, blood pressure, thermoregulation
	Neuroendocrine function

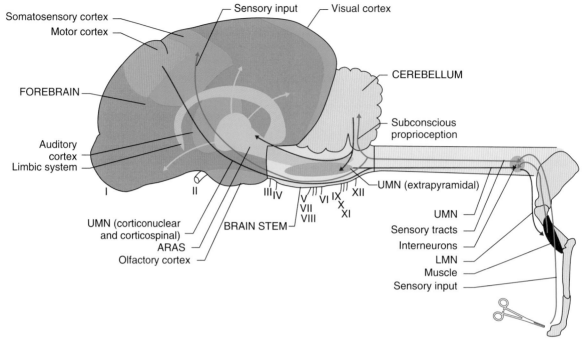

FIGURE 7.6 **Diagram demonstrating the complex interplay between various regions of the cerebral cortex and other parts of the nervous system.** (*Source:* Thomson C, Hahn C. Veterinary neuroanatomy: a clinical approach. Elsevier; 2012.)

as the hippocampus, which is involved in long-term memory and spatial navigation.

The **occipital lobe** is responsible for vision; it contains tracts that receive sensory signals from the eye and assembles this information into vision.

The **insula** (also called the Island of Reil) is an oval region buried in a deep infolding on the lateral aspect of the brain called the Sylvian fissure (or lateral sulcus), which separates the temporal lobes from the frontal and parietal lobes. The insula cortex is involved in a variety of functions, including language, decision making, self and emotional awareness, and pain perception.

Below the cortex of each cerebral hemisphere is the white matter, where myelinated nerve tracts travel upwards and downwards. Additionally, the right and left cerebral hemispheres are connected by a thick band of nerve tracts that form a bridge called the corpus callosum, which allows crosstalk between the two hemispheres. In the middle of the cerebral hemispheres are several large interconnected spaces filled with CSF (Fig. 7.7). Within the cerebrum are paired wing-like cavities called the **lateral ventricles** (or first and second ventricles). These connect in the midline and downwards into a small vertical space—the **third ventricle**—which in turn travels

via a channel called the **cerebral aqueduct** and leads downwards into the diamond-shaped larger space of the **fourth ventricle**. The fourth ventricle is located around the vicinity where the cerebellum attaches posteriorly to the brain stem and travels downwards into the middle of the spinal cord to transport CSF within the central canal. CSF communicates between the ventricular system and the subarachnoid space via specific apertures between the fourth ventricle and the subarachnoid space, called the foramina of Magendie and Luschka.

The diencephalon is located at the base of the cerebral hemispheres, adjacent to the third ventricle, which passes through the midline. It lies between the cerebral hemispheres and the brain stem underneath. It consists of several important structures, including the thalamus, hypothalamus, optic chiasma and pineal gland.

The **thalamus** and **hypothalamus** are groups of many nuclei (clusters of cell bodies). Collectively, the nuclei of the thalamus are important for transmitting sensory input towards the cerebral cortex for processing and for regulating sleep and consciousness. The thalamus on each side forms the lateral wall of the third ventricle. The hypothalamus lies below the thalamus and forms the lower portion of the third ventricle's lateral wall as

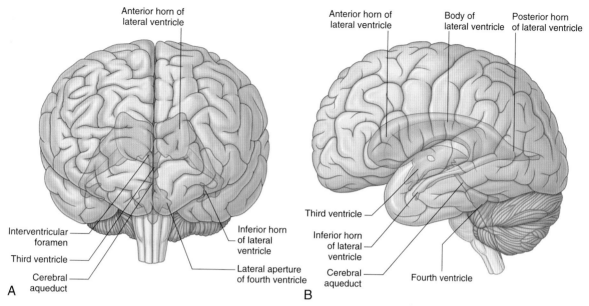

Anterior horn of lateral ventricle

Interventricular foramen

Third ventricle

Cerebral aqueduct

Inferior horn of lateral ventricle

Lateral aperture of fourth ventricle

A

Anterior horn of lateral ventricle

Body of lateral ventricle

Posterior horn of lateral ventricle

Third ventricle

Inferior horn of lateral ventricle

Cerebral aqueduct

Fourth ventricle

B

FIGURE 7.7 **The ventricular system of the brain for the production and circulation of CSF.** (*Source:* Standring S. Gray's anatomy, 41 ed. New York: Elsevier; 2016.)

well as its floor. The hypothalamic nuclei are collectively important in autonomic control of the heart rate, blood pressure, gastrointestinal activity and thermoregulation. The hypothalamus is also involved in arousal and consciousness, sleep, learning and memory. Another very important function of the hypothalamus is linking the nervous system to the endocrine system through its connection to the pituitary gland (covered in Chapter 10). The hypothalamus produces various hormones that stimulate the pituitary gland to release its hormones which target other endocrine tissue, and in turn the hypothalamus is part of a negative feedback loop that controls stimulation of the pituitary gland according to physiological needs.

The optic chiasma and pineal gland are single structures in the brain. The **optic chiasma** is an X-shaped structure where the left and right optic nerves intersect. Half of each nerve's axons cross over to the other side. The **pineal gland** is an endocrine gland that produces melatonin and therefore acts as an internal clock as melatonin regulates the sleep/wake cycle.

Below the diencephalon is the brain stem. A spherical structure is attached to the posterior aspect of the brain stem, with left and right hemispheres. This is the cerebellum and it is connected to both the cerebrum and the brain stem (Fig. 7.8). It is attached by three bridges for each hemisphere (superior, middle, inferior) which

consist of bunched nerve tracts called peduncles. The cerebellum is important for motor coordination and the control of fine movements, posture and balance; it also coordinates sensory input into the cerebrum.

Brain stem

The **brain stem** consists of three components that connect the brain to the spinal cord (Fig. 7.9). Working downwards, they are the midbrain, pons and medulla oblongata. The brain stem contains a number of critical regulatory centres that regulate body functions and it is also the origin of 10 of the 12 cranial nerves.

The **midbrain** contains the superior cerebellar peduncles which contain nerve tracts between the cerebellum, midbrain and thalamus. Centrally it contains the cerebral aqueduct, which transports CSF between the third and fourth ventricles. It also contains two nuclei on each side involved in muscular control. The red nuclei are involved in motor coordination. The substantia nigra ('dark substance' in Latin due to its dark pigmentation) contains dopaminergic neurons, and apart from motor control dopamine is involved in signalling the reward and pleasure centres of the brain, and hence regulates addictive and reward-motivated behaviour.

The **pons** is the largest portion of the brain stem and comprises the middle cerebellar peduncles containing nerve tracts between the cerebellum and the pons, and

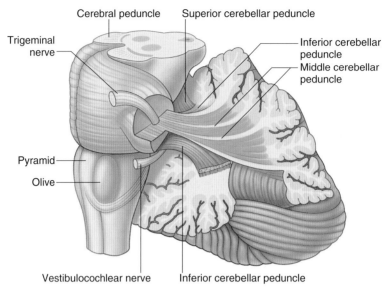

FIGURE 7.8 **Close relationship between the cerebellum and the brain stem.** (*Source:* Standring S. Gray's anatomy, 41 ed. New York: Elsevier; 2016.)

therefore it serves as the conduit between the cerebral cortex and the cerebellum. CSF runs centrally between the pons and medulla within the fourth ventricles. The pons contains the nuclei for four cranial nerves (V–VIII) and nerve tracts that control voluntary movement, as well as tactile, proprioceptive and pain sensation. It also contains the pneumotaxic centre for respiration, which prevents overdistension of the lungs and maintains the recurrent pattern of inspiration and expiration by controlling the phrenic nerve to the diaphragm.

The **medulla oblongata** contains the inferior cerebellar peduncles which communicate between the medulla,

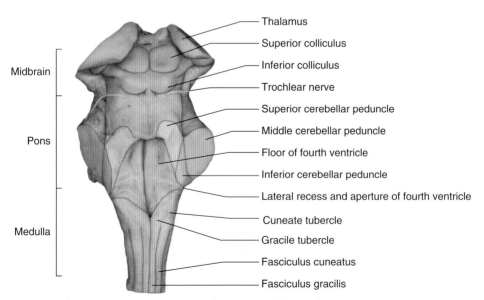

FIGURE 7.9 **Structural organisation of the brain stem.** (*Source:* Crossman AR, Neary D. Neuroanatomy: an illustrated colour text, 6 ed. Elsevier; 2019.)

spinal cord and cerebellum. The medulla has a number of centres that control the body's vital functions. Cardiac output is controlled by the cardiac centre, blood pressure is controlled by the vasomotor centre, ventilation is controlled by the respiratory centre (which receives input from chemoreceptors in the carotid artery and aorta) and vomiting, swallowing, sneezing and coughing are controlled by reflex centres.

Mechanisms of cognition and memory

Cognition and memory are complex processes governed by the interplay of several structures within the cortex and subcortical regions in the brain. The cerebral cortex can store both short- and long-term memories. Long-term memories are thought to be associated with modifications in neuronal circuitry, which may be structural changes at the junction between neurons (synapses) or changes in the neurons themselves. However, it is important to note that memory is not stored in discrete brain regions, but rather within interconnected networks. Consolidation of memory into long-term memory occurs during sleep.

The prefrontal cortex (the very anterior portion of the frontal cortex) is important in short-term memory. The left prefrontal cortex is involved in verbal working memory, while the right prefrontal cortex is involved in spatial working memory. The frontal lobe is also important in problem solving, judgement, planning, initiation, impulse control, and social and sexual behaviour (personality). The parietal lobe is important for integrating sensory information to form perception. It gives us the perception of self and spatial awareness of the environment around us. The temporal lobe is involved in recognition memory and also contains two specific structures important to memory: the amygdala and hippocampus. The amygdala is involved in emotional learning, fear and reward conditioning, as well as the consolidation of memory. The hippocampus is important in the registration of new memories, spatial learning and verbal recall. The occipital lobe is required for vision, and together with the parietal lobe is responsible for visual memory.

Other structures important for memory include basal ganglia, a group of nuclei located above the thalamus that are involved with learning, habit formation, motor memory and the coordination of motor activity. The cerebellum is important in fine motor control, and together with the basal ganglia is responsible for learned motor skills.

Spinal cord

The long column of the spinal cord contains anterior and posterior grooves: the anterior median fissure is larger and wider than the posterior median sulcus. Unlike the brain, the grey matter of the spinal cord (which contains the cell bodies) is arranged internally, surrounded by the white matter, which contains the myelinated nerve tracts that exit the spinal cord as spinal roots and continue as peripheral nerves. The spinal cord contains the central canal which transports CSF, which also flows in the subarachnoid space around the spinal cord.

Nerve fibres are bundled together into structures called **nerve roots** that enter and leave the spinal cord. For each half of the spinal cord (left or right), the dorsal (or posterior) nerve root carries sensory input into the spinal cord, and the ventral (or anterior) nerve root carries instructions out of the spinal cord for motor control. Sensory neurons in the dorsal nerve root travel upwards towards the brain via specific ascending sensory tracts, whereas motor neurons travel downwards from the brain towards the ventral nerve root in descending motor tracts. Additionally, sensory and motor neurons at each spinal level are connected via interneurons ('neurons between neurons') within the spinal cord that form a reflex arc (Fig. 7.10). Sensory input can be directly processed and converted into a motor action within this arc via an interneuron without involving the higher centres such as the cerebral cortex, thereby negating the input of cognition and conscious control. This rapid transmission of information from sensory input to motor output is commonly referred to as a **reflex**.

The dorsal sensory nerve root and the ventral motor nerve root from each end of the spinal cord (left or right) combine together to form a spinal nerve, which contains inflow and outflow neurons and is part of the peripheral nervous system. The spinal cord terminates at the level of lumbar vertebrae 1 (L1) as a tapered cone referred to as the conus medullaris. Beyond the conus medullaris the meninges continue downwards within the spinal cavity as a slender filamentous extension called the filum terminale, which continues until the sacral region to blend with the dura and periosteum of the coccyx.

Mechanism of spinal reflexes

The withdrawal reflex is a spinal reflex whereby the body instinctively withdraws from a damaging stimulus without actively thinking, in order to protect the body. For example, if you were to accidentally touch a boiling kettle with your hand this would immediately activate heat and pain receptors in your palm, which would relay sensory impulses up sensory nerves to the CNS. Within your spine, a sensory neuron would synapse with an interneuron that then connects to a motor

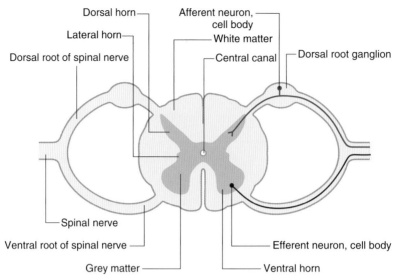

FIGURE 7.10 **A cross-section of the spinal cord demonstrating a reflex arc.** (*Source:* Standring S. Gray's anatomy, 41 ed. New York: Elsevier; 2016.)

neuron, and an impulse travelling from the sensory to the motor neuron would result in your arm immediately withdrawing your hand from the painful hot stimulus. This reflex arc with an immediate response occurs without any processing or command from your brain, particularly the cortex. However, shortly after this reflex, impulses will travel up to your brain, where information processing would lead to responses such as anger, annoyance or regret, and thought processes that reinforce the danger of hot kettles.

STRUCTURE AND FUNCTION OF THE PERIPHERAL NERVOUS SYSTEM

The PNS is the interface between the body's command centres of the brain and the spinal cord and its end targets, such as muscles or digestive organs. Apart from myelinating Schwann cells, another type of glial cell found in the PNS is satellite glial cells, which cover the cell bodies of ganglia and serve a similar function to astrocytes found in the CNS. They provide structural and metabolic support to neurons and facilitate neuronal transmission.

Spinal nerves

There are 31 pairs of spinal nerves, each pair denoted by the level of the vertebral column where it exits from the spinal cord (Fig. 7.11). This includes eight pairs of cervical nerves (C1 to C8, although note that there are

only seven cervical vertebrae). C1 spinal nerve passes between the skull and the vertebrae, C2 spinal nerve passes between C1 and C2 vertebrae, and this pattern continues downwards until C8 spinal nerve, which exits between C7 and T1 vertebrae. There are 12 pairs of thoracic nerves (T1 to T12), and the next spinal nerve (T1) exits between T1 and T2, and thereafter every spinal nerve exits below the corresponding vertebra (that is, T2 spinal nerve exits below T2 vertebra, in between T2 and T3 vertebral levels). There are also five pairs of lumbar nerves (L1 to L5), five pairs of sacral nerves (S1 to S5) and one pair of coccygeal nerves. The spinal cord ends at the level of L1 by tapering into a cone-shaped ending called the conus medullaris. Nerve roots exiting at levels below L1 descend from the conus medullaris within the spinal cavity until they reach the level of their exit. The extension of the spinal roots and their flaring out resembles a horse's tail, and so this is referred to as the cauda equina (Latin for 'horse's tail').

As described previously, dorsal and ventral spinal roots combine to form a spinal nerve with afferent (sensory) and efferent (motor) neurons. The dorsal spinal root contains a bulging cluster of cell bodies of sensory neurons known as the dorsal root ganglion. After combining the dorsal spinal root and ganglion and ventral spinal root, the spinal nerve exits the spinal cavity via an intervertebral foramen present on each side of the vertebral column (left and right) for each spinal nerve. After exiting the spinal cavity, each spinal nerve

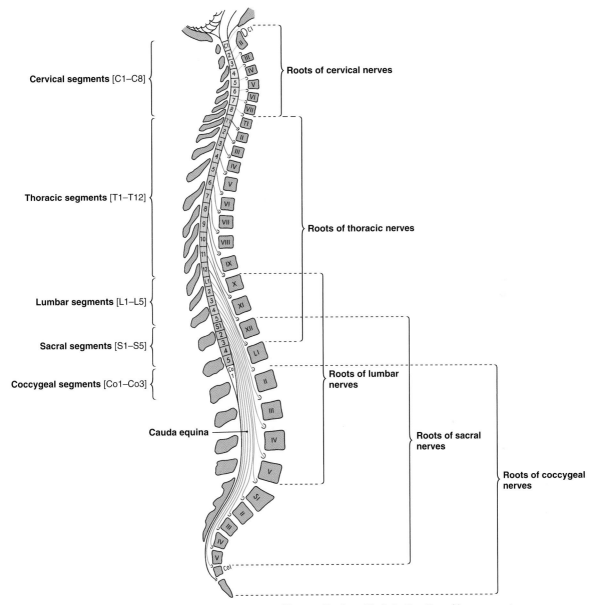

FIGURE 7.11 **The 31 pairs of spinal nerves.** (*Source:* Paulsen W. Sobotta atlas of human anatomy, 16 ed. 2018 © Elsevier GmbH, Urban & Fischer, Munich.)

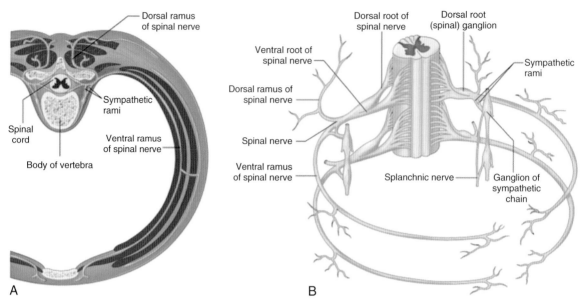

FIGURE 7.12 **Organisation of spinal nerve roots that give rise to spinal nerves.** (*Source:* Habif TP. Clinical dermatology, 2 ed. St Louis: Mosby; 1990.)

forms large branches, splitting into the distinct dorsal and ventral rami (Fig. 7.12). The dorsal rami branch into motor and sensory nerves that innervate skeletal muscles and skin. The ventral rami form the autonomic nervous system.

Peripheral nerves

The ventral rami branch into interconnecting groups of large nerves called plexuses. Each plexus contains nerves from different spinal levels to make a complex web-like network. On each side of the body, the main plexuses are the **cervical plexus** (formed by spinal nerves C1–C4, which give off sensory and motor peripheral nerves to the areas of the head, neck and upper shoulder, and the phrenic nerve, which controls the diaphragm), **brachial plexus** (formed by spinal nerves C5–T1, forming motor nerves innervating the shoulder and upper chest), **lumbosacral plexus** (formed by spinal nerves L1–S5, forming sensory nerves from the anterior abdominal wall, genitofemoral region and lower limbs, and motor nerves to the abdominal wall, lower limbs, genitalia and buttocks) and **coccygeal plexus** (formed by spinal nerve C1, forming sensory nerves that supply skin overlying the coccyx). The spinal thoracic nerves T2–T12 do not form a plexus, but rather branch into peripheral nerves that supply sensory and motor peripheral nerves to the thorax, armpit and upper limbs.

Cranial nerves

The cranial nerves are 12 pairs of peripheral nerves (I–XII) that exit the brain/brain stem and supply the head and neck region (Fig. 7.13). The first two pairs originate from the cerebrum, and the remaining 10 arise from specific parts of the brain stem. The origin, modality (sensory/motor) and specific function of each cranial nerve are outlined in Table 7.2.

Autonomic nervous system as part of the peripheral nervous system

The autonomic nervous system is responsible for **involuntary control** of the body's functions (hence its name). It contains visceral afferent (sensory) fibres that relay important information about the body's physiological parameters such as blood pH, mechanical information such as position or stretch, pain and temperature. The visceral efferent fibres elicit an autonomic effect—that is, changes in cardiac output, vascular tone and blood pressure, respiration, gastric motility, glandular secretions, genitourinary function and metabolism. These effects are administered through two important divisions of the autonomic nervous system: the sympathetic and parasympathetic divisions, which both typically innervate the same target organ/gland and act as antagonistic systems against each other.

The **sympathetic nervous system** is responsible for activating the body in situations of stress where increased

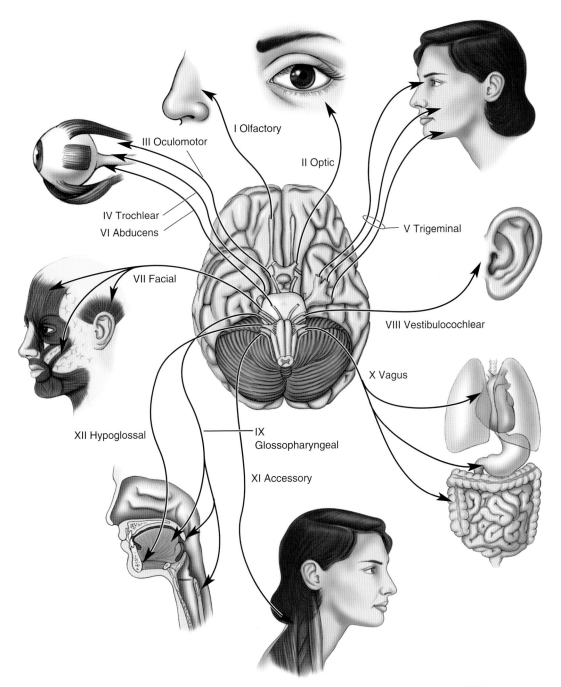

FIGURE 7.13 **Anatomy and function of the 12 pairs of cranial nerves.** (*Source:* Patton KT, Thibodeau. The human body in health and disease, 6 ed. St Louis: Mosby; 2014.)

TABLE 7.2
Outline of the 12 cranial nerves

Number	Name	Modality	Function
I	Olfactory	Sensory	Smell
II	Optic	Sensory	Vision
III	Oculomotor	Motor	Innervates muscles that control eye and eyelid movement and pupil size
IV	Trochlear	Motor	Innervates superior oblique muscle that controls eye movement
V	Trigeminal	Sensory/motor	Three branches: V1 branch (ophthalmic)—sensory input from scalp, forehead and nose region; V2 branch (maxillary)—sensory input from lower eyelids, cheeks, upper lip, upper teeth, palate and nasal mucosa; V3 branch (mandibular)—sensory input from skin over mandible and lower teeth and anterior two-thirds of the tongue, and motor input for muscles of mastication (chewing)
VI	Abducens	Motor	Innervates lacteral rectus muscle that controls eye movement
VII	Facial	Sensory/motor	Sensation to external ear, taste from anterior two-thirds of tongue and soft/hard palate; innervates muscles of facial expression and regulates tears, saliva and oral/nasal mucous secretions
VIII	Vestibulocochlear	Sensory	Hearing and balance
IX	Glossopharyngeal	Sensory/motor	Sensory input from posterior one-third of tongue (including taste), tonsils, pharynx, middle ear cavity, carotid body and sinus; innervates parotid salivary glands and stylopharyngeus muscle in pharynx
X	Vagus		Swallowing, gag reflex, phonation, involuntary control of muscles and glands (cardiorespiratory, gastrointestinal, urogenital), sensory input from cervical, thoracic, abdominal viscera, carotid and aortic bodies (chemoreceptors within the large blood vessels)
XI	Spinal accessory	Motor	Innervates trapezius and sternocleidomastoid muscles
XII	Hypoglossal	Motor	Controls tongue muscles

alertness, strength and mobility are required to respond to an emotional or a dangerous situation—the fight or flight response. It increases the activity of organs that support critical body functions during such a time, while simultaneously dampening the activity of organs that are non-critical. For example, cardiac output is increased by increased cardiac contractility; blood flow to the heart and skeletal muscles is increased by dilating blood vessels that supply them; bronchioles in the lungs dilate to increase air supply (and thus oxygen intake); and the adrenal glands are stimulated to release the stress hormones adrenaline (epinephrine) and noradrenaline (norepinephrine). In addition, the pupils dilate and sweating increases, particularly in apocrine gland-rich areas such as the palms of the hands and the armpits. Concurrently, gastrointestinal motility is inhibited, as is urine production in the kidneys. The overall effect is a catabolic system that expends energy.

In contrast, the **parasympathetic nervous system** is responsible for bodily functions in normal states and during relaxation or rest, and hence acts as the 'housekeeping system'. It is an anabolic system that conserves energy in the body. It regulates baseline heart and respiratory rates, stimulates gastrointestinal motility and the production and secretion of enzymes and saliva, and facilitates urination and defecation.

Structurally the autonomic nervous system is formed by branches of the ventral rami, which are branches of spinal nerves exiting the spinal cavity. Branches of autonomic motor fibres from the ventral rami originating from T1–L2 spinal levels form a chain of ganglia that extends upwards and downwards to cover the entire length of the spinal cord from the cervical to S1 regions. These ganglia of the sympathetic nervous system are interconnected vertically in a network known as the **sympathetic chain**, appearing like beads on a vertical chain. Within the sympathetic chain, synapses occur with autonomic neurons that form paired visceral nerves that innervate the internal organs. These visceral nerves, called **splanchnic nerves**, connect with ganglia that give off nerves that provide involuntary motor control of the visceral organs (visceral efferent fibres), as well as receive incoming sensory information from visceral organs (visceral afferent fibres). The overall structure of the autonomic nervous system is represented in Fig. 7.14.

The parasympathetic nervous system originates in cell bodies and subsequently ventral rami that exit S2–S4, as well as brain-stem nuclei associated with cranial nerves III, VII, IX and X. Unlike the sympathetic nervous system where the ganglia lie close to the spinal cord, in the parasympathetic nervous system the ganglia lie close to the effector organ, such as the heart or a kidney.

It is also worth noting that the neurotransmitters used by the sympathetic and parasympathetic nervous systems in their post-ganglionic neurons (communicating with the target organ/gland) are different. The parasympathetic nervous system mostly uses acetylcholine (and is hence called the cholinergic system), and the sympathetic nervous system uses noradrenaline (norepinephrine) (and is hence called the adrenergic system).

Control of the autonomic nervous system occurs with little processing and commanding by the cerebral cortex; it is subconscious, although some crosstalk still occurs. Many autonomic responses are based on a reflex arc, where visceral sensory input is processed into visceral effector outputs (such as increased vascular tone) at the level of autonomic ganglia, spinal cord and brain stem. Autonomic responses are associated with emotions and alertness, and therefore there is significant input from the hypothalamus, which contains several important nuclei that interact with the autonomic nervous system to exert 'central' control over this system.

Another branch of the autonomic nervous system is the **enteric nervous system**, which contains a vast network of neurons and supporting glial cells clustered into structures called enteric ganglia, which are interconnected by nerve fibres. The enteric nervous system can regulate the gastrointestinal system without relying on commands from the brain and spinal cord. It is structurally embedded within the gastrointestinal tract (discussed in Chapter 18). However, it is not completely isolated functionally and there is crosstalk between the enteric nervous system and the central nervous system through the parasympathetic and sympathetic nervous systems. Interconnected ganglia with afferent and efferent nerve fibres form networks referred to as plexuses, and reflex circuits formed with the plexuses can regulate gastrointestinal motility and secretomotor functions.

Mechanisms of wakefulness, consciousness and sleep

In clinical inpatient settings, patients often report poor sleep due to constant interruptions from clinical staff. In humans the three sleep and arousal states are wakefulness, being asleep and dreaming (while asleep). These states are regulated by a network of CNS structures known as the **reticular activating system (RAS)**. Although the mechanism of consciousness is complex and has still not been fully elucidated, what is known is that this is governed by communication between the cerebral cortex and the spinal cord via tracts that pass through and are regulated by the thalamus, hypothalamus and interconnected nuclei in the brain stem. Continued firing of impulses along the RAS is responsible for maintaining consciousness; increased signalling can act as an arousal or alerting system, and decreased signalling can lead to decreased alertness and sleep. The RAS also acts as a filter for sensory input into the cerebral cortex, allowing for prioritisation of information to enable the brain to be focused and alert.

Ordinarily, sleep is regulated by the secretion of melatonin from the pineal gland. However, this can be disrupted by CNS stimulants such as caffeine in coffee or behavioural modifications such as dancing at clubs and avoiding going to bed. Drowsiness and sleep result from suppression of the arousal centres in the brain stem and hypothalamus, filtering out of sensory input by the thalamus, and modulation of cerebral cortical activity. These events accompany changes throughout a variety of organ systems which are coordinated by the CNS. Autonomic regulation results in decreased heart rate, blood pressure, respiratory rate and gastrointestinal motility.

In the morning, in response to environmental stimuli (such as a ringing alarm clock or sunshine), decreased melatonin and increased secretion of hormones that govern wakefulness and stress (serotonin and cortisol) lead to increased firing of the RAS. This is accompanied by autonomic changes in body systems that result in increased heart rate, blood pressure and respiratory rate.

INTEGRATION OF THE NERVOUS SYSTEM WITH OTHER BODY SYSTEMS

It is important to recognise that the nervous system is closely linked to every other system in the body. It receives feedback on the body's internal parameters as well as external stimuli. It processes this information then determines a command that is relayed to the target system, be it the cardiovascular system, the gastrointestinal

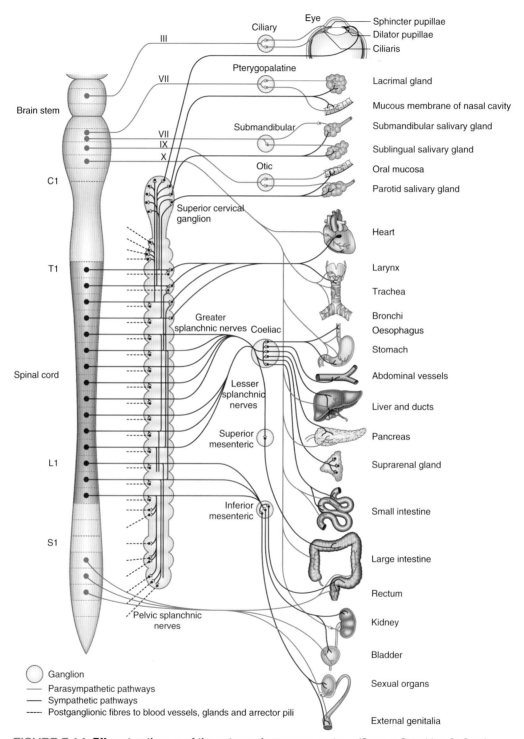

FIGURE 7.14 Efferent pathways of the autonomic nervous system. (*Source:* Standring S. Gray's anatomy, 41 ed. New York: Elsevier; 2016.)

system or an organ in the body. The nervous system works closely with the endocrine system, which also provides important hormonal signals to organs that regulate their function.

The complex networks within the brain determine human traits such as personality, emotion and memory, and our behaviour can influence our control over other body systems through processes such as movement or the voluntary actions of urination, defecation and sexual behaviour.

There are still many aspects of this incredibly complex system that remain unexplored. These include the developmental biology of neuronal circuitry and how this diverged between different species along the evolutionary pipeline; the role of stem cells in both the development and the repair of the nervous system; how the immune system helps regulate and protect the nervous system; and the role of this interplay in disease processes such as infection and cancer.

Cardiovascular system

The functional activities of the heart and blood vessels are controlled by neuronal input, which determines heart rate and contractility, as well as the vascular tone (constriction) of blood vessels, which determines blood pressure and flow. These signals are dependent on feedback from pressure and chemical (carbon dioxide/pH) receptors located within the cardiovascular system. In times of stress or activation of the body's fight or flight response, sympathetic regulation of the cardiovascular system drastically increases to ensure enough cardiac output is maintained to enable the body's response to the stressor. Additionally, CSF drains into the venous circulation, and is newly created by filtering blood plasma.

Lymphatic system

Lymphatic vessels have been known to be innervated, where autonomic regulation of the smooth muscle layer in vessels such as the thoracic duct regulates its contraction and hence lymph drainage.[4,5] In the CNS, the presence of a lymphatic drainage system is only a very recent and unexpected discovery, and this has changed our notion of CSF drainage and neuroimmunology.[6,7]

Immune system

The CNS was traditionally thought to be an immuno-privileged site, due to the blood–brain barrier preventing the migration of immune cells from blood into the CNS and the lack of lymphatic connections.[8] However, this has been completely overturned by the discovery of cerebral lymphatics, which now intimates that there is much closer integration between the nervous system and the immune system via lymphatic connections. Accounting for this may provide a better understanding of neurological disorders with an immune component such as multiple sclerosis or subtypes of epilepsy, or even how the brain and spinal cord respond and remodel after an injury such as stroke or trauma.

Respiratory system

Respiration (breathing) is a coordinated process (Chapter 17) involving the chest muscles, diaphragm, lungs and nervous system. Blood gas levels and respiratory volume are monitored by the CNS, and in turn voluntary control of respiration is exerted by the cerebral cortex, while baseline involuntary control of respiration is maintained by the respiratory centre located in the brain stem. The respiratory system is also involved in the fight or flight response, to ensure adequate oxygenation of key tissues such as the heart and skeletal muscles, and to enable excretion of carbon dioxide that increases as a result of intense metabolism.

Gastrointestinal system

Although part of the autonomic nervous system, the enteric nervous system regulates the motility and function of the gastrointestinal system without relying on commands from the brain and spinal cord. It is structurally embedded within the gastrointestinal tract (Chapter 18). There is also complex communication between the central and enteric nervous systems which controls both nervous and gastrointestinal function, and while this area is still not fully understood it is increasingly recognised that pathologies primarily thought to affect the nervous system (such as autism) have consequences in the gastrointestinal system due to the close interactions between the two systems.[9]

Integumentary system

The skin is a major sensory organ, providing a variety of senses such as touch, temperature, pain, pressure and proprioception, and a large surface area for interaction with the external environment. During times of anxiety, stress or nervousness, such as when the fight or flight response is activated, sympathetic stimulation leads to activation of sweat glands in our palms, face, feet and armpits, causing excessive sweating in these locations.

Skeletal system, joints and bone

The nervous system controls movement by coordinating the contraction and positioning of muscles, joints and bones. In turn, sensory receptors in these peripheral tissues send information regarding the body's position and movement back to the CNS. The skeletal system plays a critical role in providing a bony protective casing for the delicate CNS, comprising the skull, which protects the brain, and the vertebral column, which protects the spinal cord.

Special senses: hearing, balance and vision

Senses such as hearing, vision and proprioception are critically dependent on feedback from sensory organs being processed by the cerebral cortex into signals that enable us to perceive these senses and integrate them with higher cognitive functions such as memory and learning.

Endocrine system

The hypothalamus-pituitary axis forms a major part of the control of endocrine release in the body, and in turn the nervous system itself is regulated by a variety of hormones including melatonin, cortisol, adrenaline (epinephrine) and reproductive hormones.

One critical mechanism that depends on coordination between the endocrine and nervous systems is the fight or flight response, which is controlled by the autonomic nervous system and kicks in when we are presented with a dangerous or emotional stimulus. Several branches of the nervous system kick into action to enable us to respond in a protective manner, to fight the danger or flee from it, hence the term 'fight or flight response'. First, sensory input in the form of vision, sound or even smell is communicated to the cerebral cortex where it is processed and information regarding past experiences, emotions and memory is integrated within a complex network called the limbic system, which includes the amygdala, hippocampus, thalamus and hypothalamus. This leads to activation of the sympathetic nervous system and results in stimulation of the adrenal glands to release noradrenaline (norepinephrine) and adrenaline (epinephrine). These act on beta-adrenergic receptors in the cardiac muscle and the smooth muscle of blood vessels to cause an increased cardiac output, dilated skin, sweaty palms, trembling, increased respiration and dilated bronchioles, and decreased gastrointestinal motility. Once the danger has passed, the cerebral cortex and limbic system can override the sympathetic response and bring the body back to its normal state.

Urinary system

Urination (or micturition) involves feedback and coordination between the nervous and urinary systems. For example, the bladder sends sensory information to the brain that allows us to 'feel' a full bladder when it reaches 300–400 mL capacity. Normally, socially inappropriate urination is prevented by voluntary contraction of the external urethral sphincter, while the inner urethral sphincter remains contracted under sympathetic stimulation. However, once urination is initiated by voluntary relaxation of the external urethral sphincter, the act of urination occurs as a spinal reflex where sympathetic signals that control the internal urethral sphincter and bladder neck cause relaxation, and parasympathetic stimulation of the bladder causes its contraction and coordinated emptying. Hence this process is called the micturition reflex.

Reproductive system

Reproductive hormones are important in neural development and the regulation of sexual behaviour, and in turn the CNS controls the release of these hormones (via the hypothalamus-pituitary axis) and contributes cognition, emotion, memory, impulse control and social habits to mating behaviour. Neural innervation is important in the normal function of reproductive organs; this importance is demonstrated in situations where nerve damage in the pelvis leads to lack of sexual function—for example, after surgery for prostate cancer.

AGE-RELATED CHANGES

Following birth, infants have limited motor-neuron function, meaning that they have a limited range of motion, are aware for only short periods of time, tire easily and do not cope well with overstimulation. Within weeks, infants become more aware and start to perform more complex movements such as lifting and supporting their head, making intentional sounds, increasing their vision field and recognising when to smile. By 18 months of age, most toddlers start to develop a vocabulary, stand straight and walk, have developed good coordination, test their environment, stay awake for longer and effectively engage in play activities. These are all possible because of the complex development of neuronal pathways that support both motor-neuron function and cognitive function. If these developmental milestones are not reached, concerns are raised about the possibility of nervous system disorders.

As we age, the spinal cord and brain both undergo atrophy. Some of this is due to natural loss of neuronal cells. Neuronal cells also become less effective in transmitting neuronal impulses. Neuronal cells responsible for hearing, balance, smell and taste start to die and in time a person becomes less sensitive to these stimuli. Although loss of these cells will impact on the person's function, these changes are gradual and some people may not even notice them. The reduction in motor-neuron control means that as we get older we are not as well coordinated and are at a higher risk of falls and more serious injury.

It is important to recognise that dementia—an umbrella term that describes neurological conditions characterised by a severe decline in brain function such as thinking, memory, behaviour, understanding language and expression—is not part of the normal ageing process.

CONCLUSION

The nervous system is an incredibly complex system distributed throughout the body. The central command centres are the brain and spinal cord, which branch out into the peripheral nervous system, which includes the somatic and autonomic nervous systems. The role of the nervous system is to gather sensory information from the external environment as well as internal parameters maintained in the body such as temperature and blood pressure. This information is processed either consciously or subconsciously, and results in either voluntary movement or internal processes that regulate physiology. The nervous system and endocrine system are responsible for finely controlling all of the body's critical processes. The brain is also important in cognitive processes and behaviour that make us human. In this chapter we have described the structural and functional components of the nervous system, emphasised its central role in regulating the body and explained how this occurs via interaction with virtually every other body system.

CASE STUDY 7.1

Mary-Anne spent a long night completing an assignment and has turned up for an early morning lecture. As she sits comfortably in the chair of the lecture hall, she slowly slips into a gentle snooze. Her lecturer is not impressed.

Q1. Which gland produces melatonin?
   a. Thalamus
   b. Hypothalamus
   c. Pineal gland
   d. Brain stem

Q2. The stages of human sleep and arousal state are regulated by the:
   a. brain stem.
   b. medulla oblongata.
   c. occipital lobe.
   d. reticular activating system.

Q3. The sleep/wake cycle cannot be modified through the consumption of caffeine.
   a. True
   b. False

Q4. Which hormone is involved in regulating the sleep/wake cycle?

Q5. Describe how the nervous system regulates sleep.

CASE STUDY 7.2

Jorge is at a Halloween party when Beth, who is hiding behind the door in a ghoul costume, jumps out at him. Jorge is surprised and lets out a loud yell. He appears pale and his heart is pounding.

Q1. Which structure in the CNS has dual functions in neural function and endocrine secretion?
   a. Brain stem
   b. Thalamus
   c. Cerebral cortex
   d. Hypothalamus
   e. Corpus callosum

Q2. For a nerve impulse to be generated at the site of tissue injury and conducted to the brain, the receptor stimulation must reach a threshold needed to generate action potentials, which are then conducted across the neuronal network to the brain.
   a. True
   b. False

Q3. Why is Jorge pale?
   a. He experienced blood loss.
   b. Jorge is not receiving enough oxygen to his skin due to iron deficiency.
   c. His blood has been diverted to vital organs that have to effectively respond to danger.
   d. Jorge's paleness has nothing to do with him being frightened.

Q4. Describe neural regulation of the fight or flight response.

Q5. Which part of the CNS is responsible for increased cardiac output and blood flow to essential organs and respiration during the fight or flight response?

CASE STUDY 7.3

Zara is bustling in the kitchen to make tea for some visitors. She is distracted by the gossip at hand and without looking reaches for the kettle. She feels a hot searing pain and instinctively retracts her hand away from the kettle.

Q1. Which of the following is a reflex reaction?

   a. Withdrawing your hand due to a needle prick
   b. Moving your foot to make yourself more comfortable
   c. Putting your jumper on because you are cold
   d. Salivating

Q2. The micturition reflex is:

   a. a process that regulates bladder emptying.
   b. a process that controls the fight or flight response.

   c. a process that controls memory formation.
   d. solely responsible for maintenance of renal function.

Q3. The reflex arc involves:

   a. the input of cognition and conscious control.
   b. responses that rely on interneurons without the input of cognition and conscious control.
   c. slow transmission of impulses between the sensory input and motor output.
   d. slow response to damaging stimuli.

Q4. Describe a spinal reflex arc.

Q5. Explain how the cerebral cortex may become involved in a spinal reflex arc.

CASE STUDY 7.4

Gloria is out grocery shopping. She should have brought along her shopping list but left it on the kitchen counter. She is sure she has forgotten some items she needs for her weekend party but cannot recall what they are.

Q1. Which cells secrete insulating myelin in peripheral nerves?

   a. Astrocytes
   b. Ganglion cells
   c. Schwann cells
   d. Glial cells
   e. Oligodendrocytes

Q2. Which neurotransmitter is involved in communication in the sympathetic nervous system?

   a. Noradrenaline (norepinephrine)
   b. Serotonin

   c. Dopamine
   d. Acetylcholine
   e. Gamma aminobutyric acid (GABA)

Q3. What is the outermost covering of the CNS (brain and spinal cord) underneath the bone?

   a. Pia mater
   b. Dura mater
   c. Perineural sheath
   d. Arachnoid mater
   e. Gyrus

Q4. Name the main CNS structures involved in memory.

Q5. Explain the difference between short- and long-term memory.

REFERENCES

1. Patton KT, Thibodeau GA. Anatomy and physiology. 9th ed. St Louis: Elsevier; 2016.
2. Friede RL. The significance of internode length for saltatory conduction: looking back at the age of 90. J Neuropathol Exp Neurol 2017;76(4):258–9.
3. Hartmann P, Ramseier A, Gudat F, et al. Normal weight of the brain in adults in relation to age, sex, body height and weight. Pathologe 1994;15(3):165–70.
4. Mignini F, Sabbatini M, Cavallotti C, et al. Analysis of nerve supply pattern in thoracic duct in young and elderly men. Lymphat Res Biol 2012;10(2):46–52.
5. Mignini F, Sabbatini M, Coppola L, et al. Analysis of nerve supply pattern in human lymphatic vessels of young and old men. Lymphat Res Biol 2012;10(4):189–97.
6. Absinta M, Ha S-K, Nair G, et al. Human and nonhuman primate meninges harbor lymphatic vessels that can be visualized noninvasively by MRI. Elife 2017;6:e29738.
7. Louveau A, Smirnov I, Keyes TJ, et al. Structural and functional features of central nervous system lymphatic vessels. Nature 2015;523(7560):337–41.
8. Kipnis J, Filiano AJ. Neuroimmunology in 2017: the central nervous system, privileged by immune connections. Nat Rev Immunol 2018;18(2):83–4.
9. Rao M, Gershon MD. The bowel and beyond: the enteric nervous system in neurological disorders. Nat Rev Gastroenterol Hepatol 2016;13(9):517–28.

CHAPTER 8

Understanding the physiology of pain

CLARE FENWICK, PHD

KEY POINTS/LEARNING OUTCOMES

1. Explain how a pain impulse is generated in a process of pain transduction.
2. Describe the process of pain transmission from its origin along peripheral nerves to the central nervous system.
3. Understand why perception of pain is unique to every individual.
4. Discuss how the body modulates the pain impulse as a means of establishing homeostasis.
5. Understand why the pain experience is a whole-body experience.

KEY DEFINITIONS

- **Modulation:** occurs as the descending pain pathways are activated to change the body's awareness of pain.
- **Neurotransmitters:** chemicals produced by the brain that are released at specialised areas of the nerve cell called terminal nerve endings.
- **Nociception:** the body's response to threat resulting in the pain experience.
- **Nociceptive pain:** a neurophysiological event caused by the noxious stimulus of somatic or visceral nociceptors in an intact nervous system.
- **Nociceptor:** a sensory neuron located at the free endings of the peripheral nerve.
- **Perception:** when the individual develops a physical, emotional and cognitive awareness of pain.
- **Transduction:** occurs when a noxious mechanical, thermal or chemical event (nociception) is transferred into a pain impulse.
- **Transmission:** the movement of the pain impulse from the peripheral nervous system to the central nervous system.

ONLINE RESOURCES/SUGGESTED READINGS

- **Acute Pain Management: Scientific Evidence, 4 ed 2015** available at http://fpm.anzca.edu.au/documents/apmse4_2015_final
- **Australian Pain Management Association** available at www.painmanagement.org.au
- **Australian Pain Society** available at www.apsoc.org.au
- **National Pain Strategy** available at www.painaustralia.org.au/static/uploads/files/national-pain-strategy-2011-wfvjawttsanq.pdf
- **Pain Australia** available at www.painaustralia.org.au

INTRODUCTION

Understanding the anatomy and physiology of pain is an incomplete science due to the dynamic, complex and unique nature of the human pain experience. The physiology of pain is inherently linked to the sociocultural, behavioural, emotional and spiritual aspects of the individual.

Many theories have been proposed to explain the human pain experience, the most significant being Melzack and Wall's **gate control theory of pain**.[1] This theory suggests that the pain impulse navigates a group of neurological gates within the spinal cord before it reaches the brain.[2] These neurological gates operate in three different ways to:

1. monitor the intensity of the pain impulse
2. monitor the intensity of other sensory impulses (touch, temperature and pressure) generated at the site of injury
3. notify the brain to send messages about the pain or to ignore the message.

When an actual or a perceived threat originates, a pain impulse is generated and travels along peripheral nerves to enter the central nervous system via the dorsal horn. Imagine that a protective barrier surrounds the central nervous system with a series of gates that open or close. Melzack and Wall proposed that a noxious stimulus, such as heat or anxiety, could open a gate allowing a flood of neural messages into the spinal cord and brain.[1] Closing the gate can occur via one of two mechanisms: (1) pulling the gate closed by activating the peripheral nervous system; or (2) pushing the gate closed using the central nervous system. Activating the peripheral nervous system, through massage, vibration or applying gentle heat, stimulates the A-beta nerves to pull the gate closed and reduce the intensity of pain.[2,3] Activation of the central nervous system by distraction, meditation or release of the body's own natural pain relief (endorphins and encephalins) pushes the gate closed (Fig. 8.1).[3,4]

In 1991, Melzack moved away from the gate control theory of pain and proposed the **neuromatrix theory of pain**.[2] This theory suggests that pain perception does not occur from the brain's reflexive awareness of tissue damage; rather, the brain and spinal cord work together to produce the sensation of pain regardless of tissue damage.[5] The body is composed of a complex nervous system driving motor, sensory and cognitive activities. The neuromatrix theory of pain proposes that this complex neural network is genetically influenced and modified throughout our life by various sensory inputs, forming a body-self neuromatrix.[2,5] Inputs from cognitive-related brain areas—such as memories of past experiences, meaning and anxiety—combine with sensory signalling systems from around the body, and collectively

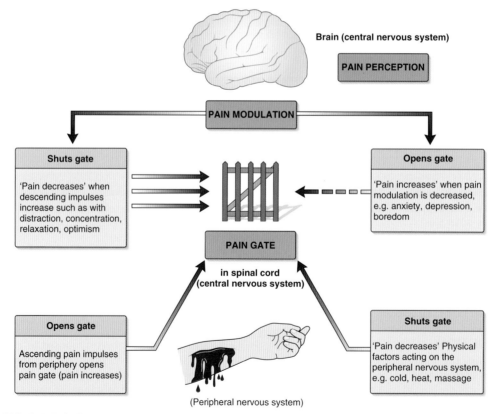

FIGURE 8.1 **Gate control theory of pain.** (*Source:* Brooker C, Waugh A. editors. Foundations of nursing practice: fundamentals of holistic care. Edinburgh: Mosby; 2007.)

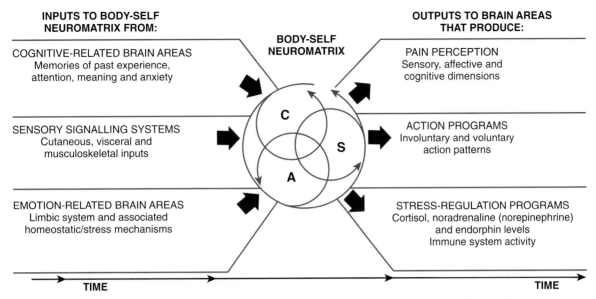

**INPUTS TO BODY-SELF
NEUROMATRIX FROM:**

**OUTPUTS TO BRAIN AREAS
THAT PRODUCE:**

**BODY-SELF
NEUROMATRIX**

COGNITIVE-RELATED BRAIN AREAS
Memories of past experience,
attention, meaning and anxiety

PAIN PERCEPTION
Sensory, affective and
cognitive dimensions

SENSORY SIGNALLING SYSTEMS
Cutaneous, visceral and
musculoskeletal inputs

ACTION PROGRAMS
Involuntary and voluntary
action patterns

EMOTION-RELATED BRAIN AREAS
Limbic system and associated
homeostatic/stress mechanisms

STRESS-REGULATION PROGRAMS
Cortisol, noradrenaline (norepinephrine)
and endorphin levels
Immune system activity

TIME   TIME

FIGURE 8.2 **Neuromatrix theory of pain.** (*Source:* Melzack R. Pain and the neuromatrix in the brain. J Dental Ed 2001;65(12):1378–82.)

these combine with emotion-related brain activities such as stress and fear (Fig. 8.2).[2] These inputs of neural messages create a pattern, or memory, of a sensory event, called a neurosignature; this neurosignature informs the brain to act.[2,5,6]

Imagine you witness a person falling over; even though you did not fall, your body stiffens and you call out. You did not sustain any injury, yet you actively responded. This phenomenon occurs because your brain has retained a memory or neurosignature of what a fall may feel like. Let's translate this concept into the pain experience. Imagine a person undergoes an amputation of a limb due to ongoing disease and pain. It is possible that the person will still experience pain in the absent limb due to their retained **memory of pain** or their **neurosignature of pain**. Every person's neurosignature of pain is reflective of that person's exclusive life experiences. Activation of this mind–body matrix will stimulate pain perception, action patterns and commence the stress regulation processes.[2] Recognising that each individual experiences pain differently will directly impact upon the clinician's ability to conduct an accurate pain assessment and initiate effective pain relief.

STRUCTURE AND FUNCTION OF PAIN

In its most basic form, pain can be classified as a threat.[7] It is normal to believe that a threat would be associated with an injury; however, not all injuries cause pain, and pain can be present without any injury.[7,8] This can be confusing and challenging for the clinician who needs to be able to interpret and respond to an individual's pain experience.

When an individual perceives a threat or noxious stimuli, a defence mechanism designed to protect the body from further noxious stimuli is activated. These noxious stimuli activate fine nerve endings located on the peripheral nerves called **nociceptors**.[9] Nociceptors send messages along the peripheral nerves into specialised nerves in the spinal cord and, in turn, these messages travel upwards to the brain. It is within the brain that the individual interprets the experience as pain and becomes aware of pain. In response to this awareness of pain another message is sent down the spinal cord to specialised nerves, causing the body to react to minimise or modify the pain experience. These ascending and descending pain pathways have evolved to detect, interpret and initiate a protective response to harmful or noxious stimuli that threaten or imply threat to the body (Fig. 8.3).[9,10]

Yet the pain experience is more complex than a neural message perceived as pain. How do we explain heartache at the death of a loved one, when no physical injury occurred? Why does a football player with a torn knee ligament continue to play despite the severe injury? Does the desire to win overrule the experience of pain? Think for a moment when you last experienced pain: what was happening within your body, what emotions were

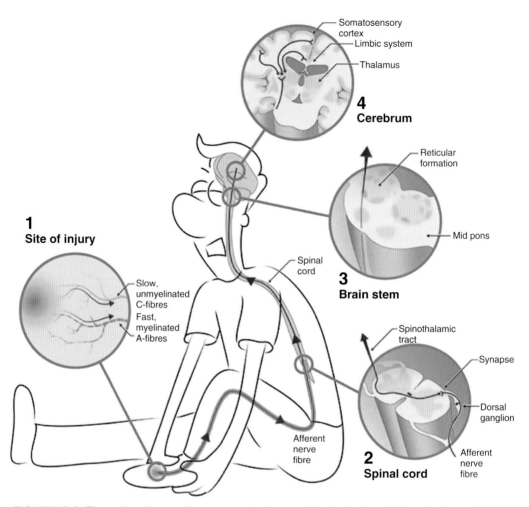

FIGURE 8.3 **The pain pathway.** (*Source:* https://neuroscience.stanford.edu/news/pain-brain. Last accessed: May 2019.)

you feeling, what social event were you participating in and what cultural expectation did you uphold? Pain is more than just a message travelling up and down pain pathways—pain is an experience of the entire person.

The neurophysiological process of pain involves three areas of the body: the peripheral nervous system, the spinal cord and the brain. Nociceptors are sensory neurons located at the free endings of the peripheral nerves.[9] **Nociception** or **nociceptive pain** is the body's response to threat, resulting in the pain experience.[11] Pain detection (transduction), pain transmission, pain modulation and pain expression (perception)[6,11] are the four distinctive processes that make up nociception. Transduction, transmission and modulation occur in the peripheral nervous system, the spinal cord and the brain.[11] Perception arises in the brain.[11]

Transduction

Transduction happens when millions of nociceptors, present throughout the body, respond to a noxious stimulus and transfer this event (nociception) into pain impulses.[9] Somatic-based nociceptors are located within the skin, muscles, connective tissue, bones and joints.[12,13] Visceral-based nociceptors are located within the thoracic, pelvic and abdominal organs.[13] Activation of somatic-based nociceptors causes pain to be described as sharp, aching or throbbing;[14] activation of visceral-based nociceptors causes pain to be described as gnawing or cramping.[14]

A noxious stimulus can be chemical, thermal or mechanical in origin and will stimulate specific types of nociceptors.[9,10] Chemical nociceptors respond to a chemical change in the environment, such as a toxic substance or the release of the inflammatory mediators

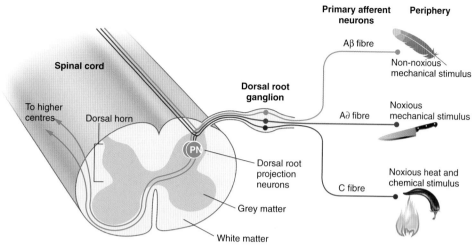

FIGURE 8.4 **Activation of nociceptors.**

bradykinin, histamine and acids.[10] Thermal nociceptors are activated by body temperatures greater than 45°C or below 5°C.[15,16] Mechanical nociceptors respond to pressure or stretching such as that associated with swelling.[15] More than one sort of nociceptor can be activated at the same time depending on the type and location of the injury (Fig. 8.4).

When an injury or a noxious stimulus occurs, damaged cells release various inflammatory mediators including prostaglandins, substance P, bradykinin, potassium, serotonin, histamine and leukotrienes.[9,10]

These mediators move through the extracellular fluid stimulating the nociceptors so that an exchange of sodium and potassium ions occurs.[17,18] This exchange results in an electrical impulse or action potential; the action potential is how the nerve carries the pain impulse along various sensory nerve fibres.[17,18] Sensory nerve fibres are responsible for carrying a variety of sensory information to the brain. How this message arrives is determined by the type of nerve fibre, the presence of a myelin sheath, how large the nerve fibre is and how fast the message is carried (Fig. 8.5).

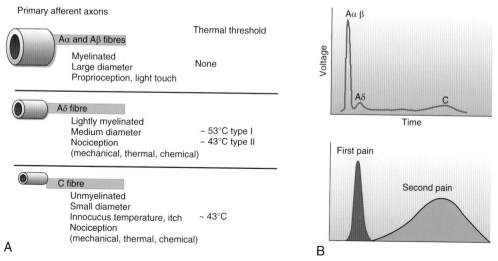

FIGURE 8.5 **Pain fibre conduction.** (*Source:* Julius D, Basbaum JD. Molecular mechanisms of nociception. Nature 2001;413:203–10.)

Sensory nerve fibres of the peripheral nervous system are divided into two categories: A fibres (A-beta and A-delta); and C fibres.[10] **A-beta fibres**, the largest and with the fastest conduction speed, carry sensory messages such as touch, pressure and vibration.[9] These sensations are classified as non-noxious stimuli and are not normally associated with pain.[19] A-beta fibres play a significant role in quietening pain sensation or pain modulation; this is discussed later in the chapter. **A-delta fibres** and **C fibres** carry noxious stimuli and will determine the type of pain sensation experienced by the individual. A-delta fibres, the second largest fibres, rapidly (5–40 m/s) carry a pain impulse along large-diameter, myelinated nerves.[9,12] A-delta fibres respond to mechanical and thermal stimuli, creating a pain sensation that is well-localised, sharp, stinging and/or pricking in sensation.[9,10,20] C fibres, the smallest fibres, slowly carry the pain impulse at a speed less than 2 m/s along unmyelinated nerve.[9,10,12] These sensory fibres are responsive to thermal, mechanical and chemical stimuli, generating pain that is diffuse, dull, long-lasting, aching and/or burning.[9] The unique characteristics of these peripheral nerves are summarised in Table 8.1.

The body's reaction to pain is complex involving many interconnecting physiological activities. The creation of a pain impulse is the first step in the individual's pain journey, the transduction of pain. The next stage is to understand how the pain impulse travels to the brain via transmission.

TABLE 8.1
A-delta and C fibres structure and function

	A-delta fibres	C fibres
Size	Large diameter	Small diameter
Structure	Myelinated	Unmyelinated
Speed of conduction	Fast (5–40 m/s)	Slow (0.5–2 m/s)
Stimulus	Responds to mechanical and thermal stimuli	Polymodal response to thermal, mechanical and chemical stimuli
Location of sensation	Well localised	Diffuse
Pain sensation	Associated with sharp, stinging and/or pricking type pain	Associated with dull, long-lasting, aching and/or burning pain

Transmission

Transmission occurs as the pain impulse moves from the peripheral nervous system into the spinal cord and brain (central nervous system). Transmission of the pain impulse occurs in three stages:

1. from the site of transduction along A-delta fibres and C fibres to the dorsal horn in the spinal cord
2. from the spinal cord to the brain stem
3. through neural connections between the thalamus, cortex and higher levels of the brain.[9]

During the first stage of transmission an 'inflammatory soup' of excitatory neurotransmitters gathers to assist movement of the pain impulse along A-delta fibres and C fibres to the dorsal horn in the spinal cord.[21] These neurotransmitters 'talk' to one another, spreading the story of pain across the body to the brain. Neurotransmitters are released at specialised areas of the nerve cell known as terminal nerve endings.[22] The characteristic of a neurotransmitter can be excitatory, inhibitory or both depending on how the body is responding to the pain impulse.[22] There are many different types of excitatory neurotransmitters including glutamate, substance P, bradykinin, nitrous oxide and calcitonin gene-related peptide.[21,23] When the pain impulse needs to be modulated or quietened, inhibitory neurotransmitters are released such as gamma aminobutyric acid (GABA), serotonin, noradrenaline (norepinephrine), endorphin, encephalin, somatostatin and dopamine (Fig. 8.6).[23,24]

The second stage of transmission occurs when excitatory neurotransmitters flood the terminal ends of the A-delta and C nerve fibres moving the pain impulse into the dorsal horn of the spinal cord.[21] The release of these neurotransmitters assists the pain impulse to cross the synaptic cleft, effectively moving the pain impulse from the peripheral nervous system to the central nervous system.[21] If we were to look at a transverse section of the spinal cord it would reveal a butterfly pattern of dark, inner **grey matter** surrounded by pale-coloured **white matter** (Fig. 8.7). Grey matter is divided into three sections: dorsal horn, lateral horn and ventral horn. Within these horns are layers of specialised cells collectively known as **rexed laminae**. There are total of 10 rexed laminae.[25] Laminae I, II and V of the dorsal horn are involved in the transmission of pain.[9,10,25] Lamina I responds to thermal or mechanical stimuli from cutaneous C, A-delta and A-beta fibres.[9] Lamina II responds to noxious and non-noxious stimuli from cutaneous and visceral C fibres,[10,25] A-delta[10] and A-beta fibres.[9] The exact function of lamina V in pain is still unclear, but pain impulses are reported to travel from A-delta and C fibres through this lamina.[9,10] A key point is that the dorsal cells have a dual role in the transmission

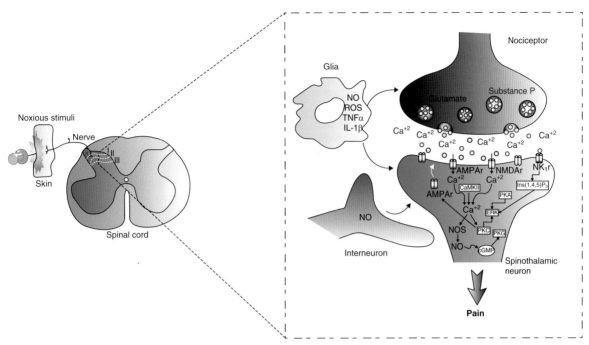

FIGURE 8.6 **Pain transmission.** (*Source:* Freire MAM, Guimaraes JS, Leal WG, Pereira A. Pain modulation by nitric oxide in the spinal cord. Front Neurosci 2009;3(2):179.)

of pain (excitatory) and modulation of pain (inhibitory) (Fig. 8.7).

As the pain impulse enters the dorsal horn it is free to travel up the ascending pain pathways—the spinothalamic tract and the spinoreticular tract.[26] The name of each tract informs us of the route the pain impulse

THE DORSAL HORN

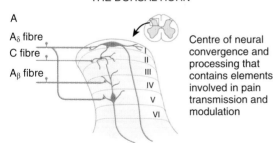

A

A_δ fibre

C fibre

A_β fibre

Centre of neural convergence and processing that contains elements involved in pain transmission and modulation

FIGURE 8.7 **Rexed laminae.** Primary afferent neurons enter the spinal cord, segregate and occupy a lateral position in the dorsal horn. Their termination in distinct zones, or laminae, is depicted. (*Source:* Davis PJ, Cladis FP. Pain management. In: Monitto CL, Yaster M, Kos-Byerly S. Smith's anaesthesia for infants and children, 9 ed. Philadelphia: Elsevier; 2017.)

travels. For example, the pain impulse travels along A-delta fibres up the spinal nerves and into the thalamus via the spinothalamic tract;[10] and travels along C fibres up the spinal nerves and into the reticular formation via the spinoreticular tract.[26] These tracts are summarised in Table 8.2. The spinothalamic tract is the main pain pathway merging into the neospinothalamic tract and the paleospinothalamic tract.[10] The neospinothalamic tract is responsible for the sensory-discriminative aspects of pain, receiving input from lamina I to the thalamus.[6,10,26] The paleospinothalamic tract is responsible for the motivational-affective aspects of the pain experience, receiving input from lamina II through the thalamus and projecting into the reticular formation, medulla, midbrain, periaqueductal grey matter and limbic system.[6,10,26] The termination of the pain impulse in the brain is when the individual will begin to perceive pain and behave accordingly.[12]

Perception

The individual's past experiences of pain, their expectations, and their emotional and cognitive responses to pain will shape their pain response (**perception**).[27] These responses in combination with neurological interactions facilitate the perception of pain. The pain impulse has

TABLE 8.2
Ascending pain pathways and their role in the pain experience

Pain fibre	Tract	Connections	Function
A-delta	Spinothalamic– neospinothalamic	Rexed laminae I Ventroposterolateral nucleus in the thalamus	Sensory-discriminative: 1. Location of stimulus 2. Is this a threat or not?
C	Spinothalamic– paleospinothalamic	Rexed laminae II Reticular formation, medulla, midbrain, periaqueductal grey matter and limbic system	Motivational-affective: 1. Emotional response 2. Do something about it
C	Spinoreticular	Reticular formation, locus coeruleus raphe, intralaminar nuclei in the thalamus, anterior cingulate cortex	Memory of pain, emotional response and descending analgesic activation

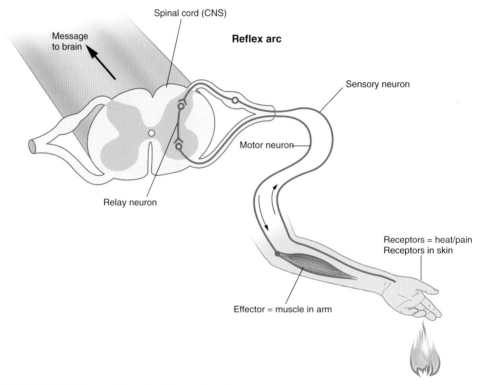

FIGURE 8.8 **Reflex response to noxious stimulus.**

travelled along the A-delta and C fibres venturing into laminae I, II and V of the dorsal horn.[10,14] The A-delta fibres rapidly ascend the neospinothalamic tract travelling to the thalamus, terminating in the somatosensory cortex.[12] Concurrently, the C fibres slowly ascend the paleospinothalamic tract, entering the pons and reticular formation, terminating in the somatosensory cortex.[26] The somatosensory cortex is where the pain impulse

becomes a meaningful, conscious awareness of pain for the individual.[28] Due to activation of the somatosensory cortex the individual will be aware of the pain before they physically react to the painful stimuli.[10] Within the reticular system the autonomic and motor response to pain is activated, resulting in the individual physically reacting to the painful stimulus, such as retracting their hand away from a hot flame (Fig. 8.8). The reticular system is also responsible for provoking the individual to observe and assess their hand to understand what happened, and to determine what the appropriate emotional response should be.[10]

The limbic system assists the somatosensory cortex in processing pain and memories of pain, and in doing so activates the individual's emotional and behavioural responses to pain.[14] It is within the limbic system where the individual will sense fear or threat of a stimulus (Fig. 8.9).[28] The somatosensory cortex facilitates the individual's understanding of the pain sensation, including pain intensity, location and type.[28] It is within the cortex that the individual links this current pain experience to past experiences of pain and their associated cognitive activities. The neurological process of sending the pain impulse to the brain is interrelated with the individual's ability to modify the pain impulse. This leads us to the final stage: modulation of pain.

Modulation

An inability to silence, soothe or modulate the experience of pain would undoubtedly lead to a miserable existence. Pain **modulation** is a multimodal process whereby descending pain pathways, inhibitory neurotransmitters and the brain itself modify the pain impulse to minimise the pain experience.[27,29–31]

When an actual or a perceived threat originates, pain impulses are sent along the A-delta and C fibres into the dorsal horn. As the A-delta and C fibres ascend the pain pathways, large-diameter A-beta fibres are activated, flooding the substantia gelatinosa of the dorsal horn with thermal and touch messages.[14] These messages activate the descending pain pathways, periaqueductal grey matter and nucleus raphe magnus, sending competing neural messages down the spinal cord to inhibit the pain impulse.[10,12,26,30] This may explain why the application of heat/cold or the action of rubbing an injury diminishes the perception of pain: the individual is

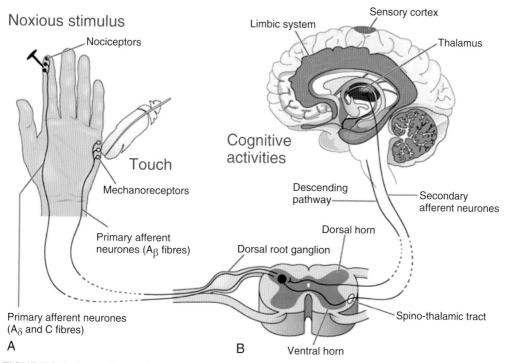

FIGURE 8.9 **Ascending and descending pain pathways.** Nociceptive nerve pathways essential for the transmission, perception and modulation of pain are depicted. **A** After an injury, nociceptive fibres carried in peripheral nerves enter the spinal cord via the dorsal horn. They are then transmitted via ascending spinothalamic, spinoreticular and spinomesencephalic tracts to the thalamus, limbic system and sensory cortex. **B** From the sensory cortex, descending control pathways modulate pain in the spinal cord and in the periphery. (*Source:* Davis PJ, Cladis FP. Pain management. In: Monitto CL, Yaster M, Kos-Byerly S. Smith's anaesthesia for infants and children, 9 ed. Philadelphia: Elsevier; 2017.)

activating competing, soothing A-beta fibres. To initiate the ascending pain pathways, excitatory neurotransmitters are released; to activate the descending pain pathways, inhibitory neurotransmitters are released.[29,30]

Inhibitory neurotransmitters—such as GABA, serotonin, noradrenaline (norepinephrine), endorphins, encephalins, dynorphins, somatostatin and dopamine—interact at a cellular level to inhibit the pain impulse.[9,14,23,24] The neurotransmitters and neuromodulators, endorphins, encephalins and dynorphins are part of the neuroendocrine system responsible for modulating the pain and stress responses.[9,10,14,29] These agents are referred to as the body's natural analgesia or opioids. Within the brain, spinal cord and digestive system are a group of opioid receptors—mu, kappa and delta.[9,10,14,29] Activation of these opioid receptors by inhibitory neurotransmitters results in pain relief for the person, a response similar to how the individual would respond to the manufactured opioids, morphine and codeine.[6,11,29]

This exchange of neurotransmitters, neural impulses and activities within the somatosensory cortex, thalamus and limbic system will be evaluated against the individual's memories of pain, learned responses to pain and emotional response to the pain event. The outcome is pain awareness and behaviours.

Referred pain

Referred pain is pain experienced not at the site of injury, but at a point some distance away.[17] For example, someone experiencing a myocardial infarction or heart attack will feel a crushing chest pain as well as pain radiating down the left arm. The pain radiating down the left arm is referred pain. It is unclear exactly how this phenomenon occurs; however, it has been proposed that nociceptors from the viscera, such as the heart muscle, and the skin travel similar pathways to the dorsal horn, and this leads to the brain recognising pain in multiple areas.[17,23]

INTEGRATION OF PAIN WITH OTHER BODY SYSTEMS

Pain does not occur in isolation from other areas of the body; rather, it causes a cascade of physiological, emotional and cognitive processes in response to a perceived threat or noxious stimuli.[27,32] Previous sections have discussed how perceived threat, recognised as pain, stimulates the pain production system. Perceived threat or pain also stimulates the stress response system.[11] Two primary mechanisms are activated in the stress response: the sympathetic nervous system and the neuroendocrine system.[32] Other secondary systems are also activated:

the motor system and the immune system.[33] The sympathetic nervous system response, known as the **sympathetic-adrenal-medullary (SAM) axis**, is responsible for the fight or flight response to a threat[34]—for example, activation of the SAM axis during an acute pain episode. In contrast, the neuroendocrine system, known as the **hypothalamic-pituitary-adrenal (HPA) axis**, is activated long after the threat has been removed[34]—for example, the HPA axis is activated when chronic pain is experienced. Chronic pain is considered a pathology or disease of the pain production system and causes a host of other pathologies for the body; as such, it is not discussed in this chapter.

Sympathetic-adrenal-medullary axis

The autonomic nervous system maintains homeostasis by regulating bodily functions such as heart rate, digestion, respiratory rate and blood pressure, without our conscious awareness. The autonomic nervous system is divided into two systems: the sympathetic nervous system and the parasympathetic nervous system.[34–36] The sympathetic nervous system is responsible for the fight or flight response, an excitatory action; whereas the parasympathetic nervous system initiates the rest-and-digest response, an inhibitory action.[34–36] In response to pain, both excitatory and inhibitory actions occur simultaneously.

Activation of the SAM axis starts when the hypothalamus stimulates the adrenal medulla to secrete the hormones adrenaline (epinephrine) and noradrenaline (norepinephrine) (Fig. 8.10).[34] Release of adrenaline (epinephrine) and noradrenaline (norepinephrine) stimulates adrenergic receptors of which there are two main types: alpha-adrenergic receptors and beta receptors. **Alpha-adrenergic receptors** are found on arteries throughout the body. When stimulated by adrenaline (epinephrine) alpha-adrenergic receptors cause the artery to constrict, placing pressure on the blood inside and resulting in elevated blood pressure or hypertension.[35,37]

Beta 1 receptors are found in heart muscle. As adrenaline (epinephrine) activates beta 1 receptors, the heart muscle contracts, causing the heart to beat harder and faster;[35,37] the heart rhythm is sinus tachycardia. **Beta 2 receptors** are found in the bronchioles of the lungs and the arteries of skeletal muscles. As adrenaline (epinephrine) stimulates the lung-based beta 2 receptors, the bronchioles dilate, allowing more air to flow in and out and increasing the breath rate;[35,38] rapid respirations are called tachypnoea. Adrenaline (epinephrine) also stimulates the skeletal muscle beta 2 receptors, causing the arteries to widen and allowing more blood to flow into the muscles, preparing the body to fight or flee.[35,37]

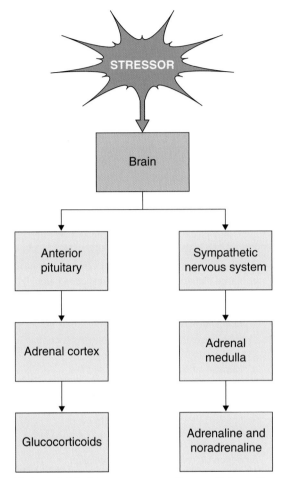

FIGURE 8.10 **Stress response.** (*Source:* Bellamy D, Pfister A. Plants, patients and people. Oxford: Blackwell; 1992.)

rate down. M3 receptors are located in the smooth muscle of bronchial tissue and cause constriction.[38] Ultimately, activation of the SAM axis is a self-limiting process whereby the sympathetic nervous system and the parasympathetic nervous system balance each other to restore homeostasis.

Hypothalamic-pituitary-adrenal axis

If an individual endures severe or prolonged pain, such as with a traumatic injury, the neuroendocrine component of the stress response will eventuate: the HPA axis.[32,39,40] The HPA axis is a cascade of interrelated hormonal events that assist the body to appropriately respond, then return to homeostasis.[39] Stimulation of the hypothalamus results in the release of corticotropin-releasing hormone (CRH), which binds to CRH receptors in the anterior pituitary gland. Stimulation of the anterior pituitary gland causes another hormone, adrenocorticotropic hormone (ACTH), to be released, which binds to receptors on the adrenal cortex, causing the release of cortisol (Fig. 8.10).[39–41] Cortisol's primary function is to facilitate the release of glucose into the bloodstream to provide a 'boost' of energy, preparing the muscles for fight or flight. Cortisol is also responsible for increasing blood pressure, reducing inflammation and suppressing memory.[41] Acquiring homeostasis post-pain event occurs through the fluidity of neurohormone and neurological activities as they work in unison, and at times in opposition, to minimise or cease the pain experience for the individual.

The chemical balancing act of the sympathetic nervous system and the parasympathetic nervous system has important implications for nurses in relation to pain assessment. Clinical observations of elevated blood pressure, rapid heart rate, fast breathing and skeletal guarding are short-lived and are not always reliable indicators that a person is in pain. The best indicator for pain assessment is to simply to ask, 'Do you have any pain?'

AGE-RELATED CHANGES

Pain perception across the life span alters with age. The human fetus is well equipped to feel pain from as early as seven weeks gestation. Cutaneous sensory receptors are present at seven weeks gestation and by full term exceed that of a full-grown adult.[42,43] Around 30 weeks gestation, A-delta and C fibres are established in the central nervous system, sending signals to the dermatomes.[42,43] A neonate exposed to multiple painful invasive procedures after birth will experience pain memory, resulting in altered pain perceptions later in life.[42,43]

Activation of the SAM axis explains why a person in acute pain will have elevated blood pressure, a rapid heart rate, fast breathing and skeletal guarding or agitation of the skeletal muscle. To counteract the agitated sympathetic nervous system in response to pain, the parasympathetic nervous system attempts to calm and soothe the nervous system through the inhibitory neurotransmitter, acetylcholine,[35] which binds to muscarinic receptors. There are five different types of muscarinic (M) receptors:[37,38] M1, M2, M3, M4 and M5, all having a different neurochemical response. M1, M4 and M5 receptors are located in the central nervous system and are responsible for memory, arousal, attention and analgesia. M2 receptors reside in the heart and reduce the contractions of the heart muscle, slowing the heart

This knowledge contradicts the once-popular belief that a human baby doesn't feel pain.

The other end of the age spectrum is no less controversial, where opposing viewpoints exist regarding the older adult's pain signalling and perception. Neurochemical deterioration and alterations in nociceptive processes in the older adult result in increased pain thresholds for non-noxious stimuli, decreased pain thresholds for pressure stimuli, with no change to thermal stimuli.[44] Contrasting evidence suggests that pain thresholds for thermal, ischaemic and mechanical stimuli decrease with age.[45] A decline in cognitive function and the presence of multiple comorbidities influence pain perception in the older adult, manifesting in specific pain behaviours.[45,46]

CONCLUSION

Pain is a complex neurophysiological event, originating in a basic awareness of impending or actual threat. This sense of threat initiates a cascade of interconnected, complementary and at times opposing neurobiological events that originate at the cellular level, interweaving neurohormones, neuromodulators and neurotransmitters and resulting in a mind–body awareness of pain. For scientists and health professionals alike, elements of the pain production system remain a mystery; yet certainty remains that the experience of pain will leave a long-lasting physical, emotional and cognitive imprint on the individual across their life span.

CASE STUDY 8.1

Samantha, a 14-year-old female, is skateboarding in the park with a group of friends. When the wheel of her skateboard hits a rock she is thrown to the ground with her arm outstretched. She hears a popping sound and feels a sharp pain shoot into her right shoulder, closely followed by a throbbing sensation. Samantha is the captain of the under-15 netball team and the semi-finals are being played tomorrow. She is worried that she won't be able to play.

Q1. How fast does A-delta fibre conduct the pain impulse?
  a. 10–20 m/s
  b. 5–40 m/s
  c. Less than 0.2 m/s
  d. Less than 2 m/s

Q2. Describe the characteristics of C fibre.
  a. Small diameter, unmyelinated, associated with dull, long-lasting aching pain
  b. Small diameter, myelinated, associated with dull, long-lasting aching pain

  c. Large diameter, myelinated, associated with sharp, long-lasting aching pain
  d. Large diameter, unmyelinated, associated with dull, short-lasting aching pain

Q3. C fibres travel through which areas of the central nervous system?
  a. Neospinothalamic and limbic system
  b. Spinoreticular and thalamus
  c. Paleospinothalamic and reticular formation
  d. Periaqueductal grey matter and neospinothalamic

Q4. Describe why Samantha feels a sharp pain sensation before the throbbing sensation.

Q5. Samantha is worried that she might not be able to play netball tomorrow. Using the pain pathways, describe where Samantha would have registered fear or worry at not being able to play netball.

CASE STUDY 8.2

Cooper, a 32-year-old male, is the manager of a busy bakery in the local shopping centre. The bakery has a large order to complete in addition to normal baking requirements. Cooper becomes distracted as a colleague calls out to him, resulting in the back of his hand brushing the hot oven tray. Feeling a sharp sensation across the back of his hand, followed by throbbing, Cooper rushes to the sink and runs his hand under cold water. Observing his hand Cooper notices that the skin is red with no signs of blistering.

His colleague asks if he is alright. Cooper gives a nod, pulls a glove over the burn and continues to work.

Q1. What group of nociceptors are activated in Cooper's injury?
  a. Mechanical and somatic nociceptors
  b. Somatic and thermal nociceptors
  c. Thermal and visceral nociceptors
  d. Thermal, mechanical and chemical nociceptors

CASE STUDY 8.2—cont'd

Q2. Which group of neurotransmitters is involved in inhibiting the pain impulse?

   a. Serotonin, noradrenaline (norepinephrine) and calcitonin gene-related peptide

   b. Bradykinins, noradrenaline (norepinephrine) and gamma aminobutyric acid (GABA)

   c. Endorphins, gamma aminobutyric acid (GABA) and encephalins

   d. Serotonin, glutamate and bradykinins

Q3. What systems are involved in the modulation of pain?

   a. Periaqueductal grey matter and neospinothalamic

   b. Spinoreticular and nucleus raphe magnus

   c. Neospinothalamic and paleospinothalamic

   d. Periaqueductal grey matter and nucleus raphe magnus

Q4. Cooper was able to modulate his pain. What is meant by the term 'pain modulation' and how does it occur?

Q5. Why was Cooper not alarmed by the pain he experienced? Explain this phenomenon using your understanding of the pain pathways.

CASE STUDY 8.3

Jane, an 81-year-old female, has fallen at home and fractured her right hip. She was taken to the emergency department for assessment and treatment. The emergency nurse, Anthony, has obtained a set of observations including blood pressure, heart rate and respiratory rate. He notices that Jane's blood pressure is 180/110 mmHg, her heart rate is 120 bpm and she has fast and shallow breathing at 22 rpm. When Anthony attempts to move Jane's right leg into a better position, Jane yells out and grabs her hip; she is visibly distressed.

Q1. Which receptor when activated is responsible for elevating the heart rate?

   a. Beta 1

   b. Muscarinic 2

   c. Beta 2

   d. Alpha adrenergic

Q2. Which part of the nervous system is primarily responsible for the rest-and-digest stress response?

   a. Sympathetic nervous system

   b. Peripheral nervous system

   c. Parasympathetic nervous system

   d. Somatic nervous system

Q3. Stimulation of the sympathetic nervous system will cause which of the following?

   a. Hypertension, bradycardia and tachypnoea

   b. Hypotension, bradypnoea and tachycardia

   c. Tachycardia, hypertension and bradypnoea

   d. Tachycardia, hypertension and tachypnoea

Q4. Jane has sustained a fractured right hip; why would her observations be elevated?

Q5. Why aren't elevated clinical observations the most reliable indicator of acute pain?

CASE STUDY 8.4

Jimmy and Makayla are 21-year-old fraternal twins. To celebrate their 21st birthday they decided to get identical tattoos on the back of their necks. Makayla already has a tattoo and was keen to get another. This was Jimmy's first tattoo and he was a bit anxious about the idea. Makayla suggested they find a tattoo parlour that can tattoo them at the same time, so she could offer support to her brother. They were lucky enough to find such a place, and the tattooist agreed to tattoo them simultaneously. Makayla hardly responded as the tattoo needle punctured her skin at 1000 pricks a minute, but Jimmy was pale, sweaty and grimacing throughout his experience. The tattooist asked Makayla and Jimmy to rate their pain, 0 being no pain and 10 being the worst pain they have experienced. Makayla scored her pain 2 out of 10 while Jimmy rated his pain 8 out of 10.

Continued

CASE STUDY 8.4—cont'd

Q1. Thermal and mechanical stimuli travel into lamina I via which group of nerve fibres?
  a. Cutaneous and visceral C, A-delta and A-beta fibres
  b. A-delta and A-beta fibres
  c. Cutaneous and visceral C fibres
  d. Cutaneous C, A-delta and A-beta fibres

Q2. Which part of Jimmy's brain alerted him to sense fear at getting a tattoo?
  a. Somatosensory cortex
  b. Limbic centre
  c. Dorsal horn
  d. Reticular system

Q3. Which group of neurotransmitters are excitatory and assist in pain transmission?
  a. Glutamate, substance P and calcitonin gene-related peptide
  b. Nitrous oxide, encephalin and calcitonin gene-related peptide
  c. Endorphin, substance P and glutamate
  d. Gamma aminobutyric acid (GABA), encephalin and substance P

Q4. Using your understanding of pain transmission, describe how the pain impulse travels from the peripheral nervous system into the central nervous system.

Q5. How can twins who have endured the same pain sensation (tattooing), at the same time, and in the same body location, experience different levels of pain?

REFERENCES

1. Melzack R, Wall PD. Pain mechanisms: a new theory. Science 1965;150(3699):971–9.
2. Katz J, Melzack R. A conceptual framework for understanding pain in the human. In: Waldman SD, editor. Pain management. 2nd ed. Philadelphia: Saunders; 2011. p. 2–9.
3. Chamley C. Pain management. In: Brooker C, Nicol M, editors. Alexander's nursing practice, 4 ed. London: Churchill Livingstone; 2011. p. 551–74.
4. Cooney MF. Nursing management of patients with pain, seizures, and CNS infections. In: Hickey J, editor. Clinical practice of neurological and neurosurgical nursing, 7 ed. Philadelphia: Lippincott Williams & Wilkins; 2014. p. 623–32.
5. Melzack R. Pain and the neuromatrix in the brain. J Dent Educ 2001;65(12):1378–82.
6. Stanos SP, Tyburski MD, Harden RN. Chronic pain. In: Cifu DX, editor. Braddom's physical medicine and rehabilitation, 5 ed. Philadelphia: Elsevier; 2016. p. 809–33.
7. Butler DS, Moseley LG. Explain pain, 2 ed. Adelaide: Noigroup Publications; 2013.
8. Merskey H, Bogduk N, IASP Task Force on Taxonomy, editors. Part III: pain terms, a current list with definitions and notes on usage. In: Classification of chronic pain, 2 ed. Seattle: IASP Press; 1994. p. 209–14.
9. Ringkamp M, Dougherty PM, Raja SN. Anatomy and physiology of the pain signalling process. In: Benzon HT, Raja SN, Fishman SM, et al, editors. Essentials of pain medicine, 4 ed. Philadelphia: Elsevier; 2018. p. 3–10.
10. Bourne S, Machado AG, Nagel SJ. Basic anatomy and physiology of pain pathways. Neurosurg Clin N Am 2014; 25(4):629–38.
11. Miner JR, Burton JH. Pain management. In: Walls RM, Hockberger RS, Gausche-Hill M, editors. Rosen's emergency medicine: concepts and clinical practice, vol. 1, 9 ed. Amsterdam: Elsevier; 2018. p. 34–51.
12. Dinakar P. Principles of pain management. In: Daroff RB, Jankvic J, Mazziotta JC, et al, editors. Bradley's neurology in clinical practice, 7 ed. London: Elsevier; 2016. p. 720–41.
13. Sikandar S, Dickenson AH. Visceral pain: the ins and outs, the ups and downs. Curr Opin Support Palliat Care 2012;6(1):17–26.
14. Montgomery R, Mallick-Searle T, Peltier CH, et al. Physiology of pain. In: Czarnecki ML, Turner HN, editors. Core curriculum for pain management nursing: American Society for Pain Management Nursing, 3 ed. St Louis: Elsevier; 2018. p. 132–69.
15. Barrett KE, Barman SM, Boitano S, et al. Ganong's review of medical physiology, 25 ed. Sydney: McGraw-Hill; 2016.
16. Solomon EP. Introduction to human anatomy and physiology, 4 ed. St Louis: Saunders; 2016.
17. Hall JE. Guyton and Hall textbook of medical physiology, 13 ed. Philadelphia: Elsevier; 2016.
18. Patton KT, Thibodeau GA. Anatomy and physiology, 9 ed. St Louis: Elsevier; 2016.
19. Mattscheck D, Law AS, Nixdorf DR. Diagnosis of nonodontogenic toothache. In: Hargreaves K, Berman LH, editors. Cohen's pathways of the pulp, 11 ed. St Louis: Elsevier; 2016. p. 684–705.
20. Patel NB. Physiology of pain (internet). In: Kopf A, Patel NB, editors. Guide to pain management in low-resource settings. International Association for the Study of Pain; 2014.

21. Nouri KH, Osugwa U, Boyette-Davis J, et al. Neurochemistry of somatosensory and pain processing. In: Benzon HT, Raja SN, Fishman SM, et al, editors. Essentials of pain medicine, 4 ed. Philadelphia: Elsevier; 2018. p. 11–20.
22. Cooper PE, Van Uum SH. Neuroendocrinology. In: Daroff RB, Jankvic J, Mazziotta JC, et al, editors. Bradley's neurology in clinical practice, 7 ed. London: Elsevier; 2016. p. 696–712.
23. Flor H, Turk DC. Chronic pain: an integrated biobehavioral approach. Seattle: IASP Press; 2011.
24. Lord B, Ramsden C. Pain management. In: Curtis K, Ramsden C, editors. Emergency and trauma care for nurses and paramedics, 2 ed. Sydney: Elsevier; 2016. p. 696–712.
25. Todd AJ, Koerber HR. Neuroanatomical substrates of spinal nociception. In: McMahon SB, Koltzenburg M, Tracey I, et al, editors. Wall & Melzack's textbook of pain, 6 ed. Philadelphia: Elsevier; 2013. p. 77–93.
26. Steeds C. The anatomy and physiology of pain. Surgery 2016;34(2):55–9.
27. Chiaramonte D, Adamo CD, Morrison B. Integrative approaches to pain management. In: Honorio BT, Rathmell JP, Wu CL, et al, editors. Practical management of pain, 5 ed. Philadelphia: Mosby; 2014. p. 658–68.
28. Heinricher MM, Cleary DR. Anatomy and physiology of pain. In: Winn RH, editor. Youmans & Winn neurological surgery, 7 ed. Philadelphia: Elsevier; 2017. p. 593–604.
29. Kirkpatrick DR, McEntire DM, Hambsch ZJ, et al. Therapeutic basis of clinical pain modulation. Clin Transl Sci 2015;8(6):848–56.
30. Westlund KN. Pain pathways: peripheral, spinal, ascending, and descending pathways. In: Honorio BT, Rathmell JP, Wu CL, et al, editors. Practical management of pain, 5 ed. Philadelphia: Mosby Elsevier; 2014. p. 87–98.
31. Geva N, Defrin R. Opposite effects of stress on pain modulation depend on the magnitude of individual stress response. J Pain 2018;19(4):360–71.
32. Hoeger Bement M, Weyer A, Keller M, et al. Anxiety and stress can predict pain perception following cognitive stress. Physiol Behav 2010;101(1):87–92.
33. Butler DS, Moseley LG. Explain pain, 2 ed. Adelaide: Noigroup Publications; 2013.
34. Everly GS, Lating JM. A clinical guide to the treatment of the human stress response, 3 ed. New York: Springer; 2013.
35. Constanzo LS. Physiology, 6 ed. Philadelphia: Elsevier; 2018.
36. Glick DB. The autonomic nervous system. In: Miller RD, editor. Miller's anaesthesia, 8 ed. Philadelphia: Elsevier; 2014. p. 346–86.
37. Ritter JM, Flower RJ, Henderson G, et al. Rang and Dale's pharmacology, 9 ed. Philadelphia: Elsevier; 2019.
38. Kramer IM. Signal transduction. Philadelphia: Elsevier; 2016.
39. Drossman DA. Biopsychosocial issues in gastroenterology. In: Feldman M, Friedman LS, Brandt LJ, editors. Sleisenger and Fordtran's gastrointestinal and liver disease, 10 ed. Philadelphia: Saunders; 2016. p. 349–62.
40. Stephens MA, Wand G. Stress and the HPA axis: role of glucocorticoids in alcohol dependence. Alcohol Res 2012;34(4):468–83.
41. Owusu MB, Chaukos DC, Park ER, et al. Mind-body medicine. In: Stern TA, Freudenreich O, Smith FA, et al, editors. Massachusetts General Hospital handbook of general hospital psychiatry, 7 ed. Philadelphia: Saunders; 2018. p. 455–60.
42. Soens M, Tsen LC. Fetal physiology. In: Chestnut D, Wong C, Tsen LC, et al, editors. Chestnut's obstetric anesthesia: principles and practice, 5 ed. Philadelphia: Saunders; 2014. p. 75–91.
43. Ranger M, Beggs S, Grunau RE. Developmental aspects of pain. In: Polin RA, Abman SH, Rowitch DH, et al, editors. Fetal and neonatal physiology, 5 ed. Philadelphia: Elsevier; 2017. p. 1390–5.
44. Hayek S, Sondhi N. Pain in the older patient. In: Argoff CE, Dubin A, Pilitsis JG, editors. Pain management secrets, 4 ed. Philadelphia: Elsevier; 2018. p. 188–95.
45. Bruckenthal P. Pain in the older adult. In: Fillit HM, Rockwood K, Young J, editors. Brocklehurst's textbook of geriatric medicine and gerontology, 8 ed. Philadelphia: Elsevier; 2017. p. 932–8.
46. Malmstrom TK, Tait RC. Pain assessment and management in older adults. In: Lichtenberg PA, editor. Handbook of assessment in clinical gerontology, 2 ed. Philadelphia: Elsevier; 2010. p. 647–77.

CHAPTER 9

Special senses: hearing, balance and vision

BRYONY A NAYAGAM, BSC (HONS), PHD • DAVID AX NAYAGAM, BSC/BE (ELECENG) (HONS), PHD

KEY POINTS/LEARNING OUTCOMES

1. Describe the different roles of the outer/middle/inner ear in the perception of sound.
2. Explain why the middle ear is important for sound conduction and the key features that enable it to do so.
3. Articulate the critical role of the inner ear hair cells in generating electrical signals that the brain can interpret into sound and position in space.
4. Discuss how the vestibular apparatus extracts information about position in space from head rotations in different planes.
5. Describe the gross anatomical structure of the eye, the basic optics of the eye and how these relate to vision.
6. Explain the basic neural mechanisms underlying the transduction of light energy into neural impulses that lead to our perception of vision.

KEY DEFINITIONS

- **Cornea:** the transparent layer forming the outermost surface of the eye.
- **External auditory canal** (i.e. the ear canal): the canal linking the outer and middle ear, which extends inwards from the pinna.
- **Fovea:** a small depression in the retina of the eye where visual acuity is at its highest.
- **Iris:** a flat, coloured, rounded membrane that lies behind the cornea of the eye; the iris has an adjustable circular opening (called the pupil) at its centre.
- **Lens:** the transparent elastic structure situated behind the iris of the eye that causes light to be focused onto the retina.
- **Middle ear:** the air-filled space between the outer and inner ear, which includes the tympanic membrane and the three auditory ossicles.
- **Ossicles:** the three smallest bones in the body, located in the middle ear space—the malleus, incus and stapes.
- **Photoreceptor:** a specialised sensory cell that is responsive to photons of light.
- **Pinna:** the external part of the ear, alternatively referred to as the auricle.
- **Retina:** a layer at the back of the eyeball that contains cells sensitive to light: these specialised cells trigger nerve impulses that pass via the optic nerve to the brain, where a visual image is formed.
- **Tympanic membrane:** the eardrum.

ONLINE RESOURCES/SUGGESTED READINGS

- **Auditory neuroscience** available at https://auditoryneuroscience.com—contains excellent videos of major concepts of auditory anatomy and physiology
- **Auditory transduction** available at www.youtube.com/watch?v=PeTriGTENoc

INTRODUCTION TO THE EAR

Take a moment to close your eyes and pay attention to the sound of the world around you. What can you hear when you are actively listening without visual input? It is impressive how much information you can gather and perceive in just a short space of time. Our ability to hear a variety of different sounds helps us to navigate our surroundings, thrive in our environment and, perhaps most importantly, underpins our ability to verbally communicate with one another. In addition, our inner ear contains another important and highly specialised sensory organ, the vestibular apparatus, which is responsible for our sense of balance, motion and position in space. Our sense of hearing and balance are integral to

our human experience and survival, and yet we often take these senses for granted until they malfunction. This chapter provides a basic introduction to the way sound and balance are encoded by the inner ear, thereby laying the foundation for the study of more complicated central auditory and vestibular processing, as relevant to the individual student.

The structure and function of the ear

In the simplest sense, we can think of the ear as having both a peripheral and a central component. The peripheral component comprises the outer ear, middle ear and inner ear (Fig. 9.1) and is critical for capturing, enhancing, decoding and sending sound and balance

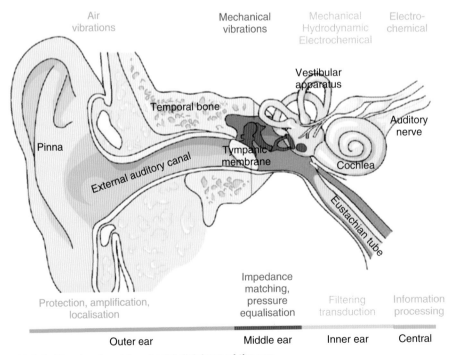

FIGURE 9.1 **Structural and functional divisions of the ear.**

information to the central component, which includes both the brain stem and the brain. The brain comprises several central processing stations where acoustic stimuli are carefully analysed, processed and re-integrated with other modalities before being perceived as sound. The external, middle and inner ear have defined and important roles in the processing of sound (external, middle and inner ear) or spatial orientation (inner ear).

The **outer ear** consists of the **pinna** and **external auditory canal**. The paired pinnae are composed of skin-covered flexible cartilage and are a common site of a variety of piercings. Unlike the pinnae of some animals (e.g. cats and dogs) the human pinnae have a fixed position on either side of the head. Approximately in the centre of each pinna is a small opening—the opening of the external auditory canal—which runs inwards ~3 cm and terminates on a very thin membrane known as the eardrum or, more correctly, the **tympanic membrane**. The outer ear can be thought of as a horizontal funnel whose primary function is to gather sound waves from our external environment and concentrate them onto the surface of the tympanic membrane.

The **middle ear** is an air-filled space between the tympanic membrane and the bony inner ear and includes the tympanic membrane and the three smallest bones in the body: the **incus**, **malleus** and **stapes** (Fig. 9.2). You may already know these bones by their common names: hammer, anvil and stirrup, respectively. The three middle ear bones are collectively termed the **auditory ossicles** and join the outer ear to the inner ear. The ossicles are interconnected to one another and to the middle ear space by a number of specialised ligaments, therefore allowing a small degree of flexibility for the transfer of vibrational sound pressure waves to the inner ear. The air-filled middle ear maintains a pressure equilibrium with the external atmosphere via the **eustachian tube**. This narrow tube connects the middle ear to the nasopharynx (the back of the throat) and runs at approximately a 45° angle. This facilitates easy drainage into the throat, and keeps the middle ear free of any fluid. The eustachian tube is closed at rest but opens to accommodate external air pressure changes. It can also be encouraged to open voluntarily by swallowing, chewing or yawning.

The **inner ear** contains an intricate labyrinth of continuous fluid-filled tubes with highly specialised sensory cells (hair cells) responsible for providing the brain with critical information regarding both sound and motion. The sensory information encoded by the inner ear is subsequently sent to the brain via the VIIIth cranial nerve, the vestibulocochlear nerve. The inner ear has a bony exterior surface, within which there reside two separate fluid-filled tubes. The outermost tube is the **bony labyrinth**, while the innermost tube is the

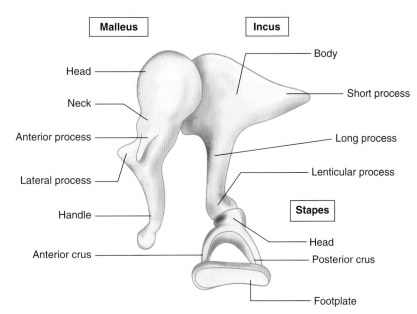

FIGURE 9.2 **Middle ear bones.** (Dhingra. Diseases of ear, nose and throat, 5 ed. Copyright © 2010 Elsevier. All rights reserved.)

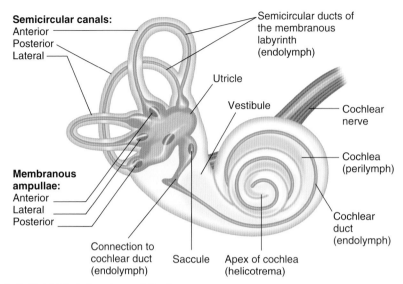

Semicircular canals:
Anterior
Posterior
Lateral

Semicircular ducts of
the membranous
labyrinth
(endolymph)

Utricle

Vestibule

Cochlear
nerve

Cochlea
(perilymph)

**Membranous
ampullae:**
Anterior
Lateral
Posterior

Cochlear
duct
(endolymph)

Connection to
cochlear duct
(endolymph)

Saccule

Apex of cochlea
(helicotrema)

FIGURE 9.3 **Fluid-filled chambers of the inner ear.**

membranous labyrinth (Fig. 9.3). The two fluids that fill these tubes are termed **perilymph** and **endolymph** and are quite different in their chemical composition. Both fluid-filled tubes are sealed from one another so that there is no mixing of the fluids. In addition, endolymph has a positive electrochemical charge of ~80 mV and is rich in potassium ions in comparison with perilymph, which is similar in composition to cerebrospinal fluid and has a resting potential of ~0 mV. The difference in electrochemical charge within endolymph is critical for the generation of nerve impulses in the inner ear.

The sensory receptors, the inner ear hair cells, reside within the endolymphatic compartments of the inner ear. They are so named for the numerous hair-like projections (called stereocilia) on their top (apical) surface. As you might imagine, these tiny hairs are very sensitive to the smallest movements of the fluid surrounding them. In the cochlea, fluid movement is produced by sound-induced mechanical vibrations from the middle ear, where the stapes ultimately causes fluid waves to be generated in the cochlea. In the vestibular system, fluid moves relative to the direction in which the head moves, thus causing movement of the hairs in the same plane.

Key functions of the outer ear
In addition to its important role in concentrating sound pressure waves onto the tympanic membrane, the outer ear serves three other key roles in hearing: protection, amplification and localisation. The long, narrow and winding external auditory canal provides protection to the more delicate structures of the middle ear and inner ear. The outer (flexible, cartilaginous) portion of the canal is lined with both lubricating (sebaceous) and wax (ceruminous) glands. The lubricating glands keep the surface of the skin from drying and cracking, thereby protecting it from invasion by microbes. The wax produced by the ceruminous glands provides a natural insecticide and in concert with the tiny hairs lining the canal that are oriented outwards, assists in trapping foreign particles and waterproofing the opening.

The funnel-like structure of the outer ear is such that its resonance properties cause a boost in sound pressure levels within the range of human speech, ~250–4000 Hz. Deformities in the anatomy of the outer ear, or indeed the auditory canal, understandably cause a reduction in the intensity of sound transmitted through the middle ear and into the cochlea. While it is ultimately neural mechanisms in the brain stem that enable the precise localisation of sound, the outer ear plays a key role in the unhindered transmission of sound signals from the environment to the brain. For instance, the way in which sound reflects off the pinna and into the external auditory canal provides the brain with critical information that enables the very precise location of sounds in the vertical plane (i.e. when sound arrives from directly in front of you, but from above or below your nose). In addition, the arrival of sound at one ear before the other—the **interaural timing difference**—provides information to the brain as to where in the horizontal plane the sound is being generated. This phenomenon works best when

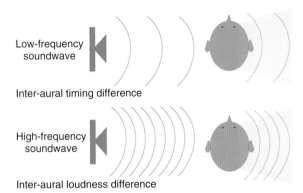

Low-frequency soundwave

Inter-aural timing difference

High-frequency soundwave

Inter-aural loudness difference

FIGURE 9.4 **Inter-aural timing and loudness differences.**

considered in terms of low-frequency sounds, which are comprised of larger, broader sound pressure waves that take longer to bend around the head. Similarly, while there is only a small difference between the ears in the arrival of high-frequency sounds, they lose some intensity (loudness) as they refract around the head. This is called the **interaural loudness difference** and it gives the brain important information as to where higher frequency sound is located in the horizontal plane. As environmental sound is not typically comprised of pure high and low tones, these circuits work simultaneously in order to give very precise localisation of sound in space (Fig. 9.4).

Middle ear physiology

Sounds are vibrations that travel through the air as fluctuating pressure waves. A vibrating sound source compresses the surrounding air molecules and then pulls them apart again, generating a regular wave of more and less compressed air. Sound can also travel as vibrations through liquids and solids. When sound pressure waves strike the eardrum they cause it to vibrate; **high-pitch sounds** (or **high-frequency sounds**) vibrate the eardrum more rapidly than **low-pitch sounds** (or **low-frequency sounds**). Louder sounds cause the eardrum to vibrate with greater intensity than softer sounds. Since the malleus is connected to the eardrum, sound pressure waves are directly relayed through the air-filled middle ear space to the fluid-filled inner ear. Impressively, the middle ear amplifies the force delivered to the inner ear using a system of leverage and decreasing surface area. The most significant increase in pressure delivered to the inner ear is caused by the transfer of vibrations from the eardrum to the stapes footplate, which is approximately 17 times smaller than the eardrum in its surface area. The amplification of sound

pressure waves by the middle ear is great enough to generate waves within the fluid of the inner ear, which the cochlea is then able to transduce into nerve impulses that can be processed by the brain.

The inner ear

The inner ear is embedded within the temporal bone of the skull and contains both the snail-shaped **cochlea** (the organ of hearing) and the semicircular hoops that comprise the **vestibular apparatus** (the organ of balance). Each organ contains thousands of specialised sensory receptors (hair cells) located within the fluid-filled chambers of the inner ear. It is these specialised hair cells that are uniquely able to provide the brain with a dynamic range of sensory information relating to both sound and position in space.

Cochlea. The cochlea is two and a half circular turns and has a length of approximately 33 mm from base to apex, but it is perhaps easier to understand as an unrolled long, straight tube (Fig. 9.5). In doing so, it is easier to appreciate several key anatomical features including the fluid vibration generated by the stapes, the arrangement of the fluid-filled compartments, the location of the sensory receptors and the way in which a fluid pressure wave is generated by the stapes.

Let us first consider the two membrane-covered openings to the cochlea—these are termed the oval window and the round window, and they are adjacent to one another in the base of the cochlea. The stapes is fused directly to the round window membrane and works in a piston-like manner to establish waves of fluid within the membranous cochlear duct. The stapes is only able to transfer middle ear vibrations due to the presence of a second flexible membrane in the base, the round window, which essentially absorbs the waves generated by the stapes. These two membranes work in opposition to one another such that when the stapes pushes inwards on the oval window, the round window membrane flexes outwards, and vice versa.

Next, let us examine the overall structure of the cochlea in this uncoiled view (Fig. 9.5). In this view, there are three fluid-filled compartments. The outermost compartments situated at the top and bottom are continuous with one another and contain the same fluid, endolymph, as described above. The innermost fluid-filled compartment is the **cochlear duct** and it contains potassium-rich endolymph. These compartments are anatomically termed the **scala vestibuli**, **scala media** and **scala tympani**. The scala vestibuli and scala media are separated by the very thin **Reissner's membrane**, while the scala tympani and scala media are separated by

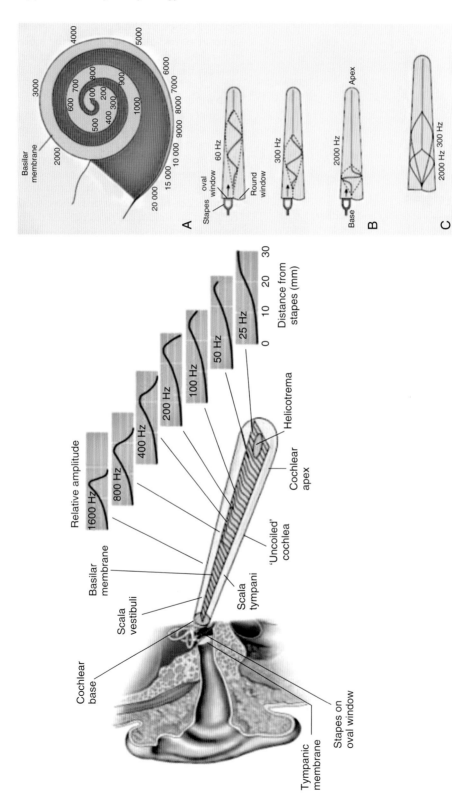

FIGURE 9.5 **Travelling wave and tonotopic organisation of the cochlea.** (*Source:* https://physics.stackexchange.com/questions/174082/physics-of-how-the-cochlea-isolates-frequencies-along-its-length/176069; www.open.edu/openlearn/science-maths-technology/science/biology/hearing/content-section-3.3)

the **basilar membrane**. The basilar membrane is highly specialised and on this membrane sit the sensory hair cells, which ultimately convert sound from a mechanical to an electrical signal that the brain can interpret.

A key feature to recognise and understand in the study of cochlear anatomy and physiology is the variable resonance properties of the basilar membrane. Variable resonance means that the membrane moves (resonates) maximally at different locations, based on the frequency of the sound vibrations received and transmitted through the vibration of the stapes. For instance, high-frequency sounds cause maximal displacement of the basilar membrane at the base of the cochlea, but sequentially lower sound frequencies cause maximal displacement at progressively more apical sites. The key features of the basilar membrane that facilitate these different resonance properties are its variable width, tension and weight. In this sense, it can be helpful to think about the properties of string instruments. What do you notice about the high-sounding strings in comparison with the low-sounding strings? High-pitched strings are narrow, tight and lighter than low-pitched strings, which are wide, loose and heavy. The same principles hold for the basilar membrane and are key in understanding its ability to separate complex sound into its component frequencies.

These anatomical features of the basilar membrane mean that different patterns of movement are produced within the cochlea in response to different sounds. If we were able to visualise the basilar membrane vibrating in response to a pure tone of ~20 000 Hz, we would observe maximal displacement towards the base of the cochlea and a discrete travelling wave of movement (Fig. 9.5). Alternatively, if we were to visualise a much lower frequency pure tone of ~200 Hz, we would see maximal displacement of the basilar membrane in the apex of the cochlea and a much broader travelling wave. Of course, it is important to remember that we do not hear speech in pure tones and most environmental sound is considered 'complex' with a number of regions of maximal displacement generated at any given time. So what we hear depends on the pattern of basilar membrane vibration produced in response to different sounds. Through experience, we learn to understand these different patterns of movement, attributing individual meanings to each. Considering the above, think about how the movement of the basilar membrane would look different under the following conditions: a pure tone, simple speech sounds, an orchestral piece of classical music.

Arguably the most critical cells underpinning our ability to hear and sense motion are the inner ear hair cells. Located in the endolymphatic compartments of the inner ear, it is these sensory receptors that convert sound or balance (travelling as a mechanical fluid wave) into an electrical signal that is sent to the brain. In the cochlea, the hair cells are located on top of the basilar membrane and therefore different populations of hair cells are activated by sounds of different frequencies. Hair cells are known as **mechano-electrical transducers**, which in the simplest terms refers to their ability to turn a sound from a mechanical signal into an electrical signal. They do this using the tiny 'hairs' (stereocilia) on their most apical surface. The stereocilia are interconnected by several mechanical channels (**mechano-electrical transduction [MET] channels**), which open and close in response to mechanical movement.

As a result of the fluid wave generated by the stapes, the hair cell MET channels open and close at frequency-specific sites along the basilar membrane. As the stereocilia are deflected in an outward motion, the MET channels are pulled open; when they are deflected inwards, the channels close. It may be helpful to visualise these channels as miniature trap doors that open and close as the basilar membrane vibrates. Recall that higher frequency sounds will cause maximal displacement of the cochlear base and that lower frequency sounds cause maximal displacement in the cochlear apex. As the MET channels open they allow potassium ions to enter the hair cells via diffusion (recall that endolymph is positively charged ~80 mV with a high concentration of potassium ions). Entry of enough potassium ions into the hair cells ultimately causes the release of neurotransmitter at the base of the hair cells. Neurotransmitter is a chemical messenger that causes the generation of an action potential in the nerve fibre attached to that hair cell. The location, timing and rate at which neurotransmitter is released from hair cells cause the activation of different populations of nerve fibres, at different periods and intensities. This code of frequency, timing and rate of nerve firing is what the brain uses to perceive and interpret the incoming sound.

Vestibular apparatus. The vestibular apparatus is commonly known as the organ of balance and it provides our brain with critical information for survival, including general motion, the position of our head and the spatial orientation of our body during movement. It consists of three interconnected hoops in the left and right inner ear (six in total) termed the **semicircular canals**. The three canals lie in the directional planes in which the head can rotate—for example, nodding up and down (as if to say 'yes'), shaking your head from side to side (as if to say 'no') or lateral bending/tilting movements

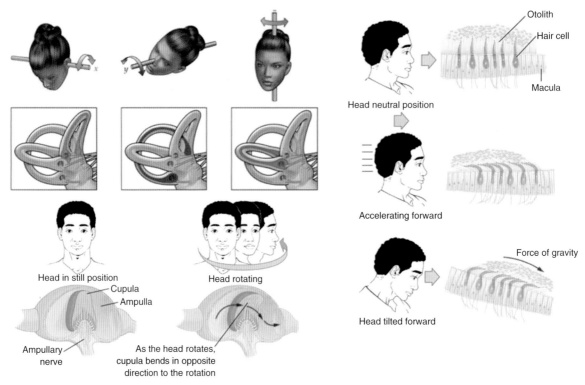

FIGURE 9.6 **Motion detection by the vestibular apparatus.** (*Source:* www.illinoisscience.
org/2018/03/how-your-ears-keep-you-balanced)

(imagine trying to touch your ear to your shoulder). The three canals are conveniently named based on their anatomical position in the inner ear: anterior, posterior and lateral. The canals are filled with endolymph; this endolymph is continuous with the cochlear endolymphatic fluid and is the reason that some rare diseases, such as Ménière's disease, can affect both hearing and balance.

As the head moves, it causes the fluid within the semicircular canals to move in a direction that corresponds to the plane of head movement. The motion of vestibular fluid is detected at the end of each canal in a region known as the **ampulla**. Consistent with the organ of hearing, each ampulla contains many hair cells with stereocilia projecting from their top surface. It is these hair cells that detect directional fluid movement and generate corresponding neural impulses (action potentials), which the brain learns through experience to interpret as various head movements/positions in space. Fig. 9.6 illustrates the directional flow of endolymph in the semicircular canals as a result of directional movement of the head. The generation of action potentials in the respective

branches of the vestibulocochlear nerve facilitate this information transfer.

The vestibular apparatus contains two further sensory structures called the **otolith organs**, which are located adjacent to the three semicircular canals. The otoliths, which specifically detect acceleration, comprise the **utricle** and the **saccule**. While it is the utricle that detects acceleration in the horizontal plane, the saccule detects acceleration in the vertical plane. The otoliths also contain sensory hair cells and are distinguished from other parts of the inner ear by the specialised calcium carbonate crystals (**otoconia**) situated near the apical surface of the hair cell stereocilia. These crystals move in response to variations in acceleration, causing the underlying hair cell stereocilia to move, and thereby generating nerve impulses specific to this directional acceleration. The vestibular apparatus is well developed to detect acceleration of the head in many directions, yet it is important to note that on its own the vestibular apparatus cannot sense velocity. With experience, and in a coordinated manner with the visual system, an approximation of velocity can be achieved. In the next section we examine the special sense of vision and the connections it shares with the inner ear.

INTRODUCTION TO THE EYE

It is said that the eyes are the windows to the soul. However, they could just as easily be described as the windows to our mind. For indeed, the delicate and specialised organ within the eye, known as the **retina**, is part of the central nervous system and provides neuroscientists with an accessible and useful insight into the mechanisms that underpin the transfer of information within the neural circuits of the brain. In the following paragraphs, we examine the specialised anatomy and physiology of the visual system that informs the way we see and perceive the world around us.

Structure and function of the eye

The eye is a highly specialised light-sensitive organ found in various classes of animals including humans. By absorbing light energy from environmentally derived incident photons, specialised cells and mechanisms within the eye extract and process relevant information about the organism's surroundings. This information is converted into electrochemical signals and rapidly conveyed to the brain, in the form of a complex neural code, for further processing—ultimately leading to the perception of vision.

Humans possess two eyes that work in concert to provide visual information and redundancy. They are located within pits in the bony skull and are oriented such that they face forwards in an arrangement typical of mammalian predators. Human eyes are often imagined to be spherical (i.e. an eyeball), but on close inspection their gross anatomy actually resembles two unequally sized spheroids concatenated and aligned roughly along an anterior–posterior axis. These structures are known as the anterior and posterior segments of the eye and they are filled with fluid—known respectively as **aqueous humour** (a thin watery fluid) and **vitreous humour** (a viscous protein-filled jelly-like material).

Cross-sectionally, the eye can be divided into three distinct layers (Fig. 9.7). The tough outermost layer, the fibrous tunic, consists of the white sclera, which forms the collagenous shell of the posterior segment. At the front of the anterior segment, continuous with the sclera, is the tough yet optically transparent outer cornea, which is where light first enters the eye. The middle layer, the vascular tunic (or uvea), includes the posterior segment's choroid (a rich meshwork of blood vessels) and retinal pigmented epithelium as well as the anterior segment's ciliary body, iris and lens (described in more detail

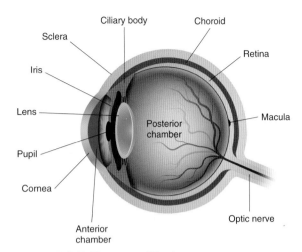

FIGURE 9.7 **Structure of the human eye.**

below). The inner layer is the retina—the complex and delicate neural tissue that provides the core visual functionality. The retina is nourished by the choroidal vessels as well as its own dedicated retinal vasculature. The entire eye (anterior and posterior segments combined) has an approximate diameter of 24–25 mm and is slightly longer in the anterior to posterior direction than it is in the vertical direction. It has a volume of ~6 cm^3 and a mass of ~6.5 g. It reaches full size by approximately 12–14 years of age in both males and females, although it is already at approximately 90% of this maximum size by age three.

Within the smaller anterior chamber is a thin mechanical structure with a central opening known as the **iris**, which acts as an optical diaphragm and opens (dilates) or closes (contracts) via activation of radial (dilator) or circumferential (sphincter) muscles attached to the multifunctional ciliary body to control the amount of light that passes through. The hole encircled by the iris is known as the **pupil** and it is the optical equivalent of the aperture of a single-lens reflex (SLR) camera. As well as controlling the light entering the eye, it also reduces spherical aberration that would otherwise occur around the periphery of the projected image and adjusts the optical depth of field in the same way as setting the f-stop on an SLR camera. Pigmentation found in the posterior layer of the iris absorbs light, allowing entry only via the pupil. It also determines eye colouring, with darker pigment probably evolving in more tropical locales to block the more intense ambient sunlight. For those students with an interest in photography, the human eye has a range of f-ratios (focal length divided by aperture) between approximately 2.3 and 8.2.

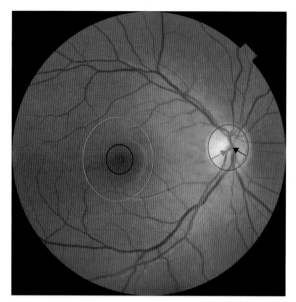

FIGURE 9.8 **Normal eye viewed through the pupil (fundus photograph) showing the central macula (green circle), fovea (black circle), central retinal artery (black arrow), central retinal vein (green arrow) and optic disc (blue circle).** (*Source:* Modified from Standring S. Gray's anatomy: the anatomical basis of clinical practice. Elsevier; 2016.)

At the posterior extent of the anterior chamber is the **lens**, fixed in position by suspensory ligaments known as the zonule of Zinn, which consist of many strands of fibres connecting the lens to the ciliary muscles. These work together to provide actuation of the lens—causing it to flatten and elongate (accommodate), thereby modulating its refractive properties to enable a variety of focal distances.

The posterior segment makes up over 80% of the volume of the eye. The key structures encapsulating the posterior chamber are the **choroid** and of course the multi-layered retina (which we cover in greater detail below). The central processes of the retina's final output cells come together in a bundle at the optic disc and form the optic nerve, which transmits information to the visual cortex via a number of preprocessing nuclei known as the **central optic pathway**. Blood vessels also enter the eye through the same port as the optic nerve and branch off to supply the inner layers of the retina with oxygen and nutrients. The outer layers of the retina receive their blood supply from the choroidal network of vessels (Fig. 9.8).

The field of view provided by a single eye (monocular vision) in the horizontal plane is roughly 95° temporal (towards the side of your head) and 60° nasal (towards your midline). It is occluded centrally by the nose and superiorly by the brow. The angles of incidence are enhanced by the refraction of light through the cornea and aqueous humour such that light may enter the pupil even at a right angle. The field of view is also increased because of the fact that both eyes work and move together to create what we call binocular vision. The typical binocular field of view in the horizontal plane, when looking straight ahead, is roughly 190° (Fig. 9.9). However, the entire eyeball is also actuated by a number of cleverly positioned extraocular muscles to shift the field of view. These muscles, known as the superior, inferior, lateral, medial and oblique rectus muscles, provide conscious and unconscious directional adjustments in azimuth and elevation planes as well as

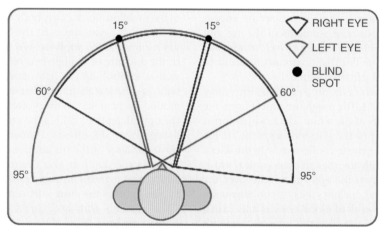

FIGURE 9.9 **Normal field of vision in the horizontal plane for both eyes.** (*Source:* www.vision-and-eye-health.com/visual-field.html)

some rotation around an axis orthogonal to the surface of the eye at the centre of the pupil.

Several associated structures surround and fringe the eyeball, including the conjunctiva, eye lids, lacrimal and sebaceous ducts and glands, eyelashes and brows. These assist in stabilising and protecting the delicate external optics and other internal structures of the eye from environmental hazards; they are not discussed further in this chapter.

Structure of the retina

The retina is a sensory organ that is responsible for transducing energy from light in the form of photons to electrochemical impulses that propagate through the optic nerve and visual pathway to the brain. It is delicate, resembling half a millimetre-thick wet tissue paper, and can easily be torn or damaged. Wrapping around the internal walls of the eye's posterior chamber, the retina comprises multiple layers with distinct cellular anatomy and physiology. Looking at a radial section of the retina, various cell types are co-located in layers that reflect stages of processing of visual information (Fig. 9.10). Proceeding from the choroid towards the

vitreous humour, these layers are as follows: Bruch's membrane (BM; the innermost layer of the choroid); retinal pigmented epithelium (RPE); photoreceptor (rod and cone) outer segments (OS); photoreceptor (rod and cone) inner segments (IS); external limiting membrane (ELM); outer nuclear layer (ONL); outer plexiform layer (OPL); inner nuclear layer (INL); inner plexiform layer (IPL); ganglion cell layer (GCL); and nerve fibre layer (NFL).

Note that the rod and cone photoreceptors are located at the posterior of the retina, meaning that incident photons must traverse the other retinal layers before striking the photoreceptors. This may seem like a counterintuitive arrangement; however, evolution has positioned the highly metabolically active photoreceptors in close proximity to the oxygen- and nutrient-rich choroidal network. As an aside, some animals, particularly nocturnal hunters, have an extra reflective layer known as the tapetum lucidum between the retina and the choroid, which bounces back photons that miss the photoreceptors on the first pass. This is essentially a biological version of night vision goggles and is why cats' eyes appear to glow when lit at night.

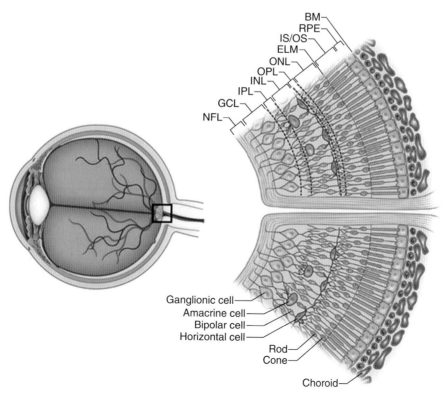

FIGURE 9.10 **Cross-section of the 10 retinal layers, taken in a region that includes the optic nerve.** (*Source:* https://www.springer.com/in/book/9781461434382)

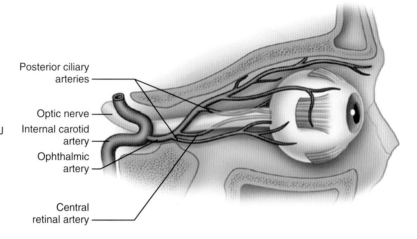

FIGURE 9.11 Arterial supply of the eye. (*Source:* Redrawn from Singh S, Dass R. The central artery of the retina I: origin and course. Br J Ophthalmol 1960;44:193–212.)

The cell bodies of the photoreceptors are located in the outer nuclear layer. It is here that the chemical depolarisation elicited by the rods and cones is integrated to form action potentials that propagate through the fibres in the outer plexiform layer to the next processing stage, the inner nuclear layer. Within the inner nuclear layer are a number of cell types: amacrine, bipolar and horizontal cells. The 'through pathway' of the retina is the photoreceptors to the bipolar cells to the retinal ganglion cells. The amacrine and horizontal cells in the inner nuclear layer modulate and refine the information flowing through the 'through pathway'. The fibre outputs of the inner nuclear layer course through the inner plexiform layer to the large retinal ganglion cells, which are the cell bodies of the optic nerve fibres that in turn course through the nerve fibre layer to a central gathering point at the optic disc. The optic disc is the nexus for the outgoing nerve fibres that form the optic nerve and exit the retina in a thick stalk-like bundle. It is also the point of entry for blood vessels that supply the inner retinal layers with oxygen and nutrients and remove waste metabolites. These blood vessels are derived from the inner carotid artery via the central retinal, ophthalmic and posterior ciliary arteries (Fig. 9.11).

The retina is not homogeneous and has an increased cell density and thickness at the centre. The central region of the retina is known as the **macula** (corresponding to central 12–13° of visual field) and at the centre of the macula is the **fovea centralis** (or foveal pit). The distribution of rod and cone density as a function of perimeter angle from the fovea is shown in Fig. 9.12. The fovea has almost exclusively cone receptors. This

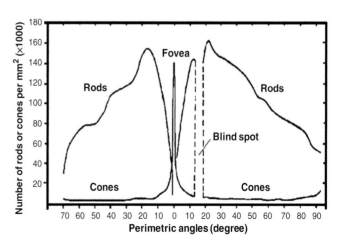

FIGURE 9.12 Cone and rod cell density as a function of perimeter angle from the fovea. (*Source:* Guenther BD, Steel DG. Encyclopedia of modern optics, 2 ed. Elsevier; 2018.)

has implications for night vision (discussed below). In addition, no nerve fibres overlay the fovea, providing a less obstructed path for incoming photons. It is here at the fovea where our highest acuity vision is achieved. Conversely, the peripheral retina is dominated by rod receptors at a lower density, which translates to lower acuity. It is important to note that at the optic disc there are no photoreceptors. This obviously means that no light transduction occurs at this point in the retina. This has implications for the continuity of the visual field, leading to a blind spot.

Visual function

The functional process of vision, where light energy is perceived consciously to gather information from the environment, is extremely complex. The main steps include eye optics, phototransduction, retinal processing and central processing. Alongside these are a number of facilitations, both mechanical and neural, which assist in extracting the most salient features of the light-derived information. Some of the key features at the subcortical level include: the ability of the eyes to move and work together to target scenes of interest and perceive depth; receptive fields within the retina that are tuned to respond to particular shapes, contrast or colours; and a self-regulating adjustment of retinal sensitivity to provide a wide dynamic range for intensity.

At the cortical level, the processing complexity increases dramatically and we do not as yet fully understand the brain's ability to perceptually bind objects, recognise motion, fill in gaps, make unconscious inferences based on subtle visual cues, recognise faces or patterns such as words, and so on. For example, yuo wlil fnid taht yuo are albe to raed tihs senetcne eevn thuohg teh letrters aer jumebld up. This is because your visual system is able to recognise the overall pattern that each word is making, and rapid coordination between visual, language and auditory centres in the brain parse and contexualise these patterns without resorting to fine interpretation of the high acuity visual input stream. Within the realm of visual neuroscience, there are many theories that seek to understand the complexities of visual processing. However, in this chapter we confine our discussion to the first two main steps: eye optics and phototransduction.

As described above, **eye optics** starts with the cornea, where light energy in the form of photons enters the eye. These incident light rays pass through the pupillary diaphragm in the centre of the iris and project onto the retina. Refraction through the lens causes inversion of the image, and as such the projection pattern of light on the retina is an inversion of the original

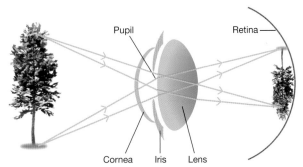

FIGURE 9.13 Why we actually see upside down: convex lens optics and image inversion.

scene, which is subsequently re-inverted by the brain (Fig. 9.13).

Once light strikes the retina the neurochemical process of **phototransduction** commences. As described above, there are two primary classes of photoreceptors: rods and cones. The outer segments of these photoreceptors are packed with photosensitive pigments in their lamellae membranes. The pigments are compound molecules comprised of a protein (opsin) and a lipid (retinaldehyde, a form of vitamin A). Rods provide monochromatic vision with high sensitivity to photonic activation across a range of wavelengths; this is particularly useful for night (scotopic) vision. Cones come in three varieties that contain pigments sensitive to the primary colours (i.e. wavelength) of light: red, blue or green. They are primarily responsible for daytime (photopic) vision. When photons of the correct wavelength are absorbed by a pigment, the retina is isomerised and this starts a cascade of molecular biological events that are beyond the scope of this chapter. Keen students looking for more information may wish to search for 'molecular cascade phototransduction' and are encouraged to review the websites provided in 'Online resources/suggested readings'.

INTEGRATION OF THE EARS AND EYES WITH OTHER BODY SYSTEMS
Immune system

The air-filled middle ear space has an important role in normal sound conduction and this can be compromised by fluid entering the space via the eustachian tube while experiencing a bad cold. The immune system is therefore important in assisting the body to return to normal homeostasis by helping to clear fluid and fight infections that may be present in the middle ear space. In cases where fluid is infected and accumulates in the middle ear space, treatment with antibiotics and decongestants is often required in order to avoid severe otitis media and resulting conductive hearing loss.

Cardiovascular system

The fine temporal and spatial representations of sound and sight by our eyes and ears have high metabolic demands and thus critically rely on a normally functioning cardiovascular system to deliver oxygen and nutrients and to remove carbon dioxide and waste. Interruptions to oxygen supply for these sensory tissues may cause lasting damage to the sensory cells responsible for hearing and vision.

Nervous system

Both the eyes and the ears are responsible for providing rich sensory information to the brain, and deprivation of this information can lead to remodelling of the brain and permanent deficits in processing. There is emerging evidence that auditory deprivation might contribute to overall cognitive decline, thus highlighting the importance of ongoing sensory input in overall brain health.

The ears and eyes are responsible for providing the central nervous system with information regarding three key senses: hearing, balance and vision. While they are 'standalone' specialist senses in their own right, here we describe perhaps the most impressive interaction between our ears and eyes: providing us with the wonderful ability to be able to stabilise our gaze while moving. This complex neural mechanism is known as the **vestibular-ocular reflex (VOR)** and is perhaps best understood by providing an example and a demonstration that you can perform yourself. Consider the acronym VOR and focus your gaze on the letters. Now, while keeping your gaze on the letters VOR, move your body from side to side and up and down. Did the letters move around or get blurry? No! The letters stayed in focus and were stable on the page, even though you were moving around. How did you do that, you ask? It is your VOR, which our inner ear, eyes and brain do automatically. You can think of it as a built-in stabilised camera in your head. When your head moves to the right, your eyes move to the left; that is, your eyes automatically compensate for your moving body. The reflex explains how we can run, dance and jump and the world doesn't spin with us. It stays perfectly stable. Together, our ears and eyes provide a huge amount of sensory information to the brain, which through several highly specialised relay stations is perceived as hearing, balance and vision.

AGE-RELATED CHANGES

As we age, so too do the specialised sensory cells within our ears and eyes. While there are a number of age-related changes to hearing, the most common occurs as a result of a lifetime of wear and tear on the tiny stereocilia on our inner ear hair cells. Without these tiny hairs, we start to lose the ability to hear clearly and at low sound intensities. **Presbycusis** is the term given to age-related hearing loss and it affects at least 25% of people over 65 years of age. Initially, presbycusis may be treated through use of a hearing aid, but once there is extensive degeneration of the inner ear hair cells, only a cochlear implant can restore a sense of hearing. Presbycusis can make it difficult to understand instructions, hear announcements and participate in routine activities.

Additionally, as we age we may start to find it difficult to hear in situations where there is a lot of background noise. This phenomenon is more commonly known as the 'cocktail party effect' and tends to manifest earlier among individuals who have been exposed to loud environments during their lifetime. Recent evidence suggests that this may be due to the preferential loss of some of the specialised synaptic connections between the inner ear hair cells and auditory neurons; it may, or may not, be recoverable with future treatments for hearing loss.

Similarly, our eyes naturally deteriorate with age and this causes a range of changes. The natural hardening of the lens that starts to occur at ~40 years of age is known as **presbyopia** and it makes it more difficult to focus on objects that are up close. It is considered a normal part of ageing and can be treated by wearing glasses. Cataracts are a leading cause of vision impairment in the elderly and cause a blurring of vision to various degrees. They are so common these days that they are currently considered to be a normal part of ageing and can be successfully treated with minor surgery. While cataracts may affect people of any age, the average age for cataract surgery in Australia is ~75 years.

More serious age-related changes to the eye occur as a result of degenerative eye disease and include glaucoma, macular degeneration and diabetic retinopathy. These have more limited treatment options and there are currently no therapies to cure or halt the progression of degeneration over time. Not surprisingly, these degenerative eye diseases are the focus of international research efforts in visual neuroscience.

CONCLUSION

This chapter introduces the basic structure and function of the auditory, vestibular and visual sense organs: the ear and the eye. It describes, in simple terms, the anatomical and physiological processes that allow us to hear, balance and see. After reading this chapter, you should have an appreciation for the different tissues, cell types and organisation of the outer, middle and inner ear and how each contributes to the amplification and transduction of mechanical vibrations in the air to electrochemical impulses within the auditory nerve. You should also understand that the inner ear provides cues to help us locate ourselves in space. Similarly, you should appreciate how the components of the eye work in harmony to focus and convert photons of incident light into a conscious representation of a visual scene. However, the exquisitely detailed biochemical and network specialisations that provide precision, discrimination and clarity as well as resilience to injury and infection remain as subjects for further learning.

ACKNOWLEDGEMENT

The authors would like to thank Dr Carla Abbott for providing helpful feedback on a draft of the manuscript.

CASE STUDY 9.1

Ellen is returning home on a flight and as her plane starts to descend for landing she feels pressure build in her ear. Ellen yawns and feels a 'popping' sensation, which seems to relieve the pressure for a moment, but it returns a few minutes later.

Q1. The middle ear lies between the outer ear and the inner ear within the temporal bone and:
   a. is air-filled.
   b. is fluid-filled.
   c. contains the semicircular canals.
   d. contains the cochlea.

Q2. Regarding the eustachian tube, which of the following is correct?
   a. The eustachian tube connects the middle ear to the laryngopharynx.
   b. The eustachian tube is open at rest.
   c. The eustachian tube has a role in keeping the middle ear free of fluid.
   d. The eustachian tube runs at a 90° angle to the throat.

Q3. Which of the following is *not* a function of the middle ear?
   a. Efficient transfer of sound vibrations between the outer and inner ear via the ossicles
   b. Maintenance of equal pressure in the middle ear space by the eustachian tube
   c. Amplification of sound pressure waves by up to 17 times
   d. Neural transduction of sound into electrical signals

Q4. Describe the underlying anatomical structures in the peripheral auditory pathway that cause a 'popping' sensation when flying.

Q5. Describe how eustachian tube function might be affected if Ellen had a cold at the time of flying.

CASE STUDY 9.2

After a late night, Dwayne decides to close his eyes during a lecture and just listen to the instructor. Even with his eyes closed, Dwayne can tell that the lecturer is walking from left to right across the front of the lecture theatre as the lecture slides are presented.

Q1. Which of the following is *not* a function of the outer ear?
   a. The outer ear acts as a funnel to concentrate sound onto the tympanic membrane.
   b. The outer ear contains ceruminous and sebaceous glands to protect the skin from infection.
   c. The outer ear helps localise the source of sound in the vertical and horizontal planes.
   d. The outer ear has a key function in maintaining balance.

Continued

CASE STUDY 9.2—cont'd

Q2. Sound travels through air as pressure waves of variable frequencies. Which of the following statements is false?

    a. High-frequency sound pressure waves vibrate the eardrum more rapidly.

    b. Low-frequency sound pressure waves vibrate the eardrum more slowly.

    c. High-intensity sound pressure waves vibrate the eardrum with a greater amplitude.

    d. Low-intensity sound pressure waves vibrate the eardrum with a greater amplitude.

Q3. Considering how sound travels through air, which of the following statements is false?

    a. High-frequency sound pressure waves arising from the left-hand side of the body will arrive at the right pinna with slightly less intensity.

    b. Low-frequency sound pressure waves arising from the right-hand side of the body will arrive at the left pinna with more intensity.

    c. High-frequency sound pressure waves arising from the right side of the body will arrive at the left and right pinnae at about the same time.

    d. Low-frequency sound pressure waves arising from directly in front of an individual will arrive at the left and right pinnae at the same time.

Q4. Describe the underlying anatomical and physiological principles behind Dwayne's ability to localise the voice of the speaker.

Q5. How would the situation change if Dwayne had an ear plug (or headphone speaker) in one ear?

CASE STUDY 9.3

On a bright summer's day to escape the heat Carter decided to watch a movie at the cinema. However, he was running late and the movie had already started when he arrived. After the movie, Carter walks out onto the street where the sun is still shining brightly. For the purposes of this case study, assume that Carter isn't wearing sunglasses (even though he should be).

Q1. When Carter's eyes are exposed to bright sunlight, which of the following statements is true?

    a. The pupils will rapidly dilate to allow less light to enter the eye, thereby protecting the retina and automatically adjusting the gain and dynamic range of vision.

    b. The photoreceptor's visual pigments are activated and broken down in the first step of a process that leads to perception of vision.

    c. The depth of field is reduced in bright light due to the smaller iris aperture.

    d. The rods are providing the most useful vision in bright light as they are less bleached than the cone photoreceptors.

Q2. When Carter is in the dark of the cinema, which of the following statements is false?

    a. Incoming photons that miss the photoreceptors on the first pass are reflected off the tapetum lucidum and have a second chance to active the retina; this improves vision in the dark.

    b. To best see in the dark, he should look slightly to the side of the target so that the image is projected away from his fovea, which only contains cone receptors that are not well suited for scotopic vision.

    c. The pupils will rapidly dilate to allow more light to enter the eye, thereby improving his night vision and automatically adjusting the gain and dynamic range.

    d. Depth of field is reduced in dim light due to the larger iris aperture.

Q3. Which of the following cells are impacted by or mediate light and dark adaptation?

    a. Photoreceptors and Purkinje cells

    b. Amacrine cells and spiral ganglion neurons

    c. Retinal ganglion cells and photoreceptors

    d. All of the above

Q4. When Carter first entered the cinema, he found it hard to read the numbers on the seat rows as everything appeared too dark. Describe the biological processes, cell types and molecular mechanisms underlying this.

Q5. When Carter exited the cinema and walked out onto the street, everything was overly bright, causing him to squint. Describe the biological processes, cell types and molecular mechanisms underlying this reaction.

CASE STUDY 9.4

Try this simple trick to find your blind spot. Sit or stand up straight. Hold both your index fingers up together (nail side towards you) directly in front of you at arm's length such that your finger tips are zeroed with your nose in both the azimuth and elevation. Close your left eye. Focus your right eye on your left index fingertip. Slowly move your right arm to the right, while keeping it parallel with the ground such that your arms resemble the hands of a clock lying flat when viewed from above. Keep focusing on your left fingertip with your right eye (your left eye should still be closed). Before your arms resemble 1 o'clock you will notice that your right fingertip disappears from sight. Repeat the process for your other eye, remembering to close your right eye and move your left arm this time.

Q1. Roughly how many degrees separation are your arms at your blind spot?

 a. 12–13° degrees

 b. 15 degrees

 c. 30 degrees

 d. Not enough information to determine

Q2. In relation to your anatomical blind spot, which of these statements is false?

 a. Your blind spot is associated with the anatomical location in the retina known as the optic disc head where there are no photoreceptors present.

 b. As a result of your eye's blind spot, you should always perform a head check before changing lanes.

 c. Your blind spot is located nasal to your fovea in your retina.

 d. Your blind spot corresponds to objects located temporal to your central visual field.

Q3. Considering this optical illusion, which of the following is true?

 a. If you had two extra arms you could find both of your blind spots simultaneously by keeping both eyes open.

 b. This trick would work just as well using your palm instead of your finger.

 c. If you used dots on a sheet of paper, instead of your fingers, this trick would still work—as long as the dots were positioned correctly with respect to your eye.

 d. All of the above are true.

Q4. Why did your fingertip disappear from sight? Why isn't there always a 'hole' in your visual field at the locations of the blind spot?

Q5. Use the technique above to explore your blind spots. Using your knowledge of lens optics and simple geometry, sketch the location and extent of your right eye's blind spot with respect to your right eye's visual field. Mark the nasal, superior, temporal and inferior sides of your sketch and indicate in degrees of arc the separation between your centre of vision (fovea) and your blind spot. Approximate the location, size and shape of your blind spot in your sketch. Bonus points if you are able to distinguish any blood vessels and their trajectories leading from your blind spot. Hint: you need to keep your eye very still to do this; it is not easy.

CHAPTER 10

Endocrine system

ZERINA TOMKINS, BAPPSC (MED LAB SCI), BAPPSC (HONS), MNSC (NURS), PHD, GRAD CERT (UNIVERSITY EDUCATION)

KEY POINTS/LEARNING OUTCOMES

1. Define what a hormone is and how hormones are classified.
2. Identify the key endocrine organs, their structure and the hormones these organs secrete.
3. Discuss the role of the endocrine system in glucose metabolism.
4. Explain the role of the endocrine system in maintaining body homeostasis such as reproductive health and calcium metabolism.
5. Identify the key structural and functional aged-related changes to the endocrine system.

KEY DEFINITIONS

- **Endocrine glands:** structures composed of highly specialised epithelial cells that secrete hormones into the blood circulation in order for the hormones to reach their target cells.
- **Endocrinology:** a discipline of science devoted to studying the function of the endocrine system.
- **Exocrine glands:** structures composed of epithelial cells that secrete predominantly enzymes into ducts opening directly into the target tissue or into other ducts in internal organs or into external body surfaces such as skin.
- **Hormone:** a substance produced by endocrine glands that acts to regulate or control specific processes, thus maintaining the body's capacity to meet daily activities of living.
- **Signalling:** a mode of cellular communication that allows cells to convey information to one another or to regulate cellular processes needed to maintain homeostasis.

ONLINE RESOURCES/SUGGESTED READINGS

- **The endocrine system** available at www.hormone.org/hormones-and-health/the-endocrine-system
- **A collection of games and activities for the endocrine system: it can be fun!** available at www.lifescitrc.org/resource.cfm?submissionID=6716
- **Endocrine system** available at www.innerbody.com/image/endoov.html
- **Endocrine system and syndromes** available at www.labtestsonline.org.au/learning/index-of-conditions/endocrine
- **Intro to the endocrine system** available at www.aptv.org/IQLEARNING/khan/video.php?readableid=intro-to-the-endocrine-system

INTRODUCTION

From conception to death, the endocrine system is involved in the regulation of nearly every cellular process in your body. It does this by releasing chemical messengers from the endocrine glands into the bloodstream and targeting cells at a distant site. A **gland** is a specialised structure that has the capacity to secrete chemical substances to regulate body function. Glands can be broadly grouped into exocrine and endocrine glands. **Exocrine glands** secrete their product through the epithelial cell surface into ducts, specialised tubular structures used as passages to move secretions to target organs. **Endocrine glands** are ductless glands that collectively form the endocrine system to control the internal body environment by secreting chemical messengers (hormones) directly into the bloodstream to reach target cells at sites distant from the site of hormone production.[1] The major endocrine glands include the hypothalamus, pituitary gland, thyroid and parathyroid glands, thymus, adrenal glands, endocrine portion of the pancreas and the gonads (ovaries in females and testes in males); the placenta is also an important endocrine organ in pregnant females (Fig. 10.1).

The primary function of the endocrine system is to maintain internal homeostasis in response to external or environmental stimuli or changes that occur within the body itself. To maintain these functions the endocrine system acts as a communication system, an integration centre (whereby several processes are integrated to achieve a specific outcome) and a control centre (where the aim is to maintain tight regulation of deviation from homeostasis).[1] Note that the chemical messenger system is not unique to the endocrine system. It is also used by the nervous system in the form of neurotransmitters and the immune system in the form of cytokines to regulate immune responses including acute inflammation.

When considered within the context of the life span, processes regulated by the endocrine system include the formation of sperm and gametes, control of the internal environment that allows implantation of the fertilised egg (zygote) and formation of the placenta to support the developing fetus. Fetal cell division and cell differentiation towards specific tissues as the embryo forms cardiovascular and nervous systems or limbs are also regulated by the endocrine system. You may recall your puberty age where boys developed broader shoulders, a deeper voice and facial hair and girls developed breasts and started to have monthly periods (menstruation). You will also be aware of menopause, when age-related changes in the endocrine and reproductive systems lead to the cessation of menstruation and eventual loss of female fertility. How does the endocrine system perform all of these functions? This chapter explores what hormones are, how they are classified and how they perform their function. We also discuss the endocrine glands that produce these hormones and how the endocrine system collaborates with other body systems to maintain body homeostasis.

STRUCTURE AND FUNCTION OF THE ENDOCRINE SYSTEM

Hormones

Hormones are chemical substances manufactured by endocrine organs (glands) in the body. They are secreted directly into the bloodstream where they travel to their target cells, often far from the gland that secreted them. These target cells have specific receptors (targets) for specific hormones (Fig. 10.2). This means that while a hormone can reach every cell in the body, it cannot exert an effect on cells unless a receptor specific for that hormone is present somewhere on that cell. For example, a receptor may be expressed on the cell surface or inside the cell. Once a hormone binds to its receptor, a series of events are activated as new messages are formed to create a cascade of signals that the cell interprets in order to generate a specific response. This is known as the **signalling** cascade or signalling transduction.[1]

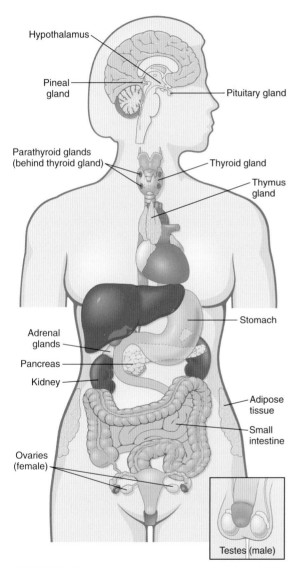

FIGURE 10.1 Endocrine system. (*Source:* Hall JE. Guyton and Hall textbook of medical physiology, 13 ed. Elsevier; 2015.)

Labels: Hypothalamus; Pineal gland; Pituitary gland; Parathyroid glands (behind thyroid gland); Thyroid gland; Thymus gland; Stomach; Adrenal glands; Pancreas; Kidney; Adipose tissue; Small intestine; Ovaries (female); Testes (male)

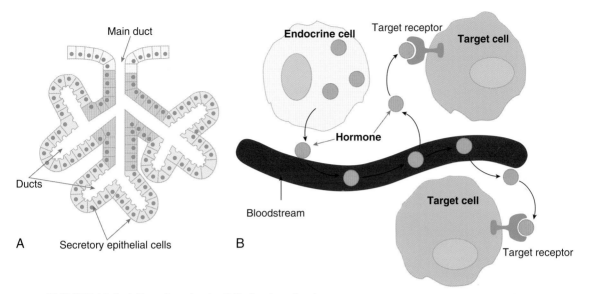

FIGURE 10.2 **A Exocrine glands. B Endocrine glands.**

Hormones act more slowly than the signals generated by the nervous system but the effect of the hormone lasts longer.[1] In addition, a hormone may exert an individual effect or act with another hormone to produce a **synergistic** (or cooperative) effect that has a greater outcome than if each hormone acted alone. It is also possible that one hormone may act in a **permissive** way—that is, one hormone permits a second hormone to exert its full effect on the target cells. Hormones may also have an antagonistic or opposing effect on another hormone; this is known as **antagonism**.

Hormones can be grouped based on their structural, functional and distance-effect characteristics (see Table 10.1 at the end of the chapter for a summary). From a structural perspective, hormones can be grouped into **steroid** hormones and **non-steroid** hormones (Fig. 10.3). Steroid hormones are manufactured by endocrine

cells from cholesterol molecules. In general, they are not stored by cells and are synthesised as needed. As cholesterol is a lipid, this gives steroid hormones lipid-soluble properties, allowing them to pass uninterrupted through the phospholipid plasma membrane of target cells. Examples of steroid hormones include cortisol, aldosterone, oestrogen, testosterone and progesterone.[1]

Non-steroid hormones comprise modified amino acids (amines), peptides (short-chain amino acids) and proteins. Examples of **non-steroid amino acid-derived hormones** include amines (melatonin, adrenaline [epinephrine] and noradrenaline [norepinephrine]) and the iodinated amino acids thyroxine and triiodothyronine. Examples of **peptide hormones** include antidiuretic hormone (ADH), oxytocin (OT), somatostatin (SS), thyrotropin-releasing hormone (TRH), melanocyte-stimulating hormone (MSH), gonadotropin-releasing

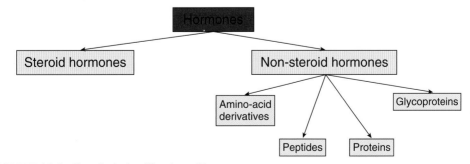

FIGURE 10.3 **Chemical classification of hormones.**

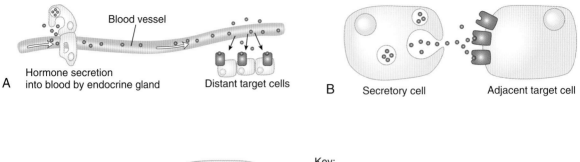

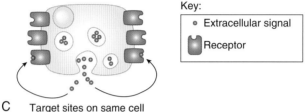

FIGURE 10.4 **Distance effect: (A) endocrine, (B) paracrine and (C) autocrine signalling.** (*Source:* Modified from www.researchgate.net/figure/Cell-communication-type-a-endocrine-signaling-b-paracrine-signaling-c-autocrine_fig2_299402847.)

hormone (GnRH) and atrial natriuretic hormone (ANH). **Glycoprotein hormones** are protein hormones that have a carbohydrate functional group joined to the polypeptide chain. This group of hormones includes human chorionic gonadotropin (hCG), follicle-stimulating hormone (FSH), luteinising hormone (LH) and thyroid-stimulating hormone (TSH). Protein hormones are complex globular structures comprised of amino acids and include growth hormone (GH), prolactin (PRL), parathyroid hormone (PTH), calcitonin (CT), adrenocorticotropic hormone (ACTH), insulin and glucagon. Non-steroid hormones tend to be synthesised as precursor molecules and processed by the endoplasmic reticulum and Golgi apparatus where the precursor molecules are stored in secretory granules.[1] When needed, the precursor molecules are released into the bloodstream and may require activation by another enzyme before they can exert their effect.

From a functional perspective, hormones can be grouped into tropic hormones, sex hormones and anabolic hormones. **Tropic hormones** target other endocrine glands and most are produced and secreted by the anterior pituitary gland. **Sex hormones** target reproductive tissues (testes in males and ovaries in female), while **anabolic hormones** stimulate anabolism in target cells (e.g. testosterone-induced stimulation of protein synthesis and muscle growth).

Finally, based on the distances they travel to their target cells, hormones can be grouped into endocrine

hormones, paracrine hormones and autocrine hormones. **Endocrine hormones** act over long distances and tend to exert a global effect, meaning that their effect may be more general and throughout the body. **Paracrine hormones** are regionally active and **autocrine hormones** act directly on the cell that secreted them or neighbouring cells. If paracrine hormone enters the bloodstream, it has no effect on other cells (Fig. 10.4).

In addition, there is a specialised group of chemicals called eicosanoids, a group of lipid molecules that include prostaglandins, thromboxane and leukotrienes, known as tissue hormones. The term 'tissue hormones' suggests that these short-lived compounds are secreted at a tissue level and diffuse a small distance within the same tissue rather than being secreted into the bloodstream to reach distant target cells.

Mechanisms of hormone release

Earlier we mentioned that the endocrine and nervous systems are very closely connected. The brain senses changes, both internal and external, through a complex set of neural sensors (receptors) and electrical impulses sent through the neuronal networks. As it interprets those sensations, the brain sends neural signals to the endocrine glands via neural networks to secrete hormones to respond to those stimuli.

In addition to control by the nervous system, the endocrine system is regulated by negative and positive feedback mechanisms. A feedback loop is a mechanism

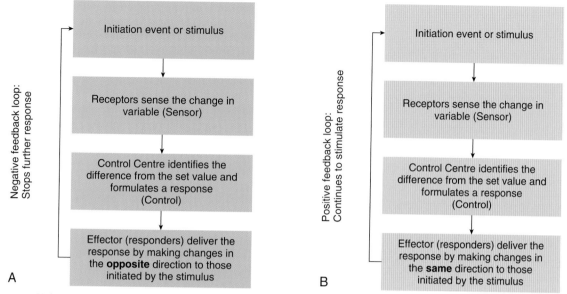

FIGURE 10.5 **A Negative feedback loop. B Positive feedback loop.**

by which information gained about a change in homeostatic balance activates a reaction that either increases the change (positive feedback) or reduces the effect to return the body back to homeostasis or equilibrium (negative effect) and keep the internal environment constant.

Thus, a **negative feedback** mechanism (Fig. 10.5A), also known as an endocrine reflex, refers to a system where loss of the initial stimulus leads to the reversed or opposite effect to maintain homeostasis. For example, blood glucose levels are maintained at a constant level, somewhere between 3.5 and 5.5 mmol/L. When you eat a meal, food is digested and carbohydrates are converted to glucose, which is absorbed into the bloodstream. The elevated level of glucose (above 5.5. mmol/L) will be detected by the pancreatic islet beta cells and they will secrete insulin to promote cellular uptake of glucose so that the blood level can return to normal (between 3.5 and 5.5 mmol/L). As the blood glucose concentration decreases, pancreatic beta cells sense this change and cease to produce and release insulin.

A positive feedback mechanism (Fig. 10.5B) refers to amplification of the initiating stimulus, which results in increased production of that hormone. Thus, the stimulus is maintained rather than abolished. An example can be seen during childbirth (Fig. 10.6). As labour begins and the baby pushes against the cervix to enter the birth canal, the cervix stretches to accommodate the baby's head. This stretch activates nerve sensory receptors located in the cervix, which fire neuronal impulses that travel to the brain. The brain stimulates the pituitary gland to release more oxytocin, which amplifies the rate of and strength of labour contractions, forcing the baby to move down the birth canal. This loop, where stretch continues, means that there is continued stimulation

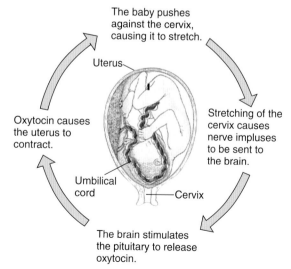

FIGURE 10.6 **An example of a positive feedback loop: childbirth.** (*Source:* https://courses.lumenlearning.com/boundless-biology/chapter/homeostasis/.)

of oxytocin secretion (**positive feedback**) until the baby is born and the stretch stimulus stops.

Mechanisms of hormone action

The mechanisms by which hormones work depend on whether a hormone is steroid-based (lipid-soluble) or amino acid-based (water-soluble). In general, steroid hormones, which are lipophilic and hydrophobic, exert their action by diffusing through the target cell plasma membrane and binding to a receptor inside the cell cytoplasm or cell nucleus to activate a series of signalling events that have a specific outcome. Non-steroid hormones, which are hydrophilic or lipophobic, attach to a receptor located on the target cell membrane. This causes a cascade of signalling events inside the cell cytoplasm, leading to a specific cellular outcome. This outcome always involves modulation of gene expression in the target cell that impacts protein synthesis (Chapter 2).

The mechanism of steroid hormone action is explained by the mobile-receptor or nuclear-receptor model (Fig. 10.7A). In this model, the lipophilic hormone diffuses through the plasma membrane and binds with a receptor that is freely moving inside the cell cytoplasm. This generates a receptor-hormone complex, which moves into the cell nucleus and binds to a specific site on the DNA molecule, thus inducing gene transcription, where DNA is transcribed into mRNA (Chapter 2). The newly formed RNA is then transported into the cell cytoplasm where it is translated into protein by ribosomes (Chapter 2). This new protein alters cell function. Because these hormones alter gene transcription through binding of the receptor-hormone complex to a designated site on the DNA molecule, these receptors are also known as **ligand-dependent transcription factors**.[1] This mechanism of action is believed to take hours to days as it takes time to transcribe the new RNA into protein. However, in another less understood model, steroid hormones can have a more rapid effect by binding to steroid hormone receptors on the plasma membrane, thus inducing or altering the signalling cascade, which then impacts how messages (chemical signals) are sent by other regulatory molecules such as other hormones or neurotransmitters.

The mechanism of non-steroid hormone action is explained through the **second messenger model** (Fig. 10.7B). In this model, the hormone (termed a first messenger) binds to the receptor spanning the plasma membrane. This is because non-steroid hormones are not lipid soluble and therefore cannot diffuse through the plasma membrane. The newly formed hormone-receptor complex leads to conformational change (change in shape) of the receptor and this leads to the generation of a chemical signal (termed a second messenger) inside the cell cytoplasm. The second messenger triggers other intracellular chemicals to produce an amplified signalling cascade that results in the desired intercellular response, such as cell proliferation, differentiation, migration, survival or death. To date, five chemicals have been identified as second messengers: cyclic adenosine monophosphate (AMP), cyclic guanosine monophosphate (GMP), inositol trisphosphate ($InsP_3$), diacylglycerol (DAG) and calcium ions-dependent complexes (Ca^{2+}).[2]

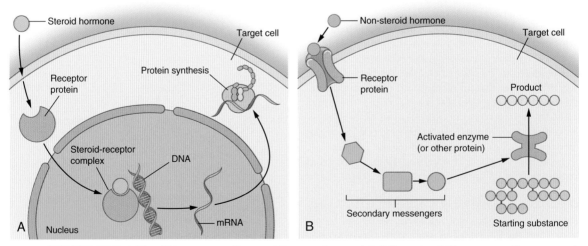

FIGURE 10.7 **A Steroid hormone action: mobile-receptor model. B Non-steroid hormone action: second messenger model.**

An example of the second messenger model is that of calcium ions responsible for muscle contraction (Fig. 10.8). In this model, a hormone (first messenger) attaches to the receptor on the plasma membrane. This leads to the opening of Ca^{2+} channels located in the plasma membrane, resulting in the rapid entry of calcium ions from the extracellular space (where concentration is higher) into the cell (where concentration is lower). Inside the cell, Ca^{2+} binds with the protein calmodulin

to form a calcium-calmodulin complex (second messenger).[1] This causes a conformational change in the calmodulin and leads to activation of enzymes called protein kinases, which collectively results in muscle contraction.

Exceptions to this view of the non-steroid hormone mechanism of action are the amino acid derivatives thyroid hormones triiodothyronine (T3) and thyroxine (T4) which, after entering the bloodstream, bind to a

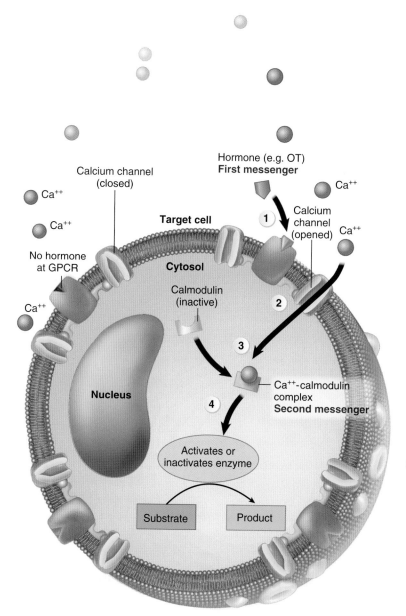

FIGURE 10.8 **Second messenger: calcium calmodulin model.** A first messenger (e.g. non-steroid hormone oxytocin) binds to a fixed receptor (G-protein–coupled receptor, GPCR) in the plasma membrane (1), which activates membrane-bound proteins (e.g. G protein) that trigger the opening of calcium channels (2). Calcium ions, which are normally at a higher concentration in the extracellular fluid, diffuse into the cell and bind to a calmodulin molecule (3). The Ca^{++}-calmodulin complex thus formed is a second messenger that binds to an enzyme to produce an effect that promotes or inhibits the enzyme's regulatory effect in the target cell (4). (*Source:* Patton KT, Thibodeau GA. Skin. In: Patton KT, Thibodeau GA, editors. Anatomy and physiology, 7 ed. London: Elsevier Health Sciences; 2010.)

plasma protein called thyroxine-binding globulin (TBG). Thyroxine is converted to T3, which enters the cell via membrane transporter proteins spanning the plasma membrane, to bind to receptors located on DNA in the cell nucleus. Like steroid hormones, thyroid hormones form a receptor-hormone complex, which then modulates gene transcription by either stimulating or inhibiting gene transcription (Fig. 10.9).[1]

It is important to understand these mechanisms from a therapeutic viewpoint as they explain how some pharmacological agents (medications) are used to treat endocrine system disorders. These disorders often arise from overproduction or underproduction of a hormone in the endocrine gland or because receptors on target cells lose their function, thus rendering the target cells unresponsive or insensitive to the effect of hormones. An example of an endocrine disorder due to overproduction of a hormone is Cushing's syndrome, a clinical manifestation arising from chronically high levels of cortisol. An example of an endocrine disorder characterised by underproduction of a hormone is hypothyroidism, which is characterised by insufficient production of thyroid hormone.

Endocrine glands

As already noted, the major endocrine glands include the hypothalamus, pituitary gland, thyroid and parathyroid glands, thymus, adrenal glands, endocrine portion of the pancreas, ovaries in females and testes in males, as well as the placenta in pregnant females. Table 10.1 (at the end of the chapter) summarises the major endocrine glands, the hormones they make and the function and structure of those hormones. Most of these glands are made of epithelial tissue, although some are made of neurosecretory tissue (also known as neuroendocrine tissue)—for example, tissue found in the hypothalamus. In this section we will start with the glands found in the head and neck region and move towards the abdominal and pelvic cavities before ending with muscle and adipose tissue.

The **hypothalamus** is comprised of numerous grey-matter nuclei clustered below the thalamus and above the pituitary gland (Fig. 10.10). Because it can release hormones and is comprised of neural tissue, the hypothalamus is the link between the endocrine and nervous systems. In addition to regulating many functions through the autonomic nervous system—such

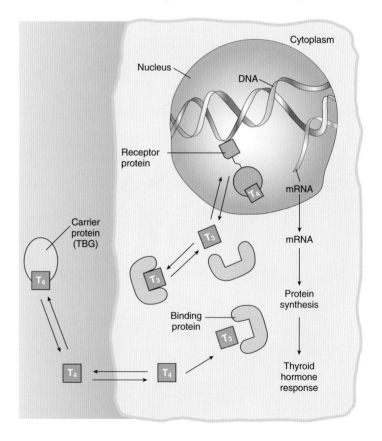

FIGURE 10.9 **Mechanism of action for T3 and T4.** TBG, thyroxin-binding globulin. (*Source:* www.78stepshealth.us/human-physiology/mechanism-of-thyroid-hormone-action.html.)

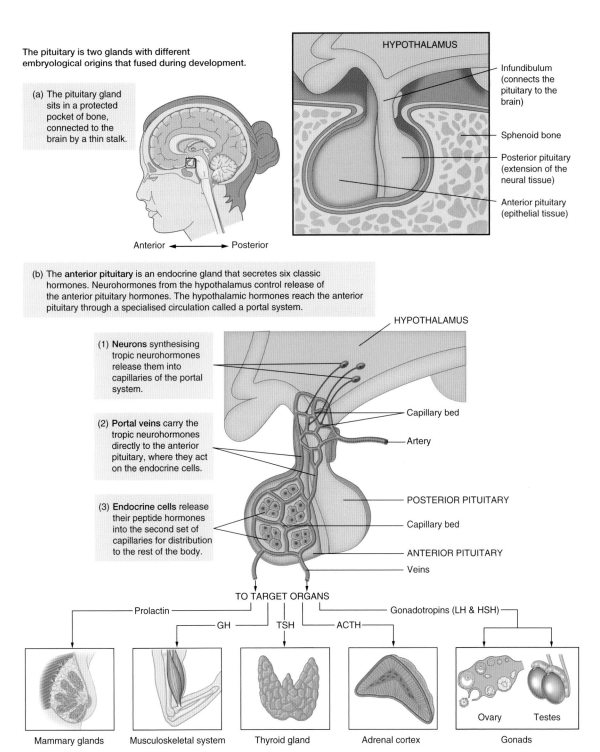

The pituitary is two glands with different embryological origins that fused during development.

(a) The pituitary gland sits in a protected pocket of bone, connected to the brain by a thin stalk.

HYPOTHALAMUS

Infundibulum (connects the pituitary to the brain)

Sphenoid bone

Posterior pituitary (extension of the neural tissue)

Anterior pituitary (epithelial tissue)

Anterior ← → Posterior

(b) The **anterior pituitary** is an endocrine gland that secretes six classic hormones. Neurohormones from the hypothalamus control release of the anterior pituitary hormones. The hypothalamic hormones reach the anterior pituitary through a specialised circulation called a portal system.

HYPOTHALAMUS

(1) **Neurons** synthesising tropic neurohormones release them into capillaries of the portal system.

Capillary bed

Artery

(2) **Portal veins** carry the tropic neurohormones directly to the anterior pituitary, where they act on the endocrine cells.

(3) **Endocrine cells** release their peptide hormones into the second set of capillaries for distribution to the rest of the body.

POSTERIOR PITUITARY

Capillary bed

ANTERIOR PITUITARY

Veins

TO TARGET ORGANS

Prolactin

GH   TSH   ACTH

Gonadotropins (LH & HSH)

Mammary glands

Musculoskeletal system

Thyroid gland

Adrenal cortex

Ovary   Testes

Gonads

FIGURE 10.10 **Hypothalamus and pituitary gland.**

as body temperature, heart rate and blood pressure, fluid and electrolyte balance, thirst mechanism and the sleep–wake cycle—the hypothalamus controls many of the pituitary gland functions. The hypothalamus secretes ADH, **GH releasing hormone**, GH inhibitory hormone or somatostatin, TRH, prolactin-inhibiting hormone, PRH, OT and CRH.

The **pituitary gland** is found in the pituitary fossa of the sella turcica (Fig. 10.10) and is covered by the dura mater called the pituitary diaphragm. This small gland is composed of two separate glands linked together by a pituitary stalk, called the infundibulum, and to the hypothalamus, which controls the capacity of the pituitary gland to inhibit or release hormones into circulation. The two glands are known as the **anterior pituitary gland (adenohypophysis)** and **the posterior pituitary gland (neurohypophysis)**. The anterior pituitary gland is made of epithelial endocrine tissue and secretes ACTH, FSH, LH, GH, PRL and TSH. The function of each of these hormones is summarised in Table 10.1 (at the end of the chapter). Hormone secretion by the anterior pituitary gland is controlled by hormones

synthesised in the hypothalamus that are released via neuronal axons into a specialised blood vessel network called the **hypophyseal portal system**. The hypophyseal portal system is unique because blood from the hypothalamus flows directly to the adenohypophysis rather than the systemic circulation. This means that the hypothalamus-synthesised hormones are delivered directly to target cells in the anterior pituitary gland. The posterior pituitary gland is composed of **neurosecretory** tissues. Neurons that synthesise ADH and OT release these hormones following neuronal stimulation into the blood circulation. See above discussion of how OT is released during labour, and how stretching of the cervix activates neuronal receptors to send impulses to the posterior pituitary gland to release more OT to increase uterine contractions.

The **pineal gland** is a pinecone-shaped gland about 1 cm in size located on the dorsal aspect of the brain. It is responsible for **melatonin**, a hormone that is produced while sleeping and inhibited by sunlight, thus regulating circadian rhythm (sleeping and feeding pattern) and mood (Fig. 10.11). The gland also forms

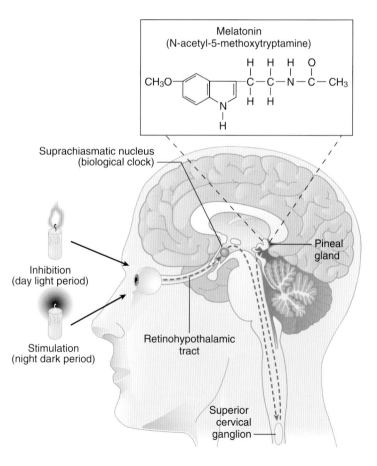

FIGURE 10.11 Pineal gland and melatonin production. (*Source:* Waldman S, Terzic A. Pharmacology and therapeutics: principles to practice, 1 ed. Elsevier; 2009.)

part of the nervous system as it receives visual stimuli from the eyes.

The **thyroid gland** is located in front of the trachea and below the larynx in the neck. It is comprised of two lobes linked together by a connective tissue called **isthmus** (Fig. 10.12). The gland is characterised by follicles lined by an epithelial cell layer with a hollow lumen filled with a thick fluid called **colloid**. Colloid contains **thyroglobulins**, which are protein-iodine complexes and the precursors of hormones T3 and T4. When T3 and T4 are needed, thyroglobulin is broken down to release T3 and T4 into the bloodstream, which then bind to thyroid-binding globulins to reach the target cells (Fig. 10.9). Both T3 and T4 are needed to regulate cell metabolism. The thyroid also produces calcitonin, which plays a part in the regulation of blood calcium levels. Thyroid gland function is controlled by the pituitary gland and hypothalamus. Reductions in thyroid hormone in the blood signal the hypothalamus to secrete TRH, which stimulates the pituitary gland to release TSH. TSH acts on the thyroid gland to stimulate the production of more thyroid hormones. Provided there is sufficient blood concentration of iodine, the thyroid will make more T3 and T4.[1]

The **parathyroid glands**, of which there are four, are located behind the thyroid gland (Fig. 10.12). They secrete **PTH**, whose major role is to regulate the body's Ca^{2+} homeostasis. Ca^{2+} is the main ion that drives muscle contractions and the conduction of neuronal impulses.

The **thymus** is an immune organ and endocrine gland located beneath the sternum. It secretes the non-steroid hormones **thymosin** and **thymopoietin**, which play a role in the production of T-cells.

The **heart** is also an endocrine organ as the heart atria have the capacity to sense the stretch inside the atria and in response the hormone-producing cells found in the upper part of the atria secrete ANP, also known as **atrial natriuretic factor (ANF)**.

The **adrenal glands** are paired organs located on top of the kidneys embedded in adipose tissue. Each gland consists of two concentric layers: the outer **adrenal cortex** and the inner **adrenal medulla** (Fig. 10.13). The adrenal cortex is composed of endocrine tissue and is organised in three distinct zones of secreting cells. The outermost layer, the **zona glomerulosa**, secretes aldosterone, a mineralocorticoid that regulates how sodium is managed in the body to maintain fluid balance and blood pressure.

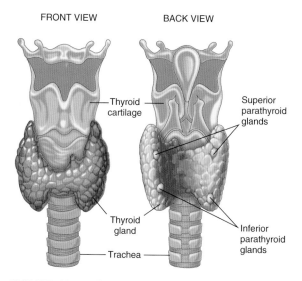

FRONT VIEW   BACK VIEW

FIGURE 10.12 **Anatomy of thyroid and parathyroid glands.**

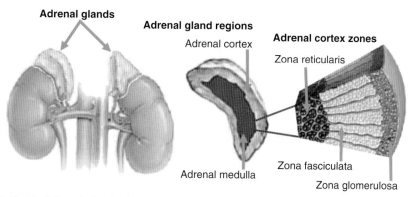

FIGURE 10.13 **Adrenal glands.** (*Source:* your hormones.com.)

The release of aldosterone is mediated by the kidneys. Cells in the middle zone, the **zona fasciculata**, secrete cortisol, a glucocorticoid that regulates food metabolism through protein and fat catabolism for gluconeogenesis, blood pressure regulation and various processes related to inflammation and immune responses. The release of glucocorticoids is regulated by the hypothalamus and anterior pituitary gland. The cells of the inner zone, the **zona reticularis**, secrete small amounts of glucocorticoids and gonadocorticoids (male sex hormones). Collectively, hormones secreted by the adrenal cortex are known as **corticosteroids**. The adrenal medulla is composed of neuroendocrine tissue that produces two important non-steroid hormones classed as **catecholamines** because they contain a catechol functional group and a side-chain amine group. These hormones are **adrenaline (epinephrine)** and **noradrenaline (norepinephrine)**. Both are released following stimulation from the sympathetic nervous system when the person is stressed or encounters a life-threatening situation. This is more commonly known as the fight or flight response.

The **kidneys** have an endocrine role as they produce **erythropoietin**, a hormone that drives the production of red blood cells. The kidneys also produce renin, which is both an enzyme and a hormone, and converts vitamin D precursor to the active form of **vitamin D**.

The **pancreas** (Fig. 10.14) is composed of both exocrine and endocrine tissue. As an **exocrine gland**, its **acinar** components produce digestive enzymes and bicarbonate (a buffering molecule) needed in the gastrointestinal tract to digest food. As an **endocrine gland**, the pancreas releases hormones needed to maintain homeostasis associated with blood glucose levels. These hormones are secreted by specialised structures inside the pancreas called islets of Langerhans that are composed of different endocrine cells. **Alpha cells (α-cells)** secrete **glucagon**, needed to increase blood glucose levels and stimulate **gluconeogenesis** through the breakdown of glycogen, and in the absence of an adequate source of glycogen, glucagon breaks down protein and fat. **Beta cells (β-cells)** secrete **insulin**, which stimulates cellular uptake of glucose, amino acids and fatty acids, thus leading to a reduction of these nutrients in the blood. **Delta cells (δ-cells)** secrete **somatostatin**, whose main role is to regulate other endocrine cells of the pancreatic islets and inhibit secretion of glucagon, insulin and **pancreatic peptide (PP)**. **F-cells or PP-cells** produce PP, a hormone that plays a role in gastrointestinal motility, function of the exocrine pancreas and the feeling of fullness or satiety. Epsilon cells (ε-cells) secrete **ghrelin**, a hormone that stimulates the hypothalamus to increase appetite and decrease the metabolic rate.

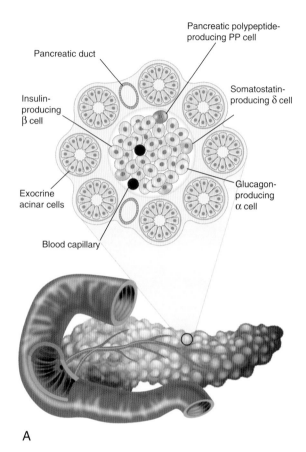

A

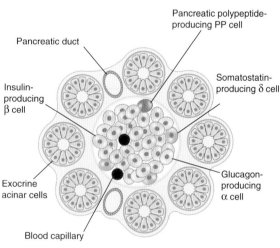

B

FIGURE 10.14 **A Anatomy of the pancreas.
B Anatomy of the pancreatic islet of Langerhans.**

Gastrointestinal mucosa secretes hormones such as gastrin, secretin and cholecystokinin, all important in the digestive process (see below).

The **testes** are paired primary male sex organs found within the scrotum. Their role is to produce **testosterone** to support the formation of new male sex cells. **Ovaries** are paired primary female gonads found in the pelvic cavity, which generate ova (eggs) and participate in the menstrual cycle. Hormones secreted by the ovaries include **progesterone**, **oestrogen** and **inhibin**.

The **placenta** forms at the time of **zygote** formation and serves to separate the fetus from maternal organs and to act as an interface between the circulatory system of the mother and the fetus. hCG is secreted by the fetal tissue component of the placenta called the **chorion**. The placenta also produces progesterone, oestrogen, relaxin and human placental lactogen (hPL), also known as somatomammotropin.

Muscles produce hormones that are collectively known as **myokines**. Examples of myokines are **irisin**, which participates in the conversion of white fat to brown fat, and **interleukin-6**, which signals to the liver to release glucose needed to meet exercise demands.

Finally, for a long time it was thought that **adipose tissue** was a site to store excess energy in the form of fatty molecules. It is only in the past three decades that it has been ascribed an endocrine role through the production of leptin, resistin and lipokine. **Leptin** has a diverse role in reproductive function, control of menstruation, immunity and energy balance. **Resistin** reduces receptor sensitivity to insulin leading to increased blood glucose levels, and lipokine increases receptor insulin sensitivity.[3]

INTEGRATION WITH OTHER BODY SYSTEMS

Endocrine glands and their hormones are linked to nearly every cell in the body. In this section we highlight the major ways in which the endocrine system acts to coordinate and maintain body homeostasis.

Integumentary system

The endocrine system plays a role in skin development, physiological function and overall skin health. Skin is a site where clinical manifestations of endocrine disorders can easily be observed, due to hypersecretion or hyposecretion of hormones. For example, loss of pigmentation may be due to reduced levels of MSH, while with the loss of pituitary gland hormones (**hypopituitarism**) clinicians are likely to observe pale skin with a yellow tinge on the palms, soles and nasolabial folds.[4]

Skin cells, namely keratinocytes and melanocytes, not only receive signals from the endocrine system, but also synthesise hormones such as catecholamines, produced by keratinocytes, ACTH, MSH and eicosanoids.[5] Skin produces and secretes testosterone and oestrogen into the blood circulation.[6] Skin also synthesises vitamin D precursor (Chapter 3) and releases it into the circulation to be converted to an active form in the kidneys. Vitamin D is fundamental to maintaining bone health.

Musculoskeletal system

Bone health relies on the appropriate regulation of calcium metabolism. As calcium is critical to the function of muscle contractions—including cardiac, blood coagulation (haemostasis) and nerve impulse conduction—its levels are tightly regulated. Calcium balance is regulated by the endocrine, digestive, musculoskeletal and urinary systems (Fig. 10.15).

The only way to obtain calcium is through the diet. It is absorbed in the gastrointestinal tract and enters the bloodstream. This leads to an increase of existing blood calcium levels, which is detected by the thyroid gland. The thyroid gland releases calcitonin from the parafollicular cells. Calcitonin acts to inhibits bone osteoclast activity and increase bone uptake of calcium, thus building the hard bone matrix. It also acts on the kidneys to decrease kidney reabsorption of calcium from the filtrate it produces during blood filtration. Collectively, this results in a decrease in blood calcium levels. A decreased dietary intake of calcium, and therefore decreased blood calcium concentration, is sensed by the parathyroid gland, which then releases PTH, which stimulates osteoclast proliferation and bone resorption by the proliferating osteoclasts, leading to bone demineralisation or breakdown of the hard matrix. Therefore, calcium and phosphate ions are released into the blood. PTH also promotes absorption of calcium from the filtrate via the kidneys back into the blood and stimulates vitamin D synthesis, also in the kidneys, to stimulate calcium absorption in the gastrointestinal tract. Note that PTH and calcitonin have opposing or antagonistic effects on calcium concentration in the blood. Collectively, these processes restore blood calcium concentration to normal, thus ensuring normal calcium-dependent processes such as nerve impulse conduction and muscular contractions.

Nervous system

The collective work of the nervous and endocrine systems allows chemical messengers and accompanied information to be communicated throughout the body. We have already mentioned how some neuronal

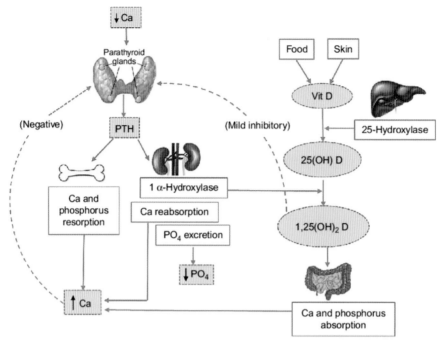

FIGURE 10.15 **Calcium homeostasis.** (*Source:* Song L. Calcium and bone metabolism indices. Adv Clin Chem 2017;82:1–46.)

tissue can also act as endocrine tissue (neuroendocrine tissue). However, in addition to this, the nervous and endocrine systems communicate with each other and this is clearly demonstrated in two specific events that have a significant impact on human health: the sleep–wake cycle and the fight or flight response. The anatomy and physiology of the sleep–wake cycle was addressed in Chapter 7.

The fight or flight response is fundamental to our survival and it simultaneously engages multiple body systems to keep us safe. When there is a perceived threat the autonomic nervous system, via the sympathetic nervous system branch, activates a cascade of events that enable a fast response. The initial threat is interpreted by the **amygdala**. From here signals are sent to the hypothalamus to stimulate the pituitary gland to release ACTH. The sympathetic nervous system activates the adrenal gland to release adrenaline (epinephrine) and noradrenaline (norepinephrine). Cortisol is also released by the adrenal gland under the influence of ACTH. This leads to an increase in blood pressure, blood glucose concentration, concentration of fatty acids in the blood and suppression of the immune system. Adrenaline (epinephrine) binds to hepatocytes and stimulates the

production and release of glucose into the blood. Adrenaline (epinephrine) and noradrenaline (norepinephrine) further act on multiple systems to induce a heightened response. For example, in the cardiovascular system there is an increase in heart contractility, dilation of coronary blood vessels and an increased heart rate. In the respiratory system bronchodilation enables the person to take more air as the rate and depth of breathing increase. There is constriction of blood vessels in the gastrointestinal tract to minimise blood flow there, and the spleen contracts to contain less blood. There is increased blood flow to the muscles and increased muscle tension needed to run, and an overall increase in nutrients to support the metabolic needs to respond to the threat.

Special senses: hearing, balance and vision

Very little is known about the effect of the endocrine system on the eyes and ears, with most information available connected to inborn genetic abnormalities or acquired conditions affecting the endocrine system. For example, mutations in a gene that encodes the growth factor receptor lead to hearing loss or abnormalities in how sound is interpreted.[7] Endocrine disorders such as chronic, poorly managed diabetes can lead to loss of both hearing and vision through changes in the structural components of the ear and eye, respectively.

Blood

The formation of new red blood cells from erythropoietic progenitors, their survival and differentiation is regulated by **erythropoietin (EPO)**, a hormone produced primarily by the kidneys, with small concentrations also produced by the liver and brain.[8] Erythropoietin synthesis is stimulated by a fall in tissue oxygen pressure, commonly known as **hypoxia**. Angiotensin II is thought to stimulate erythropoietin production and act as a growth factor for myeloid progenitors,[9] while the effect of EPO on erythropoiesis is potentiated by testosterone and somatotropin.[8] It is also proposed that oestrogen may play a role in the development of haematopoietic stem cells.[10]

Haemostasis

The link between the endocrine system and the body's capacity to form blood clots required to seal a wound occurs through regulation of calcium homeostasis, as described above. Calcium is an important cofactor in the coagulation cascade that enables formation of a fibrin clot. Endocrine disorders of the thyroid and pituitary gland are associated with clotting abnormalities, although the mechanisms as to how this occurs are not well understood.[11]

Cardiovascular system

The heart atria release ANP, a hormone that participates in homeostasis of the blood pressure (Fig. 10.16). This mechanism is activated by the atrial response to increased stretch induced by high blood pressure inside the atria. The hormone is released into circulation and targets the juxtaglomerular apparatus in the kidneys, the posterior pituitary gland via baroreceptors, and the adrenal cortex. In the kidneys, ANP reduces renin release, which leads to vasodilation. In the posterior pituitary gland, ANP causes a decrease in ADH release, which impacts on the collecting ducts in the kidneys, forcing them to decrease sodium and water reabsorption and thus reducing blood volume and therefore blood pressure. Reduction in blood volume and blood pressure decreases the atrial stretch. ANP's effect on the adrenal cortex leads to a decrease in aldosterone synthesis, thus potentiating the effect of increasing sodium and water excretion into urine, leading to reduced blood pressure due to loss of blood volume. This is an example of a negative feedback loop. Additionally, increased blood concentration of thyroid hormone levels is associated with an increased heart rate, cardiac

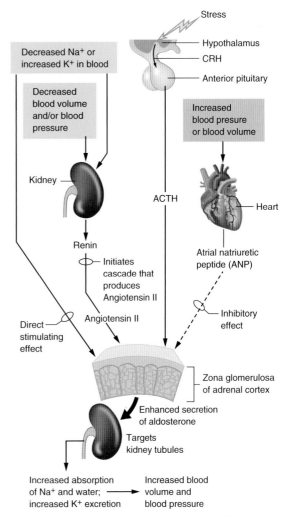

FIGURE 10.16 **Integrated communication between atrial natriuretic peptide and the renin angiotensin aldosterone system.**

contractility and cardiac output and plays a role in peripheral vasodilation, leading to increased blood organ perfusion.

Lymphatic system

The lymphatic system is intricately linked with the cardiovascular and immune systems. While some evidence exists that lymphatic vessels can respond to hormonal stimulation, such as adrenaline (epinephrine) and noradrenaline (norepinephrine), that evidence comes from animal studies and has not been confirmed in human lymphatic vessels.

Respiratory system

Hormones released by endocrine glands are delivered to lung tissue through the pulmonary circulation. The respiratory system is important in gas exchange, speech and phonation, and regulation of blood pH homeostasis. Abnormalities in hormone secretions may impact these functions.[12] For example, increased concentration of thyroid hormones and their effect on increased metabolism will be accompanied by an increased respiratory rate (number of breaths per minute). Other hormones that act in a stimulating manner include growth hormone, progesterone and testosterone, while adrenaline (epinephrine) can induce bronchodilation.[12]

Immune system

The relationship between the immune and endocrine systems is bidirectional. Evidence exists that corticosteroids inhibit immune cells from secreting cytokines such as interleukin I and II, whereas cortisol inhibits the production of interferon gamma, which increases natural killer cell activity. Similarly, the immune system, through secretion of cytokines (such as interleukin I), can impact the secretion of hormones such as ACTH through its impact on hypothalamic secretion of CRH.[13]

Gastrointestinal system

The gastrointestinal system has a role in food breakdown and absorption. This occurs in the gut and is assisted by secretions from organs such as the liver and pancreas. As described previously, as an exocrine gland the pancreas secretes enzymes needed to break down food into valuable nutrients, including glucose. As an endocrine gland, the pancreas maintains homeostatic control of glucose absorbed from the gut into the blood by secreting two antagonistic hormones: insulin and glucagon (Fig. 10.17). Thus, after a meal has been digested, when glucose is absorbed from the gastrointestinal tract into the bloodstream, there is an increase in blood glucose concentration, known as **hyperglycaemia**.[3] This is sensed in the pancreatic β-cells located in the islets of Langerhans through a specialised receptor called GLUT 2, which is a member of the glucose transporter receptors. This stimulates insulin release. Increased insulin concentration in the blood results in increased glucose uptake by the liver, muscles and other cells, thus reducing blood glucose concentration. This occurs via GLUT 4 insulin receptor, which is found on skeletal and cardiac muscle and adipose tissue. It is important to note that insulin secretion can be stimulated by other factors, such as some amino acids and the gastrointestinal hormones gastrin, secretin and cholecystokinin (CKK), although not to the same extent as blood glucose concentrations. When

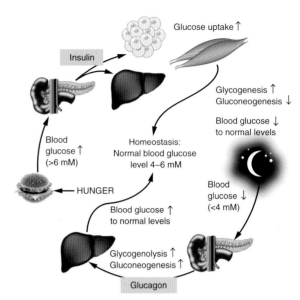

FIGURE 10.17 **Glucose homeostasis.**

insulin concentrations are high, carbohydrates are used as a source of energy rather than fats. Excess glucose is converted to glycogen and is stored in the liver and muscles as a readily available source of energy.

In contrast, when the blood glucose level falls below a certain threshold (e.g. 3.5 mmol/L), a state known as **hypoglycaemia**, insulin production is inhibited and α-cells, also found in the islets of Langerhans, secrete glucagon.[3] Glucagon acts on hepatic cells to initiate breakdown of glycogen (**glycogenolysis**) and increase **gluconeogenesis**. Both processes lead to increased availability of glucose in the blood. Somatostatin, secreted by the δ-cells of the islets of Langerhans, inhibits both insulin and glucagon production. It also decreases gastrointestinal secretion, absorption and motility.[3]

During stress, adrenaline (epinephrine) can cause glycogenolysis in the liver and mediate conversion of fat into fatty acids, leading to increased availability of resources needed to manage the situation at hand.

Nutrition and metabolism

The hypothalamus secretes TRH, which stimulates the anterior pituitary gland to secrete TSH. This hormone then binds to the receptors on epithelial cells in the thyroid gland, leading to synthesis of T3 and T4 hormones (Fig. 10.9). These hormones are released into the blood and when they reach a certain concentration signals are sent to the hypothalamus to inhibit further secretion of TRH. This negative feedback loop is constantly in action. Thyroid hormones stimulate lipid and carbohydrate metabolism, so it may not be surprising that high levels of thyroid hormone lead to an increased metabolic rate, increased rate of gastrointestinal absorption, increased body heat production and stimulation of fat mobilisation and breakdown, evident as increased levels of fatty acids in the blood. High levels of thyroid hormone also lead to gluconeogenesis and glycogenolysis and increased insulin-dependent uptake of glucose by the cells.[14]

Urinary system

The kidneys produce EPO and their function is heavily regulated by hormones. For example, kidney health is fundamental to blood pressure regulation, fluid and electrolyte balance, and systemic vascular resistance. The system responsible for this is the **renin-angiotensin-aldosterone system (RAAS)** (Fig. 10.18).

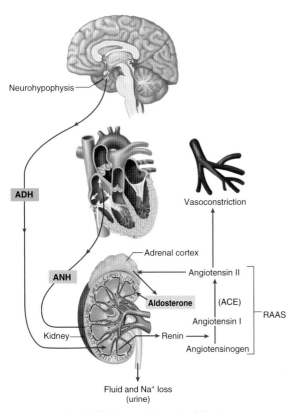

FIGURE 10.18 Renin angiotensin aldosterone system. (*Source:* Patton KT, Thibodeau GA. Skin. In: Patton KT, Thibodeau GA, editors. Anatomy and physiology, 10 ed. London: Elsevier Health Sciences; 2017.)

If there is a reduction in blood pressure, for example through loss of blood volume such as with dehydration or haemorrhage, there will be reduced blood flow to the glomerulus. This loss of blood pressure is also detected by baroreceptors in the carotid sinus. The reduction in glomerular blood pressure, described also as a loss of renal blood perfusion, is detected by specialised cells located in the juxtaglomerular apparatus located in the kidney nephrons. The juxtaglomerular apparatus produces **renin** by converting a precursor molecule, prorenin, into renin then secretes it into the blood circulation. In blood renin encounters angiotensinogen, which is produced by the liver, and converts it to angiotensinogen I. This molecule travels in the circulation and as it reaches the lung capillaries it is converted to angiotensin II by **angiotensin-converting enzyme (ACE)** found on the surface of lung capillary endothelium.

Angiotensin II exerts several powerful functions. First, it causes small-calibre vessels to narrow, leading to an increase in blood pressure. Second, it stimulates secretion of **aldosterone** from the adrenal cortex, leading to an increase in distal tubule and collecting duct absorption of sodium and water while excreting potassium, a process that leads to increased volume in the blood and therefore increased blood pressure. Third, it leads to a release of ADH, which is made in the hypothalamus and secreted by the posterior pituitary gland. ADH controls the volume of urine created by causing water reabsorption so that less volume is lost. It also exerts action on the central nervous system to stimulate the thirst centre so that the person feels the need to drink more water, to increase intravascular volume. Remember that ANP acts opposite to this process as its aim is to reduce blood pressure through increasing loss of water and sodium from the body.

As previously mentioned, PTH also acts on the kidneys to produce the active form of vitamin D, which stimulates the gut to increase intestinal absorption of calcium ions from digested food.

Reproductive system

As noted above, the gonads (testes in males and ovaries in females) are the main source of sex hormones involved in the development of male and female reproductive organs, secondary sexual characteristics and production of sperm and egg. These same hormones also play a role in breast development, menstruation and pregnancy. Hormonal control of the male and female reproductive systems is covered in Chapter 21 and the role of hormones in pregnancy is covered in Chapter 22. In this chapter, we focus on the **hypothalamic-pituitary-gonadal**

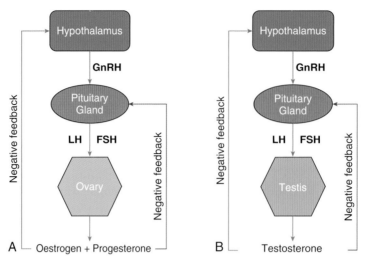

FIGURE 10.19 **Hypothalamic-pituitary-gonadal axis. A** Female. **B** Male. (*Source:* Brunton L, Hilal-Dandan R, Knollmann BC. Goodman's and Gilman's the pharmacological basis of therapeutics, 13 ed. OH: McGraw-Hill Education; 2018.)

axis (Fig. 10.19), which describes the communication system between the hypothalamus, pituitary gland and testes (in males) and ovaries (in females). Here the hypothalamus secretes GnRH, which travels into the hypophyseal portal system to the anterior pituitary gland where it stimulates endocrine cells to produce and release FSH and LH into the bloodstream. In turn FSH and LH act on the ovaries to instruct oestrogen production to regulate the ovarian cycle and the menstrual cycle. The oestrogen level forms part of a negative feedback loop, whereby it inhibits hypothalamic secretion of GnRH. The **hypothalamic-pituitary-ovarian axis** can be inhibited by hormonal contraceptives. Similarly, abnormalities in hormonal secretion that affect this axis may lead to ovulation-related disorders. To induce ovulation, for example during fertility-related treatments such as in vitro fertilisation (IVF), this axis can be affected by administering medications that stimulate an increase in FSH and therefore follicle development.

In males, LH stimulates testicular interstitial cells to produce testosterone, while FSH regulates the formation of new sperm through the process of spermatogenesis. In the male reproductive system, testosterone forms part of the negative feedback loop to shut down the production of GnRH.

Pregnancy and lactation

The endocrine system plays an important and highly complex role in pregnancy, including the development and maintenance of pregnancy, fetal health, childbirth and lactation. The mother's body, including her endocrine system, must adjust to endocrine changes associated with fetus development. We have already discussed the role of oxytocin in labour. **Oxytocin**, together with prolactin, is also directly involved in lactation and breastfeeding, another example of a positive feedback loop.

Oxytocin, released from the posterior pituitary gland in response to suckling, induces contraction of the myoepithelial cells in the breast alveoli, thus forcing milk to flow away from the alveolar epithelium towards ducts where it gathers for the next feed. Interestingly, the effect of oxytocin is driven by the mother–baby relationship, a mechanism described as the oxytocin reflex.[15] The mother's positive actions and thoughts towards her baby—such as touch, smell or seeing her baby—condition oxytocin release. This means that oxytocin, which is produced at a faster rate than prolactin, can very quickly make milk ready for the current feed and reduce the work for the baby needed to get the milk.[15]

Prolactin, released by the anterior pituitary gland in response to suckling, regulates the secretion of milk from glandular epithelial cells in the breast alveoli. Although prolactin is present during pregnancy, its effect is blocked by oestrogen and progesterone as they maintain pregnancy towards full term. After birth, progesterone and oestrogen concentrations fall rapidly and their inhibiting effect on prolactin is lost. When a newborn suckles, this acts as a stimulant to increase prolactin production and release it into the blood, in turn increasing stimulation to produce breast milk.

Interestingly, prolactin is produced at night and is stated to have a relaxing and sleepy effect on the mother, despite the fact that she is frequently awake at night to breastfeed.[15]

It is also of note that endocrine disorders can affect pregnancy. For example, during pregnancy, thyroid hormones are frequently assessed as abnormal levels of thyroid hormones are associated with fetal developmental abnormalities, including mental retardation. This is because thyroid hormones play an important role in all aspects of fetal brain development. Subsequently, iodine deficiency, seen in many underdeveloped countries, poses a significant threat to the development of a healthy baby.[16] Adequate levels of **vitamin D** are also important during pregnancy as the fetus depends on the mother for supply of vitamin D, needed for bone growth and development. Failure to obtain sufficient levels of vitamin D leads to the development of congenital rickets, which is characterised by a weakened bone structure that predisposes bones to bending as the child learns to bear weight, stand and walk.

AGE-RELATED CHANGES

With ageing there is a loss of endocrine tissue cells through atrophy, leading to decreased production of hormones—for example, oestrogen in females, growth hormone and melatonin. Older people start to have difficulties sleeping as decreased melatonin impacts on the sleep–wake cycle.

Ageing liver may offset some of these changes as the clearance of hormones also slows down. The pancreas starts to lose endocrine cells and this impacts on the secretion of hormones that control glucose metabolism, leading to a higher risk of developing diabetes. Some hormone receptors may become less sensitive, for example those for insulin. There is also disruption of the hypothalamic-pituitary-gonad axis characterised by reduced production of sex hormones in both men and women. This has an impact on fertility as well as sexual characteristics such as voice colour (tone), and facial and body hair distribution. Women's natural fertility is lost between 42 and 50 years of age due to natural declining oestrogen levels; while testosterone declines in men as they age, it seems to be a slower process as some men can father children when they are 80. Until recently, hormone replacement therapy was often used to alleviate menopause-related symptoms such as hot flushes, sudden onset of sweating and vaginal dryness. However, research has shown that this intervention may have harmful consequences in women over 60 years of age, such as coronary artery disease, stroke, blood clots and dementia, so this therapy is now used more judiciously.[17,18]

CONCLUSION

The endocrine system is a very complex regulator of cellular processes in the body. This chapter discussed the structure and function of the most important endocrine glands and their principal hormones. Most importantly, the endocrine system links several body systems together to control these processes—for example, the link between the endocrine, cardiac, nervous and urinary systems to control fluid balance and blood pressure. From a clinical perspective, you may manage patients with diabetes and assist with insulin administration during hospitalisation or in aged care settings. Furthermore, you may encounter endocrine disorders caused by hypersecretion or hyposecretion of hormones, which will impact more than one body system and manifest in complex signs and symptoms. Age-related changes dampen the endocrine system's capacity to maintain body homeostasis and these changes substantially impact our health as we get older. Resolving age-related endocrine changes with hormone replacement therapy is clinically done only if the benefits outweigh the risks.

TABLE 10.1 Major endocrine glands and hormones				
Gland	**Hormone**	**Chemical structure**	**Major function**	**Target tissue**
Hypothalamus	Thyrotropin-releasing hormone (TRH)	Peptide	Stimulates secretion of thyroid-stimulating hormone and prolactin	Anterior pituitary gland
	Corticotropin-releasing hormone (CRH)	Peptide	Causes release of adrenocorticotropic hormone	Anterior pituitary gland

Continued

TABLE 10.1
Major endocrine glands and hormones—cont'd

Gland	Hormone	Chemical structure	Major function	Target tissue
	Growth hormone (GH) releasing hormone	Peptide	Causes release of growth hormone	Anterior pituitary gland
	Growth hormone (GH) inhibitory hormone	Peptide	Inhibits release of growth hormone	Anterior pituitary gland
	Gonadotropin-releasing hormone (GnRH)	Peptide	Causes release of luteinising hormone and follicle-stimulating hormone	Anterior pituitary gland
	Dopamine or prolactin (PRL) inhibiting factor	Amine	Inhibits release of prolactin	Anterior pituitary gland
	Antidiuretic hormone (ADH) (synthesis only)	Peptide	Conserves water by preventing formation of large volume of urine; increases water permeability in distal tubules and collecting ducts of nephrons; regulates blood pressure; vasoconstriction	Kidneys Blood vessels
	Oxytocin (OT) (synthesis only)	Peptide	Causes milk ejection from lactating breast; stimulates contraction of uterine muscles during childbirth	Uterus Mammary glands
	Prolactin-releasing hormone (PRH)	Not known	This is a putative hormone in humans proposed to stimulate release of prolactin	Anterior pituitary gland
Anterior pituitary gland	Growth hormone (GH)	Protein	Stimulates protein synthesis and overall growth of most cells and tissues; stimulates fat metabolism; shifts a cell's use of nutrients away from carbohydrates to lipid catabolism; growth and development of muscle and bone	Nearly all cells in early human life span; later effect more on fat tissue, muscle, bone
	Thyroid-stimulating hormone (TSH)	Glycoprotein	Stimulates synthesis and secretion of thyroxine and triiodothyronine; promotes and maintains thyroid gland growth and development	Thyroid gland
	Melanocyte-stimulating hormone (MSH)	Peptide	Regulates skin pigmentation	Melanocytes (skin)
	Adrenocorticotropic hormone (ACTH)	Protein	Stimulates synthesis and secretion of adrenocortical hormones (cortisol, androgens and aldosterone); promotes and maintains growth and development of adrenal cortex	Adrenal cortex
	Prolactin (PRL)	Protein	Promotes development of female breasts during pregnancy and secretion of milk after childbirth	Mammary glands

TABLE 10.1
Major endocrine glands and hormones—cont'd

Gland	Hormone	Chemical structure	Major function	Target tissue
	Follicle-stimulating hormone (FSH)	Glycoprotein	*Female:* causes growth of follicles in the ovaries and oestrogen secretion *Male:* maintains spermatogenesis in Sertoli cells of testes; stimulates development of seminiferous tubules of testes	Ovaries Testes
	Luteinising hormone (LH)	Glycoprotein	*Female:* stimulates formation and activity of corpus luteum, which secretes progesterone and oestrogen in response; stimulates ovulation *Male:* stimulates testosterone synthesis in Leydig cells of testes	Ovaries Testes
Posterior pituitary gland	Antidiuretic hormone (ADH) (release)	Peptide	Conserves water by preventing formation of large volume of urine; increases water permeability in distal tubules and collecting ducts of nephrons; regulates blood pressure; vasoconstriction	Kidneys Blood vessels
	Oxytocin (OT) (release)	Peptide	Stimulates milk ejection from breasts and uterine contractions	Uterus Mammary glands
Pineal gland	Melatonin	Amine	Regulates sleep cycle (circadian rhythm)	Brain (suprachiasmatic nuclei)
Thyroid gland	Thyroxine (T4) and triiodothyronine (T3)	Iodinated amino acids	Increase the rates of chemical reactions in most cells, thus increasing body metabolic rate; regulate cell growth and cell differentiation	All cells
	Calcitonin (CT)	Protein	Promotes deposition of calcium in bone matrix; decreases blood Ca^{2+} concentration	Bone
Parathyroid gland	Parathyroid hormone (PTH)	Protein	Controls blood Ca^{2+} concentration by increasing calcium absorption by the gut and kidneys and by promoting breakdown of bone matrix, thus releasing calcium from bones into circulation; stimulates kidneys to produce active vitamin D required for gut Ca^{2+} absorption	Bone Kidneys
Thymus	Thymosin		T-cell development and maturation; immune function	Thymus
	Thymopoietin		T-cell development and maturation; immune function	Thymus
Heart	Atrial natriuretic peptide (ANP)	Peptide	Increases sodium excretion by kidneys; reduces blood pressure	Kidneys

Continued

TABLE 10.1
Major endocrine glands and hormones—cont'd

Gland	Hormone	Chemical structure	Major function	Target tissue
Adrenal cortex	Cortisol	Steroid	Multiple functions for controlling metabolism of proteins, carbohydrates and fats; reduces inflammation; dampens immune responses; increases blood glucose concentration	Almost all cells
	Aldosterone	Steroid	Increases renal sodium reabsorption, potassium secretion and hydrogen ion secretion	Kidneys
Adrenal medulla	Adrenaline (epinephrine)	Amine	Same effects as sympathetic stimulation i.e. increased blood pressure, increased heart rate, increased cell metabolism	Most organs blood vessels
	Noradrenaline (norepinephrine)	Amine	Same effects as sympathetic stimulation i.e. increased blood pressure, increased heart rate, vasoconstriction	Most organs Blood vessels
Kidneys	Renin	Peptide	Catalyses conversion of angiotensinogen to angiotensin I; renin is produced by juxtaglomerular apparatus cells and released into circulation, which is characteristic for hormones	No tissue target, acts as an enzyme
	1,25-dihydroxycholecalciferol	Steroid	Increases intestinal absorption of calcium and bone mineralisation	Bone Gut
	Erythropoietin	Peptide	Increases erythrocyte production	Bone marrow
Pancreas	Insulin (pancreatic β-cells)	Peptide	Promotes glucose entry in many cells and in this way controls carbohydrate metabolism	Nearly all cells
	Glucagon (pancreatic α-cells)	Peptide	Increases synthesis and release of glucose from liver into body fluids	Hepatocytes (liver) Muscle
	Somatostatin (SS) (pancreatic δ-cells)		Inhibits glucagon and insulin secretion; affects neurotransmission and cell proliferation	Parietal cells (stomach) Pancreatic α- and β-cells
	Pancreatic peptide (PP-cells)		Suppresses exocrine pancreatic function; decreases gastric emptying; reduces feeling of hunger	Gastrointestinal system
	Ghrelin (ε-cells)		Stimulates hunger, promotes appetite and fat storage; also produced by stomach	Brain (amygdala)
Stomach	Gastrin	Peptide	Stimulates hydrogen chloride secretion by parietal cells	Stomach
Small intestine	Secretin	Peptide	Stimulates pancreatic acinar cells to release bicarbonate and water	Pancreas
	Cholecystokinin	Peptide	Stimulates gallbladder contraction and release of pancreatic enzymes	Gallbladder Pancreas

TABLE 10.1
Major endocrine glands and hormones—cont'd

Gland	Hormone	Chemical structure	Major function	Target tissue
Testes	Testosterone	Steroid	Promotes development and maintenance of male reproductive system and male secondary sexual characteristics such as sexual drive, pubic/armpit hair; spermatogenesis	Testes Bone Skeletal muscle RBC production Anterior pituitary (negative feedback on testosterone production)
Ovaries	Oestrogens	Steroid	Promotes growth, development and maturation of female reproductive system, female breasts and female secondary sexual characteristics such as mammary glands, pubic hair; ova maturation	Ovaries Anterior pituitary (negative feedback on FSH and LH secretion) Mammary glands
	Progesterone	Steroid	Maintains lining of uterus for egg implantation; breast development	Uterus (preparation for pregnancy) Anterior pituitary (negative feedback on FSH and LH secretion)
	Inhibin		Suppresses FSH production and inhibits FSH secretion; also produced in pituitary gland, placenta and corpus luteum	Anterior pituitary gland
Placenta	Human chorionic gonadotropin (hCG)	Peptide	Promotes growth of corpus luteum and secretion of oestrogens and progesterone by corpus luteum	Ovarian corpus luteum
	Human somatomammotropin (human placental lactogen)	Peptide	Decreases maternal insulin sensitivity; decreases maternal glucose utilisation, increases fat metabolism	Mammary glands Adipose tissue
	Oestrogens	Steroid	As for ovaries	As for ovaries
	Progesterone	Steroid	As for ovaries	As for ovaries
Muscle	Irisin	Protein	Exercise-induced myokine; putative role in conversion of white fat to brown fat	Adipose tissue Muscle
	Interleukin-6		Supports anti-inflammatory reactions when secreted by muscles in response to exercise	Muscle
Adipocytes	Leptin	Peptide	Maintains body fat deposits	Hypothalamus
	Resistin	Peptide	Likely involved in insulin resistance, energy metabolism	Liver
	Lipokine	Steroid	Systemic metabolism	Muscle Liver

CASE STUDY 10.1

Ginger and Freda have been going to the gym regularly, determined to lose weight. Both women are healthy eaters and do not smoke, drink alcohol or eat junk food. While Freda has shed 5 kg in the past three months, Ginger has not lost any weight. Disappointed by this outcome, she confided to Freda that she was starting to lose her motivation to exercise. Freda suggested there might be a health-related reason why Ginger has not lost any weight and said it would be worth talking to her local health clinic. Ginger visited her local clinic where a nurse practitioner suggested that a blood test should be done to check her thyroid function.

Q1. What are hormones?

   a. Chemical messengers secreted by the exocrine system

   b. Chemical messengers secreted by the endocrine system

   c. Chemical messengers secreted by the exocrine and endocrine systems

   d. Chemical messengers secreted by the nervous system

Q2. Which endocrine gland is found in the thyroid gland?

   a. Pancreas

   b. Anterior pituitary gland

   c. Posterior pituitary gland

   d. Parathyroid gland

Q3. Thyroid hormones regulate:

   a. metabolism.

   b. growth.

   c. body temperature.

   d. all of the above.

Q4. Discuss the storage and secretion of T3 and T4.

Q5. Discuss which hormone might be responsible for Ginger's lack of weight loss despite regular exercise.

CASE STUDY 10.2

Today, your patient is 12-year-old Gabby, a bright bubbly girl who is morbidly obese for her age. She was admitted last night to the emergency department. Doctors are sure that Gabby has diabetes but are yet to define whether she has type 1 or type 2 due to the obesity factor. For the moment, while the treating team is awaiting further blood tests, you are asked to teach Gabby about the role of diet in managing diabetes. As you enter her room, you see that Gabby is eating a hamburger, with her mum by her side. You also notice that on Gabby's table there is an open block of chocolate, a bag of sweets and an open can of soft drink.

Q1. Which hormone is responsible for regulating glucose levels following meal ingestion?

   a. Glycogen

   b. Glucagon

   c. Insulin

   d. Parathyroid hormone

Q2. Which hormone is produced by pancreatic α-cells?

   a. Somatostatin

   b. Insulin

   c. Ghrelin

   d. Glucagon

Q3. When a person starts to feel hungry, which hormone signals to the brain to feel hunger?

   a. Somatostatin

   b. Ghrelin

   c. Glucagon

   d. Insulin

Q4. Should you be worried that Gabby is eating a hamburger and that there is an open block of chocolate, a bag of sweets and a can of soft drink on her bedside table? Provide a rationale for your answer.

Q5. If Gabby's pancreas does not make insulin, what effect will this have on glucose homeostasis?

CASE STUDY 10.3

Georgia, who is 12 weeks pregnant, visited her doctor to review the blood tests that were taken as part of the routine check on the mother's health. Her doctor told Georgia that her vitamin D levels are very low and that she needs to start taking supplements immediately, as vitamin D deficiency may impact on the bone development of her unborn child.

Q1. Which hormone is made by the thyroid gland?
   a. Testosterone
   b. Parathyroid hormone
   c. Calcitonin
   d. Adrenaline (epinephrine)

Q2. Calcitonin can be structurally classified as:
   a. steroid hormone.
   b. glycoprotein hormone.
   c. protein hormone.
   d. amino acid derivative.

Q3. As parathyroid hormone acts on bone cells, it can be classified as:
   a. exocrine hormone.
   b. paracrine hormone.
   c. endocrine hormone.
   d. autocrine hormone.

Q4. Discuss how low levels of maternal vitamin D may impact on the bone development of an unborn child.

Q5. Propose what might be the long-term consequences for infant growth and development if vitamin D levels continue to be insufficient to meet the needs of the growing infant.

CASE STUDY 10.4

A young couple has been trying for a baby for three years without success. They contact a fertility specialist who runs a series of tests to determine why they cannot conceive. These tests investigate their levels of various reproductive hormones.

Q1. Which of the following hormones are produced by the ovaries?
   a. Oestrogen, progesterone and inhibin
   b. Oestrogen, follicle-stimulating hormone and inhibin
   c. Luteinising hormone, oestrogen and inhibin
   d. Progesterone, oestrogen and luteinising hormone

Q2. The placenta is an endocrine organ because it produces:
   a. human chorionic gonadotropin (hCG) and relaxin.
   b. follicle-stimulating hormone.
   c. atrial natriuretic peptide.
   d. erythropoietin.

Q3. Which hormone can be used as a blood test to determine the viability of a fetus in the first three months of pregnancy?
   a. Oestrogen
   b. Testosterone
   c. Oxytocin
   d. Human chorionic gonadotropin (hCG)

Q4. Suggest which hormones would be tested to determine causes of infertility in males and females.

Q5. Propose how hormonal insufficiency might lead to issues with infertility in males and females.

REFERENCES

1. Hall JE. Introduction to endocrinology. In: Hall JE, editor. Guyton and Hall textbook of medical physiology. Philadelphia: Saunders; 2011. p. 881–93.
2. Pollard TD, Earnshaw WC, Lippincott-Schwartz J, et al. Second messengers. In: Pollard TD, Earnshaw WC, Lippincott-Schwartz J, et al, editors. Cell biology. Philadelphia: Elsevier; 2017. p. 443–62.
3. Hall JE. Insulin, glucagon and diabetes mellitus. In: Hall JE, editor. Guyton and Hall textbook of medical physiology. Philadelphia: Saunders; 2011. p. 939–54.
4. Demirkesen C. Skin manifestations of endocrine diseases. Turk Patoloji Derg 2015;31(Suppl.):145–54.
5. Zouboulis CC. Human skin: an independent peripheral endocrine organ. Horm Res 2000;54:230–42.
6. Orfanos CE, Adler YD, Zouboulis CC. The SAHA syndrome. Horm Res 2000;54(5–6):251–8.
7. Cherian KE, Kapoor N, Mathews SS, et al. Endocrine glands and hearing: auditory manifestations of various endocrine and metabolic conditions. Indian J Endocrinol Metab 2017; 21(3):464–9.
8. Jelkmann W. Regulation of erythropoietin production. J Physiol 2011;589(6):1251–8.

9. Freudenthaler SM, Schreeb K, Korner T, et al. Angiotensin II increases erythropoietin production in healthy human volunteers. Eur J Clin Invest 1999;29(10):816–23.

10. Heo HR, Chen L, An B, et al. Hormonal regulation of hematopoietic stem cells and their niche: a focus on estrogen. Int J Stem Cells 2015;8(1):18–23.

11. Kyriakakis N, Lynch J, Ajjan R, et al. The effects of pituitary and thyroid disorders on haemostasis: potential clinical implications. Clin Endocrinol (Oxf) 2016;84(4):473–84.

12. Lencu C, Alexescu T, Petrulea M, et al. Respiratory manifestations in endocrine diseases. Clujul Med 2016;89(4):459–63.

13. Chryssikopoulos A. The relationship between the immune and endocrine systems. Ann N Y Acad Sci 1997;816:83–93.

14. Bowen R. Mechanism of action and physiologic effects of thyroid hormones. Available from: www.vivo.colostate.edu/hbooks/pathphys/endocrine/thyroid/physio.html.

15. World Health Organization. The physiological basis of breastfeeding. In: Infant and young child feeding: model chapter for textbooks for medical students and allied health professionals [Internet]. Geneva: World Health Organization; 2009.

16. Brent GA. The debate over thyroid-function screening in pregnancy. N Engl J Med 2012;366(6):562–3.

17. Wentzensen N, Trabert B. Hormone therapy: short-term relief, long-term consequences. Lancet 2015;385(9980):1806–10.

18. National Cancer Institute. Menopausal hormone therapy and cancer. Available from: www.cancer.gov/about-cancer/causes-prevention/risk/hormones/mht-fact-sheet.

CHAPTER 11

Blood

PETER HAYWOOD, BNURS

KEY POINTS/LEARNING OUTCOMES

1. Identify the main components of blood.
2. Discuss the basic functions of erythrocytes and leucocytes.
3. Understand and interpret a complete blood count report.
4. Explain how and why the body maintains blood concentrations of leucocytes and erythrocytes.

KEY DEFINITIONS

- **Erythrocyte:** a red blood cell; its predominant function is to transport oxygen and carbon dioxide.
- **Erythropoietin:** an erythrocyte growth factor, released by the kidneys at levels that depend on the amount of oxygen in the blood.
- **Haemoglobin:** the protein in erythrocytes that binds to oxygen and carbon dioxide.
- **Leucocyte:** a white blood cell; many different types of leucocytes make up the cellular component of the immune system.
- **Phagocytosis:** the process that some types of white blood cells use to engulf and ultimately destroy infectious organisms, cells or cell debris.

ONLINE RESOURCES/SUGGESTED READINGS

- **Australian and New Zealand Society of Blood Transfusion, links and resources** available at https://anzsbt.org.au/resources/links-resources
- **Australian Red Cross Blood Service** available at www.donateblood.com.au
- **Blood Matters Program, Victoria State Government**, available at www2.health.vic.gov.au/hospitals-and-health-services/patient-care/speciality-diagnostics-therapeutics/blood-matters
- **Haematology Society of Australia and New Zealand Nurses' Group** available at www.hsanz.org.au/hsanz-nurses-group.asp
- **Lab Tests Online** available at labtestsonline.org.au

INTRODUCTION

The five litres of blood in the average human body make up a vital transportation and communication system between body organs. Blood is comprised of a liquid portion, known as **plasma**, and a cellular component that encompasses red blood cells (RBCs, known as erythrocytes), white blood cells (collectively termed leucocytes) and platelets (known as thrombocytes). **Erythrocytes** in blood participate in the exchange of oxygen and carbon dioxide between the lungs and nearly all cells of the body. **Leucocytes** form the cellular component of the immune system, preventing infections or controlling the extent of an infection once it occurs. Blood cells are predominantly generated and developed in the bone marrow, though certain types of leucocytes can divide and differentiate within the bloodstream or organs, such as the spleen, lymph nodes and thymus. In the event of a skin infection, for example, the leucocyte division can occur at the site of infection.

In healthcare we often think of blood in the context of blood tests. The **complete blood count (CBC)**, sometimes called a **full blood count (FBC)** or **full blood examination (FBE)**, is a commonly requested blood test that looks at the number and composition of erythrocytes and leucocytes. When we discuss blood within a professional context, or with patients, it is usually in reference to these blood results. For this reason, this chapter addresses the function of erythrocytes and leucocytes in the context of the CBC.

STRUCTURE AND FUNCTION OF BLOOD

If a blood sample were to be spun at high speed (e.g. in a centrifuge) it would separate into distinct layers, each

of which has a different composition (Fig. 11.1). The bottom layer is red and is comprised of erythrocytes. Atop of the erythrocyte layer is a fine wispy layer of leucocytes and platelets, whereas the uppermost layer is a yellowish liquid called plasma.[1] When blood tests are run, each laboratory will present the CBC results slightly differently, as different geographical regions use different measuring units as well as different instruments to measure those values. However, those results will always contain haemoglobin, erythrocyte cell count, leucocyte cell count (also known as the white cell count, WCC), platelets and a breakdown of the different types of leucocytes.[2] In the following sections, we examine these components to help you understand why these parameters are so important to measure and interpret correctly.

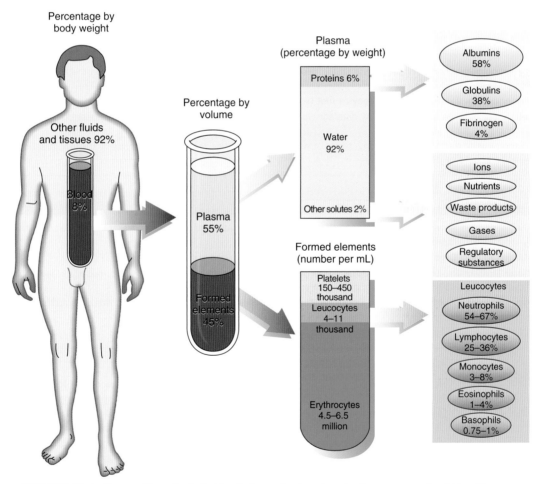

FIGURE 11.1 **Composition of whole blood.** Approximate values for the components of blood in a normal adult. (*Source:* Craft JA, Gordon CJ, Huether SE, McCance KL, Brashers VL, Rote NS. Understanding pathophysiology, 2 ed. Sydney: Elsevier; 2015.)

Haemoglobin

Haemoglobin (Hb) is a protein made up of four smaller protein chains (globins) and a non-protein pigment called a haem (Fig. 11.2).[1] Within each haem molecule there is an iron ion in the form of ferrous ion, or Fe^{2+}. This is a site where oxygen reversibly binds to the haem ring once it is diffused from the lungs into the blood circulation. The oxygenated haem carries oxygen from the lungs to the tissues. Within the capillaries haemoglobin releases oxygen and then reversibly binds to carbon dioxide. Oxygen binding to haemoglobin is dependent on the concentration of oxygen in the local environment. For example, in an area of high altitude, where there is decreased partial pressure of oxygen in the air (and therefore fewer molecules of oxygen to breathe in), the body needs to generate more erythrocytes to maximise oxygen-binding capacity.[1,3,4] The carbon dioxide binds to the globin proteins of haemoglobin, which the erythrocytes then carry back to the lungs to be breathed out.

There are about 280 million haemoglobin molecules in a single erythrocyte.[5] There are 135–175 grams of haemoglobin in each litre (L) of blood for men and 115–155 g/L for women. The amount of haemoglobin is a measure of the ability of blood to bind and transport oxygen to tissue peripheries. As clinicians, we are always interested in how much haemoglobin is available to a person in terms of both the number of erythrocytes in the blood and the amount of haemoglobin in each erythrocyte. This is because it tells us whether the person can meet the metabolic demands of their own body and respond to challenges to that function. For example, people deficient in haemoglobin due to a diet lacking in iron will not have a sufficient amount of haemoglobin to oxygenate the tissues so that they can perform their function.[1] Similarly, someone with fewer erythrocytes than expected may be short of breath on exertion, as their body is working hard trying to bring more oxygen to help the muscles do their work. Small blood losses are tolerated reasonably well by the body, but losses greater than 20% are likely to activate the protective mechanisms that supply blood only to the most important organs.[1] The more severe the blood loss, the more likely the person is to experience haemorrhagic shock.

Whenever iron binds to oxygen, erythrocytes become a brighter shade of red, as evident after they have been through the lungs and are in the peripheral arteries.[1] After delivering oxygen to the tissues, and returning to the heart via veins, erythrocytes appear a darker shade of red. This characteristic was used in early clinical assessments of blood samples where the shade of red was compared to a standard to estimate the level of haemoglobin.[6]

Erythrocyte count

It is estimated that adult human blood contains about 5.4 million erythrocytes for every microlitre, with men having slightly higher concentrations than women, which is attributed to physical and physiological differences. The word 'erythrocyte' is derived from the Greek word for 'red' (*erythro*).

It is estimated that it takes about 20 seconds for an erythrocyte to make a full trip around the body.[5] This journey is undertaken continuously for approximately 120 days before the erythrocyte is sequestered then destroyed by the spleen and liver.[1] The spleen contains a very fine sieve structure (trabeculae) only 3 micrometres wide, much narrower than the 7-micrometre diameter of an erythrocyte. While young, healthy erythrocytes are highly flexible, as evidenced by their capacity to bend and squeeze through very narrow capillaries (with a diameter of 5–7 micrometres), older, more fragile erythrocytes lose that elasticity. As aged erythrocytes pass through narrow capillaries they burst and eventually die. These damaged cells are recognised in the spleen, which prevents them from continuously circulating. To keep up with the natural death rate the body produces about two million erythrocytes per second.[7,8] The body requires a great amount of iron to meet this production demand. Fortunately, we do not need to eat this much iron as macrophages in the liver and spleen break down haemoglobin and release iron into the bloodstream to be used again by the bone marrow when making new erythrocytes.

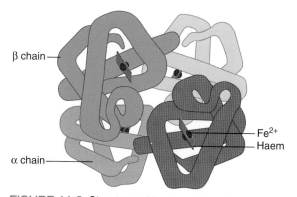

FIGURE 11.2 **Structure of haemoglobin.** There are four globin chains (two alpha [α] and two beta[β]), each containing a haem molecule and an iron (Fe^{2+}) atom. (*Source:* Hudnall SD. Hematology: a pathophysiologic approach, 1 ed. Philadelphia: Mosby; 2012.)

β chain

α chain

Fe^{2+}
Haem

Packed cell volume

Packed cell volume (PCV), sometimes called the **haematocrit (Hct)**, is the proportion of erythrocytes in the blood. Just under half the volume of blood is made up of erythrocytes, the other half mainly being plasma.[1] A person who has lost erythrocytes, for instance through increased bleeding (haemorrhage), or who cannot make enough due to underlying pathology, will have a decreased PCV. However, it is important to recognise that PCV is also a measure of plasma, levels of which can be affected by many factors. For example, fluid loss without blood loss as observed in cases of dehydration: a dehydrated person has effectively lost some plasma due to fluid loss, such as perspiration on a very warm day, so their blood will have more erythrocytes per millilitre of blood. On a blood test, their PCV and haemoglobin will be higher, even though they do not actually have an increased number of erythrocytes in their body. If a person has consumed a large volume of fluid, such as water, the PCV will decrease, even though the total number of erythrocytes within their body has not changed. This highlights that when interpreting this result it is important to have the patient's presentation in mind and to correlate those numbers back to the patient's history.

Mean cell volume

To travel through the vascular system and to perform their oxygen-delivery function, erythrocytes need to be both strong and flexible.[5] They measure about 7 micrometres in diameter and have a biconcave disc shape (Fig. 11.3). This shape enables them to travel through small capillaries, which are often smaller than their diameter. It also allows them to line up in the capillary lumen so that diffusion of oxygen and carbon dioxide can take place at the most effective rate of exchange. Mature erythrocytes lack a nucleus and mitochondria and consequently cannot reproduce or use the aerobic pathway to generate their own energy. Instead, erythrocytes employ the anaerobic pathway, importantly not consuming any of the oxygen they carry.

The **mean cell volume (MCV)** represents the measurement of the volume or size of erythrocytes. Young erythrocytes tend to be a little larger than old erythrocytes. This is because older erythrocytes undergo cell shape and size changes due to the natural ageing process and accompanying deformation that takes place as erythrocytes pass through narrow capillaries. It is proposed that erythrocytes lose around 10% of their size in their first week in the bloodstream, and around 20% over their lifetime.[8]

From a clinical perspective, changes in the MCV can indicate several conditions. Decreased MCV is reflective of conditions such as an iron deficiency. Iron is a major constituent of haemoglobin and therefore significantly contributes to erythrocyte size. Thus, in the presence of iron deficiency when there are inadequate levels of iron to form erythrocytes, they mature at a smaller size. In contrast, increased MCV reflects a deficiency in vitamins such as folate or vitamin B12 that are needed for correct DNA synthesis; in such conditions erythrocytes may be larger than usual.

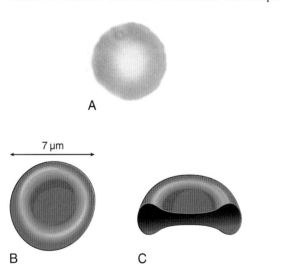

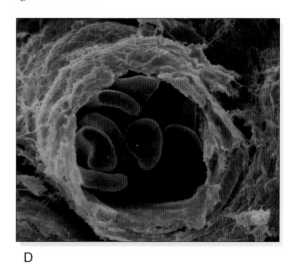

FIGURE 11.3 **Red blood cell. A** Under light microscope. **B** Drawn from the front. **C** Drawn in section. **D** Coloured scanning electron micrograph of a group of red blood cells travelling along an arteriole. (*Source:* Waugh A, Grant A. Ross & Wilson anatomy and physiology in health and illness, 13 ed. Elsevier Ltd; 2018.)

Mean cell haemoglobin

The **mean cell haemoglobin (MCH)**, or mean corpuscular haemoglobin, represents a calculated value that is an average quantity of haemoglobin present in one erythrocyte. As previously mentioned, the amount of haemoglobin in each erythrocyte is influenced by the amount of iron available for the formation of a fully functional haemoglobin molecule. Large erythrocytes tend to have more haemoglobin, and small cells' erythrocytes tend to have fewer. The MCH value is derived from the MCV and mean cell haemoglobin concentration.

Mean cell haemoglobin concentration

The **mean cell haemoglobin concentration (MCHC)** is calculated by dividing the haemoglobin level by the PCV. It is the amount of haemoglobin in a given volume of erythrocytes. Although very similar to the MCH, MCHC takes into account the size of erythrocytes. Large erythrocytes (high MCV), such as those found in vitamin B12 or folate deficiency, have a high MCH but the MCHC is likely to be within the normal range.

Reticulocyte count

Reticulocytes are immature erythrocytes, which are rarely seen in a healthy individual.[4] High numbers are seen only in conditions that require rapid production of erythrocytes and in some forms of blood cancers (leukaemias). In a healthy adult, erythrocytes are made in the bone marrow, through a process called **erythropoiesis**. The main growth factor that prompts stem cells to grow and differentiate into erythrocytes is a hormone called **erythropoietin**. Erythropoietin is mainly produced by the kidneys.[5] As blood flows through the kidneys, the oxygen sensors in the kidneys detect oxygen levels in the blood. When the amount of oxygen is sensed to be low, the kidneys will produce more erythropoietin.

Erythropoietin travels to the bone marrow and stimulates resident stem cells to reproduce and form new erythrocytes from haematopoietic stem cells. Stem cells are cells capable of becoming any cell in the body. These stem cells go through different stages of differentiation and maturation into erythrocytes. The nucleated precursors of erythrocytes in the marrow gradually accumulate iron to make haemoglobin and increase in size. At this point these cells are known as a **pronormoblasts**. Eventually, the nucleated cells lose their nucleus; this form of erythrocyte is considered immature and they are called **reticulocytes**. A reticulocyte contains some RNA that can be identified under the microscope if stained with special tissue dyes. It takes two to three days for these cells to lose their RNA and become a mature erythrocyte. Reticulocytes are structurally flexible and can squeeze their way out of the bone marrow and into the bloodstream. Healthy blood rarely contains reticulocytes: their presence is more accentuated in conditions that require increased volume of erythrocytes due to increased need for oxygenation, a primary function of erythrocytes. For example, acute blood loss during trauma would lead to increased release of reticulocytes into the bloodstream to help compensate for the blood volume lost and to meet the tissues' need for oxygen.

White cell count

A healthy person lives in a peaceful coexistence (symbiosis) with many species of microorganisms such as bacteria, yeast and viruses. However, some microorganisms are capable of causing harm to the human body. Through evolutionary adaptation, the body has developed a capacity to defend itself against these invaders. The major contributors to the defence system are **leucocytes** (*leuko-* from the Greek word for 'white'). In a centrifuged sample, leucocytes appear as a fine wispy white line between the erythrocytes and the clear yellowish plasma.

There are approximately 5000–10,000 leucocytes per microlitre in adult blood.[5] Unlike erythrocytes, they do not contain haemoglobin. They do, however, contain a nucleus and organelles, which means that they can reproduce.

Given their role in controlling and preventing infections, in times of stress the total number of leucocytes will increase. For example, a person with influenza is likely to have a higher than normal leucocyte count. This is often referred to as a 'reactive' response, as the body is appropriately 'reacting' to the influenza. A decreased leucocyte number is a sign of a pathology that is a result of either the body's decreased capacity to produce these cells in the bone marrow or the cells dying faster than biologically destined. Rarely, the bone marrow will make great numbers of specific leucocytes or leucocyte precursors, a condition associated with leucocyte cancers, known as **leukaemia**.

All leucocytes start as stem cells in the bone marrow. It is a similar process to erythrocyte formation: cells in a very immature state reproduce and differentiate into mature cells in the bone marrow. In fact, erythrocytes and leucocytes share the same ancestor cell: the **pluripotent haematopoietic stem cell** (Fig. 11.4). This cell family tree branches off into different types of blood cells. Along the path of maturation, the cells will structurally (morphologically) look different at different stages. An immature cell is often referred to as a **blast** (the Greek word for 'sprout'). This process occurs in the bone marrow and so these cells would not normally appear in the blood. If the bone marrow is trying to make more leucocytes than is usually required, there may be an abundance of blasts and some will go into the

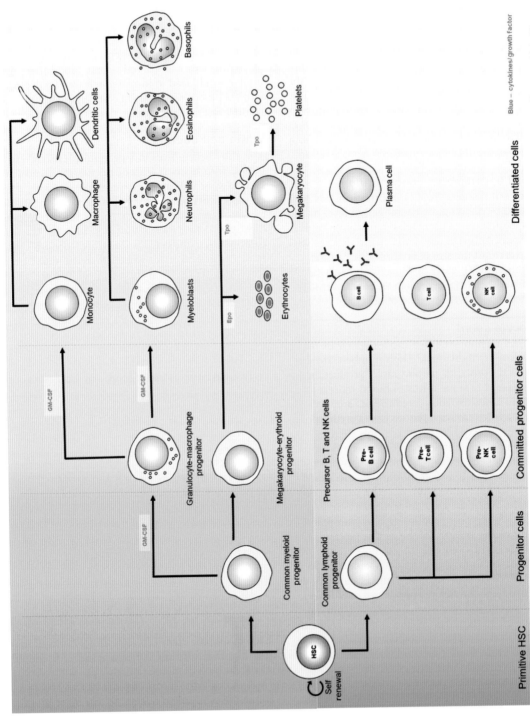

FIGURE 11.4 Diagram of haematopoiesis shows derivation of cells from the pluripotent haematopoietic stem cell. (*Source:* Alvin Bacero Bello, Hansoo Park, Soo-Hong Lee. Current approaches in biomaterial-based hematopoietic stem cell niches. Actbio. Acta Materialia Inc.; 2018.)

bloodstream and will be detected during a blood test. It is also worthwhile mentioning that lymphoid organs such as the spleen, thymus and lymph nodes are sites of maturation for some leucocytes, such as lymphocytes.

Neutrophils

The most common type of leucocyte in the blood is the **neutrophil**.[5] Under a microscope it appears to be a 'neutral' colour as it is stained by similar amounts of acidic and basic types of tissue stain used to stain blood films.

Neutrophils are one of the main cells that first respond as part of the immune response to kill invading bacteria. They do this by effectively eating them: the medical term is **phagocytosis** (*phago* from the Greek word 'to eat'). To do this, neutrophils extend part of their outer membrane to eventually engulf the bacteria, then release bactericidal enzymes that break down the ingested bacteria. Another way that neutrophils kill engulfed bacteria is by releasing toxic chemicals (such as hydrogen peroxide and superoxide) (Fig. 11.5).

Although they are the most common leucocyte, neutrophils actually spend only 4–8 hours within the bloodstream. After being released by the bone marrow into the circulation, neutrophils migrate into tissues throughout the body. When there is an infection neutrophils act swiftly, but as the act of phagocytosis is a suicide mission, neutrophils induce their own death through **apoptosis**, or programmed cell death. This process increases the likelihood that the bacteria will die within the neutrophil. Neutrophil death releases pro-inflammatory chemicals that encourage other leucocytes to the area to combat the injurious stimuli.[9] In a homeostatic state (i.e. no inflammation), it is estimated

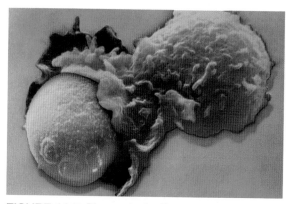

FIGURE 11.5 **Phagocytosis.** (*Source:* Waugh A, Grant A. Ross & Wilson anatomy and physiology in health and illness, 13 ed. Elsevier Ltd; 2018.)

that neutrophils will survive in the tissues for only four or five days. This means there is quite a high turnover of neutrophils and to meet the demand of maintaining homeostasis the bone marrow needs an equally high production, in the order of one million cells per second.[10]

The main growth factor needed for neutrophil development is **granulocyte colony stimulating factor**, often abbreviated as GCSF. GCSF is produced by many different cells (such as macrophages, epithelial cells and fibroblasts) under different circumstances and for different purposes, one of which is to stimulate neutrophils to grow and differentiate.[11] It can be made synthetically and given to people when they have low numbers of neutrophils, such as when they have received chemotherapy for cancer treatment.

Lymphocytes

Bacteria differ from human cells in structure and function and neutrophils have evolved to recognise and eliminate bacteria. However, neutrophils may occasionally be overwhelmed by the number of bacteria present and they also generally do not recognise viruses or damaged body cells that require elimination so that they do not turn into a harmful cell (i.e. by becoming a cancer cell). This deficiency is compensated for by another subset of leucocytes known as **lymphocytes**.[5] Lymphocytes operate in response to bacterial infections, either in a supportive or a directional role. There are many subtypes of lymphocytes, but they are broadly classified into two main groups: **B-lymphocytes** and **T-lymphocytes**. Although all lymphocytes ultimately originate from the bone marrow, T-lymphocytes migrate from bone marrow to the thymus in order to differentiate into fully functional T-cells. T-cells derive their name from this process, as the 'T' stands for thymus. Similarly, B-cells undergo their maturation process mainly in the bone marrow, and to a lesser extent the spleen and lymph nodes.[5] While it is tempting to consider that the 'B' is for bone marrow it actually signifies bursa of Fabricius, an organ in birds where B-cells were first discovered.

Monocytes/macrophages

Another type of cell that can perform phagocytosis is macrophages.[1] They develop in the bone marrow and spend very little time in the bloodstream. During this time, they are referred to as **monocytes**. Once they migrate from the bloodstream into the tissues, they become **macrophages**. They survive in the tissues much longer than neutrophils and are morphologically larger in size. Like neutrophils, macrophages ingest bacteria. However, unlike neutrophils, macrophages survive and can go on to ingest many bacteria. They can manipulate the ingested bacteria for presentation to lymphocytes in order to activate **adaptive immune responses** (discussed in Chapter 15). Macrophages also ingest dead erythrocytes and therefore actively participate in iron recycling in the body. They can perform these functions for months, although their survival is likely to be dictated by the material they ingest.[12]

Macrophages are scattered throughout the body but have a heavier presence in locations where bacteria are more likely to enter the body, such as the upper respiratory tract, the digestive system and the skin. Macrophages in the spleen and lymph nodes participate in capturing bacteria arriving through the bloodstream.

When large numbers of bacteria in one area of the body have been digested, there will also be dead neutrophils and macrophages that form a white material, commonly known as **pus**. The pus will gradually break down and be reabsorbed by the local lymphatic vessels and transported via the lymph system into circulation and excretion via the kidneys and liver.[1] This is an important process in wound healing. Different types of macrophages, both pro-inflammatory and anti-inflammatory, play a very important role in regulating the wound-healing process.[13]

Eosinophils

Eosinophils are less common in the bloodstream.[5] Their number increases when the body is infected by parasitic worms. Here, the eosinophils release chemical mediators able to destroy a parasite. Their numbers are also increased in association with allergic conditions such as pollen-induced asthma.

Basophils

Basophils are also quite rare.[5] They contain high amounts of histamine, a chemical that will cause vasodilation and results in increased blood flow to the affected region. This is the same chemical that is released in hay fever, commonly treated with an anti-histamine medicine. Basophils are very similar to mast cells, which also contain a high level of histamine, but research suggests that these two cells are very distinct entities.[14]

Platelets

Platelets (Plt), or **thrombocytes**, are not actually cells, but 2–3 micrometre fragments of cell cytoplasm that participate in blood clot formation.[5] In inactivated form, platelets assume a lens-shaped structure, similar in appearance to a dinner plate. However, following injury, they change shape to become rounder and form projections that help them stick to structures such as endothelial cells or collagen fibres in the injured area.

This change of shape also facilitates further binding of platelets to form a multi-layered plug that can withstand blood flow pressure.

Platelets are also made in the bone marrow, where they start off as large cells called **megakaryocytes**. Each megakaryocyte can make 1000–3000 platelets. Although they do not have a nucleus, platelets contain 'granules' that have components that will affect the shape and behaviour of other platelets and cells during a bleeding event. Platelet production is regulated by **thrombopoietin**, which is synthesised by the liver. People with low amounts of platelets, known as **thrombocytopenia**, may use synthetically manufactured thrombopoietin to stimulate the bone marrow to make more platelets. Platelets typically live about 10 days.[15]

Mean platelet volume

Like erythrocytes, young platelets tend to be larger than older platelets. **Mean platelet volume (MPV)** is a calculated measurement that estimates the average size of platelets in a blood sample. Increased presence of large platelets may signify premature death of platelets and indirectly demonstrate that the bone marrow may be compensating for this by making more platelets.

Fig. 11.6 and Table 11.1 illustrate the different classes of blood cells.

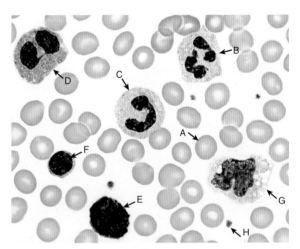

FIGURE 11.6 **Normal cells in peripheral blood.** **A** Erythrocyte (red blood cell, RBC). **B** Neutrophil (segmented neutrophil, NEUT, SEG, polymorphonuclear neutrophil, PMN). **C** Band (band neutrophil, BAND). **D** Eosinophil (EO). **E** Basophil (BASO). **F** Lymphocyte (LYMPH). **G** Monocyte (MONO). **H** Platelet (PLT). (*Source:* Keohane E, Otto C, Walenga J. Rodak's hematology, 6 ed. Saunders; 2019.)

TABLE 11.1
Classes of blood cells

Blood cell	Diagram	Description	Approximate diameter	Approximate life span	Concentration in blood
Erythrocyte		Biconcave disc that is able to squeeze through small capillaries; transports oxygen and carbon dioxide	7 μm	120 days	$3.8–6.5 \times 10^{12}$/L (Haemoglobin 115–180 g/L)
Neutrophil		Spherical shape; most common type of white blood cell; attacks infectious microbes	12–15 μm	6 hours in blood, 3 days in tissues	$1.5–7.5 \times 10^{9}$/L
Platelet		Uneven disc shape; changes shape when activated to form blood clots	3 μm	7 days	$150–400 \times 10^{9}$/L
Lymphocyte		Spherical shape; produces antibodies, directs other components of the immune system; categorised into B- and T- lymphocytes	6–14 μm	Up to several years depending on type	$1–4 \times 10^{9}$/L
Monocyte		Spherical shape; becomes macrophage when leaving the bloodstream; capable of ingesting multiple microbes	12–17 μm	Months in the tissues	$0.2–0.8 \times 10^{9}$/L
Eosinophil		Spherical shape; attacks parasitical worms; involved in inflammatory responses	10 μm	10 days	$0.1–0.4 \times 10^{9}$/L
Basophil		Spherical shape; involved in inflammatory responses; releases histamine	11 μm	3 days	$0.02–0.1 \times 10^{9}$/L

Source: Patton K, Thibodeau G. Anatomy and physiology, 9 ed. St Louis: Mosby; 2016. The Royal College of Pathologists Australia. Full blood count. Available from: www.rcpa.edu.au/Library/Practising-Pathology/RCPA-Manual/Items/Pathology-Tests/F/Full-blood-count on 9 June 2018.

Blood group

Various components of blood can be donated and transfused to other people. However, the immune system is finely tuned to attack foreign substances such as bacteria and transfused erythrocytes might be recognised as 'foreign' by lymphocytes. This would prompt an immune response that if widespread enough could become life-threatening. Human beings are similar enough to each other that there are a limited number of types or groups of erythrocytes that could prompt such an immune response. There are in fact many hundreds of potential combinations of antigens and antibodies that are involved in blood grouping.[1] The most common, and in some ways the most important for transfusion, are the **A**, **B** and **O** blood groups:

- People with type A blood have 'anti-B' antibodies. These antibodies identify B group erythrocytes as foreign, and interact with lymphocytes to mount an attack against them.
- In a similar way, type B blood has 'anti-A' antibodies.
- Type O blood is slightly different, as it has both 'anti-A' and 'anti-B' antibodies, and these would mount an attack against either group A or group B erythrocytes. However, type O blood has the advantage of not having either A or B antigens on the surface of the erythrocytes. Consequently, type O blood can be transfused to someone with A, B, AB or O blood.
- In type AB blood, the erythrocytes have both A and B type antigens, but the blood has no 'anti-A' or 'anti-B' antibodies. A person with type AB blood can safely receive a transfusion from any of the other groups, but their blood cannot be transfused to someone with any of the other blood groups.

Another important blood grouping system is the **Rh**, or **rhesus**, **grouping**.[1] There are several antigens within the Rh groups, with **Rh(D)** being the most relevant. People with the Rh(D) antigen are said to be '**positive**'; those without it are '**negative**'. So, a person who knows their blood group to be 'A negative' has A group antigens but not Rh(D) antigens on the surface of their erythrocytes.

INTEGRATION OF BLOOD WITH OTHER BODY SYSTEMS

Blood links all body systems through transport of oxygen and nutrients needed for survival and removal of waste products that in excess can be harmful.[1] The adaptations and feedback systems needed to maintain healthy blood are extremely intricate and complex. An example where this is easily evident is that of a volunteer blood donor. In the absence of needed elements of blood to carry out its numerous functions, patients experience significant complications. However, a healthy volunteer blood donor can donate blood as their body can activate adaptive mechanisms and compensate for a loss of blood with minimal physiological cost to self.

Respiratory system

A volunteer blood donor will usually donate around 500 mL of blood at a time (approximately 10% of their total amount of blood). After donation, fluid intake may increase the blood volume, but the number of erythrocytes will be lower, as will the concentration of haemoglobin per unit of volume of blood. Subsequently, the same amount of blood will deliver slightly less oxygen than before. This effect can be so subtle that the donor does not notice it. Nevertheless, donors are generally advised not to undertake vigorous exercise immediately after donating blood. During exercise, the oxygen requirements of the muscles increase. Oxygen leaves the haemoglobin for redistribution to tissue cells. Subsequently, the haem has less oxygen bound to it, and the globin has slightly more carbon dioxide bound to it. For a blood donor, this effect will be accentuated. Various nerves throughout the body and the respiratory centre in the brain detect the increased carbon dioxide levels in the blood and this leads to the sensation of shortness of breath and light-headedness, and an increase in the respiratory rate.

Cardiovascular system

To maintain a safe blood pressure, the heart will compensate for the 500 mL of blood donated by increasing the heart rate. The peripheral vascular system will constrict to increase the volume in the blood vessels and keep a constant blood pressure. Decreased blood pressure may lead to decreased blood supply to the brain and further contribute to the sensation of light-headedness. Donors are warned of this potential side effect and are required to rest and drink something before leaving the donation centre. Some people also feel colder after donating blood. This is because blood has an important role in maintaining body temperature and distributing heat. For example, blood vessels near the skin can constrict to reduce the amount of blood that is being cooled down by the environment. Similarly, when there is too much heat, the body uses the blood to transfer heat to the vessels near the skin so that the heat can evaporate.

Urinary system

The receptors in the blood donor's kidneys will detect decreased blood volume and precipitate the response of the cardiovascular system. With fewer erythrocytes, the kidneys detect a decreased level of blood oxygen. In response, the kidneys produce erythropoietin, the primary growth factor that stimulates the bone marrow to produce more erythrocytes. There will be noticeably more reticulocytes in the bloodstream, as the newly produced erythrocytes leave the bone marrow with some remaining RNA strands. Slight changes may be present on the CBC: a marginally lower haemoglobin, red cell count and PCV, and a marginally higher MCV and reticulocyte count. The white cell count is unlikely to be noticeably affected, as the white blood cells exist in a much smaller proportion in the bloodstream.

Gastrointestinal system

The gastrointestinal system is important in supplying and maintaining vital nutrients, such as iron, vitamin B12 and folate, needed to produce blood cells. Although mechanisms exist to enable the body to recycle iron, the body itself cannot synthesise iron. Over time, some iron is permanently lost and so the ability of the gastrointestinal system to effectively absorb dietary iron is essential in maintaining erythrocyte production and therefore body homeostasis. Blood loss during menstruation is a frequent reason for iron-deficiency anaemia in females and is a rationale for educational advice on increasing dietary iron intake for menstruating women compared with men of the same age.

A month after donating blood haemoglobin and erythrocytes may have been replaced, but it is unlikely that sufficient iron will have been absorbed from the gastrointestinal tract to replace lost iron. Continued blood donations will further challenge existing iron stores. In the absence of iron, new erythrocytes would have less haemoglobin (lower MCH) and be smaller (lower MCV). Over time, even the total haemoglobin level of the blood would be lower. This physiological response is the reason why blood donors are limited to making four blood donations per year: a three-month gap is considered a realistic time to obtain enough replacement iron in the diet. Donors who deliberately supplement their diet with iron replace their erythrocytes faster than those who do not.[16]

Folate and vitamin B12 are two nutrients that are needed for any cell to make DNA during cell division. As these vitamins are modified in the process of producing DNA and cannot be recycled, continuous supply arriving via the gastrointestinal tract is vital. Cells formed in the absence of vitamin B12 and folate are not efficient in their function.

The liver also participates in the breakdown of old erythrocytes and the storage of erythrocytes. In addition, it produces the platelet growth factor thrombopoietin and many of the clotting factors that interact with platelets to form a clot. Recycled iron is stored in the liver.

AGE-RELATED CHANGES

Age-related changes in the haematopoietic system impact the formation of all blood cells and platelets. It is proposed that there is a decline in the production of stem cells and progenitor cells as well as loss of functional capacity. This has been linked to changes and decline in hormonal production associated with age. Furthermore, genetic changes that result in mutations likely to lead to blood cancers such as leukaemia are more common. There is also a decline in leucocyte immunological function, with decline suggested for both innate and adaptive immunity. It is these changes that are responsible for public health campaigns promoting vaccinations to the elderly.[17]

CONCLUSION

Blood is vital to so many organs, through its role in oxygen and nutrient supply, removal of waste products, heat management, prevention of infection and prevention of blood loss. The cellular elements of the blood are erythrocytes, leucocytes and platelets. Each of these cells undertakes a specific function that collectively enables body homeostasis. Inadequate formation of these cells leads to functional decline that in some cases can be compensated for—for example, in the case of the blood donor. However, if these mechanisms fail, blood components cannot maintain homeostasis and this may lead to blood cancers or failure of organs to survive, such as during significant blood loss. While many body systems can survive because of the role of blood in delivering vital ingredients needed for their function, those systems have a reciprocal effect on the blood by providing the nutrition it needs to effectively form its cellular elements.

CASE STUDY 11.1

Tom is a farmhand who lost a lot of blood in a workplace accident. In hospital he had many blood tests. At its lowest, his haemoglobin was 78 g/L. He makes a good recovery and leaves hospital two days after admission with his arm fully functional but has been given a medical certificate for the rest of the week off. He often feels fatigued and gets a bit short of breath when he walks a lot. When discharged his haemoglobin is 85 g/L.

Continued

CASE STUDY 11.1—cont'd

Q1. When Tom lost blood he lost erythrocytes, platelets, leucocytes and plasma. List these in order from most to least in terms of the volume that appear in blood.

  a. Platelets, leucocytes, erythrocytes, plasma

  b. Plasma, platelets, erythrocytes, leucocytes

  c. Plasma, erythrocytes, platelets, leucocytes

  d. Erythrocytes, plasma, platelets, leucocytes

Q2. What is the main organ that regulates how many erythrocytes are produced by making erythropoietin?

  a. The liver

  b. The kidneys

  c. The bone marrow

  d. The pancreas

Q3. A reticulocyte is:

  a. a white blood cell that fights viral infections.

  b. a platelet that has been 'activated' and helps form a blood clot.

  c. an immature erythrocyte that contains remnant RNA.

  d. a mature erythrocyte that is old and will soon be destroyed by the spleen.

Q4. Discuss how Tom's haematopoietic system responded to the blood loss experienced following his injury.

Q5. Considering the level of injury and the blood loss experienced, why does Tom require time off work?

CASE STUDY 11.2

Mingdi is a student nurse who lives with his grandfather. His grandfather goes to the doctor often and frequently gets blood tests including a CBC. Mingdi focuses on three parameters, haemoglobin (Hb), platelets (Plt) and white cell count (WCC), and wants to help his grandfather by interpreting these blood results.

Q1. What is the normal haemoglobin concentration in blood, for males?

  a. 90–110 g/L

  b. 120–150 mg/L

  c. 135–175 g/L

  d. 135–175 mg/L

Q2. What is the normal platelet count in blood?

  a. $150–450 \times 10^9$ per L

  b. $100–130 \times 10^9$ per L

  c. $50–150 \times 10^9$ per L

  d. $10–50 \times 10^9$ per L

Q3. What is the most common type of white blood cell?

  a. Lymphocytes

  b. Neutrophils

  c. Macrophages

  d. Monocytes

Q4. What are these three parameters (Hb, Plt, WCC) and why is it important to know that they are not too low?

Q5. Discuss how different body systems contribute to maintaining Mingdi's grandfather's constant blood cell numbers in the circulation.

CASE STUDY 11.3

Hazel is a three-year-old girl who enjoys exploring. Two days ago, while walking in the park barefoot, she kicked her toe against a fallen tree branch, breaking the skin. Yesterday, the toe was swollen and red and there was some pus where the skin had broken. Today, the toe is bruised and the tip is red, but the skin is not broken.

Q1. Which cells do most of the work of digesting and killing bacteria during bacterial infections?

  a. Neutrophils and macrophages

  b. Platelets and neutrophils

  c. Neutrophils and lymphocytes

  d. Lymphocytes and erythrocytes

CASE STUDY 11.3—cont'd

Q2. When all the bacteria at the site of an infection have been killed, what will the remaining pus contain?

  a. Connective tissue cells

  b. Dead tissue, dead bacterial fragments and dead inflammatory cells

  c. Erythrocytes

  d. Platelets

Q3. In the case of a serious infection, we would expect the number of neutrophils in the blood to:

  a. be reduced, as neutrophils leave the bloodstream to get to the site of infection.

  b. not change much, as leucocytes in the tissues will replicate if more of them are needed.

  c. be increased, as the bone marrow releases more neutrophils in response to infection.

  d. not change much, as most infection fighting is done by erythrocytes.

Q4. What is the role of leucocytes in the pus formation seen on Hazel's toe?

Q5. What is causing the bruising of Hazel's toe?

CASE STUDY 11.4

Jonathan sometimes donates blood, around 500 mL at a time. He feels no adverse effects but the nurse always cautions him to avoid strenuous exercise afterwards, asks him to drink plenty of fluids both before and after donating and warns him that he may get light-headed after donating. The nurse also reminds him that he is not allowed to donate for three months afterwards.

Q1. The most important nutrients we get from our diet that we need to produce red cells are:

  a. iron, folate, vitamin B12.

  b. iron, vitamin C, GCSF.

  c. folate, vitamin C, erythropoietin.

  d. vitamin B12, GCSF, vitamin D.

Q2. Which of the following would you expect to make someone feel tired?

  a. A low level of white blood cells in the blood

  b. A low level of red blood cells in the blood

  c. A low level of platelets in the blood

  d. A low level of plasma in the blood (i.e. a high number of red blood cells)

Q3. To reproduce enough blood cells to make up for blood donation will take about:

  a. 3 hours.

  b. 3 days.

  c. 1 month.

  d. 3 months.

Q4. On a physiological level, how can Jonathan donate blood without feeling any obvious side effects?

Q5. Why would the nurse caution Jonathan to avoid exercise and drink plenty of fluids, and remind him that he may feel light-headed and not to donate blood for three months?

REFERENCES

1. Patton K, Thibodeau G. Blood. In: Anatomy and physiology. 9th ed. St Louis: Mosby; 2016.

2. The Royal College of Pathologists Australia. Full blood count. Available from: www.rcpa.edu.au/Library/Practising -Pathology/RCPA-Manual/Items/Pathology-Tests/F/Full-blood-count [Accessed 9 June 2018].

3. Hudnall SD. Hematology: a pathophysiologic approach. 1st ed. Philadelphia: Mosby; 2012.

4. Helms CC, Gladwin MT, Kim-Shapiro DB. Erythrocytes and vascular function: oxygen and nitric oxide. Front Physiol 2018;9. https://doi.org/10.3389/fphys.2018.00125.

5. Hoffman R, Benz E, Silberstein L, et al. Hematology: basic principles and practice. Chicago: Elsevier; 2018.

6. Wintrobe MM. The direct calculation of the volume and hemoglobin content of the erythrocyte: a comparison with color index, volume index and saturation index determinations. Am J Clin Pathol 1931;1(2):147–66. https://doi .org/10.1093/ajcp/1.2.147.

7. Waugh A, Grant A. Ross and Wilson anatomy and physiology in health and illness. 12th ed. Edinburgh: Elsevier; 2014.

8. Higgins JM. Red blood cell population dynamics. Clin Lab Med 2015;35(1):43–57. https://doi.org/10.1016/j.cll.2014 .10.002.

9. Kobayashi SD, Malachowa N, DeLeo FR. Influence of microbes on neutrophil life and death. Front Cell Infect Microbiol 2017;7:159. https://doi.org/10.3389/fcimb.2017 .00159.

10. Summers C, Rankin SM, Condliffe AM, et al. Neutrophil kinetics in health and disease. Trends Immunol 2010;31(8):318–24. https://doi.org/10.1016/j.it.2010.05.006.

11. Bendall LJ, Bradstock KF. G-CSF: from granulopoietic stimulant to bone marrow stem cell mobilizing agent. Cytokine Growth Factor Rev 2014;25(4):355–67. https://doi.org/10.1016/j.cytogfr.2014.07.011.

12. Zent CS, Elliott MR. Maxed out macs: physiologic cell clearance as a function of macrophage phagocytic capacity. FEBS J 2017;284(7):1021–39. https://doi.org/10.1111/febs.13961.

13. Krzyszczyk P, Schloss R, Palmer A, et al. The role of macrophages in acute and chronic wound healing and interventions to promote pro-wound healing phenotypes. Front Physiol 2018;9:419. https://doi.org/10.3389/fphys.2018.00419.

14. Fang Y, Xiang Z. Roles and relevance of mast cells in infection and vaccination. J Biomed Res 2016;30(4):253–63. https://doi.org/10.7555/JBR.30.20150038.

15. Mason KD, Carpinelli MR, Fletcher JI, et al. Programmed anuclear cell death delimits platelet life span. Cell 2007;128(6):1173–86. https://doi.org/10.1016/j.cell.2007.01.037.

16. Kiss JE, Brambilla D, Glynn SA, et al. Oral iron supplementation after blood donation. JAMA 2015;313(6):575. https://doi.org/10.1001/jama.2015.119.

17. Henry CJ, Marusyk A, DeGregori J. Aging-associated changes in haematopoiesis and leukemogenesis: what is the connection? Aging 2011;6:643–56.

CHAPTER 12

Haemostasis

FIONA NEWALL, PHD, RN • ZERINA TOMKINS, BAPPSC (MED LAB SCI), BAPPSC (HONS), MNSC (NURS), PHD, GRAD CERT (UNIVERSITY EDUCATION)

KEY POINTS/LEARNING OUTCOMES

1. Explain primary and secondary haemostasis.
2. Differentiate between extrinsic and intrinsic pathways involved in the coagulation pathway.
3. Describe how platelet activation and the coagulation pathway are regulated.
4. Describe how blood clots are dissolved.
5. Link age-related changes to haemostasis.

KEY DEFINITIONS

- **Common coagulation pathway:** a mechanism by which the initial platelet plug is fortified by the deposition and integration of fibrin to strengthen and amplify the plug and enable injured vessels to repair themselves.
- **Extrinsic coagulation pathway:** also known as the tissue factor pathway, this refers to the process where exposure of subendothelial tissue factor due to loss of endothelial cell integrity leads to activation of clotting mechanisms aimed at fortifying the platelet plug and the fibrin clot.
- **Haemostasis:** the process of forming blood clots to stop bleeding after injury. It requires vascular response, platelet plug formation, deposition of a fibrin clot on the platelet plug and dissolution of the clot when it is no longer needed.
- **Intrinsic coagulation pathway:** also known as the contact activation pathway, this refers to the process of initiating deposition of the fibrin matrix in the platelet plug through activation of the clotting pathway following the interaction of subendothelial collagen and blood-circulating clotting factors that will result in the formation of fibrin.
- **Platelet activation:** a process that leads to a change in platelet shape from spherical to star-shaped, which enables platelets to express receptors to adhere to injured blood vessels to seal an injured site.

ONLINE RESOURCES/SUGGESTED READINGS

- **Thrombosis & Haemostasis Society of Australia and New Zealand** available at www.thanz.org.au
- **A practical guide to laboratory haemostasis** available at www.practical-haemostasis.com
- **Haemostasis** available at https://courses.lumenlearning.com/ap2/chapter/hemostasis

INTRODUCTION

Blood volume is a highly preserved function of the human body due to the important role that blood plays in the delivery of oxygen and nutrients to tissues, immune function and maintenance of blood pressure. Thus, any loss of blood is undesirable. The human body has developed sophisticated mechanisms, collectively termed **haemostasis**, that are activated to prevent further blood loss after injury by forming a seal at the site of injury in the form of a clot. Collectively, these mechanisms balance the body's innate capacity to initiate, amplify, propagate and ultimately resolve blood clots when no longer needed, as the process of haemostasis also ensures that blood moves through the body in a fluid state.[1] The clot itself stabilises injury in blood vessels and facilitates the vascular healing process at the site of injury. The clot that is formed in blood vessels is also known as a **thrombus**. If a thrombus breaks apart, pieces can

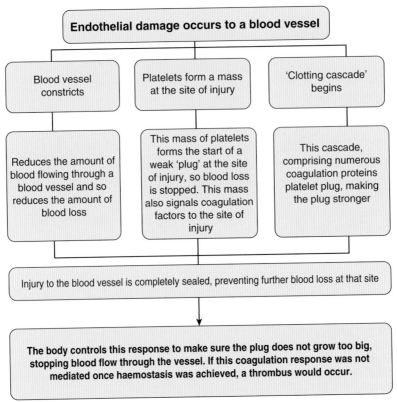

FIGURE 12.1 **Haemostasis response to endothelial damage to a blood vessel.**

travel throughout the body. These pieces are known as **emboli** (singular = embolus).

The sequence of interrelated processes that occur to maintain haemostasis in the setting of endothelial damage occurring to a blood vessel wall are summarised in Fig. 12.1 and discussed in greater detail throughout this chapter. Specifically, this chapter focuses on the structure and function of platelets; the intrinsic, extrinsic and common coagulation pathways; intravascular, vascular and extravascular components of haemostasis; and the difference between primary and secondary haemostasis. We also introduce mechanisms responsible for clot breakdown and discuss the most common coagulation blood tests likely to be encountered in clinical settings.

STRUCTURE AND FUNCTION OF PLATELETS

Platelets are irregularly shaped cell fragments of 2–5 micrometres in size (Fig. 12.2). They constitute less than 1% of blood volume, with a range of 150,000–400,000

platelets/mm³ being considered normal. From a structural perspective, platelets have a plasma membrane that encloses platelet cytoplasm. The plasma membrane is surrounded by a glycocalyx covering and it expresses receptors important for adhesion to injured vessels and other platelets. These include glycoproteins Ib/IX and IIb/IIIa receptors; coagulation factors I, II, VII, IX and X; phospholipids; structural proteins; and ion channels and pumps.[2] The plasma membrane also provides structural support (as platelets change shape during the activation process) and release of granules stored inside platelets through the open canalicular system. A dense tubular system serves as a site for calcium storage and production of compounds such as prostacyclin and thromboxane.

Platelet cytoplasm contains the Golgi apparatus, glycogen particles, peroxisomes, lysosomes and mitochondria that provide energy in the form of adenosine triphosphate (ATP), alpha granules that contain components needed for effective clotting and platelet adhesion to injured vessel and other platelets, and dense granules that contain calcium and serotonin, which is

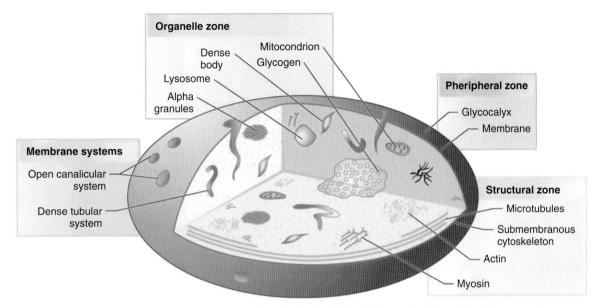

FIGURE 12.2 Simplified structure of a blood platelet. A platelet is oval in shape. Platelet structural compartments can be divided into the peripheral zone (which consists of plasma and the associated glycocalyx layer), the membrane system (which comprises the open canalicular system and dense tubular system), the organelle zone (which contains mitochondria, glycogen particles, dense body, lysosome and alpha granules) and the structural zone (which contains microtubules, submembranous skeleton and myofilaments: actin and myosin). (*Source:* McKenzie SB, Williams JL. Clinical laboratory hematology, 2 ed. Modified, with permission, from Thompson AR, Harker LA. Manual of hemostasis and thrombosis, 3 ed. Philadelphia: FA Davis; 1982.)

important for vessel constriction. **Alpha granules** contain platelet-derived growth factor, which plays a role in endothelial cell division and repair.[3] Platelet cytoplasm contains a dense tubular system and sub-membranous filaments that act as contractile proteins and assist in platelet shape changes as platelets become activated.

Platelets are formed through the process of **thrombopoiesis** (Fig. 12.3). Precursor cells, **megakaryoblasts**, reside in the red bone marrow, lungs and to a lesser extent the spleen.[4] As megakaryoblasts mature they migrate towards sinusoidal blood vessels in the bone marrow to extend cytoplasmic cell processes, known as **proplatelets**, into vessel lumen. At this point the proplatelets are shed as fragments of cell cytoplasm into the blood (Fig. 12.4).[5] Platelets are therefore cellular fragments and have an estimated life span of seven days. While most are circulating in the blood, about one-third of platelets are stored in the spleen.

Clotting factors

Clotting factors, also known as **coagulation proteins**, are a group of proteins found in the blood plasma. They are involved in the formation of the fibrin mesh that reinforces the initial platelet plug formed at the site of injured endothelium. The formation of the fibrin mesh is a result of a series of predictable reactions that involve coagulation factors, non-enzymatic cofactors, calcium (Ca^{2+}), fibrinogen and phospholipid. **Phospholipid** is found in platelets, whereas coagulation factors, except tissue factor, are present in blood circulation. Clotting factors are named by roman numerals but may also have a common name. For example, the common name for factor I is fibrinogen. The naming of clotting factors by roman numerals helps us to visualise how coagulation factors are activated in sequence by acting upon each other. These events are arbitrarily termed the **intrinsic coagulation pathway**, the **extrinsic coagulation pathway** and the **common coagulation pathway**.[6]

Most clotting factors circulate as zymogens or proenzymes. **Zymogens** are inactive precursors of an enzyme that require activation by another enzyme to become active. Except for factors III, IV and VIII, the rest are produced in the liver. Factor III is synthesised by endothelial cells and vascular smooth muscle cells of

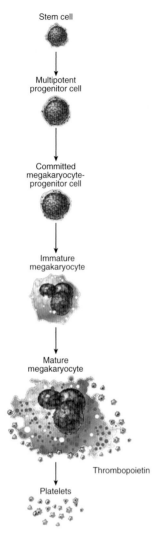

Stem cell

Multipotent
progenitor cell

Committed
megakaryocyte-
progenitor cell

Immature
megakaryocyte

Mature
megakaryocyte

Thrombopoietin

Platelets

FIGURE 12.3 **Platelet formation.** (*Source:* Modified from www.researchgate.net/publication/5418847 _Thrombocytopenia_associated_with_chronic_liver _disease/figures?lo=1.)

the blood vessels;[7] factor IV (calcium) is obtained from the diet; and the site of synthesis of factor VIII is unknown. When depicting the role of coagulation factors in clot formation, abbreviations are used to simplify the reactions. Thus, clotting factor VIII is abbreviated to FVIII. Furthermore, when a clotting factor is activated, the abbreviation is followed by 'a' for activation—for example, FVIIa.

Clotting factors are outlined below and in Table 12.1:

- **Clotting factor I** (fibrinogen) is a precursor protein of fibrin. Fibrin is a polymer that strengthens the platelet plug at the site of injury.
- **Clotting factor II** (prothrombin) is a relatively unstable protein that is split into smaller proteins, one of which is thrombin.[8]
- **Clotting factor III** (tissue factor or thromboplastin) is found in the tissue underneath the endothelial cell layer in the tunica media and tunica adventitia. Under homeostatic conditions it is not in contact with blood unless the endothelial cell layer is injured.
- **Clotting factor IV** (calcium) is required at multiple points in the coagulation cascade where it plays a role in the activation of other coagulation factors or facilitates the processes needed to form a clot.
- **Clotting factor V** (proaccelerin or labile factor) is a cofactor that binds to platelets and is activated by thrombin. It is also required by activated factor X, together with calcium, to convert prothrombin to thrombin.[9]
- **Clotting factor VI** is not assigned.
- **Clotting factor VII** (proconvertin) is a vitamin K-dependent factor that initiates the coagulation process in collaboration with tissue factor.
- **Clotting factor VIII** (anti-haemophilic factor A) is a cofactor of activated factor IX. Although primarily synthesised by the liver, the lungs and spleen also contribute to the circulating level of this factor.[10] Deficiency of factor VIII results in a condition known

FIGURE 12.4 **Release of platelets into bone sinusoidal blood vessels for distribution in the systemic circulation.** (*Source:* www.hematology.org/ Thehematologist/Diffusion/6102.aspx.)

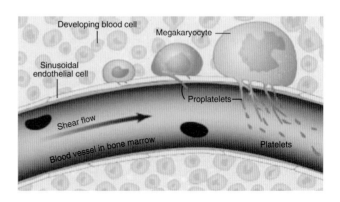

Developing blood cell

Megakaryocyte

Sinusoidal
endothelial cell

Proplatelets

Shear flow

Blood vessel in bone marrow

Platelets

TABLE 12.1
Coagulation proteins: class of action

Clotting factor number	Clotting factor name	Function	Classification
I	Fibrinogen	Fibrin clot formation	Fibrinogen family
II	Prothrombin	Fibrin clot formation; activation of factors I, V, VII, VIII, XI and XIII	Vitamin K-dependent family
III	Tissue factor or thromboplastin	Cofactor to factor VIIa	Cofactor
IV	Calcium	Required for coagulation reactions involving phospholipids	Cofactor
V	Proaccelerin or labile factor	Cofactor required for FX-mediated conversion of prothrombin to thrombin; binds platelets	Fibrinogen family
VI	Not assigned	Not assigned	Not assigned
VII	Proconvertin	Initiates the coagulation process in collaboration with factor III (tissue factor); activates factors IX and X	Vitamin K-dependent family
VIII	Anti-haemophilic factor A	Cofactor of activated factor IX	Fibrinogen family
IX	Anti-haemophilic factor B or Christmas factor	Activates factor X and forms dense complex with factor VIII	Vitamin K-dependent family
X	Stuart–Prower factor	Requires activation by factor IX; activates factor II	Vitamin K-dependent family
XI	Plasma thromboplastic antecedent	Activates factor IX	Contact family
XII	Hageman factor	Activates factors XI and XIV	Contact family
XIII	Fibrin-stabilising factor	Stabilises the fibrin clot by cross-linking fibrin	Fibrinogen family
XIV	Prekallikrein or Fletcher factor	Travels in blood as a complex with cofactor high-molecular-weight kininogen (HMWK)	Contact family
XV	High-molecular-weight kininogen (HMWK) or Fitzgerald factor	Travels as an inactive protein in blood; acts as a cofactor	Contact family
XVI	von Willebrand factor (vWF)	Binds to factor VIII; facilitates platelet adhesion to subendothelium	Glycoprotein
XVII	Anti-thrombin III	Inactivates enzymatic activity of thrombin; activates factors XII, XI, X and IX	
XVIII	Heparin clotting factor II	Naturally occurring inhibitor of coagulation; inhibits factor IIa	
XIX	Protein C	Inactivates factors Va and VIIIa	
XX	Protein S	Cofactor for protein C; protein C-S complex destroys activated factors V and VIII	Cofactor

as haemophilia A, which is characterised by loss of capacity to form clots when physiologically needed (e.g. during wound healing).

- **Clotting factor IX** (anti-haemophilic factor B or Christmas factor) deficiency results in a condition known as haemophilia B or Christmas disease, which is characterised by prolonged bleeding time.

- **Clotting factor X** (Stuart–Prower factor) is a vitamin K-dependent enzyme produced in the liver. It is activated by factor IX with its cofactor factor VIII, and factor VII with its cofactor factor III. Factor X cleaves prothrombin. Lack of vitamin K leads to loss of production of inactive factor X, which negatively affects clotting capability.

- **Clotting factor XI** (plasma thromboplastic antecedent) circulates in blood as an inactive factor that plays a role in activation of factor IX.
- **Clotting factor XII** (Hageman factor) is activated by negatively charged surfaces such as glass.[7] In a glass test tube, once activated factor XII goes on to activate factor XI and prekallikrein.
- **Clotting factor XIII** (fibrin-stabilising factor) is an enzyme called transglutaminase that fortifies the fibrin clot by crosslinking the deposited fibrin. It is activated by thrombin and requires calcium as a cofactor in order to fulfil its intended function. This factor is found in both plasma and platelet alpha granules.[11]
- **Clotting factor XIV** (prekallikrein or Fletcher factor) circulates in plasma as a complex with cofactor high-molecular-weight kininogen (HMWK). It is activated to form kallikrein by activated factor XII, plasmin and HMWK. Kallikrein then coverts HMWK to kinins and accelerates factor XII activation. Kallikrein and activated factor XII form a complex known as plasminogen activator, which converts plasminogen to plasmin, whose function is to dissolve formed clots.
- **Clotting factor XV** (HMWK or Fitzgerald factor) circulates in plasma as an inactive protein. During injury, it binds to the injured vessel wall and as it becomes activated it gains the capacity to initiate blood coagulation and to form bradykinin, a vasodilator.
- **Clotting factor XVI** (von Willebrand factor, vWF) is a glycoprotein produced by both endothelial cells and platelets that facilitates platelet adhesion to the injured vessel wall. vWF is also a carrier protein for factor VIII.[12] von Willebrand disease is an inherited disorder characterised by either insufficient or ineffective production of vWF.
- **Clotting factor XVII** (anti-thrombin III) is a glycoprotein whose role is to inactivate the enzymatic activity of thrombin, activated factors XII, XI, X and IX. Anti-thrombin III is therefore a naturally occurring inhibitor of coagulation.
- **Clotting factor XVIII** (heparin clotting factor II) is another naturally occurring inhibitor of coagulation employing similar mechanisms to anti-thrombin III but focused on thrombin.
- **Clotting factor XIX** (protein C) is a vitamin K-dependent glycoprotein that exists free in plasma. It is activated by thrombin.

- **Clotting factor XX** (protein S) is also a vitamin K-dependent glycoprotein. When activated protein C is complexed with protein S and they become potent inhibitors of coagulation by destroying activated factors V and VIII.[7]

Coagulation factors may be broadly classified into the **fibrinogen family** (fibrinogen, factors V, VIII and XIII), **vitamin K-dependent proteins** (factors II, VII, IX and X) and the **contact family** (factors XI and XII, HMWK and prekallikrein).[13]

Extrinsic coagulation pathway

The term 'extrinsic' refers to the tissue factor location being in the subendothelial layer rather than the blood circulation. The **extrinsic coagulation pathway** (Fig. 12.5) starts with injury-induced exposure of tissue factor in the subendothelial layer as well as in the plasma membrane of nearby endothelial cells.[14] As tissue factor has a high affinity for factor VII, any exposure of tissue factor to plasma factor VII will initiate formation of a calcium bridge between tissue factor-factor VII complex on the cell surface. The resulting tissue factor-calcium-factor VIIa complex then converts factor X to Xa in the common pathway. The same complex also activates factor IX to IXa in the intrinsic coagulation pathway.

Intrinsic coagulation pathway

The term '**intrinsic**' refers to all components required for the coagulation process being present in the blood. It includes contact family activation factors prekallikrein, HMWK, factors XII and XI; vitamin K-dependent factor IX; and fibrinogen family factor VIII. The **intrinsic coagulation pathway** (Fig. 12.5) is initiated when factor XII is activated following damage to the endothelium. Recall that injured endothelium has a thrombogenic surface. Activated factor XII (factor XIIa) in the presence of HMWK then activates factor XI to XIa. This cascade continues as factor XIa together with calcium ions converts factor IX to IXa. Factor IXa—which in the presence of platelet phospholipid, calcium ions and cofactor factor VIIIa—converts factor X to Xa in the common pathway.

Common coagulation pathway

The **common coagulation pathway** starts with activation of factor X to Xa (Fig. 12.5), by either the extrinsic or intrinsic pathway. At this point, factor Xa, cofactor Va, phospholipid and calcium ions convert factor II (prothrombin) to factor IIa (thrombin). Factor IIa then polymerises fibrinogen to fibrin while factor XII acts to further stabilise the polymerised network. It is important to highlight that the intrinsic and extrinsic pathways do

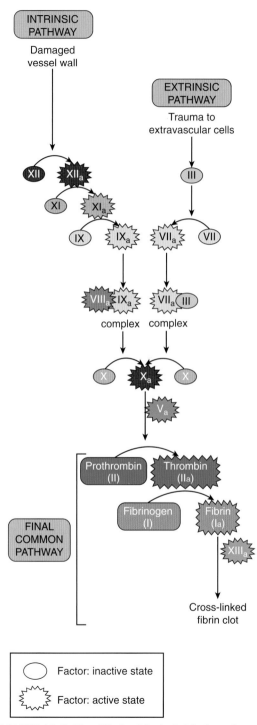

not occur as singular entities. Rather, the two pathways interact and seem to be activated around the same time.

Blood vessels and their role in intravascular, vascular and extravascular haemostasis

Blood—comprised of a liquid portion called plasma and cellular elements such as red blood cells, leucocytes and platelets—circulates in a closed system of blood vessels. When we refer to the intravascular component of haemostasis, we refer to platelets and many components in the plasma that are involved in either the formation of a clot or the dissolution of the formed clot, a process called **fibrinolysis**. This closed unidirectional pathway can be visualised with the flow of blood starting from the left heart ventricle through the aortic system to arteries, capillaries, venules and veins, returning to the right side of the heart.

Regardless of vessel type, arteries, veins and capillaries share common structural components and each is composed of three layers: the tunica intima, tunica media and tunica adventitia. Hence when we refer to the vascular component of haemostasis we refer to blood vessels through which blood flows. The inner layer, the **tunica intima**, is composed of endothelial cells lining the vessel lumen and the underlying basement membrane. Endothelial cells of the tunica intima come into direct contact with blood. However, as the intact endothelial layer is anti-thrombotic in nature due to endothelial release of anti-thrombotic substances such as nitric oxide and **prostacyclin I2**,[15] it will not randomly activate the platelets flowing in blood or initiate and promote coagulation through engagement with coagulation factors carried in blood.

The middle layer, the **tunica media**, is composed of vascular smooth muscle cells and their associated basement membrane that includes collagen molecules and an occasional fibroblast, a connective tissue cell. When the tunica intima is damaged these components are exposed to blood flow and the surfaces becomes **thrombogenic**. This means that platelet activation will be initiated as well as activation of clotting factors aimed at forming a clot.

The outermost layer, the **tunica adventitia**, is composed of loose connective tissue, fibroblasts and mesenchymal cells, the last of which seem to have progenitor/stem cell-like properties and can participate in vessel repair. This layer anchors the vessel to the surrounding tissue. The tunica adventitia and surrounding tissue (extracellular matrix) is referred to as the **extravascular component**. This component is important in wounds where the damage goes beyond one injured vessel to affecting a large area needing repair.

FIGURE 12.5 **Simplified extrinsic, intrinsic and common pathways of coagulation.** (*Source:* Modified from https://courses.lumenlearning.com/ap2/chapter/hemostasis.)

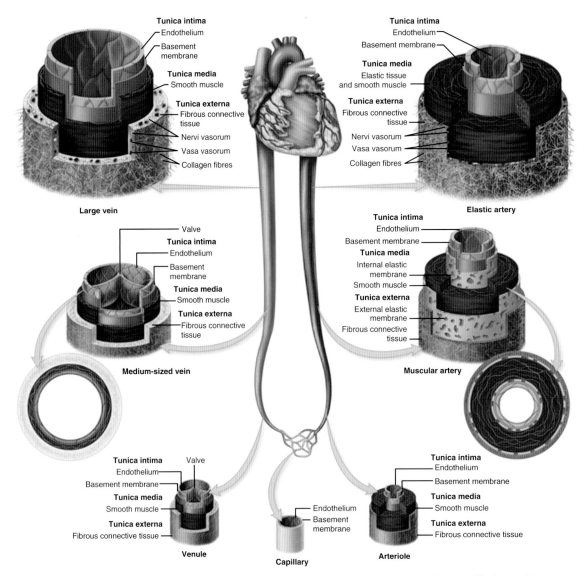

FIGURE 12.6 **Blood flows in a closed system that comprises the heart, arteries, capillaries and veins.** (*Source:* Patton KT, Thibodeau GA, editors. Anatomy and physiology, 9 ed. London: Elsevier Health Sciences; 2015.)

Fig. 12.6 outlines the basic structural components of arteries, veins and capillaries to help you to visualise these three layers and how they may play a part in haemostatic mechanisms.

Haemostatic mechanisms: primary and secondary haemostasis

When an injury results in loss of blood vessel integrity—for example, a vessel is severed or part of it is damaged—and blood leaves the closed circuit, haemostasis will occur in two stages: primary and secondary. During primary haemostasis a weak platelet plug is formed to act as 'first aid' and close the initial bleeding site in the injured vessel. This plug is then reinforced by a fibrin network and additional platelet integration so that it can withhold the pressure exerted by the blood flow. This second step constitutes **secondary haemostasis**.

Primary haemostasis

During primary haemostasis (Fig. 12.7) four overlapping events take place: contraction of vessel walls (vasoconstriction), platelet adhesion to the injured vessel, platelet

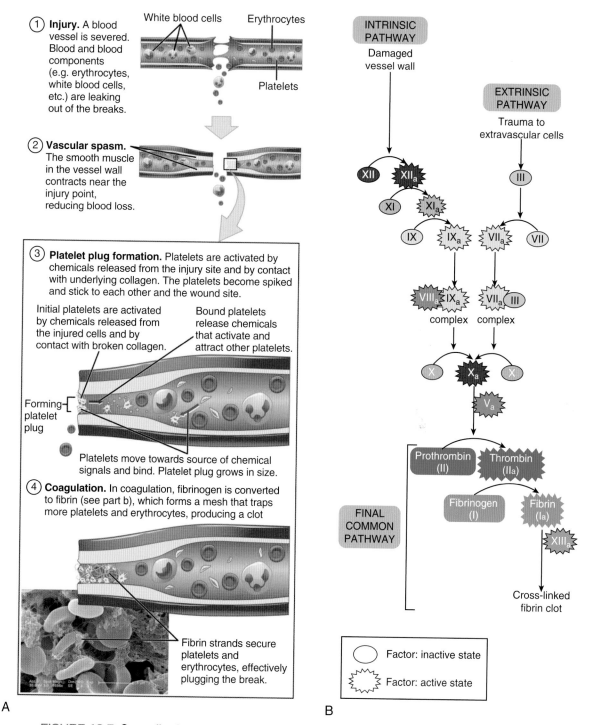

FIGURE 12.7 **Generalised representation of primary and secondary haemostasis. A** Primary haemostasis: platelet plug formation. **B** Secondary haemostasis: formation of fibrin clot. (*Source:* Modified from https://courses.lumenlearning.com/ap2/chapter/hemostasis.)

activation and platelet aggregation leading to formation of the platelet plug. After injury, a vessel will spasm, which will lead to **vasoconstriction**. The purpose of vasoconstriction is to reduce blood flow and therefore reduce the volume of blood lost from circulation. This is mediated by endothelin-1, a molecule secreted by injured endothelial cells and acting on the vascular smooth muscle cells, forcing them to contract.[16] The endothelial lining will be either damaged or lost, exposing the collagen that is a constituent of the endothelial basement membrane and is found around the vascular smooth muscle cells of the tunica media. Under normal conditions, endothelial cells produce vWF, which is stored

in the endothelial basement membrane matrix where it binds to subendothelial collagen. vWF is also produced by platelets and is stored in platelet alpha granules. The role of vWF is to act as a link between the injured vessel and the platelet, thus facilitating formation of the platelet plug (Fig. 12.8).

Platelets, or thrombocytes, are produced in the bone marrow under the regulation of the hormone thrombopoietin through the process of megakaryocyte fragmentation. On the platelet surface specific glycoproteins are expressed that are important in the adhesion and aggregation of platelets. With respect to **platelet adhesion** to collagen, **glycoprotein (GP)** Ia is important. Adhesion

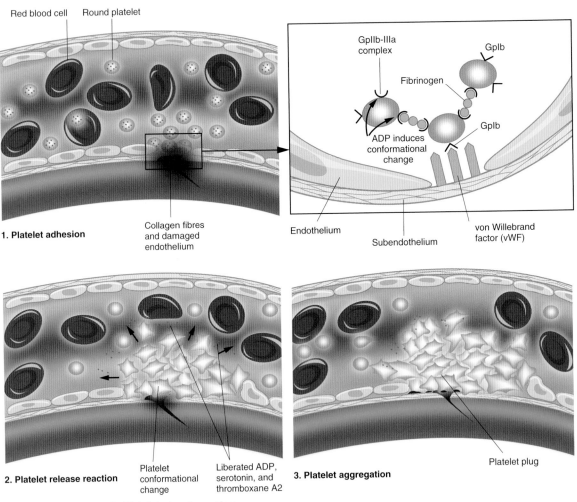

1. **Platelet adhesion** — Red blood cell, Round platelet, Collagen fibres and damaged endothelium

GpIIb-IIIa complex, GpIb, Fibrinogen, GpIb, ADP induces conformational change, Endothelium, Subendothelium, von Willebrand factor (vWF)

2. **Platelet release reaction** — Platelet conformational change, Liberated ADP, serotonin, and thromboxane A2

3. **Platelet aggregation** — Platelet plug

FIGURE 12.8 **Platelet plug formation.**

to vWF expressed by the subendothelial layer is mediated by GP Ib, IIb and IIIa. The binding site for GP IIb–IIIa is also the receptor for fibrinogen, an important component needed for platelet aggregation. Thus, during vessel injury, once the endothelial cells are damaged, collagen and vWF become exposed. Circulating platelets will slow down and start to roll along the vessel wall until they encounter collagen, to which the platelets bind via GP Ib, and vWF, to which the platelets bind via GPIIb–GP IIIa. This results in platelet adhesion. As platelets adhere to the injured vessel, they also undergo shape transformation, from discoid to star-shaped, whereby they develop pseudopodia-like structures that allow them to increase their surface area and enhance interactions between neighbouring platelets. This is known as **platelet activation**. In addition to being activated by adhesion to collagen, platelets can be activated by platelet agonists such as thrombin, an enzyme that plays a principal role in secondary haemostasis. Following their change of shape, platelets release the contents of their alpha granules such as vWF, adenosine diphosphate (ADP), calcium, thrombin, serotonin, fibrinogen and thromboxane A2, with the latter acting as a vasoconstrictor (and it is also produced by endothelial cells).[7] ADP further activates platelets by interacting with ADP receptors on the platelet surface. The intrinsic system is activated by the contact of coagulation factor XII, HMWK and prekallikrein with subendothelial collagen, which then sets off the secondary haemostatic mechanism.

Secondary haemostasis

During secondary haemostasis, the initial platelet plug is reinforced with fibrin mesh, which is formed by polymerisation of fibrinogen, a protein found in the blood circulation. The formation of fibrin is driven by the coagulation process consisting of the intrinsic, extrinsic and common coagulation pathways responding to vessel injury.

Fibrinolysis

As the blood vessel heals and endothelial cell layer integrity is re-established—that is, the endothelial cells migrate from either side of the injury to form a single layered tunica intima—the endothelium starts to secrete substances that act to further restore the endothelial cell surface towards being anti-thrombogenic. For this purpose, endothelial cells secrete tissue plasminogen activator (tPA) to initiate the breakdown of the fibrin clot that has formed at the site of the injury (Fig. 12.9). Endothelial cells also provide an adhesion site for anti-thrombin III, which then permits anti-thrombin III to exert its inhibitory effects on thrombin. Furthermore, endothelial cells synthesise thrombomodulin, which binds thrombin. This reaction allows activation of protein C, which binds with protein S to form protein C-S complex, which inhibits coagulation and enhances fibrinolysis. **Tissue factor pathway inhibitor (TFPI)** is another inhibitor of coagulation that is secreted by endothelial cells and platelets and can be found travelling in plasma. It acts by preventing the formation of tissue

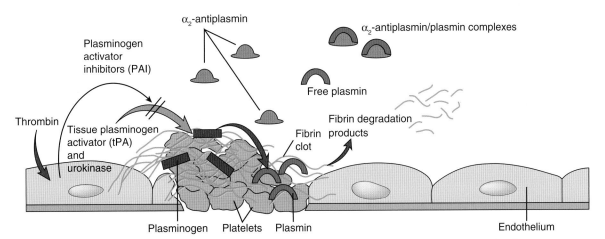

FIGURE 12.9 Fibrinolysis. Fibrinolysis is a process that involves endothelial cells and blood anti-coagulation proteins. The aim is to dissolve a blood clot and return the blood vessel to homeostatic state. (*Source:* https://vet.uga.edu/ivcvm/courses/VPAT5200/01_circulation/hemostasis/hemostasis06.html.)

factor FVIIa complex, thus interfering with the intrinsic coagulation process.[17]

At the same time, fibrin in the clot adsorbs the plasminogen from the circulation. Once inside the clot, plasminogen is converted to plasmin, which then starts to cleave the fibrin clot. Any excess plasmin found in the circulation will be managed by the molecules that destroy plasmin, known collectively as **anti-plasmins**. Examples of anti-plasmins include α_2-macroglobulin, α_1-anti-trysin, α_2-anti-plasmin and anti-thrombin III. α_2-macroglobulin also inhibits thrombin and kallikrein, while anti-thrombin III also inhibits thrombin, factors XIIa, XIa, Xa and IXa and kallikrein. This means that in addition to having a role in the lysis of the fibrin clot, these two anti-plasmins interrupt the coagulation cascade pathway. Anti-plasmins are therefore naturally occurring inhibitors of fibrinolysis which is necessary to maintain the positive effect of wound healing, as excessive fibrinolysis would lead to opening of the wound due to premature loss of the protective clot.

Blood tests for haemostasis

If it is suspected that a person may have an abnormality in forming clots when physiologically needed—for example, during wound healing—blood tests may be ordered. Such abnormalities can be grouped broadly into **bleeding disorders** and disorders that lead to **excessive blood clot formation**.

If a person has experienced prolonged bleeding or they bruise easily, one or more of their clotting factors may be missing, which impacts the coagulation pathway. A blood sample will be collected in a tube that contains a special anticoagulant (3.2% sodium citrate, which is equivalent to 109 mM sodium citrate) to test the **clotting profile**, sometimes also requested as **clotting studies**. Sodium citrate is a chelator, meaning that it will bind Ca^{2+} ions in the blood sample, thus preventing clotting from occurring in the test tube.[18] Blood tests will also be used to determine how long it takes blood to clot. Examples of tests that may be taken include platelet count, factor V, fibrinogen levels, prothrombin time (PT, the time it takes to form a blood clot), activated partial thromboplastin time (aPTT) and thrombin time (TT, which indirectly estimates the capacity of fibrin to form clots). A less frequent test may be **bleeding time**.[18] The PT test checks for defects in the extrinsic coagulation pathway. Simply, a reagent containing thromboplastin (an enzyme that converts prothrombin to thrombin), tissue factor, calcium and phospholipid is added to the blood sample, initiating blood clotting. Remember that extrinsic pathway activation commences with tissue factor expression. In the aPTT test, coagulation is assessed by

activating the intrinsic coagulation pathway. In this case, negatively charged silica and phospholipids are added to plasma. Recall that factor XII can be activated by negatively charged surfaces like glass.[18]

Rare blood test requests are associated with hereditary conditions affecting coagulation. For example, testing for factor V Leiden is used to identify a variant of factor V, which leads to failure to have this factor inactivated by protein C and therefore places the person at increased risk of venous thromboembolism. Deficiencies in protein S and protein C are other rare disorders that result in abnormalities in the function of coagulation factors V and VIII.[18]

Another test you may encounter is the D-dimer test. Here the aim is to identify a specific fragment of fibrin clot, known as **D-dimer**, which is generated as the clot is being lysed by fibrinolysis. It is used as an indicator of whether clot lysis is taking place in the body.

INTEGRATION WITH OTHER BODY SYSTEMS

Cardiovascular system

In this chapter we have highlighted the important role that blood vessels play in primary and secondary haemostasis. When injured, blood vessel endothelium secretes factors that attract platelets as well as initiating the coagulation cascade. Once the endothelial cells re-establish endothelial cell integrity in the blood vessels, they secrete fibrinolytic factors that lead to dissolution of the formed clot. Failure to dissolve a vascular clot can lead to deep vein thrombosis, myocardial infarction and stroke due to emboli lodging in the smaller vessels.

Gastrointestinal system

The gastrointestinal system is where vitamin K, a fat-soluble vitamin, is formed by bacteria residing in the gut. Vitamin K does not play a direct role in coagulation, but it is fundamental to the synthesis of coagulation factors II, VII, IX and X, protein C and protein S. In adults vitamin K deficiency is very rare but it is observed in infants, where it leads to excessive bleeding.

At birth, newborns are relatively deficient in vitamin K, meaning that all proteins that require vitamin K-induced activation to reach an 'active' state are in lower abundance. This is due to two factors: vitamin K cannot cross the placenta and breast milk is low in vitamin K. Without the administration of vitamin K at birth, the rate of haemorrhagic disease of the newborn is approximately 0.17% of all births, but this falls to less than 0.0001% when parenteral vitamin K is administered.[19] Parental refusal of vitamin K injection does occur and is often associated with concomitant vaccine hesitancy or refusal. A Canadian study reported that rates of vitamin K injection refusal range from 0.2% in hospital births to 14.5% in planned home births, demonstrating a marked variation in the prevalence of this decision, which can have significant negative health-related outcomes for the infant.[20]

In Australia, at birth all infants receive an intramuscular injection of vitamin K to prevent the possibility of vitamin K-associated bleeding disorders. For neonates under 1500 grams in weight the dose is 0.5 mg given as a single dose at birth; for neonates weighing more than 1500 grams, the dose is 1 mg given as a single dose at birth.[21]

A healthy liver is essential for an effective coagulation system as nearly all coagulation factors are made in the liver. Chronic liver diseases can impact the synthesis of coagulation factors and inhibitor factors as well as lead to decreased clearance of activated clotting factors. Furthermore, chronic liver diseases are associated with defective platelets as well as increased risk of excessive fibrinolysis.[22]

Skeletal system

The bone marrow of long bones such as the femur is home to haematopoietic cells. These cells, under the influence of many growth factors, differentiate into different lineages of blood cells. One of those factors is **thrombopoietin**, which helps differentiate bone marrow megakaryoblasts into megakaryocytes and then facilitates the disintegration of these cells into cell fragments and thus platelets.

Pregnancy

As described in Chapter 22, significant alterations in the haemostatic system occur during pregnancy. These changes are physiological, aimed at optimising placental blood flow and minimising the risk of haemorrhage during delivery. Nonetheless, for some women changes in haemostatic proteins during pregnancy can confer an increased risk of thrombosis, particularly if they have a pre-existing thrombophilia. This is due to the balance between procoagulant and anticoagulant proteins becoming disregulated, fostering a pro-thrombotic state that cannot be adequately compensated for.

AGE-RELATED CHANGES

Normative coagulation reference ranges for Australian children using current laboratory methods have provided conclusive evidence that the haemostatic system is dynamic and constantly evolving from birth through to adulthood.[23] The resultant balance between pro-coagulant and anticoagulant proteins in infants and children renders them relatively thrombo-protected. For example, for the same insult (e.g. surgery, prolonged bed rest) children are far less likely to develop thrombotic complications compared with adults.

Table 12.2 presents the age-related differences in coagulation parameters in a cohort of Australian children. There are significant differences between many coagulation parameters determined for infants, children and adults. Of note, the levels of coagulation factors II and X in newborn babies are 50% lower compared with levels in healthy adults. Similarly, levels of AT are significantly reduced at birth, but increase rapidly during infancy. Throughout infancy and childhood, the ability of plasma to generate thrombin is approximately 50% lower than that of adults. Monagle and colleagues were the first to demonstrate that individual age-related variations in coagulation parameters have a cumulative effect on thrombin generation.[23]

Andrew and colleagues reported on an in vitro study of thrombin regulation in children compared with adults in the presence and absence of unfractionated heparin (UFH).[24] This study demonstrated that the ability of children's plasma to generate thrombin was significantly reduced compared with that of adult plasma. Andrew and colleagues further demonstrated that increased levels of α_2-macroglobulin present throughout childhood result in a greater proportion of thrombin inhibition in plasma from children being mediated by α_2-macroglobulin compared with that observed in adult plasma.

CONCLUSION

Haemostasis is a complex physiological process with the primary aim of maintaining blood in a fluid state until such time that thrombus propagation at a site of endothelial damage is necessary to prevent blood loss. Through formation of a platelet plug (primary haemostasis) and activation of the coagulation pathway to form a fibrin mesh to fortify the platelet plug (secondary haemostasis) vascular injury is stabilised to allow vessel healing. This healing process is further facilitated by collaborative interaction between the endothelium and blood to lyse the clot once it is no longer needed through fibrinolysis. Age-related research in haemostasis clearly indicates that children differ from adults in many ways, including being protected from thrombotic processes in the early years of their lives.

TABLE 12.2
Haemostasis reference ranges for Australian children

			Age				
	1 day	3 days	1 month–1 year	1–5 years	6–10 years	11–16 years	Adults
Coagulation test							
aPTT (sec)	38.7* (34.3–44.8)	36.3* (29.5–42.2)	39.3* (35.1–46.3)	37.7* (33.6–43.8)	37.3* (31.8–43.7)	39.5* (33.9–46.1)	33.2 (28.6–38.2)
TCT (sec)	Not available	Not available	17.1* (16.3–17.6)	17.5* (16.6–18.2)	17.1 (16.1–18.5)	16.9 (16.2–17.6)	16.6 (16.2–17.2)
PT (sec)	15.6* (14.4–16.4)	14.9* (13.5–16.4)	13.1 (11.5–15.3)	13.3* (12.1–14.5)	13.4* (11.7–15.1)	13.8* (12.7–16.1)	13.0 (11.5–14.5)
INR	1.26* (1.15–1.35)	1.20* (1.05–1.35)	1.00 (0.86–1.22)	1.03* (0.92–1.14)	1.04* (0.87–1.20)	1.08* (0.97–1.30)	1.00 (0.80–1.20)
Fibrinogen (g/L)	2.8 (1.9–3.7)	3.3 (2.8–4.0)	2.4* (0.8–1.2)	2.8* (1.6–4.0)	3.0 (2.0–4.9)	3.2 (2.1–4.3)	3.1 (1.9–4.3)
Coagulation factor (%)							
II	54* (41–69)	62* (50–73)	90* (62–103)	89* (70–109)	89* (67–110)	90* (61–107)	110 (78–138)
V	81* (64–103)	122 (92–154)	113 (94–141)	97* (67–127)	99* (56–141)	89* (67–141)	118 (78–152)
VII	70* (52–88)	86* (67–107)	128 (83–160)	111* (72–150)	113* (70–156)	118 (69–200)	129 (61–199)
VIII	182 (105–329)	159 (83–274)	94* (54–145)	110* (36–185)	117* (52–182)	120* (59–200)	160 (52–290)
IX	48* (35–56)	72* (44–97)	71* (43–121)	85* (44–127)	96* (48–145)	111* (64–216)	130 (59–254)
X	55* (46–67)	60* (46–75)	95* (77–122)	98* (72–125)	97* (68–125)	91* (53–122)	124 (96–171)
XI	30* (7–41)	57* (24–79)	89* (62–125)	113 (65–162)	113 (65–162)	111 (65–139)	112 (67–196)
XII	58* (43–80)	53* (14–80)	79* (20–135)	85* (36–135)	81* (26–137)	75* (14–117)	115 (35–207)
Coagulation inhibitors							
AT	76* (58–90)	74* (60–89)	109* (72–134)	116* (101–131)	114* (95–134)	111* (96–126)	96 (66–124)
Protein C chromogenic	36* (24–44)	44* (28–54)	71* (31–112)	96* (65–127)	100 (71–129)	94* (66–118)	104 (74–164)
Protein C clotting	32* (24–40)	33* (24–51)	77* (28–124)	94* (50–134)	94* (64–125)	88* (59–112)	103 (54–166)
Protein S clotting	36* (28–47)	49* (33–67)	102* (29–162)	101* (67–136)	109* (64–144)	103* (65–140)	75 (54–103)
TFPI free (ng/mL)	Not available	Not available	7.13* (5.63–8.44)	6.80 (5.06–10.07)	6.69* (4.29–9.31)	7.66* (5.15–8.74)	10.7 (6.12–12.34)
TFPI total (ng/mL)	Not available	Not available	77.49 (69.42–85.58)	76.33 (61.27–89.8)	73.99 (59.13–88.02)	74.09 (61.63–87.36)	87.49 (63.64–104.34)
ETP (pM.min)	Not available	Not available	4865* (2653–7162)	4429* (2537–6084)	5365* (2719–8938)	7593 (3373–8930)	8475 (7043–10205)

Note: Results presented as mean (95% of population);*p<0.05.
aPTT = activated partial thromboplastin time; AT = anti-thrombin; ETP = endogenous thrombin potential; INR = International Normalised Ratio; PT = prothrombin time; TCT = thrombin clotting time; TFPI = tissue factor pathway inhibitor
Source: Adapted with permission from Monagle P, Barnes C, Ignjatovic V, Furmedge J, Newall F, Chan A et al. Developmental haemostasis: impact for clinical haemostasis laboratories. Thrombosis Haemost 2006;95:362–72.

CASE STUDY 12.1

Josie is a 28-year-old schoolteacher pregnant for the first time and in her second trimester of pregnancy. She has recently been diagnosed with a deep vein thrombosis. Her mother and maternal aunt both developed deep vein thromboses during pregnancy. Josie's unborn baby is a girl.

Q1. Injury to a blood vessel is repaired through:
   a. primary and secondary haemostasis.
   b. proliferation of endothelial cells at the site of injury.
   c. removal of endothelial cells from the tunica intima.
   d. both a and b are correct.

Q2. The initiation of fibrin clot formation in the injured blood vessel is due to:
   a. activation of cell-death processes.
   b. absence of platelets from circulation.
   c. reduced levels of clotting factors in circulation.
   d. activation of the coagulation pathway.

Q3. During pregnancy changes in the haemostatic system:
   a. promote placental blood flow.
   b. reduce the risk of haemorrhage during childbirth.
   c. increase the risk of thrombosis.
   d. all of the above.

Q4. Why might three members of Josie's family all have developed thromboses during pregnancy?

Q5. Josie is worried about the risk of her unborn baby girl developing a thrombosis after birth. Is this a likely outcome?

CASE STUDY 12.2

Peter was born by vaginal delivery at 39 weeks gestation following an uncomplicated pregnancy. His father was present during the labour and delivery, and both parents cuddled Peter immediately after birth. While still in the delivery suite, Peter's parents were told that it was time for him to have his vitamin K injection.

Q1. Which coagulation protein/s require vitamin K to reach their 'active' state?
   a. Coagulation factors II, VII, IX and X
   b. Anti-thrombin
   c. Tissue factor pathway inhibitor
   d. Fibrinogen

Q2. What is the risk of haemorrhagic disease of the newborn if vitamin K is not given?
   a. 17%
   b. 7%
   c. 1%
   d. 0.17%

Q3. Why are neonates deplete of vitamin K at birth? (Select all that apply)
   a. Breast milk does not contain vitamin K.
   b. Vitamin K doesn't cross the placenta during pregnancy.
   c. The mother didn't drink enough orange juice during pregnancy.
   d. They aren't; there is no need for vitamin K to be given to neonates.

Q4. Propose why adults do not require vitamin K injections to keep their coagulation pathway functioning well.

Q5. Discuss why a healthy liver is needed to maintain a healthy coagulation pathway.

CASE STUDY 12.3

Billy is a 16-year-old boy with hobbies including mountain-biking, skateboarding and rock-climbing. He has no significant past medical history, beyond the expected cuts and scrapes associated with childhood and adolescence. He was at his local skate park this morning when he sustained a 5 cm laceration to his right knee after landing awkwardly.

Q1. What physiological process is involved in ensuring that Billy's body mounts an appropriate response to this injury to prevent excessive blood loss?
   a. Homeostasis
   b. Haemostasis
   c. Revascularisation
   d. Metabolism

Continued

CASE STUDY 12.3—cont'd

Q2. What is the first physiological response initiated by the body to minimise blood loss after an injury?
  a. Increase in blood pressure
  b. Reduction in temperature
  c. Vasoconstriction
  d. Vasodilation

Q3. The subendothelial layer can activate platelet adhesion to the site of an injury as well as the coagulation pathway to deposit fibrin mesh.
  a. True
  b. False

Q4. Why is platelet aggregation at the site of an injury not a sufficient response to minimise blood loss?

Q5. Discuss the role of endothelial cells in clot dissolution.

CASE STUDY 12.4

Jonathon is an 85-year-old man who has no previous history of poor health. On his drive home from the shops he was involved in a multi-vehicle accident that resulted in him sustaining major abdominal, head and lower limb injuries. He was transported very quickly via ambulance to his closest emergency department, where he was assessed and referred to surgery.

Q1. On arrival, Jonathon had a platelet count of 28,000 per microlitre of blood. The reference range is usually 150,000–450,000. Why might this be the case?
  a. Due to the prolonged response to injury, his platelets were mobilised to the site of his injuries and consumed in building clots as a response to his significant injuries.
  b. He was deficient in platelets prior to his injuries.
  c. Platelets were destroyed in the spleen.
  d. Platelets self-destructed at the time of his injuries.

Q2. Considering his age, Jonathan:
  a. will be protected from thrombophilic conditions.
  b. may experience an increased risk of thromboembolism.
  c. may have decreased capacity to make new platelets.
  d. both b and c are correct.

Q3. Considering that Jonathan requires surgery and his platelet count is low, to reduce the risk of complications associated with bleeding, which of the following treatments may be planned?
  a. Platelet transfusion
  b. Anti-thrombin III
  c. Thrombin
  d. Red blood cell transfusion

Q4. Jonathon is in significant pain and has been administered narcotic analgesia to help ameliorate this. What part of the normal haemostatic response might this impact?

Q5. Jonathon's injuries include significant disruption to his vascular endothelium at multiple sites. Why is this significant with respect to his ability to mount an appropriate response to his injuries in terms of minimising blood loss?

REFERENCES

1. Lewis S, Bain B, Bates I. Practical haematology, 10 ed. Philadelphia: Churchill Livingstone Elsevier; 2001.
2. Giglia TM, Massicotte MP, Tweddell JS, et al. Prevention and treatment of thrombosis in pediatric and congenital heart disease: a scientific statement from the American Heart Association. Circulation 2013;128(24):2622–703.
3. Brummel KE, Jenny NS, Mann KG. Molecular and cellular hemostasis and fibrinolysis. In: Lanzer P, Topol EJ, editors. Pan vascular medicine: integrated clinical management. Berlin: Springer Berlin Heidelberg; 2002. p. 287–318.
4. Afdhal N, McHutchison J, Brown R, et al. Thrombocytopenia associated with chronic liver disease. J Hepatol 2008;48(6):1000–7. doi:10.1016/j.jhep.2008.03.009.
5. Machlus KR, Italiano JE Jr. The incredible journey: from megakaryocyte development to platelet formation. J Cell Biol 2013;201(6):785–96.
6. Palta S, Saroa R, Palta A. Overview of the coagulation system. Indian J Anaesth 2014;58(5):515–23. doi:10.4103/0019-5049.144643.
7. Lanzkowsky P, editor. Manual of paediatric haematology, 5 ed. Elsevier; 2011.

8. Stubbs MT, Bode W. A player of many parts: the spotlight falls on thrombin's structure. Thromb Res 1993;69(1):1–58.

9. Duga S, Asselta R, Tenchini ML. Coagulation factor V. Int J Biochem Cell Biol 2004;36(8):1393–9.

10. Lenting PJ, van Mourik JA, Mertens K. The life cycle of coagulation factor VIII in view of its structure and function. Blood 1998;92(11):3983–96.

11. Komáromi I, Bagoly Z, Muszbek L. Factor XIII: novel structural and functional aspects. J Thromb Haemost 2011; 9(1):9–20.

12. Palta S, Saroa R, Palta A. Overview of the coagulation system. Indian J Anaesth 2014;58(5):515–23. doi:10.4103/0019-5049.144643.

13. Palta S, Saroa R, Palta A. Overview of the coagulation system. Indian J Anaesth 2014;58(5):515–23. doi:10.4103/0019-5049.144643.

14. Price GC, Thompson SA, Kam PCA. Tissue factor and tissue factor pathway inhibitor. Anaesthesia 2004;59(5):483–92.

15. Mitchell JA, Ali F, Bailey L, et al. Role of nitric oxide and prostacyclin as vasoactive hormones released by the endothelium. Exp Physiol 2008;93(1):141–7.

16. Marasciulo FL, Montagnani M, Potenza MA. Endothelin-1: the yin and yang on vascular function. Curr Med Chem 2006;13(14):1655–65.

17. Mast AE. Tissue factor pathway inhibitor: multiple anticoagulant activities for a single protein. Arterioscler Thromb Vasc Biol 2016;36(1):9–14.

18. Harris NS, Bazydlo LAL, Winter WE. Coagulation tests. A primer on hemostasis for clinical chemists. Available from: www.aacc.org/publications/cln/articles/2012/january/coagulation-tests.

19. Phillippi JC, Holley SL, Morad A, et al. Prevention of vitamin K deficiency bleeding. J Midwifery Women's Health 2016;61(5):632–6.

20. Sahni V, Lai FY, MacDonald SE. Neonatal vitamin K refusal and nonimmunization. Pediatrics 2014;134(3):497–503.

21. South Australian Neonatal Medication Guidelines. Vitamin K. Available from: www.sahealth.sa.gov.au/wps/wcm/connect/b02d36804cd80dd3bbf9bba496684d9f/VitaminK_Neo_v2_0_24042018.pdf?MOD=AJPERES&CACHEID=ROOTWORKSPACE-b02d36804cd80dd3bbf9bba496684d9f-mJLhmrX.

22. Amitrano L, Guardascione MA, Brancaccio V, et al. Coagulation disorders in liver disease. Semin Liver Dis 2002;22(1):83–96.

23. Monagle P, Barnes C, Ignjatovic V, et al. Developmental haemostasis: impact for clinical haemostasis laboratories. Thrombosis Haemost 2006;95:362–72.

24. Andrew M, Mitchell L, Vegh P, et al. Thrombin regulation in children differs from adults in the absence and presence of heparin. Thrombosis Haemost 1994;72(6):836–42.

CHAPTER 13

Cardiovascular system

STEVEN NELSON, GDCE • ZERINA TOMKINS, BAPPSC (MED LAB SCI), BAPPSC (HONS), MNSC (NURS), PHD, GRAD CERT (UNIVERSITY EDUCATION)

KEY POINTS/LEARNING OUTCOMES

1. Describe the main anatomical structures of the heart and blood vessels.
2. Describe the components of the electrical conducting system of the heart and of a normal electrocardiograph.
3. Link the heart contraction event with the cardiac conduction system.
4. Discuss the concept of cardiac output and blood pressure and how this adapts to meet functional demands.
5. Discuss how the function of the cardiovascular system affects other body systems and how those systems impact cardiac output and blood pressure.

KEY DEFINITIONS

- **Afterload:** the force that opposes the heart's ventricle ejection of blood.
- **Blood pressure:** the pressure in the aorta and arteries measured at peak contraction of the left ventricle and relaxation in between contractions.
- **Cardiac output:** measure of the amount of blood ejected from the left ventricle over the span of one minute.
- **Contractility:** the ability of cardiac muscle to contract through the shortening of muscle fibres.
- **Heart rate:** the number of times the heart beats in one minute.
- **Preload:** the stretching force that distends the cardiac ventricular muscle just before contraction.
- **Stroke volume:** the amount of blood ejected from the ventricle in a single contraction.

ONLINE RESOURCES/SUGGESTED READINGS

- **Cardiovascular system: coronary arteries** available at www.youtube.com/watch?v=R_x_AaRxrol
- **ECG interpretation** available at www.racgp.org.au/education/professional-development/online-learning/webinars/heart-health/ecg-interpretation
- **Flow through the heart** available at www.khanacademy.org/science/health-and-medicine/circulatory-system/circulatory-system-introduction/v/flow-through-the-heart
- **Heart Foundation Online Learning** available at www.heartfoundation.org.au/for-professionals/online-learning
- **Meet the heart!** available at www.khanacademy.org/science/high-school-biology/hs-human-body-systems/hs-the-circulatory-and-respiratory-systems/v/meet-the-heart
- **The heart: anatomy and function** available at www.coursera.org/lecture/infarction/the-heart-anatomy-and-function-hnfHS

INTRODUCTION

The cardiovascular system, also known as the circulatory system, is made up of the heart, blood and blood vessels—a network of pipelines that conduct blood throughout your body. The cardiovascular system can be further divided into the **pulmonary circulation**, where blood is oxygenated (discussed in Chapter 17), and the **systemic circulation**, which refers to the circulation found in the rest of the body. The **heart** is a hollow muscular organ that pumps blood via the blood vessels

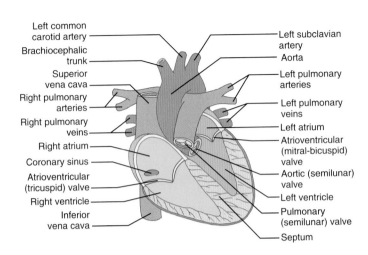

FIGURE 13.1 Anatomy of the heart.
(*Source:* Jones M, Harvey A, Main E. Anatomy and physiology of the respiratory and cardiac systems. In: Main E, Denehy L, editors. Cardiorespiratory physiotherapy: adults and paediatrics. Elsevier; 2016.)

to tissues, where the blood supplies tissue cells with nutrients and oxygen and removes cellular waste and carbon dioxide. Blood is composed of plasma, leucocytes, erythrocytes and platelets (see Chapter 11). While erythrocytes continuously supply oxygen and nutrients to the cells and remove cellular metabolic waste products for excretion via the kidneys and lungs,[1] leucocytes play a role in immunity (Chapter 15) and platelets participate in blood clotting (Chapter 11). Blood also transports hormones and electrolytes, and helps maintain temperature homeostasis and pH levels. There are three types of blood vessels: arteries, capillaries and veins. In general, arteries conduct blood away from the heart towards the smaller diameter capillaries then to veins, which merge into a great vein known as the vena cava to return blood to the heart.

The focus of this chapter is the main anatomical components and physiological functions of the heart and blood vessels that are responsible for continuous and effective circulation of blood through the vascular network to maintain the body's homeostatic functions. In addition, the chapter demonstrates the close link between cardiac function and the vascular system, and how adaptations in these two components in cooperation with feedback from other body systems enable you to quickly react and adapt to the demands of the environment, such as running.

STRUCTURE AND FUNCTION OF THE HEART

The heart is made up of four chambers: the **right** and **left atria** and the **right** and **left ventricles** (Fig. 13.1).[2] The right and left atria are separated by the **interatrial septum**, and the right and left ventricles are separated

by the **interventricular septum**. The left ventricle has a thicker muscular wall than the right ventricle as it must generate greater pressure to pump the blood into the systemic circulation, whereas the right ventricle only pumps the blood into the pulmonary circulation, which requires less effort. The atria and ventricles are made up of myocardium (heart muscle) designed to contract and relax with precise timing to maximise flow of blood through the heart.[2]

The heart has three layers: the endocardium, myocardium and pericardium (Fig. 13.2).[3] The **endocardium**

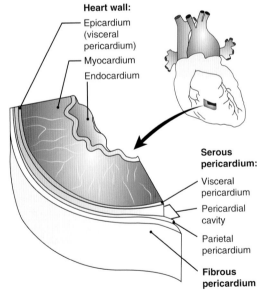

FIGURE 13.2 Layers of the heart. (*Source:* Cohen BJ, Hull K. Memmler's the human body in health and disease, 13 ed. Philadelphia: Lippincott Williams & Wilkins; 2015.)

is an internal thin layer composed of endothelial-like cells that provides a non-thrombogenic surface, thus allowing blood to move through the heart easily. The middle layer is the **myocardium**, which is made up of cardiac muscle cells known as cardiomyocytes that contract and relax to pump blood through the heart and into the body. The myocardium of the ventricles is thicker with muscle than that of the atria.[3] The third layer is the double-layered **pericardium**, which is composed of fibrous and serous pericardium. These two layers are separated by serous fluid, which acts as a shock absorber, thus protecting the heart from external shock. The pericardium is designed to decrease friction from the motion of the pumping heart and the pericardial sac the heart sits within.[3]

There are four one-directional valves that prevent backflow of blood and allow the heart to pump blood continuously in one direction. These valves are connected to the heart through structures called chordae tendineae. The valves are made of flaps or cusps composed of fibrous connective tissue covered by specialised endothelium. The right atrioventricular valve, also known as the **tricuspid valve**, and the left atrioventricular valve, also known as the **mitral (or bicuspid) valve**, control blood flow between the atria. The **pulmonary** and **aortic valves** (also known as the semilunar valves) are made up of three cusps. The pulmonary valve is in the right ventricle and blood pumped from the right ventricle goes through this valve and into the pulmonary artery. The aortic valve is in the left ventricle and blood pumped from the left ventricle goes through this valve and into the aorta (Fig. 13.3).[2,3]

Gaining an understanding of the structure of the heart will help you to understand how the anatomical

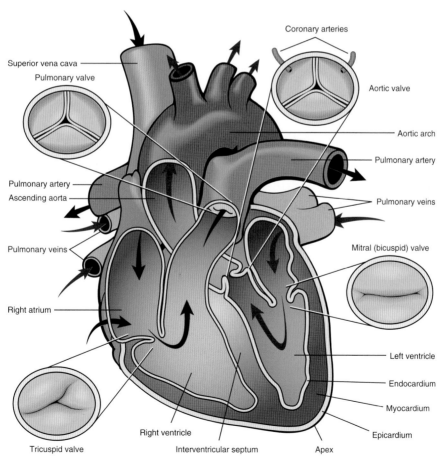

FIGURE 13.3 Location of the four heart valves. (*Source:* Damjanov I. Pathology for the health professions, 4 ed. Elsevier; 2012.)

parts of the cardiovascular system function together to propel blood around the body. In view of this, the first concept to discuss is the flow of blood through the heart as it relates to the conduction system of the heart, cardiac output and regulation of blood flow and blood pressure homeostasis.

Blood flow through the heart

Starting with blood returning to the heart (Fig. 13.4), carbon dioxide-rich blood enters the heart via the inferior and superior venae cavae pouring into the right atria. This occurs during the heart's relaxation stage, also known as diastole. At first, the right atrioventricular (tricuspid) valve is closed. As the pressure from the blood builds up inside the right atria and it starts to exceed the pressure existing in the right ventricle, the blood pushes the leaflets of the right atrioventricular valve to open and funnel blood into the ventricle.[4] As the blood volume fills the ventricle, its circular movement inside the ventricle, combined with the increase in blood volume and pressure inside the ventricle, pushes the leaflets to close. When the ventricle contracts, this contraction forces blood to push against the tricuspid valve, thus sealing it completely and preventing backflow, while opening

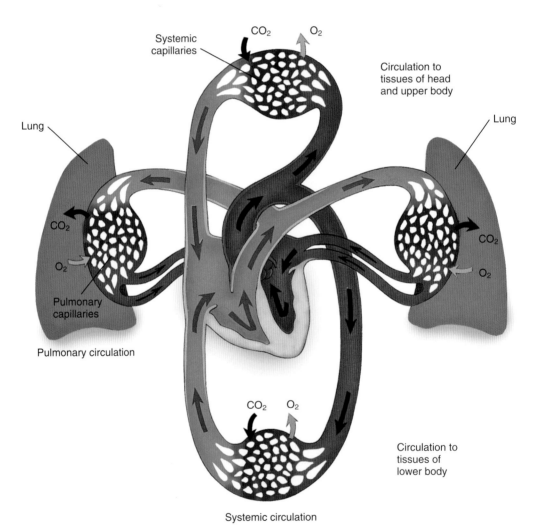

FIGURE 13.4 Blood flow through the heart and body. (*Source:* Rodriguez NE. Egan's fundamentals of respiratory care, 11 ed. St Louis; Elsevier; 2017.)

the pulmonary valve and pushing blood into the pulmonary artery, an area with lower blood pressure than that observed in the ventricle at this point. Deoxygenated blood is conducted away from the heart into pulmonary arterioles and then pulmonary capillaries.[4] The main pulmonary artery is the only artery that does not carry oxygenated blood (Fig. 13.4). In the lungs, gas exchange occurs between the capillaries and the alveoli of the lungs, with carbon dioxide released to the alveoli by diffusion and oxygen taken up by the red blood cells from the alveoli, also by diffusion (as explained in Chapter 17). This now-oxygenated blood leaves the pulmonary capillaries to enter small-diameter pulmonary venules, eventually emptying into the left atria via the main pulmonary vein. From the left atria blood is pumped, using the same principles as above, to the left ventricle via the mitral valve and through contraction of the right ventricle out through the aortic valve and into the aorta for distribution to the systemic circulation.[4]

Coronary circulation

The heart is responsible for pumping blood to all parts of the body to meet the functional demands of cells in the tissues. This includes the supply of blood through the **coronary circulation** (Fig. 13.5), the vessels that supply and drain blood from the heart. The left and right coronary arteries—the two main arteries that branch to supply the heart—arise from the left and right aortic sinuses within the aorta. Blood flows into the left and right coronary arteries when the heart is relaxed and allows backflow of blood into these arteries. The left coronary artery branches into the left anterior descending artery, also known as the anterior interventricular artery, the marginal artery and the left circumflex artery. The right coronary artery branches into the right marginal artery. These arteries give rise to smaller arteries that eventually become capillaries densely dispersed throughout the myocardium. In the capillaries, blood delivers oxygen and nutrients required by the cardiomyocytes to perform required functions. In return, cardiomyocytes release carbon dioxide and metabolic waste into the blood circulation.

Blood then converges towards the coronary venules which merge into larger veins that empty into the coronary sinus, which runs between the left atrium and the left ventricle then drains into the right atrium. The clinical relevance of the coronary circulation is best seen in individuals who suffer a sudden heart attack (myocardial infarction) due to blockage in the coronary vessels. For example, a blockage of the left anterior descending artery is likely to cause damage to the right and left ventricles and the anterior two-thirds of the intraventricular septum.

The heart sounds

When you use your stethoscope to listen to someone's healthy heartbeats, what you hear are two distinct sounds, 'lub' and 'dub', that repeat. These sounds are generated as blood flows through the heart. The **lub** sound (S_1 sound) reflects closure of the tricuspid and mitral valves, whereas the **dub** sound (S_2 sound) reflects closure of the aortic and pulmonary valves.

Conduction system of the heart

The heart contracts rhythmically through a tightly controlled generation of impulses (also known as action potentials) that trigger contraction of the myocardium. The electrical conduction system of the heart (Fig. 13.6) includes four main structures: the **sinoatrial (SA) node**, **atrioventricular (AV) node**, **atrioventricular (AV) bundle** (also known as the bundle of His) and **Purkinje fibres** (also known as subendocardial branches). Each of these structures is composed of specialised cardiac cells that are not contractile but instead generate and rapidly conduct action potentials through the heart.

The SA node, often called the pacemaker of the heart, is the master regulator of the rate of electrical impulses arising from this structure.[3] While the SA node receives

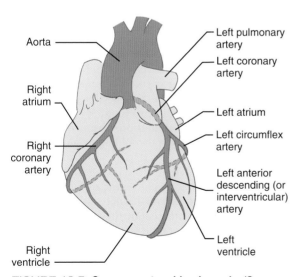

FIGURE 13.5 Coronary artery blood supply. (*Source:* Modified from Jones M, Harvey A, Main E. Anatomy and physiology of the respiratory and cardiac systems. In: Main E, Denehy L, editors. Cardiorespiratory physiotherapy: adults and paediatrics. Elsevier; 2016.)

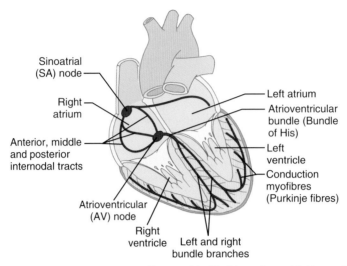

FIGURE 13.6 **Cardiac conduction system.** (*Source:* Modified from Jones M, Harvey A, Main E. Anatomy and physiology of the respiratory and cardiac systems. In: Main E, Denehy L, editors. Cardiorespiratory physiotherapy: adults and paediatrics. Elsevier; 2016.)

feedback external to the heart to speed up and slow down the heart rate depending on the body's needs, the actual signal that starts each heartbeat is generated within the SA node's own specialised cells. Therefore, the SA node controls both heartbeat formation and the rate of that formation.[3]

The action potential generated by the pacemaker fibres is a very complex event. The simplest description is that during the resting membrane potential of a pacemaker fibre, potassium (K^+) leaks out of the cell while sodium (Na^+) and calcium (Ca^+) ions rush across the membrane into the fibre.[2,3] This leads to slow depolarisation of the membrane and a build-up of the potential towards a threshold to trigger the action potential.

Prior to the initiation of the electrical impulse, the atria are relaxed and blood flows into the atria. As the wave of electrical impulse generated from the SA node travels through the atrial myocardium, travelling from cardiomyocytes to cardiomyocytes, it causes a wave of contraction evident as the pumping motion of the atria, or atrial contraction. This is possible because each cardiomyocyte is linked to another cardiomyocyte by specialised **electrical junctions**. The electrical impulse then reaches the AV node located between the atria and the ventricle (Fig. 13.6).[2,3] The AV node is the only way for an electrical impulse to travel between the atria and the ventricle. Here, the action potential pauses slightly

before the impulse continues to travel through to the ventricle. This is to allow for contraction of both atria, opening of the atrioventricular valves and for blood to flow into their respective ventricles (known as ventricular filling time). Once this pause has finished, the impulse continues down into the ventricle.[3] Stimulation of the AV node to allow for faster conduction through the AV node from the atria and the ventricle is called **dronotropy**. This is closely associated with the timing of the heart rate as each impulse generated from the SA node needs to travel through to the ventricle at a matching rate.

The electrical impulse travels along conduction pathways and through the ventricle to maximise coordination of the contraction. From the AV node the impulse travels down the AV bundle and separates down the bundle branches (Fig. 13.6). The left bundle branch travels into the left ventricle and the right bundle branch into the right ventricle. Coming off the bundle branches are the Purkinje fibres, which terminate in the subendocardium, sending the electrical impulse further into the muscle of the ventricle so that the timing of the contraction of muscle is as efficient as possible.[3] As the electrical impulse terminates, ventricular contraction occurs. At this point, the atrioventricular valves are closed (to prevent blood backflow into the atria) and blood is ejected via the semilunar valves into the systemic circulation. The cardiac muscle or force of contraction of the cardiac muscle in the ventricles is called **inotropy**.[2,3]

Myocardial contraction is caused by electrical impulses travelling through cardiac muscle cells and can be monitored and interpreted using an **electrocardiograph (ECG)**. To perform an ECG, electrodes are placed on the wrists, ankles and chest to create a representation of heart muscle contraction and relaxation. ECG waveform can be seen in a real-time display on a monitor or printed out as a snapshot and is a common method of measuring a person's heart rate.[5] Fig. 13.7 shows the various parts that make up an ECG waveform, labelled P, Q, R, S and T as they relate to contraction and relaxation of the atria and ventricles. The P wave represents contraction of the atria; the QRS wave represents contraction of the ventricles; and the T wave represents relaxation of ventricular muscle in between contractions.[6,7]

Following impulse conduction through the conduction system gives you an understanding of how the timing of contraction of the myocardium is coordinated and how changes in the actions of the SA node, AV node and cardiac muscle alter cardiac output or the amount of blood ejected from the left ventricle over the span of one minute. Understanding the components of a normal ECG helps you to recognise when abnormalities may lead to cardiac dysfunction; for example, that associated with myocardial infarction.

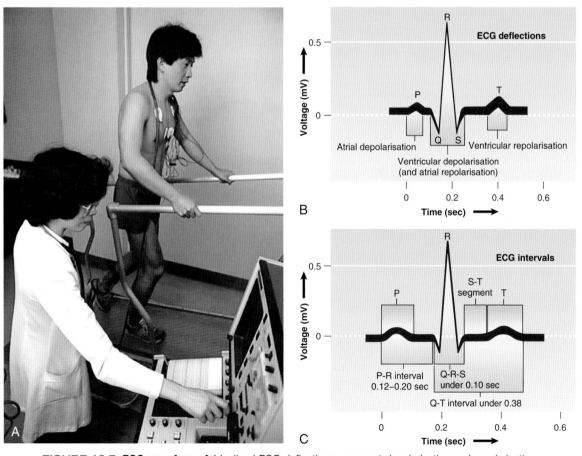

FIGURE 13.7 **ECG waveform. A** Idealised ECG deflections represent depolarisation and repolarisation of atria and ventricle. **B** Principal ECG intervals P, QRS, and T waves. The P-R interval is measured from the start of the P wave to the start of the Q wave. **C** ECG waveform with respect to an electrical signal travelling through the heart. (*Source:* Modified from Patton KT, Thibodeau GA, editors. Anatomy and physiology, 9 ed. London: Elsevier Health Sciences; 2015.)

Cardiac cycle

An important part of the cardiac system is the **cardiac cycle** (Fig. 13.8). The cardiac cycle consists of all the physiological events that occur in the heart within a single heartbeat. This includes the electrical impulse and associated contraction events, mechanical factors (blood volume and blood pressure) and heart sounds. The cycle is divided into two main events: contraction (**systole**) and relaxation (**diastole**) of the atria and the ventricles.[4,8,9]

During atrial diastole, blood flows passively from the systemic veins, such as the inferior and superior venae cavae and coronary sinus, into the right atria and from four pulmonary veins into the left atria. This flow is due to the higher pressure that exists in the systemic veins when compared with the atria. At this point, the right and left atrioventricular valves are open. As blood fills in the atria, the pressure within the atria increases and it is felt by the atrial myocardium. Two events occur. The first event is characterised by passive blood flow

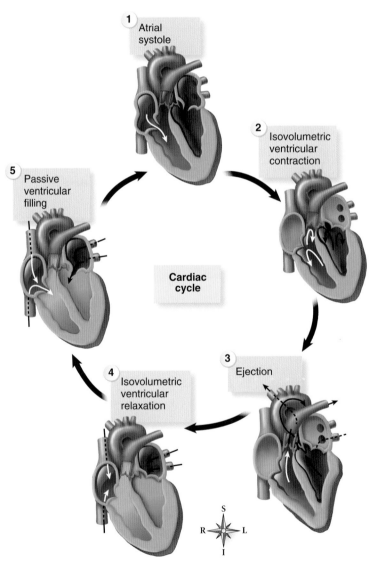

FIGURE 13.8 **Cardiac cycle.** (*Source:* Patton KT, Thibodeau GA, editors. Anatomy and physiology, 10 ed. London: Elsevier Inc.; 2019.)

from the atria through the open atrioventricular valves into the ventricles due to the pressure being lower in the ventricles. During this time the pulmonary and aortic valves are closed, preventing backflow from the pulmonary artery and aorta into their respective ventricles. The second event is when the heart impulse is generated, causing myocardial contraction leading to atrial systole. This, combined with the remaining blood volume and associated pressure, forces the remaining blood volume into the ventricle, which at this time is in late diastole. Atrial contraction occurs after depolarisation of the myocardium and it is represented by a P wave on the ECG.

During ventricular systole when the myocardium contracts due to ventricular depolarisation, the pressure inside the ventricle increases to a point where it is greater than in the atria, which are now in diastole. This also results in blood backflow which seals the atrioventricular valves. At this stage, the ventricle is not ready to eject the blood as there is not enough pressure due to the blood volume being constant. This stage of the initial phase of ventricular systole is known as **isovolumic contraction** or isovolumetric contraction. The **end diastolic volume (EDV)**, more commonly known as **preload**, is the volume of blood found in the ventricle at the end of atrial systole, just prior to atrial contraction.[4,8,9]

In the next stage of ventricular systole, a further increase in the blood pressure in the ventricular space results in the ventricular blood pressure being greater than the pressure in the pulmonary trunk and aorta. This, combined with ventricular contraction, forces the pulmonary and aortic semilunar valves to open. As the pressure needed to push the blood into the aorta is greater than that required to push the blood into the lungs, the pressure generated by the contraction of the left ventricle will be greater, even though the volume of blood ejected is the same. This volume of ejected blood is known as the **stroke volume**. The volume of blood remaining in the ventricle following ventricular contraction is known as the **end systolic volume (ESV)**.[4,8,9]

During ventricular diastole, when the ventricle is relaxing, repolarisation of the cell membrane takes place, and this is evident as a T wave on the ECG. In the early phase of ventricular relaxation, there is a decrease in ventricular blood pressure below that seen in the aorta and the pulmonary arteries. To prevent the subsequent backflow of blood from the aorta and the pulmonary artery back to the heart, the pulmonary and aortic valves are shut closed. At this time, the atrioventricular valves are also closed, and no new blood is introduced into the ventricle. This phase of ventricular diastole is called the **isovolumic** (or isovolumetric) **ventricular relaxation phase**.[2,9]

As diastole progresses there is further relaxation of the ventricular myocardium and a decrease in ventricular blood pressure to a point where it falls below the blood pressure in the atria. This difference in blood pressure allows the atrioventricular valves to open and blood passively flows from the atria to the ventricle. The decrease in ventricular pressure also enables passive blood flow from the systemic veins, including the pulmonary veins, into the atria. At this stage both the atria and the ventricle are in diastole, and the semilunar valves are closed, thus marking completion of the cardiac cycle lasting one complete heartbeat.

Cardiac output, preload, afterload and contractility

The heart is often described as a house where the chambers are the rooms, the valves are the doors and the conduction system is the electrical wiring. Everything can be linked to either the pumping of the heart or the electrical/conduction system of the heart. Here we examine concepts that are core to understanding the mechanics of the pumping function of the heart, starting with cardiac output.

Cardiac output (CO) is the amount of blood that the heart pumps into the body within one minute. Two factors influence cardiac output: **stroke volume (SV)**, the amount of blood pumped out of the heart in a single contraction; and **heart rate (HR)**, the number of times the heart beats in one minute. This can be represented by the equation **SV × HR = CO**.[2,4,9] Change either the heart rate or the stroke volume and this will influence the CO. Understanding how CO changes will help you to understand how the body responds to imbalances between demand and supply of blood and oxygen throughout the body.[4]

For example, when running a runner needs more blood to be supplied to organs and tissues, causing the body to send signals via neuronal pathways to the heart that it needs to increase both the heart rate and the force of contraction, thus increasing both the SV and HR components of the equation, which increases CO and therefore systemic blood and oxygen supply. When there is no longer a need for this increased demand of oxygen delivery, for example when the runner ends their run, the body sends signals to the heart, again via neuronal pathways, that it is time to slow the heart rate and decrease the force of contraction.[4] These signals directing the heart to work harder or to decrease its work are mediated by the sympathetic and parasympathetic nervous systems.

Preload is the stretch of the wall of the ventricles or filling of blood into the ventricles, both left and right (Fig. 13.9). An increase in filling or stretch is described as increased preload.[2,4,9] For example, when a person is dehydrated, a decreased intravascular blood volume means a reduced flow of blood returning to the ventricles. This leads to a lower demand on the heart to accommodate that volume and stretch. Reduced filling and stretch result in decreased preload.[4]

Afterload is the force against which the heart has to eject blood out of the left ventricle through the aortic valve and out of the right ventricle through the pulmonary valve.[2,4,9] As described above, prior to ventricular contraction the aortic and pulmonary valves are closed while the ventricles fill, thus ensuring one-directional blood flow between ventricular contractions. Once the left and right atria have emptied into their respective ventricles, the tricuspid and mitral valves close and ventricular pressure builds until the pressure inside the ventricles is higher than that beyond the closed valves. It is this difference in pressure that forces the aortic and pulmonary valves to open.[2,4,9] The ventricles contract and blood is pumped through the valves into the pulmonary and systemic circulation. The pressure that the ventricle must build up to is the afterload. In terms of effort, the higher the pressure that is required to force that valve to open, the higher the afterload.[4] An example of this is vasoconstriction of the peripheral arteries as part of the body's natural mechanism to reduce heat loss when exposed to the cold. This response causes the

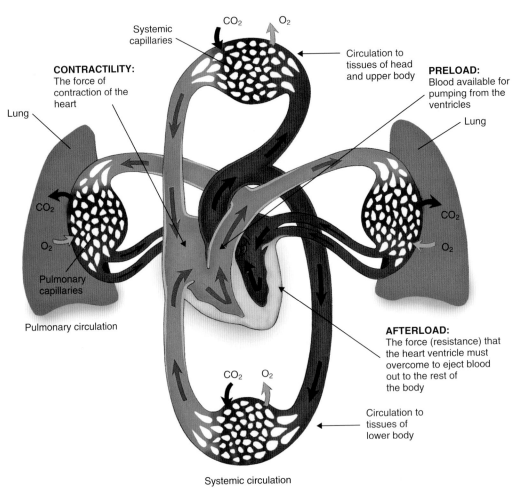

FIGURE 13.9 **Preload, afterload and contractility.** (*Source:* Modified from Rodriguez NE. Egan's fundamentals of respiratory care, 11 ed. St Louis; Elsevier; 2017.)

blood vessels to constrict, creating a smaller space within the vessels with the same fluid volume within. This increases pressure in the arteries that the ventricle must push against, and therefore an increase in afterload is observed.

Contractility is the force of contraction of the muscles of the ventricles (Fig. 13.9).[2,4,9] An increased force of contraction results in an increased stroke volume, increasing CO. The harder the cardiac muscle contracts, the more blood is pumped out of the ventricle. Increased contractility is stimulated by the body to increase CO when an increase in demand arises. Think of a runner going from standing still to commencing their run: this would cause stimulation to make the ventricles increase their force of contraction in order to supply the increased demand for blood to parts of the body working harder to maintain a running pace. Factors that influence preload, afterload and contractility can substantially alter blood flow through the heart.[4] The Frank–Starling law captures this in terms of contractility: the more stretched the heart fibres at the beginning of contraction, the stronger the contraction. This law takes into consideration that cardiac fibres can reach maximum capacity to stretch but, in reality, the heart will pump out what it receives.

Blood pressure

Blood pressure is a common term that most people are familiar with, but what do the numbers relating to blood pressure mean? A blood pressure reading has two numbers, a larger number over a smaller number—for example, 120/80. The top number is the **systolic blood pressure** and the bottom number is the **diastolic blood pressure**. Systolic blood pressure is the peak pressure on the wall of the aorta during ventricular contraction, while diastolic blood pressure is the pressure on the walls of the aorta in the relaxation phase between ventricular contractions.[9] It is worth noting at this point that filling of the coronary arteries takes place in diastole.

Another factor influencing blood pressure is **peripheral vascular resistance (PVR)**. PVR is created by the friction caused by blood on the artery walls as it flows through the lumen of those vessels. Factors that affect PVR, and therefore blood flow, are blood viscosity (the stickiness of blood) and vessel length and diameter. Blood viscosity and vessel length are relatively constant and do not change much in a healthy, well-hydrated adult, meaning that vessel diameter is an important variable relating to blood flow. The narrower the vessel, the greater the friction and the greater the resistance of blood flow through the arteries. Hence the smaller the vessel, the greater the PVR it generates and subsequently

the greater the alteration of the blood pressure.[2,4,9] In the next section, we take a closer look at blood vessel structure to help you to visualise the heart's capacity to deliver blood around the body.

Blood vessels

While the heart pumps blood through the body, blood flow depends on the type of blood vessel (Fig. 13.10).[1,2,4,9] As oxygenated blood is carried away from the heart via the aorta, the aorta branches into arteries. The arteries have a smaller vessel diameter as they move further away from the heart. The arteries then branch into arterioles and metarterioles so that blood can be ferried to the capillary network, specialised blood vessels that permit close interaction of blood and the surrounding tissues. It is at this level that erythrocytes and tissue cells exchange oxygen and carbon dioxide and that nutrients are delivered to tissue cells and metabolic waste is removed. It is important to note that capillary structure differs greatly in different organs as it has developed to serve the functions of each organ—for example, the continuous capillaries in the skin, the specialised fenestrated capillaries in kidney nephrons that have evolved to assist blood filtration, and liver endothelial sinusoids that have evolved to facilitate the liver's detoxifying function (Fig. 13.11).[2,4,9] Deoxygenated blood then travels from the capillary network to the small-calibre venules, which coalesce into larger veins until they all unite into the inferior and superior venae cavae and deliver blood to the right ventricle.

Arteries, veins and capillaries differ in structure, elasticity, diameter and function.[10] **Elasticity** is associated with the larger arteries and provides them with the capacity to stretch to accommodate blood arriving with ventricular contractions, increase the pressure and return to their original diameter between contractions.[10] In general, blood vessels have three layers. The internal layer facing the blood flow, the **tunica intima**, is lined with endothelial cells, which provide a non-thrombogenic surface that stops erythrocytes from adhering to the surface, thus enabling a flow that is in parallel down the length of the blood vessel (laminar blood flow).[1] The middle layer, the **tunica media**, is comprised of concentrically arranged smooth muscle cells that control the vessel's ability to contract and modify the blood flow.[1] An example of this is contraction of blood vessels in order to preserve heat when exposed to severe cold. This layer is thickest in the aorta, as it must withstand the greatest blood pressure as the blood is ejected from the left ventricle. The aortic tunica media also contains many elastic fibres that further aid its capacity to stretch and recoil in response to blood flow from the heart. The

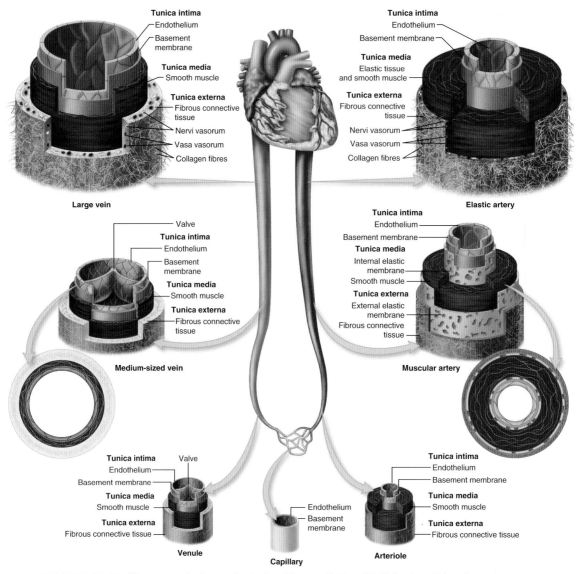

FIGURE 13.10 **Structure of veins and arteries.** (*Source:* Patton KT, Thibodeau GA, editors. Anatomy and physiology, 9 ed. London: Elsevier Health Sciences; 2015.)

tunica media thins out as the aorta branches out and is further away from the heart. This is because the further blood is from the heart, the lower the blood pressure. The third layer, the **tunica adventitia**, is composed of connective tissue and anchors the vessel to the rest of the surrounding tissue.

As noted above, how blood flows through the vessels depends on vessel type and blood viscosity. As blood flows through a vessel it exerts force on the walls of

that vessel. The vessel's resistance to that force is the PVR. Increased PVR means that there will be a need to increase blood pressure to overcome that resistance in order to push blood towards the capillary network where the cells are waiting for oxygen and nutrients to be delivered.[9] Contraction of arteries is another of the body's mechanisms to maintain homeostasis by changing their diameter to maintain optimal blood pressure. The mechanisms that control contraction and

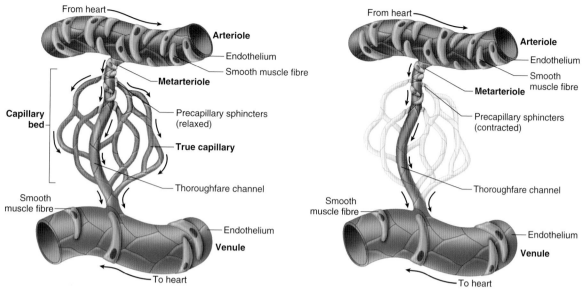

FIGURE 13.11 **Structure of capillaries.** (*Source:* Patton KT, Thibodeau GA, editors. Anatomy and physiology, 9 ed. London: Elsevier Health Sciences; 2015.)

relaxation of arteries are controlled by the autonomic nervous system.[1,2,4,9]

To assist in returning deoxygenated blood to the heart, skeletal muscle contractions compress the veins within the muscle, pressing blood towards the heart.[2] This external pressure is required for two reasons: (1) blood pressure in the veins is low and the veins cannot constrict sufficiently to push blood against gravity back to the heart; and (2) to enable the closure of the semilunar valves, thus enabling blood flow in one direction. Thus when skeletal muscles compress the vein, the semilunar valves are closed, backflow is prevented and blood is conducted back to the heart.[11]

INTEGRATION OF THE CARDIOVASCULAR SYSTEM WITH OTHER BODY SYSTEMS

All organs and nearly all tissue types in the body are vascularised. This is because the cells that reside in these structures need oxygen and nutrients to perform their function, and require carbon dioxide and metabolic waste to be removed, as high concentrations are detrimental to cell survival. Meeting these metabolic needs is further supported by adequate blood pressure, which ensures adequate tissue perfusion with blood. Adequate blood pressure is dependent on the heart's ability to alter its rate and output in communication with the autonomic nervous system.[12]

Integumentary system

The relationship between the cardiovascular system and the integumentary system is evident in thermoregulatory function, which exists to control heat loss from the body when the core body temperature rises above a set value—under healthy conditions this is between 36.5 and 37.5° Celsius. At this point, the heat produced by metabolic reaction is in balance with the heat lost to the environment. Using our example of the runner, as the runner increases their musculoskeletal work, which requires increased amounts of adenosine triphosphate (ATP) to maintain the mechanical work of the muscles, the muscles generate heat and metabolic waste, including carbon dioxide.[1,13] This heat is transferred to blood in the blood vessels and carried through the cardiovascular system to the skin, where it is actively removed through secretion of sweat to prevent an excessive rise in body temperature (see Chapter 3).

Muscular system

Skeletal muscles enable you to walk, maintain your posture, swim and breathe; smooth muscles enable you to empty your bowels and for urine to be moved along in your body; and cardiac muscle enables your heart to pump. To do these functions at rest or during stress, muscles require high levels of oxygen and ATP. At rest, it is estimated that 20% of cardiac output goes to muscles to sustain their function. This output is even greater during exercise. It has been estimated that up to 80% of cardiac output could be directed to skeletal muscles during extreme physical exercise.[13] How blood is distributed in the skeletal muscle at that time while maintaining the functions of the rest of the body is controlled by the autonomic nervous system through sympathetic innervation, which produces vasoconstriction through alpha[1] and alpha[2] adrenoceptors found in the cell membranes of vascular smooth muscle cell. The effect of adrenaline (epinephrine) on beta[2] adrenergic receptors, also found on the cell membranes of vascular smooth muscle, is thought to be responsible for vasodilation effects.[13]

Nervous system

A significant influence on the workings of the cardiovascular system is the autonomic nervous system. The autonomic nervous system, a branch of the peripheral nervous system, is used for regulation of and feedback to the cardiovascular system, and this is performed by parts of the autonomic nervous system known as the sympathetic nervous system (SNS) and the parasympathetic nervous system (PSNS).[4]

The action of the SNS is often described by the phrase 'fight or flight' while the action of the PSNS is described by the phrase 'rest and digest'. As these phrases suggest,

the SNS is responsible for stimulation of various parts of the body to meet an increased demand for blood and oxygen—this may be related to physical exertion or emotional stress. The PSNS provides neuronal input aimed at returning to a relaxed state after the increased demand, or stressful event, has passed.[8]

With respect to control of the heart rate, the SNS is connected to the SA node, the AV node and the ventricular myocardium via the sympathetic cardiac nerve (see Fig. 13.12). Stimulation of the SNS results when the body requires a greater output of blood because of increased oxygen demand. A simple example of this is exercise or playing sport, resulting in an increased requirement for blood flow to the parts of the body that are working harder. An increase in oxygen demand means the body works to increase CO; remember CO equals SV multiplied by HR (for one minute). SNS stimulation will increase both HR and SV to create this increase in CO.[4,8] SNS stimulation leads to increased SV and HR through the chronotropic and inotropic effects of sympathetic stimulation.[14]

Sympathetic chronotropic stimulation causes an increase in the rate of the SA node firing electrical impulses and therefore increases HR. This stimulation also causes faster conduction across the AV node from the atria to the ventricle. Regulation of the HR and AV

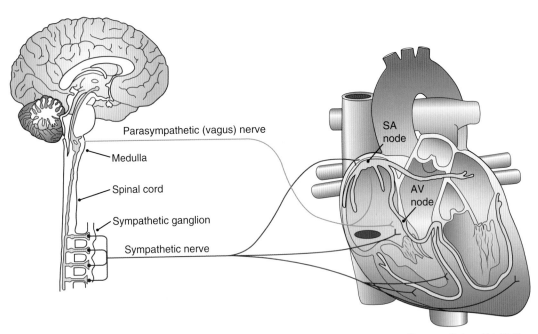

Parasympathetic (vagus) nerve

Medulla

Spinal cord

Sympathetic ganglion

Sympathetic nerve

SA node

AV node

FIGURE 13.12 **Sympathetic and parasympathetic connection to the heart.** (*Source:* Cohen BJ, Hull K. Memmler's the human body in health and disease, 13 ed. Philadelphia: Lippincott Williams & Wilkins; 2015.)

node conduction are connected in this way as each impulse generated from the SA node needs to travel through to the atria to the AV node and then to the ventricle at a matching speed to the HR. Inotropy relates to the force of contraction of the cardiac muscle: sympathetic inotropic stimulation increases the force of contraction and therefore the SV or amount pumped out of the ventricle with each contraction.[3,8] Sympathetic chronotropic and inotropic stimulation occur simultaneously as they work together to increase CO when it is required.

Autonomic nervous system sympathetic regulation of the cardiovascular system's response to physical exertion or emotional stress is the release of adrenaline (epinephrine) by the adrenal gland. Once released into the bloodstream adrenaline (epinephrine) circulates through the body, stimulating the adrenoceptors. Adrenoceptors can be divided into two categories: alpha-adrenergic or α_1 and α_2 located primarily in the peripheral vasculature, and beta-adrenergic or β_1 and β_2 located in the heart.[14] Sympathetic stimulation of β_1 and β_2 receptors causes an increase in chronotropic and inotropic effects increasing CO. The response of α_1 and α_2 receptors to sympathetic stimulation causes vasoconstriction of the large and terminal arterioles.

PSNS stimulation is connected to the SA and AV nodes via the vagus nerve (cranial nerve X) so it affects only chronotropy but not inotropy. Parasympathetic stimulation of chronotropy decreases SA node firing, decreasing the rate of impulses to make the heart beat at a slower rate as well as decreasing the rate of conduction across the AV node.[4,8] There is no parasympathetic connection to ventricular muscle and therefore no parasympathetic stimulation can occur. Instead, once sympathetic stimulation stops, ventricular muscle returns to a baseline contraction strength rather than an increased force that SNS stimulation creates. Ventricular muscle always contracts with the same force unless stimulated by the SNS to work harder. Once SNS stimulation ceases, the increased force of contraction ceases.[4]

Another example of neuronal involvement in the function of the cardiovascular system is its role in blood pressure control. The cardiovascular system, in conjunction with other systems, acts to maintain homeostasis through manipulation of blood pressure. Several factors that affect our blood pressure are regulated by the body to maintain an ideal blood pressure. Different parts of the vasculature have different pressures; for example, the veins work at significantly lower pressure than the arteries. When talking about blood pressure it is related to the pressure in the aorta and major arteries.[4,10] An adequate blood pressure in the aorta and major arteries

suggests that the pressure will be adequate to maintain perfusion throughout the body, meaning the pressure is adequate to meet the metabolic demands of the body.[4]

When an increase or a decrease in blood pressure is detected, the body uses several mechanisms to bring it back to a normal level.[4,10] Rising or declining blood pressure is recognised when the arterial pressure rises above or falls below the normal range, triggering what is known as the baroreceptor reflex.[4] **Baroreceptors** (Fig. 13.13), specialised nerve structures located in the carotid sinus and the aortic arch, are part of the body's efforts to maintain an ideal blood pressure.

When there is an increase in blood pressure in the aorta above the normal range, baroreceptors are stimulated through sensing the aortic stretch. This stimulation causes an increase in impulses sent from baroreceptors that stimulate the **cardio-inhibitory centre** in the brain.[4] This causes a decrease in sympathetic impulses sent to the heart, decreasing the heart rate and the contractility of ventricular muscle, thus causing a decrease in CO. Baroreceptor stimulation also causes vasodilation of the arteries. A decrease in CO and vasodilation causes less blood to enter the arteries, which now have a larger diameter, causing a decrease in blood pressure.

When there is a decrease in blood pressure in the aorta below the normal range, baroreceptors are inhibited. This inhibition causes a decrease in impulses sent from baroreceptors that stimulate the **cardio-acceleratory centre** in the brain.[4] This causes increased sympathetic impulses to be sent to the heart, increasing the heart rate and the contractility of the ventricular muscle and causing an increase in CO. Baroreceptor inhibition also causes vasoconstriction or constriction of the arteries. An increase in CO and vasoconstriction causes more blood to enter the arteries, which now have a smaller diameter, causing an increase in blood pressure.[4,10]

Endocrine system

The link between the endocrine system and the cardiovascular system is bidirectional. The organs and glands of the endocrine system are highly vascularised. Hormones are secreted by the endocrine glands into the local vasculature then transported either as free forms (water-soluble hormones) or bound to carrier proteins (lipid-soluble forms) effectively through the whole body so that the hormones reach the target cells. While hormones have complex actions on many tissues, some of these actions are directed to the cardiovascular system.[15] For example, adrenaline (epinephrine) and noradrenaline (norepinephrine), secreted by the adrenal medulla, impact every heart function, while at the level of

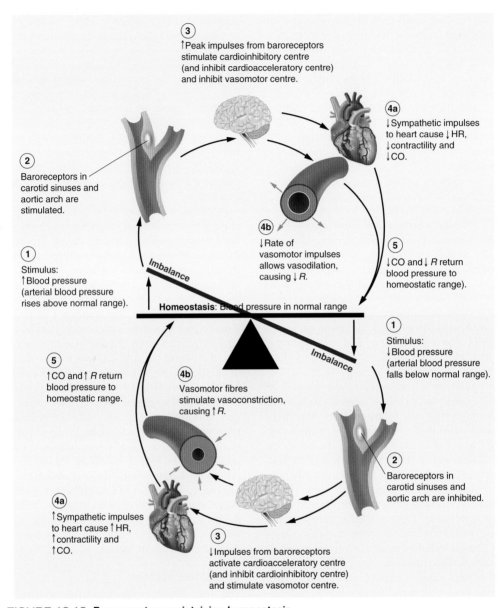

③ ↑Peak impulses from baroreceptors stimulate cardioinhibitory centre (and inhibit cardioacceleratory centre) and inhibit vasomotor centre.

④a ↓Sympathetic impulses to heart cause ↓HR, ↓contractility and ↓CO.

② Baroreceptors in carotid sinuses and aortic arch are stimulated.

④b ↓Rate of vasomotor impulses allows vasodilation, causing ↓R.

⑤ ↓CO and ↓R return blood pressure to homeostatic range).

① Stimulus: ↑Blood pressure (arterial blood pressure rises above normal range).

Imbalance

Homeostasis: Blood pressure in normal range

Imbalance

① Stimulus: ↓Blood pressure (arterial blood pressure falls below normal range).

⑤ ↑CO and ↑R return blood pressure to homeostatic range.

④b Vasomotor fibres stimulate vasoconstriction, causing ↑R.

② Baroreceptors in carotid sinuses and aortic arch are inhibited.

④a ↑Sympathetic impulses to heart cause ↑HR, ↑contractility and ↑CO.

③ ↓Impulses from baroreceptors activate cardioacceleratory centre (and inhibit cardioinhibitory centre) and stimulate vasomotor centre.

FIGURE 13.13 **Baroreceptors maintaining homeostasis.**

blood vessels these hormones control PVR by controlling vasoconstriction and vasodilation. Parathyroid hormone, secreted by the parathyroid gland, controls blood levels of calcium ions, which are fundamental to heart function. Abnormalities in the hormones renin, aldosterone, antidiuretic hormone and angiotensin II have an impact on cardiovascular function, as discussed below in the section on the urinary system. Abnormalities in hormones secreted by the thyroid gland—triiodothyronine (T_3) and

thyroxine (T_4)—also negatively impact on cardiovascular function in terms of heart rate, heart contractility, cardiac output and peripheral vasodilation, which can lead to increased supply of blood to many organs as well as reduced systemic peripheral resistance.[15]

Heart atria produce the **hormone atrial natriuretic peptide (ANP)**, which responds to increased stretch in the atria induced by high pressure inside the atria. The hormone is released into the circulation and acts on the kidneys to influence the glomerular filtration rate (GFR, discussed in Chapter 20) with the intent to reduce blood pressure and therefore decrease atrial stretch.[1]

Blood

The volume of circulating blood is a determining factor in regulatory mechanisms controlling the heart and vascular functions. Blood (discussed in detail in Chapter 11) is composed of cellular elements (including red blood cells, white blood cells, platelets and a very small percentage of circulating progenitor cells) and plasma. Plasma contains thousands of proteins, including hormones, and carbohydrate-based molecules, fatty acids and nucleic acids. General blood loss as seen in trauma will initiate compensatory mechanisms that integrate the urinary, cardiovascular, nervous and hormonal systems to preserve blood pressure. Overall, the greater the blood loss, the greater the response in preserving the blood pressure to maintain homeostasis. Loss of a smaller volume of plasma due to dehydration will also result in compensatory mechanisms being activated to maintain blood pressure. Loss of red blood cells alone will result in decreased capacity of the cardiovascular system to deliver oxygenated blood and remove carbon dioxide. Loss of platelets in the blood will lead to reduced capacity of the injured endothelium to form a platelet plug and prevent further blood loss.

Lymphatic system

Perhaps the closest connection between the cardiovascular system and the lymphatic system is observed during embryonic development when the cardinal vein wall gives rise to a lymph sac comprised of early precursors of lymphatic cells. These cells undergo significant anatomical and physiological changes to fully form the lymphatic system.[16] Both the lymphatic system and the cardiovascular system are comprised of networks of vessels that together maintain tissue fluid homeostasis. As the unidirectional initial lymphatic vessels collect excess interstitial fluid from peripheral tissues, they merge into lymphatic veins which terminate in lymphatic ducts that empty into the left and right subclavian veins. This process is discussed in more depth in Chapter 14. To carry lymph to the blood circulation, lymphatic vessels actively overcome pressure gradients that oppose flow, a function that is facilitated by the intraluminal lymphatic valves, which prevent lymph backflow, and periodic contraction of the lymphatic smooth muscle cells. Extrinsic compression of lymphatic vessels by the surrounding tissue that arises from muscular activity and breathing facilitates propulsion of lymphatic fluid towards the heart.[17] Lymph returning to the blood circulation is rich in fatty acids

and chylomicrons absorbed from the gastrointestinal tract (see Chapter 18).

Immune system

Cells of the immune system (discussed in Chapter 15) are distributed throughout the body by the cardiovascular system. This is best seen in the migration of leucocytes to an injured area during acute inflammation (see Chapter 16). At this point, close interaction between the endothelial cells lining the tunica intima and the receptors on the leucocyte cell surface allow leucocytes to slow down, attach to these receptors, then roll over the endothelial layer until they reach the area where they can transmigrate across the endothelium into the injured tissue under the guidance of the chemokine gradient present in the injured tissue. Lymphoid organs such as the spleen and lymph nodes also contain unique capillary networks that enable immune functions to occur. For example, in the spleen, spleen marginal artery branches into smaller vessels towards the spleen marginal sinus, an open-ended vascular structure that allows blood to arrive into the spleen marginal zone and be screened for infectious agents. If encapsulated bacteria arrive in the spleen marginal zone via the marginal sinus, they will be detected by the spleen marginal zone B cells, which then transmigrate into the spleen marginal zone and differentiate into plasma cells to produce the antibodies needed to combat the bacterial infection.[12]

Respiratory system

The cardiovascular and respiratory systems are linked through the gas exchange and acid–base balance functions (see Chapters 17 and 19 for more detail), with the circulatory system responsible for the delivery of oxygenated blood to tissues.[8] The function of the cardiovascular system itself is heavily dependent on the adequate supply of oxygen and effective removal of waste products. The heart is a highly metabolic organ that due to its constant pumping function demands high supply of oxygen and nutrients to produce ATP using aerobic metabolism. Interruption of blood flow leads to anaerobic metabolism and formation of lactic acid, which can result in chest pain. In the case of complete obstruction of the vessel, a heart attack or acute myocardial infarction can occur.[1] The larger blood vessels (e.g. aorta) have their own vascular supply in the form of a network of small blood vessels known as the **vasa vasorum**, which ensures that the larger vessels are well supplied with oxygen and nutrients as they are not thin enough to allow diffusion of oxygen and nutrients to vascular cells.[4]

Gastrointestinal system

Blood vessels are distributed throughout the gastrointestinal system (discussed in Chapter 19) where they have three main roles: to transport nutrients absorbed by the gastrointestinal system to the rest of the body; to deliver hormones secreted by the endocrine glands required for food digestion in different parts of the gastrointestinal system; and to supply gastrointestinal organs with oxygen and nutrients and remove cellular metabolic waste, including carbon dioxide.[4]

Urinary system

The kidneys are the major constituents of the urinary system and play a fundamental role in maintaining blood pressure by changing the volume of fluid in the circulation as needed. The kidneys regulate blood volume via a direct or an indirect mechanism.[4] The direct mechanism involves regulation of the filtration and excretion rate of fluid out of the circulating blood. If the blood pressure increases, the kidneys filter out more fluid from the blood and excrete this excess fluid as urine. If the blood pressure drops, this filtered fluid is retained and returned to the bloodstream, increasing circulating volume and thus increasing blood pressure.[4]

The indirect mechanism is mediated by the **renin-angiotensin-aldosterone system (RAAS)** (Fig. 13.14). Effects of arterial hypotension (decreased blood pressure) are felt by the juxtaglomerular apparatus, a

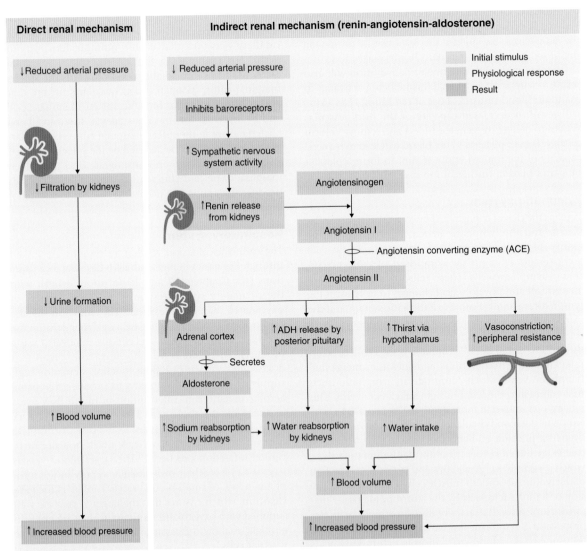

FIGURE 13.14 **Renin-angiotensin-aldosterone system (RAAS) in the regulation of blood pressure.**

specialised structure formed by the distal convoluted tubule and the glomerular afferent arteriole in the kidneys. This leads to the release of the enzyme renin into blood. Renin converts angiotensinogen to angiotensin I, a weak vasoconstrictor. Angiotensin I circulates through the bloodstream, where angiotensin-converting enzyme (ACE) in blood capillaries, located mostly in the lungs, forms angiotensin II molecules. Angiotensin II causes vasoconstriction of all blood vessels. Angiotensin II also circulates to the adrenal cortex where it stimulates the secretion of aldosterone. Aldosterone increases sodium reabsorption in the kidneys from urine to blood in exchange for potassium and hydrogen ions, which also causes increased water retention and therefore increased intravascular blood volume. In this way, aldosterone also affects blood pH levels (loss of H^+).

Loss of blood volume leads to increasing osmolarity of tissue fluid, leading to release of antidiuretic hormone (ADH) from the hypothalamus. This activates the thirst mechanism, constricting peripheral vessels, and leads to increased water reabsorption in the kidney tubules to increase blood volume.[4]

Reproductive system

Male and female reproductive organs are highly vascularised. Blood vessels deliver sex hormones secreted by the endocrine glands that regulate the reproductive function (discussed in Chapter 21) and supply reproductive organs with oxygen and nutrients while removing cellular metabolic waste, including carbon dioxide.[4] In the female reproductive system, blood vessels play a crucial role during menstruation, a complex event regulated by the endocrine system (see Chapter 21 for details). The endometrium, an outer layer of the uterus, contains unique blood vessels called **spiral arterioles**.[18] Following menstruation, as the endometrium renews, the cells of the spiral arterioles proliferate and the arterioles grow longer and more coiled. Following ovulation, in anticipation of possible embryo implantation, the arterioles cease to proliferate. If implantation occurs, the arterioles undergo changes that enable the uterus to support development of the placenta and the embryo within. If implantation fails to occur, a decrease in progesterone initiates constriction in the spiral arterioles leading to endometrial ischaemia and death of the surrounding tissue. It is this tissue that is sloughed off during menstruation. This leads to the formation of a denuded bleeding area in the endometrium. Following menstruation, a clotting process takes place at the ends of the spiral arterioles to cease the bleeding and enable the spiral arterioles to regenerate in time for the new ovulation cycle.[18]

Pregnancy

During pregnancy (discussed in Chapter 22), the female cardiovascular system undergoes major changes. By the eighth week of pregnancy CO is estimated to increase by 20% and by week 20–28 it is estimated to increase by 40%.[19] This increase in CO as the pregnancy progresses is thought to be due to peripheral vasodilation regulated by the hormone oestrogen. An increase in SV (likely caused by an increase in ventricular wall muscle mass and end diastolic volume seen in pregnancy) and to a lesser extent HR is thought to be the driving force behind the increased CO in response to increased peripheral vasodilation. SV is thought to decline towards the end of the third trimester, while the HR increase is maintained, which preserves increased CO. Overall, blood pressure is decreased in the first and second trimesters and returns to pre-pregnancy levels closer to labour (birth).[19]

Also significant is the maternal/fetal haemodynamic profile. In the supine position (lying on the back), pressure from the pregnant uterus compresses the inferior vena cava leading to a reduction in venous return to the heart and a decrease in SV and CO. It is for this reason that pregnant women are advised to rest and be nursed in the left or right lateral position. If a pregnant woman must be kept on her back, her pelvis needs to be rotated to tilt the uterus to the side in order to reduce the pressure on the inferior vena cava thus improving cardiac output and the blood flow to the placenta and the fetus. A recent study on still births linked that a pregnant woman's sleeping position as supine, which would lead to the reduction on uterine blood and subsequent loss of placental blood perfusion, was associated with an increased risk of stillbirths.[20–23]

Following birth, cardiovascular function is thought to return to pre-pregnancy levels in a healthy female.

AGE-RELATED CHANGES

The cardiovascular system is affected by the ageing process, which each of us experiences at a different rate. These changes are distinct from disease-related changes and therefore must be distinguished from cardiovascular diseases. Ageing heart is characterised by changes in the conduction of the heart impulses thus affecting the heart rate. In some cases there is a loss of self-paced pacemaker cells, while in other cases deposition of fat and fibrous tissue may interfere with conduction. Deposition of the pigment lipofuscin takes place[4] and heart cells start to degenerate. The valves inside the heart harden due to a build-up of calcium (calcification), which impacts on their capacity to fully open and close.

With age, baroreceptors become less sensitive, compromising the body's capacity to effectively respond to sudden changes in blood pressure.[1,2,9] There is decreased responsiveness to beta-adrenergic receptor stimulation and an increase in catecholamine secretions. The aorta and the arterial vascular tree lose their elastin and become less elastic. This affects vessel elasticity and the capacity to accommodate the blood volume ejected from the ventricles. In return, this leads to increased left ventricular afterload and left ventricular hypertrophy and places an increased demand on the heart to pump harder, thus resulting in increased systolic blood pressure.[1,2,4,9] Age-related changes of hormones involved in regulation of blood pressure further impact the health of the cardiovascular system. Collectively, these changes increase an older person's risk of developing cardiovascular dysfunctions.

CONCLUSION

The cardiovascular system regulates blood flow and blood pressure and this function is executed in close collaboration with the urinary and endocrine systems. Furthermore, the cardiovascular system enables oxygenated, nutrient-rich blood to reach the cells, while removing metabolic wastes to sites where they can be effectively disposed. This is possible due to the close interaction between the cardiovascular system and the respiratory system. Furthermore, a link exists between normal physiological cardiovascular responses to increasing and decreasing demands of other body systems, such as the integumentary system, muscular system and reproductive system, and complex feedback mechanisms exist between these systems aimed at the body's ever-changing blood flow and blood pressure requirements.

CASE STUDY 13.1

Alex was running late and trying to get to work as quickly as possible. He heard the train coming and ran as fast as he could towards the station to catch the next train.

Q1. Which of these statements best describes the equation to measure cardiac output?

   a. The amount of blood ejected from contraction of the left ventricle multiplied by 60.

   b. The total amount of blood in the left ventricle in diastole multiplied by the heart rate measured over 60 seconds.

   c. The amount of blood ejected from contraction of the left ventricle multiplied by the heart rate measured over 60 seconds.

   d. The amount of blood left in the left ventricle after contraction multiplied by the heart rate measured over 60 seconds.

Q2. The sympathetic nervous system response known as 'fight or flight' is triggered:

   a. by a physical and/or emotional stressor to meet the demands of increased activity or preparing for the potential of increased physical activity.

   b. only as a response to increased physical activity occurring after exertion has commenced.

   c. after a significant amount of physical exertion has taken place to meet significantly increased demand.

   d. as a response to relax and slow down the heart rate and force contraction of the heart.

Q3. Sympathetic chronotropic and inotropic stimulation of the heart can be most accurately described as:

   a. an increase in the speed of conduction through ventricular muscle.

   b. an increase in SA node firing, the speed of AV node conduction and the force of contraction of the ventricles.

   c. a decrease in SA node firing, the speed of AV node conduction and the force of contraction of the ventricles.

   d. increased cardiac output through increasing the force of contraction of the ventricles.

Q4. Describe what happens to stroke volume and heart rate when the cardiac output required is increased because of this sudden exertion.

Q5. Describe the sympathetic nervous system's role when increased cardiac output is required.

CASE STUDY 13.2

After running as fast as he could to the train station, Alex got on the train just as the doors closed. Finding a seat Alex started to relax as his half-hour train journey began.

Q1. The parasympathetic nervous system response known as 'reset and digest' is triggered:

a. by a physical and/or emotional stressor to meet the demands of increased activity or preparing for the potential of increased physical activity.

b. only as a response to increased physical activity occurring because of prolonged exertion.

c. after a significant amount of physical exertion has taken place to meet significantly increased demand.

d. once physical or emotional stressors are no longer occurring to slow down the heart rate.

Q2. The effect of parasympathetic stimulation on the SA node, AV node and ventricular muscle contraction can most accurately be described as:

a. an increase in the force of contraction of the ventricular muscle.

b. a decreased rate of SA node firing and the speed of AV node conduction with no increase in the force of contraction of the ventricles.

c. a decrease in SA node firing and the speed of AV node conduction.

d. an increase in SA node firing and the speed of AV node conduction with an increase in the force of contraction of the ventricles.

Q3. When blood pressure in the aorta is higher than normal, baroreceptors will:

a. stimulate the cardio-inhibitory centre of the brain, causing decreased heart rate, stroke volume and vasodilation.

b. stimulate the cardio-inhibitory centre of the brain, causing increased heart rate, stroke volume and vasoconstriction.

c. stimulate the cardio-acceleratory centre of the brain, causing increased heart rate, stroke volume and vasoconstriction.

d. stimulate the cardio-acceleratory centre of the brain, causing decreased heart rate, stroke volume and vasoconstriction.

Q4. Describe what happens to stroke volume and heart rate when the cardiac output required is decreased.

Q5. Describe how moving to a resting state after running will cause the baroreceptors to regulate the blood pressure.

CASE STUDY 13.3

On a hot day Caitlin spent a few hours playing soccer with her friends. When she finished playing she realised that she had not had anything to drink for several hours and felt very thirsty.

Q1. In Caitlin's case, dehydration will cause:

a. a decrease in preload, a decrease in afterload and no change in cardiac output.

b. an increase in preload, a decrease in afterload and no change or a drop in cardiac output.

c. a decrease in preload, an increase in afterload and no change or a drop in cardiac output.

d. an increase in preload, a decrease in afterload and a decrease in cardiac output.

Q2. The actions of angiotensin II in the setting of dehydration is best described as:

a. angiotensin II causes vasoconstriction of all blood vessels to increase blood pressure.

b. angiotensin II causes vasodilation of all blood vessels to decrease blood pressure.

c. angiotensin II directly causes sodium and water reabsorption.

d. angiotensin II converts into 'angiotensinogen' I.

Q3. The actions of aldosterone in the setting of dehydration can be best described as aldosterone:

a. increases potassium reabsorption from urine to blood to increase water retention and intravascular blood volume.

b. causes vasoconstriction to increase blood pressure.

c. increases sodium reabsorption from urine to blood to increase water retention and intravascular blood volume.

d. converts angiotensin I into angiotensin II.

Q4. Discuss how dehydration affects preload, afterload and blood pressure.

Q5. Describe the compensatory mechanisms related to the kidneys that will activate to maintain normal blood pressure in this situation.

CASE STUDY 13.4

Sonia sat down preparing to give a presentation in front of a large group of people; she was feeling very nervous. Sonia noticed that her heart rate had increased significantly.

Q1. The effect of adrenaline (epinephrine) on the conduction system is best described as:

    a. an increase in SA node firing and a decrease in AV node conduction.

    b. an increase in SA node firing and an increase in AV node conduction.

    c. a decrease in SA node firing and an increase in AV node conduction.

    d. a decrease in SA node firing and a decrease in AV node conduction.

Q2. The effect of adrenaline (epinephrine) on blood vessels and afterload is best described as:

    a. vasodilation and a decrease in afterload.

    b. vasodilation and an increase in afterload.

    c. vasoconstriction and an increase in afterload.

    d. vasoconstriction and a decrease in afterload.

Q3. Adrenoceptors alpha and beta are primarily located:

    a. α_1 and α_2 in the heart and β_1 and β_2 in the blood vessels.

    b. α_1 and α_2 in the blood vessels and β_1 and β_2 in the heart.

    c. α_1 and α_2 in the blood vessels and β_1 and β_2 in the kidneys.

    d. α_1 and α_2 in the kidneys and β_1 and β_2 in the heart.

Q4. Describe the parts of the conduction system that are stimulated to increase the heart rate in this situation.

Q5. Describe the role of adrenaline (epinephrine) in this situation and its effect on the heart and blood vessels.

REFERENCES

1. Patton K, Thibodeau G. Anatomy and physiology. London: Elsevier Health Sciences; 2015. p. 699–727.
2. Jones M, Harvey A, Main E. Anatomy and physiology of the respiratory and cardiac systems. In: Cardiorespiratory physiotherapy: adults and paediatrics. Philadelphia: Elsevier; 2016. p. 1–46.
3. Huszar R. Huszar's ECG and 12-lead interpretation. St Louis: Elsevier; 2017. p. 1–15.
4. Marieb E, Hoehn K. Human anatomy and physiology. Boston: Pearson; 2013. p. 658–750.
5. Porritt K. Tabbner's nursing care. Sydney: Elsevier; 2016. p. 636–706.
6. Buckley T. The structure and function of the cardiovascular and lymphatic systems. In: Craft JA, Gordon CJ, Huether SE, et al, editors. Understanding pathophysiology, ANZ ed. Sydney: Elsevier; 2019. p. 563–609.
7. Wagner G, Strauss D. Marriott's practical electrocardiography. Philadelphia: Wolters Kluwer; 2014.
8. Rodriguez NE. The cardiovascular system. In: Kacmarek RM, Stoller JH, Albert J, editors. Egan's fundamentals of respiratory care. St Louis: Elsevier; 2017. p. 207–29.
9. Pappano A, Gil Wier W. Cardiovascular physiology. Philadelphia: Elsevier; 2013. p. 237–62.
10. Jonson Cohen B, Hull K. Memmler's the human body in health and disease. Philadelphia: Wolters Kluwer; 2015. p. 338–61.
11. Phillips N. Berry & Kohn's operating room technique. St Louis: Elsevier; 2017. p. 909–12.
12. Lokmic Z, Lämmermann T, Sixt M, et al. The extracellular matrix of the spleen as a potential organiser of immune cell compartments. *Semin Immunol* 2008;20(1):4–13.
13. Klabunde RE. Cardiovascular physiology concepts. Available from: www.cvphysiology.com/Blood%20Flow/BF015.
14. Vanputte C, Regan J, Russo A. Seeley anatomy & physiology. New York: McGraw-Hill; 2014. p. 547–68.
15. Biondi B, Palmieri EA, Lombardi G, et al. Effects of thyroid hormone on cardiac function: the relative importance of heart rate, loading conditions, and myocardial contractility in the regulation of cardiac performance in human hyperthyroidism. *J Clin Endocrinol Metab* 2002;87(3):968–74.
16. Srinivasan RS, Dillard ME, Lagutin OV, et al. Lineage tracing demonstrates the venous origin of the mammalian lymphatic vasculature. *Genes Dev* 2007;21:2422–32.
17. Aspelund A, Robciuc MR, Karaman S, et al. Lymphatic system in cardiovascular medicine. *Circulation Res* 2016;118: 515–30.
18. Maybin JA, Critchley HOD. Menstrual physiology: implications for endometrial pathology and beyond. *Hum Reprod Update* 2015;21(6):748–61.
19. Soma-Pillay P, Nelson-Piercy C, Tolppanen H, et al. Physiological changes in pregnancy. *Cardiovasc J Afr* 2016; 27(2):89–94.
20. Stacey T, Thompson JM, Mitchell EA, et al. Association between maternal sleep practices and risk of late stillbirth: a case-control study. *BMJ* 2011;14(342):d3403.
21. Gordon A, Raynes-Greenow C, Bond D, et al. Sleep position, fetal growth restriction, and late-pregnancy stillbirth: the Sydney stillbirth study. *Obstet Gynecol* 2015;125:347–55.
22. Owusu JT, Anderson FJ, Coleman J, et al. Association of maternal sleep practices with pre-eclampsia, low birth weight, and stillbirth among Ghanaian women. *Int J Gynaecol Obstet* 2013;121:261–5.
23. Heazell AEP, Li M, Budd J, et al. Association between maternal sleep practices and late stillbirth: findings from a stillbirth case-control study. *BJOG* 2017;doi.org/10.1111/ 1471-0528.14967.

CHAPTER 14

Lymphatic system and tissue fluid balance maintenance

ZERINA TOMKINS, BAPPSC (MED LAB SCI), BAPPSC (HONS), MNSC (NURS), PHD, GRAD CERT (UNIVERSITY EDUCATION) • JANE PHILLIPS, BAPPSCI (PHYSIO)

KEY POINTS/LEARNING OUTCOMES

1. Describe the structure and function of the lymphatic system.
2. Discuss the formation, flow direction and drainage of the lymph.
3. Explain how the structure of lymphatic vessels and the direction of lymph flow regulate tissue fluid homeostasis.
4. Link the structure and function of the lymphatic system to the function of other body systems.

KEY DEFINITIONS

- **Endothelium:** a single layer of cells, known as endothelial cells, that lines the inner surface of blood and lymphatic vessels. Endothelial cells are in direct contact with circulating blood and lymph separating them from the vessel's smooth muscle and the remaining extravascular tissue.
- **Lymph:** a proteinaceous interstitial fluid drained from interstitial tissue.
- **Lymph node:** a small, bean-shaped lymphoid organ that contains different types of immune cells and acts as a surveillance centre that screens lymph transiting through the lymph node.
- **Lymphangion:** a functional unit of a collecting lymphatic vessel that lies between two lymphatic valves. These valves are semilunar in shape and facilitate one-way flow of lymph from tissue periphery towards the central vascular circulation.
- **Lymphatic vessels:** tube-like structures that conduct lymph from tissue periphery to systemic circulation.

ONLINE RESOURCES/SUGGESTED READINGS

- **Lymphatic Education & Research Network** available at https://lymphaticnetwork.org
- **Lymphatic filariasis** available at www.who.int/news-room/fact-sheets/detail/lymphatic-filariasis
- **Lymphatic system** available at www.myvmc.com/medical-centres/cancer/lymphatic-system
- **The Royal Children's Hospital Melbourne Clinical Practice Guidelines: Snakebite** available at www.rch.org.au/clinicalguide/guideline_index/Snakebite

INTRODUCTION

The lymphatic system is comprised of lymphatic vessels, lymph, lymphoid tissues and lymphoid organs. Lymphoid organs include the lymph node, thyroid gland, spleen, colon, tonsils, intestinal Peyer's patches and thymus (Fig. 14.1A). In simplest terms, we can think of it as a drainage system organised to transport fluid, called lymph, which has been filtered out of the blood at the arterial end of the vessels (Fig. 14.1B) back to the central circulation. In particular, this fluid passes into the closed-ended initial lymphatic capillary vessel, then drains via connecting vessels to lymph collecting vessels, along which it travels, passing through one or more lymph nodes before returning to the venous system and thus the blood circulation. **Lymph** is a colourless and odourless fluid that contains proteins, immune cells, antigens,

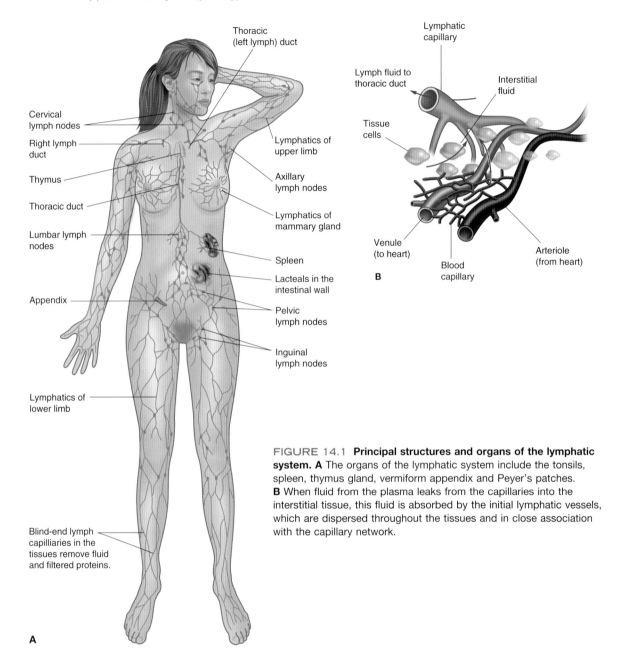

Cervical lymph nodes

Right lymph duct

Thymus

Thoracic duct

Lumbar lymph nodes

Appendix

Lymphatics of lower limb

Blind-end lymph capilliaries in the tissues remove fluid and filtered proteins.

Thoracic (left lymph) duct

Lymphatics of upper limb

Axillary lymph nodes

Lymphatics of mammary gland

Spleen

Lacteals in the intestinal wall

Pelvic lymph nodes

Inguinal lymph nodes

A

Lymphatic capillary

Lymph fluid to thoracic duct

Tissue cells

Interstitial fluid

Venule (to heart)

Blood capillary

Arteriole (from heart)

B

FIGURE 14.1 **Principal structures and organs of the lymphatic system. A** The organs of the lymphatic system include the tonsils, spleen, thymus gland, vermiform appendix and Peyer's patches. **B** When fluid from the plasma leaks from the capillaries into the interstitial tissue, this fluid is absorbed by the initial lymphatic vessels, which are dispersed throughout the tissues and in close association with the capillary network.

lipids, macromolecules and particulate matter.[1] An exception to this appearance is the lymph arriving from lymph vessels of the small intestine. Here, the lymph is milky and dense as it contains lipid globules derived from fats absorbed in the small intestine.[2]

Lymphatic vessels or 'lymphatics' are present wherever blood vasculature is present. So it is not surprising that lymphatic capillaries are absent from avascular structures such as the epidermis, cornea, hair, nails and cartilage. Until 2015 it was thought that lymphatics were also absent from the central nervous system. However, in the last few years lymphatic vessels have been found to line the dural sinuses,[3] thus dispelling the myth of the central nervous system lacking lymphatic drainage.

Initial lymphatic vessel (lymphatic capillary)   Collecting lymphatic vessel

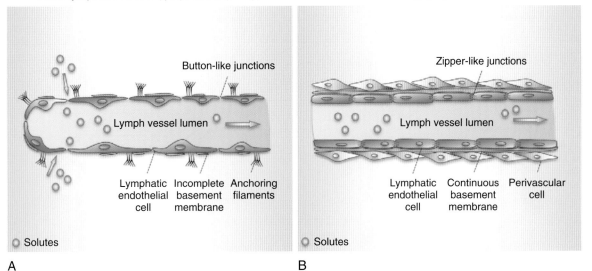

FIGURE 14.2 The cellular structures of initial lymphatic vessel and collecting lymphatic vessel.
A The initial lymphatic vessel is characterised by overlapping endothelial cells that contain flap-like structures that enable the fluid and solutes dissolved in that fluid to flow into the lymphatic vessel. Once the vessel is full, the flaps are closed by the internal pressure formed by the fluid (lymph). Note that these same endothelial openings are sites where immune cells would enter the lymphatic vessel and travel to lymph nodes where the immune response can take place. From here, the fluid would be propelled into the collecting lymphatic vessel. **B** Note that the collecting lymphatic vessel does not contain openings that would allow interstitial fluid to enter the lymphatic vessel. (*Source:* Kalucka J, Teuwen L-A, Geldhof V, Carmeliet P. How to cross the lymphatic fence. Circ Res 2017;120:1376–8.)

The lymphatic system maintains homeostasis by: (1) transporting fluid that filters from the capillaries into the interstitial tissue back to the cardiovascular system; (2) absorbing and transporting dietary fats from the gastrointestinal system to the cardiovascular circulation; and (3) assisting the capture, transport, identification and destruction of foreign antigens. The focus of this chapter is on fluid transport. The role of the lymphatic system in the absorption and transport of dietary fats from the gastrointestinal system to the cardiovascular circulation is covered in Chapter 13, while the role of the lymphatic system in assisting the capture, transport, identification and destruction of foreign antigens is covered in Chapter 15.

STRUCTURE AND FUNCTION OF THE LYMPHATIC SYSTEM

Lymphatic vessels

The adult human lymphatic system starts with closed-ended thin-walled channels lined with endothelial cells. When examined under the microscope, these channels—**initial lymphatic capillaries** (Figs 14.2 and 14.3)—have an irregular appearance, with a diameter of 20–70 μm. Uniquely, the endothelial cells lining the initial lymphatic capillaries are shaped like an oak leaf, and each oak flap overlaps with another[4] to form fluid inlets. These flaps are joined together by the cell junction molecules located along the sides of the flaps.[5] Initial lymphatic capillaries have a discontinuous basement membrane and are held in place by anchoring filaments. The capacity of the initial lymphatic capillaries to collect and conduct lymph up the lymphatic vessel tree depends on gravity, atmospheric pressure and the physical activity of the muscles (muscle pump) and diaphragm (respiratory pump), which helps controls breathing.[1,6,7,8]

The initial lymphatic capillaries merge into the **collecting lymphatics** (Fig. 14.2). The endothelial cells are connected to one another by cell junctions that now appear in zipper-like format.[5] The vessel is lined with a layer of continuous smooth muscle cells and continuous

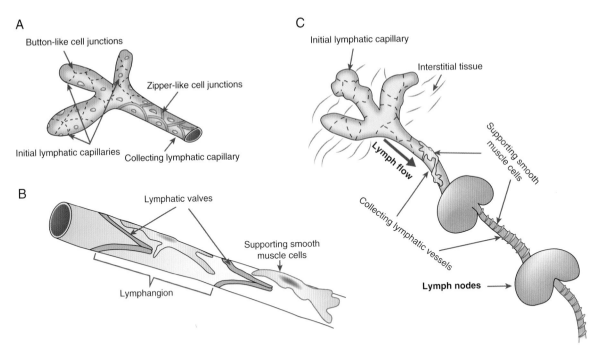

FIGURE 14.3 **Lymphatic fluid circulation. A** The initial lymphatic vessel is characterised by overlapping endothelial cells that contain flap-like structures and button-like junctions. **B** The collecting lymphatic vessel, which is characterised by zipper-like cell junctions tightly connecting lymphatic endothelial cells, enables the fluid and solutes dissolved in that fluid to flow into the lymphatic vessels that will eventually converge to empty into the venous circulation. **C** Lymph uses the network of lymphatic vessels to travel through a network of lymph nodes, where the immune system can screen the lymph for foreign particles and mount an appropriate immune response.

basement membrane. Inside the collecting lymphatic capillary, paired intraluminal semilunar valves are present. An area between two consecutive lymphatic valves is called a **lymphangion**. The smooth muscle within the walls of the lymphangion contracts when distended, causing the lymph to be propelled proximally. This movement is also facilitated by adrenergic, cholinergic and peptidergic nerves.[1] The function of the lymphatic valve (Fig. 14.3) is to prevent the backward flow of lymph between neighbouring lymphangions,[9] further ensuring proximal movement towards the systemic circulation.

Lymph flow

Collecting or afferent lymphatics drain the lymph into lymph nodes (Fig 14.1A). In lymph nodes the immune system scrutinises the lymph for foreign antigens. If an antigen is detected, an appropriate immune response will be activated. Following this surveillance point, lymph exits the lymph nodes into efferent (exiting) collecting lymphatics to travel to the cervical lymphovenous portals, which empty the lymph into the venous blood circulation.[6] On the right side of the body, the right jugular trunk, right subclavian trunk and right bronchomediastinal trunk can either individually drain into the right subclavian vein, or converge into the right lymphatic duct, which empties into the right subclavian vein. The left jugular trunk, left subclavian trunk and left bronchomediastinal trunk can empty into the junction of the internal jugular and subclavian veins or converge into the thoracic duct, which empties into the junction of the internal jugular and subclavian veins.[1,6]

Lymphatic vessel structure and function differ from tissue to tissue. This heterogeneity is not surprising as the tissues and organs where these lymphatic vessels reside have unique structures and functions. As such they place differing demands on the regional lymphatic system. This complexity is further enriched by the fact that lymphatic vessels from different organs may converge to a common lymphatic vein that is not located in any of the parent organs. From a clinical perspective, when lymphatic vessels are chronically obstructed, the tissue they drain becomes swollen and distended due to local accumulation of the protein-rich fluid. This is known as **lymphoedema**.

Damage to a collecting lymphatic vessel can lead to the formation of chyle fistulas, whereby lymph leaks from the injured vessel and accumulates in the surrounding cavities. If this occurs in the abdomen it is known as **chyloperitoneum**, and if it occurs in the thoracic cavity it is known as **chylothorax**.[10] Arguably the most important reason for knowing lymphatic vessel drainage patterns, including the distribution of associated lymph nodes, is their role in spreading cancer cells throughout the body, a process called **metastasis**. An example of this is secondary malignancies or metastases of the lungs that have arisen due to spread from gastrointestinal cancers via lymphatic channels shared between the two organs.

Formation of lymph

Blood flows from the heart through the systemic circulation back to the heart because there is a difference in pressure between the aorta and the vena cava (Fig. 14.4).[11] As blood is pumped from the heart through the aorta into arteries and arterioles, it does so under an estimated pressure of 100–120 mmHg. As the aorta branches into arteries and branches that have a smaller diameter, that pressure decreases due to increasing peripheral resistance. By the time the blood reaches the arterioles, it is estimated to be 50 mmHg. Arterioles give rise to meta-arterioles. Blood flow from meta-arterioles can move in two ways: (1) into a capillary bed, if the pre-capillary sphincter, a layer of smooth muscle formed in the transition zone between an arteriole and a capillary, is relaxed; (2) if the pre-capillary sphincter is constricted, the blood will bypass the capillary bed and enter the venous circulation (Fig. 14.4).[12]

The capillary structure is characterised by a single layer of endothelial cells supported by a basement

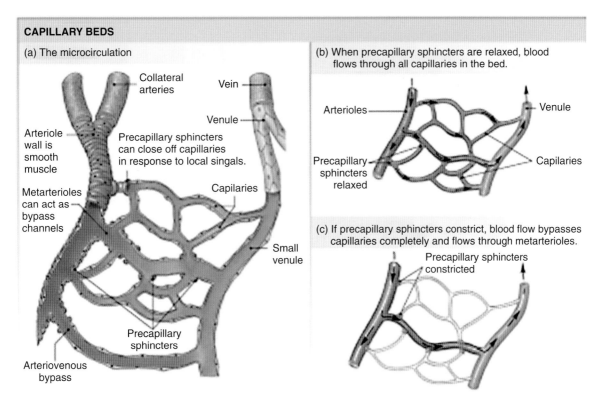

FIGURE 14.4 Blood flow through the blood capillary network and formation of interstitial fluid.
(*Source:* Silverthorn D. Human physiology: an integrated approach, 7 ed. Austin, TX: Pearson; 2016.)

membrane and contractile cells that are very similar to smooth muscle cells and are called **pericytes**.[12] At this level there is an exchange of oxygen and nutrients for carbon dioxide and metabolic waste. After the exchange has taken place, the blood enters the venules and moves into the venous system.

At the blood–tissue interface of small-calibre vessels (microvessels), there are two blood vascular forces that dictate the movement of water and solutes between the blood and tissue spaces (Fig. 14.5). These forces are hydrostatic pressure and osmotic pressure.[11] Hydrostatic pressure is pressure exerted by the blood against the wall of the capillary. As fluid exits the capillary into the interstitial tissue it also increases the interstitial fluid hydrostatic pressure. Osmotic pressure, also known as oncotic pressure and colloid osmotic pressure, is pressure that drives the movement of fluid from the interstitial tissue (an area of relatively low protein concentration) back into the capillary lumen (an area of relatively high protein concentration). Osmotic pressure is determined by the difference in the protein-to-water concentrations in the blood and the interstitial tissue fluid.

Blood flow in capillaries is slow.[11] This is because the total surface area covered by the capillary network is large, hence blood arriving from meta-arterioles is distributed across a greater total cross-sectional area. This reduction in flow contributes to effective exchange of materials at the capillary bed between blood plasma and the cells external to the capillary, and diffusion of smaller dissolved solutes and gases, such as oxygen and carbon dioxide. Another form of capillary exchange is **bulk flow**. Here, due to differences in osmotic pressure gradients, the movement is in the direction from higher to lower pressure. Movement out of a capillary is called **filtration**; movement into a capillary is called **absorption**.

During capillary filtration, at the end closer to the arterial network, the net hydrostatic pressure is higher in the capillary vessel lumen and as such it forces fluid out of the capillary into the interstitial spaces through the endothelial cell junctions.[11] Hydrostatic pressure tends to decrease along the length of the capillary. Hence in a capillary at the venous end, it is expected that the osmotic pressure will be higher due to water lost at the arterial end of the capillary; that is, there will be a high concentration of protein present in a lower concentration of water. There is a gradual decline in filtration over the length of the capillary, with net filtration into the tissues/

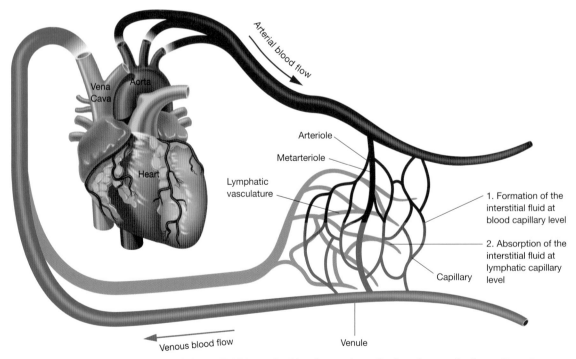

FIGURE 14.5 **Movement of tissue fluid from the blood vessels to the lymph vessels: formation of interstitial fluid.**

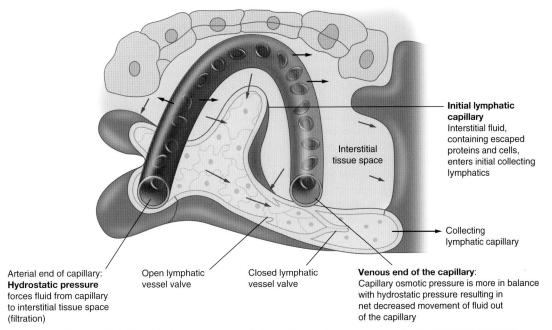

Initial lymphatic capillary
Interstitial fluid, containing escaped proteins and cells, enters initial collecting lymphatics

Interstitial tissue space

Collecting lymphatic capillary

Arterial end of capillary: **Hydrostatic pressure** forces fluid from capillary to interstitial tissue space (filtration)

Open lymphatic vessel valve

Closed lymphatic vessel valve

Venous end of the capillary: Capillary osmotic pressure is more in balance with hydrostatic pressure resulting in net decreased movement of fluid out of the capillary

FIGURE 14.6 **Relationship between hydrostatic and oncotic pressure in driving the formation of interstitial fluid from the blood capillaries to the lymphatic capillaries.**

interstitial spaces.[13] Previously it was thought that there would be a reabsorption event at the post-capillary level, on the venous side.[12] This movement would have been dictated by the rate and direction of fluid movement at the capillary level and would be proportional to the difference in hydrostatic pressure and colloidal osmotic pressure (known as Starling's principle).[14,15] However, since the early 1990s a series of experiments[16] has shown that Starling's principle does not hold, as continuous reabsorption at the venous end was unlikely to occur. Instead, it is now thought that all interstitial fluid is returned to the systemic circulation via the lymphatic vessels (Fig. 14.6).[14–16] Absorption of such a large volume of interstitial tissue is feasible when it is considered that the initial lymphatic vessels have specialised oak-leaf-like cell junctions that act as opening pores to allow fluid influx.[4,5,17]

Regulation of lymph flow in lymphatic vessels

When interstitial fluid enters the initial lymphatic vessels it does so because there is a pressure gradient between the interstitial tissue and the lymphatic capillary. The literature suggests that the pathway to the lymphatic vessels is earmarked by anchoring filaments, which extend deeply into connective tissue and connect to the network

of elastic fibres, thus permitting them to control their own diameter.[1] Once the fluid is inside the initial lymphatic vessels, the internal pressure exerted by that fluid is sufficient to close the junctions of the oak-leaf-shaped endothelium. This effectively seals the entry sites to prevent further fluid entry. Lymph in the initial lymphatic vessels is under the influence of tissue pressures at this stage, as lymph may move in either direction at this level, before it enters the collecting vessels which have lymph valves to ensure one-way movement. Once inside the collecting vessels, lymph is further propelled by intrinsic and extrinsic lymphatic pumps. The extrinsic pump refers to cyclical compression and expansion of the lymphatics by surrounding tissue forces, such as the contraction and relaxation of skeletal muscles (known as the **muscle pump**), breathing (known as the **respiratory pump**) and blood flow through the venous system (known as the **venous pump**). The intrinsic pump refers to rapid/phasic contractions of lymphatic vessel smooth muscle cells, thought to be due to innervation by adrenergic, cholinergic and peptidergic neuronal fibres.[18]

Lymphangiogenesis

The lymphatic system develops early during embryogenesis through the complex interplay of stem and progenitor cells, growth factors and the local environment. Genetic abnormalities of the lymphatic system lead to failure of tissue fluid homeostasis and some abnormalities are incompatible with life.[1] The process of how new lymphatic vessels form is called **lymphangiogenesis**.[19] Lymphangiogenesis can occur in adulthood when there is an injury such as a wound, or chronic obstruction of the lymphatic system, and new vessels enable new draining pathways to form. Obstruction of the lymphatic vessels may be caused by an infection such as roundworm (a parasitic nematode, resulting in the infection known as filariasis), lymph node dissection, inborn errors that lead to failure to develop functional lymphatics, or growth of tumour cells (metastasis). Overgrowth or impaired growth of lymphatic vessels has been associated with many disease processes including rheumatoid arthritis, psoriasis and chronic wound healing.[7]

INTEGRATION OF THE LYMPHATIC SYSTEM WITH OTHER BODY SYSTEMS

Most of the time you will be unaware that the lymphatic system exists, until some form of insult or injury results in increased strain on lymphatic vessel function. For example, the presence of dysfunctional lymphatic vessel drainage is noted in a blister, where due to burn damage to lymphatic vessels, lymph is noted in the form of the blister. If you have had knee surgery or an ankle sprain, you would have noticed the swelling that remains around the joint for a prolonged period. After the injury has resolved the residual fluid needs to be drained away by lymphatics that are either recovering from the surgery/injury or are overwhelmed by the volume of fluid to be returned to the circulation. This section examines how the lymphatic system contributes to homeostasis of other body systems.

Integumentary system

The lymphatic vessels have been best studied in the skin. This is due to ease of accessibility to tissue material and because of the rich supply of lymphatic vessels found in the skin. The initial lymphatic capillary vessels, found just beneath the papillary dermis, are known as the **superficial plexus**. The epidermis is devoid of lymphatic vessels. As initial lymphatic capillaries coalesce into collecting lymphatic vessels, the fluid is drained vertically into the deeper lymphatic vessel plexus found at the junction of the reticular dermis and the subcutis.

In addition to tissue fluid balance, lymphatic vessels play an important role in facilitating the movement of Langerhans cells from the skin to the lymph nodes where they present foreign antigens for immune responses. **Lymphangitis**, an inflammation of the lymphatic vessels

which occurs mostly as a result of a bacterial infection, can be easily observed in the skin as red linear streaks that extend from the site of infection to the regional lymph nodes. Impaired lymphatic function in the skin is evident as **oedema** and can lead to impaired immune responses and fibrosis of the local skin tissue.[20] Lymphoedema is a chronic condition of lymph stasis where there is an accumulation of lymph in the tissues;[16] it can result from cancer-related treatment (where it is known as secondary lymphoedema) or a genetic mutation evident early in life (where it is known as primary lymphoedema, a condition without a cure). In both types of lymphoedema, the application of multi-layer bandaging (compression therapy) is used as a management strategy. Bandaging increases tissue pressure, resulting in reduced capillary filtration and therefore less lymph is produced. Bandaging is one factor, along with exercise, recommended to improve lymph movement, to maximise uptake into lymphatic vessels by the changes in pressure with muscle movement.[20]

Musculoskeletal system

Skeletal muscles are responsible for movement, heat production and maintenance of posture (Chapter 6). This highly vascularised tissue also has a lymphatic network that is reported to follow arcading and transverse arterioles and is surrounded by muscle fibres.[8] The arterial pulsations and changes in muscle contraction and relaxation (the muscle pump) facilitate opening and closing of the lymphatic capillaries and movement of lymph along the vessel. Hence, when a muscle is stretched, it helps facilitate the opening of the initial capillaries so that the interstitial fluid can enter the lymphatic vessel lumen. Muscle contraction leads to increased pressure in the filled lymphatic vessel, causing lymph to be propelled uni-directionally forwards.[10] This physiological control of lymph movement is one reason why physiotherapists and lymphoedema therapists advise physical activity, as it will lead to increased lymph flow peripherally in the collecting lymphatic vessels and move lymph centrally to draining lymphatic ducts. Bone tissues do not contain lymphatic vessels. However, fractured bone will cause inflammation and tissue oedema and, in some cases, injury to the local lymphatic vessels—responses that require the lymphatic system to react and assist in fracture repair.

Joints

Joints (Chapter 5) are broadly divided into fibrous, cartilaginous and synovial joints. Lymphatic vessels are present in adipose, areolar and fibrous types of the normal synovial joint membrane, with fewer lymphatic vessels present in the superficial subintima and greater numbers found in the deep subintima and underlying fibrous tissue of the joint capsule.[21] Joint cartilage is an avascular structure and it does not contain lymphatic vessels.

Nervous system

The central nervous system has a specialised drainage system called the paravascular or **glymphatic system**. The glymphatic system consists of a para-arterial influx route for cerebrospinal fluid (CSF) to enter the brain parenchyma, and it is coupled to a clearance mechanism for the removal of tissue fluid from the brain and spinal cord interstitium.[22] The movement of CSF is dependent on arterial pulsation.[23] The dural sinuses and meningeal arteries are also lined with lymphatic vessels.[3,24] This lymphatic vasculature, connected directly to the glymphatic system, facilitates immune cell trafficking and drains into deep cervical lymph nodes.[3,24]

Special senses: hearing, balance and vision

In the eye ball (Chapter 9), a specialised structure referred to as **Schlemm's canal** collects aqueous humour (formed from blood in the capillaries) from the anterior eye chamber and delivers it to the episcleral blood vessels via aqueous veins. In so doing, Schlemm's canal regulates intraocular pressure. For a long time it was thought that Schlemm's canal was a type of venous vessel (venous sinus), but Schlemm's canal has characteristics and features more common with lymphatic vessels than venous vessels.[25]

The human ear is composed of the external, middle and inner ear (Chapter 9). A dense lymphatic network is prominent in the skin of the external ear but not in the cartilage component of the external ear. The lymphatic system of the outer and middle ear drains into the cervical lymph nodes, while lymphatic vessels have not been identified in the inner ear. The middle ear and the middle ear mucosa contain submucosal lymphatic pathways that drain into the upper cervical lymph nodes. It is therefore not surprising that if you have a cold that also affects your ears, the lymph nodes in your neck will be swollen.

Cardiovascular system

The heart has a very rich network of lymphatic vessels that form three plexuses: subendocardial, myocardial and subepicardial. The subendocardial and myocardial plexuses drain into the subepicardial plexus.[6] The efferent vessels arising from the subepicardial plexus form the left and right cardiac collecting trunks. The left trunk usually empties into the inferior tracheobronchial node,

whereas the right trunk drains into the brachiocephalic node. Lymphatic vessels also appear in cardiac valves but their role there is not known. Heart lymphatic vessels function to tightly maintain cardiac tissue fluid homeostasis and therefore contribute to normal cardiac output.[26] There is some suggestion that the heart's lymphatic vasculature could be therapeutically targeted to promote healing following myocardial ischaemia and infarction.[27] Cardiac surgery often produces damage to the lymphatic vasculature that can lead to oedema and impair ventricular function.[26,28]

The lymphatic system also contributes to the maintenance of blood volume and blood pressure through its capacity to effectively absorb and transport the interstitial fluid from the tissue periphery to the central venous circulation. If blood pressure is very low and the heart requires an increased volume of blood to maintain blood circulation, a compensatory mechanism will be activated that will instruct the lymphatic system to absorb more interstitial fluid for return to the venous circulation, thus contributing to increased intravascular blood volume.[6]

Immune system

It is important to distinguish between the lymphatics and lymphoid tissue. Lymphatic vessels are uni-directional tube-like structures lined with endothelial cells that collect and drain tissue fluid present in the interstitial spaces. They are also conduits for lymphocytes, antigen-presenting cells and soluble foreign particles (Fig. 14.3).[10] Lymphoid tissue (e.g. lymph nodes) is an organ structure consisting of large aggregates of lymphocytes, supporting cells such as fibroblasts and a unique extracellular matrix that often provides cues about cell 'home' so that circulating lymphocytes can recognise a site where they should home themselves.[29] The role of lymphatic vessels within the immune system is to facilitate the immune responses (Chapter 15) by acting as freeways or conduits for antigens and antigen-presenting cells travelling uni-directionally from the tissue periphery to lymphoid organs, such as lymph nodes, where the adaptive immune response can generate a plethora of immune functions aimed at combating foreign invaders. How lymph nodes and their resident immune cells participate in the immune response is covered in Chapter 15.

Respiratory system

The respiratory system helps regulate lymph flow. Breathing, a passive process that enables air exchange in the lungs, is characterised by pressure changes during inhalation and exhalation. These pressure changes affect lymph return by propelling lymph forwards. When thinking about how the lymphatic system contributes to fluid homeostasis of the lungs, the first thought is often pulmonary oedema. This condition is characterised by the lungs filling with interstitial fluid, which prevents oxygen exchange and the person struggles to breathe. Lymphatic vessels are essential in keeping fluid away from lung tissues by draining excess interstitial fluid. The structure of the lymphatics of the respiratory system is considered from two perspectives: the intrathoracic respiratory tract, which encompasses the trachea, bronchi, lungs and pleura; and the thoracic wall. Lymphatic vessels of the pulmonary system originate in a superficial subpleural plexus and drain into a deeper plexus that accompanies the branches of pulmonary vessels and bronchi. The deeper plexus runs in submucosal and peribronchial parts of larger bronchi with the plexus extending down to the bronchioles. Lung alveoli do not have lymphatic vessels.[6]

The lymphatics of the lungs and visceral pleura empty into the bronchopulmonary lymph nodes at the bifurcations of the larger bronchi[30] (Fig. 14.7). From here, the lymphatic vessels empty into tracheobronchial nodes, which drain into the bronchomediastinal trunk on each side. The bronchomediastinal trunk usually empties directly into the junction of the internal jugular and subclavian veins. Less commonly, the right

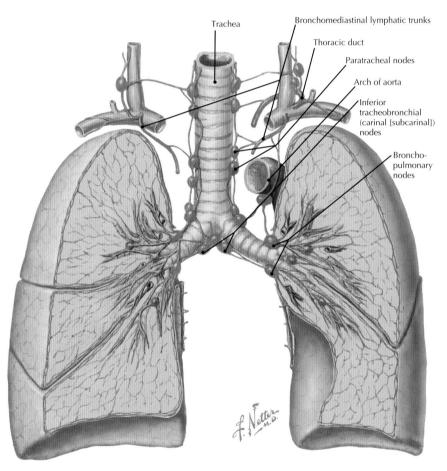

FIGURE 14.7 **Lymph drainage of the lung.** The lymphatics of the lungs empty into the bronchopulmonary lymph nodes at the bifurcations of the bronchi. Lymph travels the tracheobronchial nodes, which drain into the left and right bronchomediastinal trunks. The bronchomediastinal trunks usually empty into the junction of the internal jugular and subclavian veins or, less commonly, into the right duct. The left lymph duct can also drain into the thoracic duct. (*Source:* Netter Image ID 20645, Reg ID: 02783.)

bronchomediastinal trunk drains into the right lymph duct and the left drains into the thoracic duct.[6,30]

The lymphatics of the thoracic wall comprise the anterior thoracic wall and the posterolateral thoracic wall. The anterior thoracic extends craniocaudally from the level of the clavicle and jugular notch to the level of the xiphisternal joint and extends bilaterally from one anterior axillary line to the other.[6]

While the function of the lymphatic system in the lungs revolves around tissue fluid balance and immune functions, recently it has been proposed that the lymphatic vasculature may play a role in preparing the fetal lung for inflation at birth.[31]

Gastrointestinal system

Gastrointestinal lymphatics are essential for immune surveillance, regulation of gut interstitial fluid balance and transport of absorbed lipids to the bloodstream. As the gastrointestinal system is densely colonised by commensal bacteria and has a large absorptive surface area, the lymphatic vessels also play a role in innate immunity and tolerance.[2] If the gastrointestinal surface, which is also a barrier to bacteria into the systemic circulation, was compromised, it would be easy for bacteria to gain access to the bloodstream and cause systemic infection or **sepsis**.

Increased lymph flow in the gastrointestinal organs is observed after feeding, in cases of acute and chronic inflammation and during intestinal obstruction.[2] The small intestine, large intestine, oesophagus, stomach and accessory digestive organs such as the salivary glands, liver, pancreas and gallbladder have lymphatic networks. While in most gastrointestinal organs the lymphatic vessels conduct interstitial fluid back to the bloodstream, a subset of specialised lymphatics exists in the small intestinal villi, known as **lacteals** (Fig. 14.8), which are fundamental to efficient absorption and transport of absorbed lipids, a function performed by small intestine epithelial cells, enterocytes. Similar to skin lymphatics, the lymphatic vessels of the small intestine are arranged

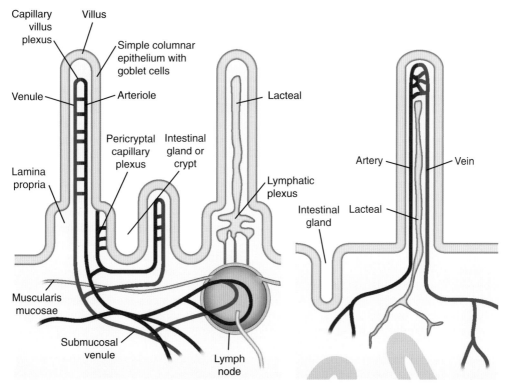

FIGURE 14.8 **Lacteals of the small intestine.** The wall of the small intestine comprises folds (plicae) of mucosa, which are covered with villi. Each villus contains lacteals, which assist with the absorption of food. (*Source:* Redrawn from Kierszenbaum A. Histology and cell biology: an introduction to pathology. Philadelphia: Mosby; 2002.)

in superficial and deep plexuses that carry lymph to the mesentery.[6] In the large intestine there are no lacteals and lymphatic vessels there are more involved in innate immunity, tolerance and immune surveillance. Surgical disruption to colon lymphatics can cause colon oedema, which may resolve once new lymphatic vessels develop and become functional; alternatively, if the lymphatic system cannot repair its function, the oedema becomes permanent, thus impairing the function of this organ.[2] Interestingly, intestinal Peyer's patches lack afferent lymphatic vessels. Instead, Peyer's patches receive an antigen through antigen-presenting cells, such as dendritic cells, located in gut mucosa.[2] Mesenteric lymph nodes are also associated with the intestine and they receive antigens through afferent lymphatic vessels in the mesentery.

Urinary system

The lymphatics of the urinary system are instrumental in tissue fluid balance. However, little is understood how lymphatics function in this system. Ureteric lymphatic vessels start in submucosal, intramuscular and adventitial plexuses and tend to drain into either renal collecting lymphatics or lateral aortic lymph nodes. Urethral lymphatic vasculature is not well described. However, these vessels drain into internal iliac nodes or deep inguinal nodes.[6]

The distribution of lymphatics in the normal human kidney has been demonstrated around the intrarenal arteries/veins, in the interstitial tissue around the glomeruli and renal tubules. The uni-directional flow of lymph is proposed to start with the initial lymphatic capillaries found in the cortical interstitial tissue around the glomeruli and renal tubules.[32] More lymphatic vessels have been reported in cortex than medulla and may contain erythrocytes, which is an unusual observation as erythrocyte presence in lymphatics of other tissues, such as mesentery, is usually associated with micro-thrombi formation.[1,32]

Reproductive system

The female reproductive system consists of essential and accessory reproductive organs (Chapter 21). The essential reproductive organs are ovaries, and the accessory reproductive organs are the uterine tubes, uterus, vagina, vulva and mammary glands. It has been suggested that there are three drainage pathways shared by the ovaries, uterine tubes and upper part of the uterus. The first pathway involves drainage through the ovarian ligament towards the lymph nodes in the obturator fossa and the internal iliac artery. The second pathway drains lymph through the suspensory ligament towards the para-aortic

and para-caval lymph nodes. The third pathway drains the ovaries into the inguinal lymph nodes.[6] Vaginal lymphatic vessels link with those of the cervix. Lymphatic vessels of the lower uterine body and the cervix drain mostly into the external iliac nodes.[6] Uterine lymph vessels enlarge greatly during pregnancy.[33]

The organs of the male reproductive system are also divided into essential and accessory reproductive organs. The essential reproductive organs are the testes, and the accessory reproductive organs are the genital ducts (epididymis, vas deferens and ejaculatory duct), glands (seminal vesicles, prostate gland, bulbourethral glands) and supporting structures (scrotum, penis and spermatic cords). The testicular lymphatic system starts in the superficial plexus under the tunica vaginalis and drains into the deep plexus found in the testes and epididymis. Lymphatic vessels from the ducts drain into the external iliac nodes, whereas those from seminal vesicles drain into the internal iliac nodes. Prostate lymphatic vessels drain into the internal iliac and sacral nodes. Lymphatic vessels of the glans penis drain into the deep inguinal and external iliac nodes, whereas vessels from erectile tissue and the penile urethra drain into the internal iliac nodes.[6] For both male and female reproductive systems, the removal of local lymph nodes and damage to the lymphatic system through cancer-associated treatment can lead to the development of secondary lymphoedema.

AGE-RELATED CHANGES

Little is known about age-related changes of the lymphatic system. Animal studies suggest that the ageing process affects the capacity of the lymphatic system to transport lymph due to a reduction in lymphatic vessel contractility leading to increases in tissue oedema.[34] The issues with contractility may be associated with impaired lymphatic smooth muscle contractility and loss of skin elasticity, which can lead to changes in the structure and capacity of the initial lymphatic capillaries to uptake the interstitial fluid. There may be decreased capacity to transport pathogens to lymph nodes due to loss of capacity to regulate endothelial opening in the initial lymphatic capillaries and subsequent propulsion of the lymph to lymph nodes, meaning that in these cases there would be an increased capacity for pathogens to invade the surrounding tissue.[34] Overall, this would contribute to an impaired immune response.

CONCLUSION

The lymphatic system is integral to the maintenance of tissue fluid homeostasis through the collection of excess interstitial fluid and transport of that fluid (lymph) through the initial lymphatic capillaries, collecting lymphatic vessels and lymphatic trunks for emptying into the venous blood circulation. Lymphatic vessels exist in all vascularised body systems and their structure and function are heavily influenced by the organs they serve. This dynamic system is also essential to the capacity of immune cells to form appropriate immune responses, for tissue metabolic products to be cleared and for fats absorbed during the digestive process to be transported to the blood circulation. Injury to lymphatic vessels can lead to lymphangiogenesis. Age-associated changes in the lymphatic system are poorly understood but it has been suggested that increased lymphatic vessel permeability leads to tissue oedema and reduced capacity to transport the antigen or pathogen to the lymph node for the appropriate immune response, thus impairing homeostasis.

CASE STUDY 14.1

Anne, who is 25 years old, frequently flies overseas to attend research conferences. This year she has taken four overseas trips, with each flight being a minimum of eight hours in duration. The last flight she took was to Iceland. After these trips, she noticed that her shoes did not fit so well and her ankles were a little swollen, taking several days to return to normal and being a little worse each time. She has decided that the next time she goes overseas, she will do more exercise during the flight.

Q1. The lymphatic system is composed of:
   a. lymphatic vessels, lymph nodes, lymphoid organs and lymph.
   b. lymphatic vessels, lymph nodes, blood and lymph.
   c. arteries, veins, capillaries and lymph.
   d. thymus, spleen, lymph nodes and blood.

Q2. Lymph flow is:
   a. uni-directional from the collecting lymphatic capillaries towards the systemic venous circulation.
   b. uni-directional and it starts from the collecting lymphatic veins.
   c. characterised by direct drainage of the lymphatic capillaries into the arteries.
   d. bi-directional as it flows from the arteries to the veins.

Q3. The purpose of lymph flow through the lymph nodes is to:
   a. accumulate in lymph nodes.
   b. be returned to the initial site of the formation of lymph in the tissue periphery.
   c. be surveyed by the immune cells located in the lymph nodes for the presence of foreign antigens.
   d. collect foreign antigens and deliver them to the central nervous system.

Q4. What factors might have contributed to the development of swelling in Anne's feet?

Q5. List the factors that assist lymph to return from the extremities to the circulation. For each factor, comment why air travel would affect lymph flow.

CASE STUDY 14.2

Tom, a 45-year-old carpenter, has returned from a volunteer trip to Central America where he has spent the last six weeks building a school for local children. Towards the end of his stay in Central America, Tom noticed that his legs were quite swollen below the knees and were getting bigger. At the local clinic, the doctor explained that Tom might have filariasis, a parasitic disease that occurs when filarial larvae (classified as nematodes or roundworms) enter the lymphatic system and develop into adult worms. The doctor also explained that this can lead to obstruction of the infected vessel and tissue swelling.

Q1. The general structure of the initial lymphatic capillary includes:
   a. continuous endothelial cells connected with zipper-like cell junctions, intact basement membrane, uni-directional lymphatic valve and coverage by smooth muscle cell.
   b. discontinuous endothelial cell layer, discontinuous basement membrane, uni-directional lymphatic valve and lack of smooth muscle cell support.

Continued

CASE STUDY 14.2—cont'd

c. discontinuous endothelial cell layer containing specialised button-like cell junctions, discontinuous basement membrane and lack of smooth muscle cell support.

d. continuous endothelial cell layer, continuous basement membrane and lack of smooth muscle cell support.

Q2. The general structure of the lymphatic collecting vessels includes:

a. endothelial cells connected tightly with cell junctions, intact basement membrane, uni-directional lymphatic valve and coverage by smooth muscle cell.

b. discontinuous endothelial cell layer, discontinuous basement membrane, uni-directional lymphatic valve and lack of smooth muscle cell support.

c. discontinuous endothelial cell layer, intact basement membrane and uni-directional lymphatic valve.

d. continuous endothelial cell layer, continuous basement membrane and lack of smooth muscle cell support.

Q3. Lymphangitis vessels can effectively drain the tissue fluid and return it back to systemic circulation because:

a. the lymphatic capillary vessel structure contains specialised endothelial cell junctions that allow endothelial cells to expand and accommodate incoming tissue fluid.

b. there is a pressure gradient difference between tissue fluid and the lymphatic vessel, which permits the flow of fluid into the vessel lumen.

c. lymphatic fluid flow is uni-directional, with tissue fluid moving from the tissue periphery to the systemic blood circulation via the thoracic duct.

d. all the above.

Q4. What is the normal function of the lymphatic system?

Q5. Explain the presence of swelling in Tom's legs.

CASE STUDY 14.3

Tom and Jack are walking in the bush when Jack suddenly feels a sharp scratch on his ankle and realises on looking back that the stick he just trod on wasn't a stick but a brown snake, which arched up to bite his ankle. Jack shouts to warn Tom, who is behind him, but notes the snake has quickly shot off into the bush, thankfully disappearing for now. Jack tells Tom that he has been bitten by the snake and Tom administers first aid.

Q1. Which statement below best describes the relationship between the lymphatic system and the cardiovascular system?

a. The lymphatic system maintains tissue fluid balance, which impacts on blood volume and blood pressure maintenance.

b. The lymphatic system helps formation of the heartbeat.

c. The lymphatic system controls the opening and closing of the heart valves.

d. The lymphatic duct drains into the aorta.

Q2. What is the area between two consecutive lymphatic valves called?

a. The left bronchomediastinal trunk

b. A lymphangion

c. The right jugular trunk

d. The right subclavian trunk

Q3. Lymphangitis of the skin is evident as:

a. enlarged lymph nodes.

b. tissue fibrosis.

c. red linear streaks that extend from the site of infection to the regional lymph nodes.

d. bruise.

Q4. Assuming the fangs of the snake have grazed or punctured the skin, what is the most likely pathway for the venom to reach the cardiovascular system, where it will cause the most danger to Jack?

Q5. Which factor that assists the movement of lymph is the most controllable/preventable, thus potentially protecting Jack's cardiovascular system from the venom?

CASE STUDY 14.4

A group of geology researchers were given information that a meteorite had disintegrated in an area of the Snowy Mountains. Armed with a geological map and an estimate of where the meteorite fragments might have fallen, the team set out to retrieve the fragments. The journey started early in the morning with the team splitting into several groups to cover a greater search area. During the expedition, the team soon established that the terrain was difficult due to tall grass and meandering creeks, and a radio warning was issued by the team leader for all members to be careful of where they walked. Just as the announcement was made, one of the team, Kaia, fell into a wombat hole. She called out to her team member, Andy, who walked over to help her out. As Kaia stepped onto her left leg, pain shot through it. Rolling her trousers up, she noticed a protrusion in the middle part of her shin bone and swelling but no broken skin. Concerned that Kaia had broken her leg, Andy called headquarters and asked for a car to be sent over. At the local hospital, it was confirmed that Kaia had fractured her tibia and that casting would be required.

Q1. Lymphangiogenesis is the process of:

a. developing new lymphatic vessels in response to injury.

b. synthesis of new bone tissue needed to support lymphatic vessel structure.

c. developing new blood vessels.

d. increase in lymphatic vessel diameter due to increased functional demand.

Q2. Lymph flow is facilitated by which of the following mechanisms?

a. Thoracic pressure changes during breathing

b. Contraction of lymphatic smooth muscle cells

c. Movement of skeletal muscles

d. All of the above

Q3. When the lymphatic structure of a limb is obstructed due to injury, the result is:

a. increased localised tissue swelling distal to the site of injury.

b. increased localised tissue swelling proximal to the site of injury.

c. decreased localised tissue swelling proximal to the site of injury.

d. decreased localised tissue swelling distal to the site of injury.

Q4. Suggest why there would be swelling associated with a bone fracture.

Q5. What response would you expect from the lymphatic system in this case?

REFERENCES

1. Lokmic Z. Utilizing lymphatic cell markers to visualize human lymphatic abnormalities. J Biophotonics 2017;11(8).

2. Alexander JS, Ganta VC, Jordan PA, et al. Gastrointestinal lymphatics in health and disease. Pathophysiol 2010;17(4): 315–35.

3. Louveau A, Smirnov I, Keyes TJ, et al. Structural and functional features of central nervous system lymphatic vessels. Nature 2015;523(7560):337–41.

4. Zoltzer H. Initial lymphatics: morphology and function of the endothelial cells. Lymphol 2003;36(1):7–25.

5. Baluk P, Fuxe J, Hashizume H, et al. Functionally specialized junctions between endothelial cells of lymphatic vessels. J Exp Med 2007;204(10):2349–62.

6. Gabella G. Cardiovascular system. In: Williams PL, Bannister LH, Berry MM, et al, editors. Gray's anatomy: the anatomical basis of medicine & surgery. London: Churchill Livingstone; 1995. p. 1605–26.

7. Alexander JS. Editorial: lymphatic vessel functions in health and disease. Pathophysiol 2010;17(4):225–7.

8. Havas E, Parviainen T, Vuorela J, et al. Lymph flow dynamics in exercising human skeletal muscle as detected by scintography. J Physiol 1997;504(1):233–9.

9. Petrova TV, Karpanen T, Norrmen C, et al. Defective valves and abnormal mural cell recruitment underlie lymphatic vascular failure in lymphedema distichiasis. Nat Med 2004;10(9):974–81.

10. Patton KT, Thibodeau GA. Lymphatic system. In: Anatomy and physiology, 9 ed. St Louis: Elsevier; 2016. p. 728–48.

11. Patton KT, Thibodeau GA. Circulation of blood. In: Anatomy and physiology. St Louis: Elsevier; 2016. p. 700–27.

12. Patton KT, Thibodeau GA. Blood vessels. In: Anatomy and physiology. ed 9. St. Louis: Elsevier; 2016. p. 665–98.

13. Mortimer PS, Rockson SG. New developments in clinical aspects of lymphatic disease. J Clin Invest 2014;124(3): 915–21.

14. Adamson RH, Lenz JF, Zhang X, et al. Oncotic pressures opposing filtration across non-fenestrated rat microvessels. J Physiol 2004;557(3):889–907.

15. Michel CC. Fluid exchange in the microcirculation. J Physiol 2004;557(3):701–2.

16. Levick JR. Revision of the Starling principle: new views of tissue fluid balance. J Physiol 2004;557(3):704.

17. Zöltzer H. Morphology and physiology of lymphatic endothelial cells. In: Shepro D, editor. Microvasculature research: biology and pathology. San Diego: Elsevier; 2006. p. 535–44.

18. Planas-Paz L, Lammert E. Mechanosensing in developing lymphatic vessels. Adv Anat Embryol Cell Biol 2014;214: 23–40.

19. Alitalo K. The lymphatic vasculature in disease. Nat Med 2011;17(11):1371–80.

20. Australasian Lymphology Association. Lymphoedema management. Available from: www.lymphoedema.org.au/about -lymphoedema/lymphoedema-management.

21. Xu H, Edwards J, Banerji S, et al. Distribution of lymphatic vessels in normal and arthritic human synovial tissues. Ann Rheum Dis 2003;62(12):1227–9.

22. Iliff JJ, Wang M, Liao Y, et al. A paravascular pathway facilitates CSF flow through the brain parenchyma and the clearance of interstitial solutes, including amyloid beta. Sci Transl Med 2012;4(147):147ra111.

23. Kiviniemi V, Wang X, Korhonen V, et al. Ultra-fast magnetic resonance encephalography of physiological brain activity: glymphatic pulsation mechanisms? J Cereb Blood Flow Metab 2016;36(6):1033–45.

24. Aspelund A, Antila S, Proulx ST, et al. A dural lymphatic vascular system that drains brain interstitial fluid and macromolecules. J Exp Med 2015;212(7):991–9.

25. Aspelund A, Tammela T, Antila S, et al. The Schlemm's canal is a VEGF-C/VEGFR-3-responsive lymphatic-like vessel. J Clin Invest 2014;124(9):3975–86.

26. Mehlhorn U, Geissler HJ, Laine GA, et al. Myocardial fluid balance. Eur J Cardiothorac Surg 2001;20(6): 1220–30.

27. Huang LH, Lavine KJ, Randolph GJ. Cardiac lymphatic vessels, transport, and healing of the infarcted heart. JACC Basic Transl Sci 2017;2(4):477–83.

28. Ullal SR, Kluge TH, Gerbode F. Functional and pathologic changes in the heart following chronic cardiac lymphatic obstruction. Surgery 1972;71(3):328–34.

29. Lokmic Z, Lammermann T, Sixt M, et al. The extracellular matrix of the spleen as a potential organizer of immune cell compartments. Semin Immunol 2008;20(1):4–13.

30. Ellis H. Lungs: blood supply, lymphatic drainage and nerve supply. Anaesth Intensive Care Med 2008;9(11):462–3.

31. Jakus Z, Gleghorn JP, Enis DR, et al. Lymphatic function is required prenatally for lung inflation at birth. J Exp Med 2014;211(5):815–26.

32. Ishikawa Y, Akasaka Y, Kiguchi H, et al. The human renal lymphatics under normal and pathological conditions. Histopathol 2006;49(3):265–73.

33. Kleppe M, Kraima AC, Kruitwagen RF, et al. Understanding lymphatic drainage pathways of the ovaries to predict sites for sentinel nodes in ovarian cancer. Int J Gynecol Cancer 2015;25(8):1405–14.

34. Zolla V, Nizamutdinova IT, Scharf B, et al. Aging-related anatomical and biochemical changes in lymphatic collectors impair lymph transport, fluid homeostasis, and pathogen clearance. Aging Cell 2015;14(4):582–94.

CHAPTER 15

Immune system

AMANY ABDELKADER, PHD • MICHAEL SALVATORE BARBAGALLO, PHD

KEY POINTS/LEARNING OUTCOMES

1. Describe the various components that make up the innate and adaptive immune system.
2. Discuss how adaptive and innate immunity function to protect the body from pathogens.
3. Link how the immune system and its various components interact with the whole body in order to maintain systemic defence.
4. Understand the balance of a normal functioning immune system in maintaining homeostasis.

KEY DEFINITIONS

- **Adaptive immunity:** immunity that is acquired and highly specialised.
- **Antibody** (or immunoglobulin): a large Y-shaped protein that enables the immune system to neutralise pathogens and viruses.
- **Antigen:** a foreign molecule that induces an immune response.
- **Inflammation:** a physical condition of the body in response to infection (or injury) that involves generation of heat and swelling.
- **Innate immunity:** non-specific immune responses to attack invading pathogens.
- **Major histocompatibility complex (MHC):** a cell surface protein responsible for the immune system's ability to determine cells of 'self' and 'non-self'.
- **Memory cells:** lymphocyte cells that are able to trigger an immune response to particular antigens after a period of time from initial exposure.
- **Phagocytosis:** the process whereby cells engulf pathogens and cells marked for destruction.

ONLINE RESOURCES/SUGGESTED READINGS

Hendry C, Farley A, McLafferty E, Johnstone C. Function of the immune system. Nurs Stand 2013;27(19):35–42.

INTRODUCTION

The major role of the immune system is the recognition of infectious and cellular abnormalities from normal functioning cells. In this chapter we explore the immune system and its interactions within the body to maintain internal protection. While the immune system is mainly cellular based, it protects the body by two distinct mechanisms: the *innate* (non-specific or first line of defence) response, which includes physical barriers and other responses to rapidly protect; and the *adaptive* (specific) response, where immune cells target specific pathogens. Combined, the innate and adaptive immune responses provide a significant degree of protection from external pathogens and abnormalities. In this chapter we explore both of these mechanisms and the means by which they maintain protection and hence homeostasis of the whole body by integration with other systems.

STRUCTURE AND FUNCTION OF THE IMMUNE SYSTEM

The immune system plays a crucial role in being able to recognise cells that are not our own, have been altered

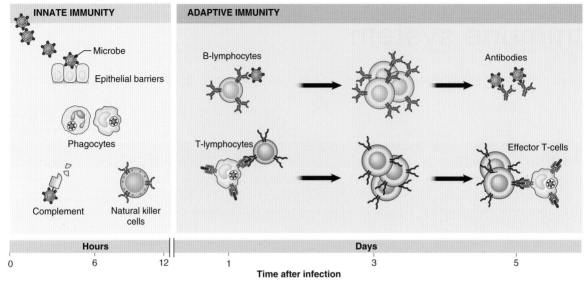

FIGURE 15.1 **The differences between innate and adaptive immunity.** (*Source:* Patton KT, Thibodeau GA, editors. Anatomy and physiology, 10 ed. London: Elsevier Health Sciences; 2017.)

or are no longer 'normal'. The cell surface protein, **major histocompatibility complex (MHC)**, is unique to individuals and allows recognition of the body's own cells from that of others.

The immune system has several layers of defence from invading pathogens, toxins and abnormal cells. In this chapter we consider the immune system's innate and adaptive responses (Fig. 15.1). The key to understanding these is that the system can respond in stages depending on the 'invader' (pathogen). In the first layer of defence, the innate immune response sees the invader removed or weakened. This response occurs in several stages. In the first stage bodily fluids destroy the pathogen or a physical barrier (skin or membrane) prevents access. Examples include saliva containing enzymes able to kill some bacteria in food. The second stage includes the ability to recognise pathogens as not being a part of 'own self' or as being foreign. This process is dependent upon a recognition process that activates cells of the innate immune system to target and remove them. The second layer of defence is the adaptive immune response. Here, a specific pathogen is targeted via a specialised set of immune cells. The key difference is, unlike the innate response, immune cells multiply and become active and targeting is highly specific (hence the term adaptive). Table 15.1 summarises the key differences between innate and adaptive immune responses.

TABLE 15.1
Summary of innate and adaptive immunity

Characteristics	Innate immunity	Adaptive immunity
Specificity	Not specific	Specific
Speed	Rapid: immediate, up to several hours	Slower: several hours to several days
Memory	None	Yes
Does not react to self	Yes	Yes

Innate immunity: the non-specific immune response

Innate immunity is the first line of defence as well as the fastest means to respond to pathogens and potential infections. The response is the same for each exposure; hence it is also known as the non-specific response because it reacts the same regardless of the pathogen. In this section we focus on the mechanisms of the innate response, including physical and biochemical barriers of defence (skin and membrane linings), phagocytosis and the various cells of the innate system (see Fig. 15.2 for a summary), immune surveillance, the role of

Neutrophil

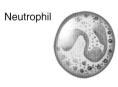

Basophil

Eosinophil

Lymphocyte

Monocyte

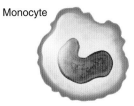

FIGURE 15.2 **White blood cells.** (*Source:* Patton KT, Thibodeau GA, editors. Anatomy and physiology, 10 ed. London: Elsevier Health Sciences; 2017.)

TABLE 15.2	
Physical and biochemical barriers of the innate immune system	
Location	**Barrier defence mechanism**
Skin	Keratinised cells of the skin ensure that it is too tough for pathogens to gain entry to the body
Respiratory tract Bronchi	Ciliated cells push particles that are inhaled up the tract; mucus produced assists in trapping pathogens for phagocytosis
Stomach Small intestine Gastrointestinal tract	Hydrochloric acid kills pathogens Peyer's patches keep microbes controlled Inhabiting bacteria (normal flora) of the gut stimulate gut mucosa to produce antibodies to pathogens
Urinary tract	High acidity of urine assists in keeping pathogens out

TABLE 15.3	
Phagocytic cells throughout the body	
Location	**Phagocyte**
Bloodstream	Circulating phagocytes
Bone	Osteoclasts
Central nervous system	Microglia
Connective tissues	Histiocytes
Epidermis	Langerhans cells
Liver	Kupffer cells
Lung	Alveolar macrophages
Lymph nodes	Lymphoid macrophages
Serous fluids	Pleural macrophages
Spleen	Splenic macrophages

interferon and the complement system, and the process of inflammation.

Physical and biochemical barriers

Physical barriers play a pivotal role in preventing or minimising entry of pathogens into the body. There are many variations as to how the body naturally does this—for example, the skin is thick enough to prevent pathogen entry, and sweat glands secrete chemicals that naturally inhibit some bacteria. The respiratory system is lined with goblet cells that create a thick mucus to trap pathogens. These physical and biochemical barriers to infection are summarised in Table 15.2.

Phagocytosis

A **phagocyte** is a white blood cell that is able to engulf and destroy pathogens through the process of **phagocytosis**. During this process, the phagocytic cell detects a pathogen and small 'detectors' or receptors on the

surface signal it to engulf the entire pathogen. Once the phagocyte has engulfed the pathogen, a host of killing mechanisms can be used. There are many types of phagocytic cells with different names depending on their identification and location in the body; some of these are outlined in Table 15.3. **Macrophages** (a type of phagocytic cell) have the added ability to function as antigen-presenting cells, by displaying small parts of the digested proteins (peptides) from the pathogen on the surface; we will look at the importance of this in triggering an adaptive immune response in the coming sections.

Some cells of the innate immune response can be grouped under the classification of **granulocytes**. These cells contain granules or 'sacs' of cytotoxic chemicals that assist in the destruction of pathogens. These cells include **mast cells**, **basophils** and **eosinophils**. Mast cells are vital for attacking pathogens that are too large for phagocytes to engulf. They secrete enzymes onto the surface of the pathogenic cell to degrade it. Eosinophils and basophils both play a role in the allergic response and inflammation. Eosinophils contain cytotoxic contents and basophils contain large amounts of histamine to trigger an inflammatory response.

Immune surveillance

Natural killer (NK) cells target cells infected by viruses (or that are cancerous) for destruction. They are known as surveillance cells as they monitor and target cells that have become abnormal. In order to do this they rely upon recognition of the MHC cell surface molecule (class I), which during viral infection or cancer is altered. Once they recognise these cells they release perforin to destroy the cells (Fig. 15.3). Perforin is a protein that sticks to the surface of the target cell and induces the process of automated cell death, otherwise known as **apoptosis**. Importantly, not all viruses and cancers can be detected by NK cells, particularly if they do not produce surface molecule alterations or if they are somehow masked to avoid detection.

Interferon

Cells have the ability to communicate with each other by releasing chemicals called cytokines. An important example in the immune system is **interferon**—a small protein released by cells infected by viruses (or by the phagocytic cells that have engulfed them). Interferon binds to receptors on normal healthy cells to activate production of antiviral proteins to prevent viral replication. Interferon further activates macrophages and NK cells to assist. There are three different forms of interferon:

1. interferon alpha, involved in the activation of NK cells
2. interferon beta, involved in slowing the rate of inflammation
3. interferon gamma, involved in the activation of macrophages.

The complement system

The **complement system** is another protein-based innate immune response. This form of protection relies on complement proteins released via a number of different pathways. All variations of the complement pathway require activation via surface receptors on the pathogen. This activation results in a series of chain reactions that eventuate in complement proteins forming membrane attack complexes that result in cell lysis of the pathogenic cell, enhanced phagocytosis or the release of histamine (mast cells and basophils) to increase inflammation.

Inflammation and fever

Inflammation is the body's response to tissue damage and includes a defined response in order to assist in counteracting the damage. The triggers are many, including high-impact or tissue abrasions and cuts, irritation, contact with chemicals, pathogens and environmental changes such as hot or cold temperatures. The key feature is the damage or death of cells, with the contents of the cells being released. This changes the chemical balance of the interstitial fluid and activates mast cells to release histamine, heparin and prostaglandins (among others). These have several downstream effects in the

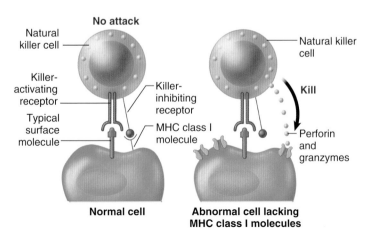

FIGURE 15.3 **Natural killer cells.** (*Source:* Patton KT, Thibodeau GA, editors. Anatomy and physiology, 10 ed. London: Elsevier Health Sciences; 2017.)

inflammatory response. There are two simultaneous phases that occur:

1. Vascular phase: redness, swelling and pain. Histamine makes capillaries more permeable, thus blood flow is increased (redness). Local sensory neurons are stimulated, resulting in pain.
2. Cellular phase: activation of phagocytes. This further triggers release of cytokines.

Further to the inflammatory response, a fever (body temperature greater than 37.2°C) is a whole-body response and can be triggered by pyrogens. Pyrogens are small proteins that are produced by many pathogens and released into the bloodstream. They induce production of prostaglandins, which in turn act upon the temperature-regulating portion of the hypothalamus and change the body set-temperature thermostat. Pyrogens are not only produced by many pathogens, but also released from healthy cells that have been damaged. Fever can also play a beneficial role in inhibiting some pathogens by raising temperature, as can the cellular metabolism process, which can result in some immune defences occurring more quickly.

Adaptive immunity: the specific immune response

Unlike the innate immune response the adaptive response is highly specific. The adaptive response is reliant upon recognition of **antigens**, small chemical 'parts' or products of pathogens. **Antibodies** (or immunoglobulins) are glycoproteins produced by lymphocytes that recognise antigens, binding with them to aid in their inactivation. This portion of the immune system relies heavily on the bone marrow and thymus, where two types of cells (B- and T-cells) are formed. These cells have several forms:

1. B-lymphocytes (B-cells) are formed in the bone marrow and can mature into:
   - plasma cells that are used to form antibodies to react with antigens
   - memory cells that express antibodies on the cell surface and live long lives to assist in antigen recognition and production of antibodies.
2. T-lymphocytes (T-cells) are formed in the bone marrow but mature in the thymus into:
   - helper T-cells that enhance the efficiency of other immune cells (B-cells)
   - cytotoxic T-cells that kill infected cells via the process of cell-mediated immunity
   - regulatory T-cells that assist in control of other lymphocytes
   - memory T-cells that assist in rapid activation upon repeat exposure to pathogens.

There are two different types of adaptive immune response: cell-mediated and antibody-mediated (humoral). Fig. 15.4 summarises these different responses. The overall importance and benefits of the adaptive immune response include its high specificity (to antigens), versatility to combat and adapt to the array of antigens it will be exposed to, and its memory to reactivate in instances of re-exposure.

Cell-mediated immunity

Cell-mediated immunity relies on antigens being presented to T-cells, which can occur by two distinct mechanisms:

1. MHC presentation, whereby viruses integrate into the cell, affect the structure of the MHC and produce 'tagged' MHC structures for T-cells to recognise as 'non-self' and target for destruction.
2. Cluster of differentiation (CD) markers, whereby a large group of different proteins present on the T-cell surface assist in antigen recognition.

Once a T-cell has recognised an antigen, it needs to activate a response, which it does by dividing and producing clones to assist with inactivation of the pathogen. Typically this is completed by a cytotoxic T-cell, which secretes toxins (perforin or lymphotoxin) or cytokines (helper T-cells) that instruct the target cell to die. Fig. 15.5 provides a schematic of how T-cells carry out the process of cell-mediated protection.

Antibody-mediated immunity

Antibody-mediated immunity involves B-cells detecting antigens and responding by producing antibodies specific to the target antigen. This is like a 'lock and key' with each antibody specific to its antigen. Once this recognition occurs, the activated B-cell triggers cell division, whereby two cells form either plasma cells, used to mass produce antibodies, or memory B-cells, reserved for re-exposure with the same antigen (Fig. 15.6).

It is important that we consider the importance of antibody production. As already mentioned, antibodies are specific to the antigen that is presented. Once the antibody and antigen form a complex, it can be attacked by **neutralisation** (turning off the active portion of the pathogen) or **agglutination** (whereby the clumping of large numbers of antigens and antibodies stimulates the complement system, activation of phagocytes and the inflammatory response).

Various classes of antibodies or immunoglobulins (Ig) have roles in the immune response:

- IgG: the largest class of antibodies responsible for viral, bacterial and toxin protection; can be passed from mother to child across the placenta.

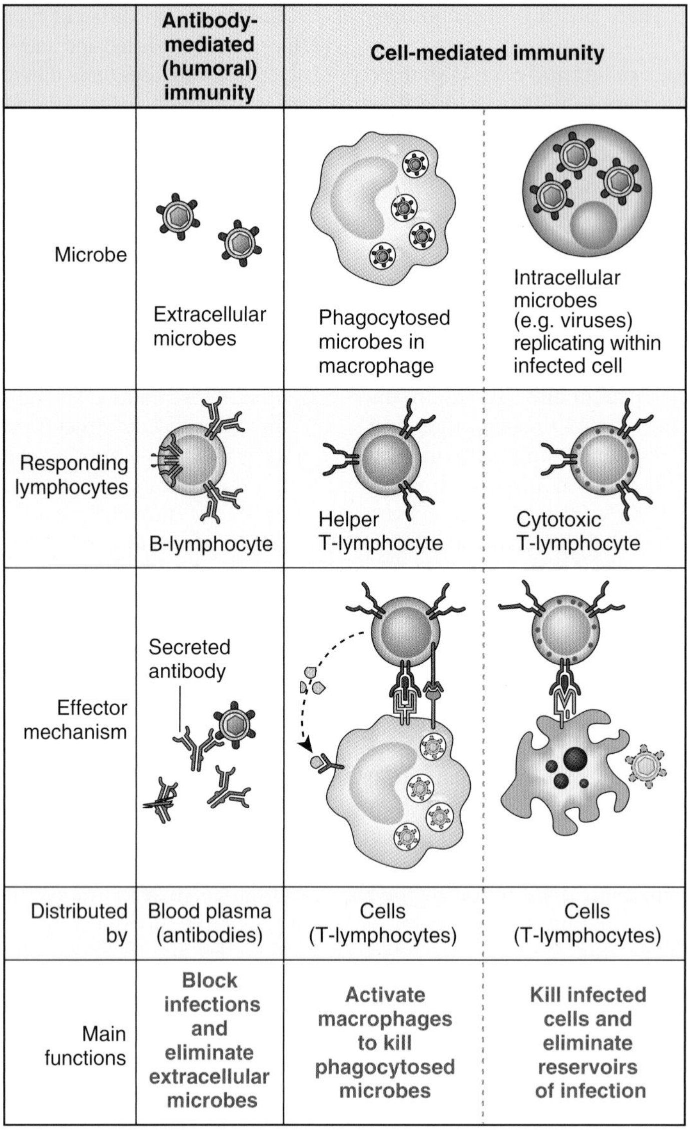

	Antibody-mediated (humoral) immunity	Cell-mediated immunity	
Microbe	Extracellular microbes	Phagocytosed microbes in macrophage	Intracellular microbes (e.g. viruses) replicating within infected cell
Responding lymphocytes	B-lymphocyte	Helper T-lymphocyte	Cytotoxic T-lymphocyte
Effector mechanism	Secreted antibody		
Distributed by	Blood plasma (antibodies)	Cells (T-lymphocytes)	Cells (T-lymphocytes)
Main functions	**Block infections and eliminate extracellular microbes**	**Activate macrophages to kill phagocytosed microbes**	**Kill infected cells and eliminate reservoirs of infection**

FIGURE 15.4 **Cell-mediated and antibody-mediated responses of the adaptive immune system.** (*Source:* Patton KT, Thibodeau GA, editors. Anatomy and physiology, 10 ed. London: Elsevier Health Sciences; 2017.)

- IgE: important in allergic responses; responds to basophils and mast cells and activates release of histamine and inflammation-inducing chemicals.
- IgD: antigen receptor on B-cells.
- IgM: first class of antibody secreted after antigen exposure; responsible for blood type.
- IgA: can be either circulatory in the blood or secretory (mucus, breast milk, saliva, tears, semen) and attack pathogens before internal entry.

Immunocompetence and maintenance of normal immune function

Immunocompetence or the development of immunity or resistance to infection by a pathogen occurs via the innate or adaptive response. However, this process can be considered as either active (that is, developed by the body in response to antigens) or passive (when antibodies are delivered to the body, such as from mother to child).

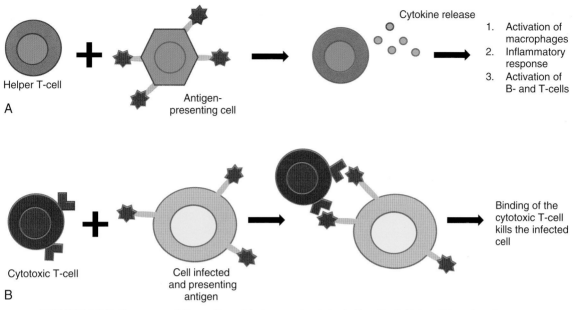

FIGURE 15.5 **Summary of the action of helper and cytotoxic T-cells. A** Helper T-lymphocyte. **B** Cytotoxic T-lymphocyte.

As outlined in Table 15.4 active and passive immunity can occur naturally or artificially. When a child is born they receive immunity passively from the mother and actively via exposure and vaccination. As the body ages and is exposed to antigens, further immunity develops. The balance of homeostasis and the functioning of the normal immune system can be tipped by three different means:

- **Hypersensitivity** can occur when there is a delay in reaction to exposure to antigens.
- **Autoimmunity** can occur when antibodies are produced and act against antigens of the 'self', leading to tissue damage.

- **Immunodeficiency** can occur when immunity is impaired, leading to a heightened risk of attack as there is less protection in place.

INTEGRATION OF THE IMMUNE SYSTEM WITH OTHER BODY SYSTEMS

The survival of any organism depends on the development of 'barriers' to prevent pathogens from gaining access. The immune system plays a crucial role in maintaining and restoring homeostasis.[1] In order to do this, there are many lines of defence within the

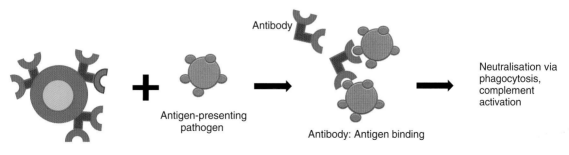

FIGURE 15.6 **Action of B-cells in antibody-mediated immunity.**

TABLE 15.4
Development of immune system

Type	Example
NATURAL IMMUNITY	
Active (exposure)	A child develops chickenpox (varicella) and acquires immunity to any subsequent infections
Passive (exposure)	An infant receives protection via breastfeeding from the mother's milk
ARTIFICIAL IMMUNITY	
Active (exposure)	Injection of the causative agent, such as vaccination against polio, confers immunity
Passive (exposure)	Injection of protective material (antibodies)

body requiring integration with other body systems (Table 15.5).

Integumentary system

As mentioned above, one of the first lines of defence is the existence of a physical barrier to prevent entry of pathogens. The skin not only senses and responds to stimuli from the external environment but also provides physical barrier protection. All layers of the skin are densely populated with nerve fibres and communicate with different cells. Nerve endings closely interact with the epidermis and dendritic cells within the epidermis and macrophages in the dermal layer of the skin resist infection. In response to a foreign body, mast cells trigger inflammation and mobilise cells of the lymphatic system in a process that is highly complex and not yet fully understood.[2]

Skeletal system

It is now well known that bone remodelling is continuously carried out to maintain bone function and homeostasis. The skeletal system is no longer considered a metabolically inert organ, but in fact is critical in that bone provides the microenvironment required for the development of immune cells, which are derived from haematopoietic cells. Osteoclasts, which can differentiate into macrophages or dendritic cells, originate from haematopoietic cells and are important in the repair of bone following injury. Conditions such as rheumatoid arthritis, where destruction of articular cartilage and bone are evident, appear to be mediated by inflammatory processes and driven by infiltration and activation of T-lymphocytes.[3]

Muscular system

The muscular system provides a protective role for superficial lymph nodes and the lymphatic vessels. Apart from providing this physical protection, the muscular system aids in propelling lymph along lymphatic vessels. Skeletal muscle accounts for approximately 40% of body mass and is susceptible to injuries in daily life. The process of muscle regeneration is divided into several stages in which acute inflammation and immune cells are critical. Following injury, damaged membranes of muscle fibres release cellular contents and chemotactic factors into the extracellular space. This leads to infiltration of immune cells, such as mast cells and neutrophils.[4] These cells help to clear damaged myofibrils and can also secrete various cytokines, recruiting more immune cells to the site. The lymphatic system plays a major role in circulating the cells required.

Respiratory system

The respiratory system is constantly exposed to potentially dangerous environmental factors. To protect the respiratory system from these pathogens, several lines of defence exist, and as with response to injury in other locations, macrophages play a role in healing injured lung tissue. Alveolar macrophages protect the epithelial surface and engulf foreign particles. The respiratory mucosa lines the conducting portion of the respiratory system and acts as a filtration system. The mucosa and cilia in some portions of the respiratory system prevent entry of harmful pathogens.[5]

Gastrointestinal system

The digestive tract possesses a mucosal lining able to secrete acids and enzymes. Within the stomach wall, gastric glands made up of two types of cells (parietal cells and chief cells) secrete gastric juice. Parietal cells can also indirectly secrete hydrochloric acid, by increasing the concentration of H^+ and Cl^-. The hydrochloric acid produced can kill most microorganisms ingested, denaturing proteins and inactivating most enzymes.

The human microbiome is made up of microbes and their genes that live on and within the body. In the large

TABLE 15.5
Integration of the immune system with other body systems

Body system	Means of integration
Cardiovascular system	• Endothelium initial site of interaction • Circulating pro-inflammatory cytokines may lead to increases in nitric oxide in conditions such as septic shock
Digestive system	• Mucosal lining secretes acids and enzymes that kill microorganisms ingested and denatures proteins • Human microbiome is crucial to the development of our immune system
Endocrine system	• Thymus produces thymosins required for the development of T-lymphocytes • Thymosins, important in coordinating and regulating the immune response, are circulated by the lymphatic system • Release of glucocorticoids which are anti-inflammatory and inhibit the activity of white blood cells and other immune system components
Integumentary system	• Provides a physical barrier • Macrophages in dermal layer of the skin resist infection and present antigens • Mast cells trigger inflammation and mobilise cells of the lymphatic system • Lymphatic system provides IgA antibodies secreted onto integumentary surfaces
Lymphatic system	• Provides adaptive defences • Responsible for production, maintenance and distribution of lymphocytes
Muscular system	• Protects superficial lymph nodes and lymphatic vessels • Aids in propelling lymph along the lymphatic vessels • Lymphatic system circulates immune cells required to combat muscular injuries and regenerate damaged cells
Nervous system	• Noradrenaline (norepinephrine) released to lymphoid organs, which can affect lymphocytic traffic, circulation and proliferation • Can also affect cytokine production and activity of lymphoid cells • Microglia, local macrophages, are highly phagocytic antigen-presenting cells
Reproductive system	• During pregnancy, immunoglobulins that recognise antigens the mother has been exposed to (primarily IgG) are transferred from the mother to the fetus via the placenta • Following delivery, IgA is transferred from the mother to the baby in breast milk
Respiratory system	• Alveolar macrophages patrol the epithelial surface and engulf foreign particles • Fibroblasts and macrophages facilitate restoration of the epithelial barrier following injury • Mucosa and the presence of cilia provide a physical defence against harmful pathogens
Skeletal system	• Provides microenvironment for immune cell development • Osteoclasts can differentiate into macrophages or dendritic cells and are important in bone repair
Urinary system	• Lined with epithelial cells and resident immune cells that provide protection • Acidic nature of urine contributes to the innate defence system

intestine, gut bacteria break down nutrients that are not absorbed elsewhere and produce vitamins. The existence of this microbiome contributes to the development of the immune system.

Urinary system

The urinary system is constantly exposed to microorganisms that inhabit the gastrointestinal tract. However, the urinary system is protected by various defences. For example, the urinary system is lined by epithelial cells and immune cells that provide protection against infection.[6] The majority of urinary tract infections arise from bacteria that originate in the gut. Typically, the urinary tract resists infection due to the resident cells which have a unique antimicrobial property. The acidic nature of urine also provides innate (non-specific) defence against infections. However, once bacteria are able to evade the barriers, infections occur.

Reproductive system

The immune system plays a crucial role in reproduction not only before but also during pregnancy. During ovulation, a number of inflammatory mediators migrate to the ovulation site, including granulocytes, macrophages and T-lymphocytes, and are activated locally. The maternal immune response is thought to protect the mother from over-invasion of trophoblasts, allowing acceptance of the fetal-placental unit at the same time. The mucosal surfaces of the female reproductive tract are lined with a thin layer of fluid that contains an array of antimicrobials—these provide the first line of defence against pathogens.[7–12] Both the female and the male reproductive tracts are protected by innate and adaptive immune responses.

During pregnancy, immunoglobulins are transferred from mother to fetus. These immunoglobulins recognise antigens the mother has been exposed to. IgG is the main form transferred across the placental barrier. Following delivery, IgA is transferred to the baby via breast milk.

Cardiovascular system

Within the cardiovascular system, the endothelium is an essential selective barrier that regulates movement of water, solutes, gases and cellular components of blood.[13] The vascular endothelium plays an active role in the inflammatory response seen in conditions such as septic shock. Endothelial cells are normally in a state of homeostasis, with a range of inflammatory mediators and innate immune and coagulation systems orchestrating the host response to septic shock.[13–15] Disturbances in the endothelium can alter homeostatic balance and open the door to infection. The endothelium is also the initial site of interaction with immune cells that enter tissues in response to damage and acts to facilitate the actions of the innate and adaptive immune systems.[16]

Elevated levels of circulating pro-inflammatory cytokines are observed in septic shock. There is evidence demonstrating that cytokines, such as interleukin-6 (IL-6) and tumour necrosis factor-alpha (TNF-α), involved in septic shock lead to an increase in nitric oxide (NO). This suggests that cytokines produce their cardio-depressant effects, seen in septic shock, via a NO dependent mechanism,[17,18] leading to a reduction in cardiac output, increasing vasodilation and reducing blood pressure.

Endocrine system

The endocrine system is an essential 'partner' to the immune system in that the thymus produces a number of hormones (thymosins) involved in the development and maintenance of T-lymphocytes. Thymosins are responsible for coordinating and regulating the immune response within the body. The lymphatic system is involved in circulating thymosins throughout the body to areas of need.

The adrenal gland releases glucocorticoids (steroid hormones) from the cortex that are important in glucose synthesis and the formation of glycogen. Glucocorticoids also have anti-inflammatory properties and inhibit the activity of white blood cells and other components of the immune system. Glucocorticoids slow the migration of phagocytic cells to injury sites, and mast cells are less likely to release histamine and other chemicals that are pro-inflammatory.

Nervous system

During an immune response the brain and the immune system 'communicate' to maintain homeostasis. Lymphoid organs, upon stimulation, release noradrenaline (norepinephrine) from sympathetic nerve terminals. Immune cells express receptors specific for noradrenaline (norepinephrine) and can affect lymphocyte traffic, circulation and proliferation. Receptor stimulation can also affect production of cytokines and the activity of lymphoid cells. The main aim of activation of the sympathetic nervous system during an immune response may be to localise the inflammatory response through induction of neutrophils.[19,20] However, activation of the sympathetic nervous system during an immune response suppresses T-helper cells, preventing the effects of pro-inflammatory cytokines.

The nervous system also contains microglia, which are the macrophages of the central nervous system. Microglia are highly phagocytic, antigen-presenting cells that are important during development and stimulate adaptive defences.

Lymphatic system

The lymphatic system is responsible for providing adaptive defences against infection for all systems throughout the body. This system is even more widespread than first thought, with recent evidence of large areas of fluid-filled spaces in between tissues, the interstitium.[21,22] This suggests that immunological interactions occur within this space.

Without the lymphatic system, which is responsible for the production, maintenance and distribution of lymphocytes, the body would not be capable of returning fluid or solutes from the periphery to the blood. The lymphatic system also plays a crucial role in distributing hormones and nutrients and removing waste products from tissues to the circulation.

AGE-RELATED CHANGES

As we age, our immune system ages and starts to lose its capacity to provide protection against infections and optimal surveillance for cancer cells. Thus, older people are more susceptible to infections, such as respiratory infections, and more likely to be diagnosed with cancers.[23] Older people are also more likely to have an impaired response to a vaccine and to develop an inflammatory disease such as osteoarthritis. All this contrasts with the fetus, whose immune system is needed to tolerate the mother's alloantigens. Once a baby is born and encounters environmental antigens, the immune system has to learn to recognise each of these antigens and mount appropriate self-limiting immune responses. The immune system continues to evolve through childhood through active exposure to antigens (e.g. via vaccinations) or by picking up germs through exposure to infected individuals.

CONCLUSION

The immune system plays a pivotal role in recognising infectious and cellular abnormalities from normal functioning cells. The two mechanisms by which the immune system functions are the innate (non-specific) immune response, which includes physical barriers and other responses to rapidly protect the body, and the adaptive (specific) response, whereby immune cells target specific pathogens. What is evident is that no one system works alone in maintaining body homeostasis, but rather all body systems work in unison to maintain protection of the body.

CASE STUDY 15.1

While walking home, Alyson received a bite from a mosquito. She felt a sting, and there was redness where the mosquito had bitten her. She didn't think much more of the bite, and went to bed soon after returning home. During the night the bite became very itchy and sore, and she noticed a large red lump at the site.

Q1. What is the purpose of increased capillary permeability?
   a. Allow cells to travel to the area of damage
   b. Attract histamine to the area of damage
   c. Engulf any venom present
   d. Stop itchiness

Q2. Itchiness after a mosquito bite is caused by:
   a. increased capillary permeability.
   b. histamine release in the area.
   c. skin growing back.
   d. venom engulfed by phagocytes.

Q3. Skin is an important part of the innate immune system because:
   a. histamine is released from skin cells.
   b. it allows phagocytosis to occur.
   c. it is a barrier to foreign substances.
   d. most insects cannot penetrate skin.

Q4. What is the role of phagocytes in the innate immune response?

Q5. How does the vascular system enable the cells of the immune system to respond?

CASE STUDY 15.2

Bob's son was born via caesarean section two weeks ago. Bob's friend Paul says that Bob should be very careful that his son does not get infections because he 'missed out' on his mother's immunity when he was born via caesarean section.

Q1. What are the most predominant antibodies secreted in breast milk?
   a. IgG
   b. IgE
   c. IgD
   d. IgM
   e. IgA

Q2. Infants are not efficient at producing antibodies of their own until approximately 6 months of age, thus the _____ immune response of their own is not fully functioning at birth.
   a. Adaptive
   b. Innate

Continued

CASE STUDY 15.2—cont'd

Q3. If Bob's son was born 3 months premature:

    a. there would be no difference in his immune function.

    b. breast milk will not be produced by his mother.

    d. antibodies may not have been passed from mother to child via the placenta.

    d. there would be no exposure to intestinal flora from the mother.

Q4. What is Paul worried about in terms of Bob's son 'missing out' on his mother's immunity?

Q5. How is immunity passed from mother to child via breast milk?

CASE STUDY 15.3

Freddy had an influenza vaccination at his workplace. Later that day his housemate Kelly asked how he was feeling, to which Freddy responded that his arm was sore and he felt tired, like he was coming down with something. Kelly said he was probably reacting to the effect of the vaccine and that he should rest.

Q1. The vascular phase of inflammation includes redness, swelling and pain. It is due to:

    a. irritation from the healthcare workers' hands.

    b. release of histamine from damaged cells.

    c. antibodies being produced by the body.

    d. infection with the influenza virus.

Q2. Antigens trigger the production of antibodies to fight the reoccurrence of infection. Which cell type triggers the production of antibodies?

    a. Macrophages

    b. Natural killer (NK) cells

    c. Eosinophils

    d. B-cells

Q3. Fever is an important mechanism in the production of antibodies from a vaccine. What is its role?

    a. Destroy or kill the vaccine

    b. Speed the process of antibody production

    c. Slow the process of antibody production

    d. Prepare the body for the virus

    e. Protect the body from other pathogens

Q4. Which aspect of the immune system is involved in protecting Freddy from the influenza virus post vaccination?

Q5. Why does Freddy experience the symptoms he details to Kelly post vaccination?

CASE STUDY 15.4

Mary is 78 years old. Her appetite has declined in the last few years; she mostly eats dry toast at night and sometimes has a snack during the day. Mary struggles to complete some daily tasks but loves gardening. Two weeks ago she received a cut from a rose thorn that still has not healed. She now has a weeping wound on her forearm, and feels tired and run down.

Q1. As Mary ages she has a reduced immune system due to reduced lymphocytes in:

    a. lymphoid tissue.

    b. bone tissue.

    c. blood.

    d. thymus.

    e. All the above.

Q2. Cytokines are much higher in concentration in the elderly; their ability to enable cell-to-cell communication is:

    a. enhanced.

    b. diminished.

    c. not affected.

Q3. If Mary were to improve her diet this would:

    a. have no effect on her immune system.

    b. strengthen her immune system.

    c. improve her gut microbiome and improve the breakdown nutrients.

    d. both B and C.

Q4. Explain why Mary's immune system might have contributed to delayed wound healing.

Q5. How does Mary's reduced appetite affect her immune system?

REFERENCES

1. Sattler S. The role of the immune system beyond the fight against infection. Adv Exp Med Biol 2017;1003:3–14.
2. Choi HW, Abraham SN. Mast cell mediator responses and their suppression by pathogenic and commensal microorganisms. Mol Immunol 2015;63(1):74–9.
3. Grcevic D, Katavic V, Lukic IK, et al. Cellular and molecular interactions between immune system and bone. Croat Med J 2001;42(4):384–92.
4. Chazaud B, Sonnet C, Lafuste P, et al. Satellite cells attract monocytes and use macrophages as a support to escape apoptosis and enhance muscle growth. J Cell Biol 2003;163(5):1133–43.
5. Hsia BJ, Ledford JG, Potts-Kant EN, et al. Correction notice for TNF-R on mast cells regulate airway responses to *Mycoplasma pneumoniae*. J Allergy Clin Immunol 2016;137(1):336.
6. Abraham SN, Miao Y. The nature of immune responses to urinary tract infections. Nat Rev Immunol 2015;15(10):655–63.
7. Wira CR, Ghosh M, Smith JM, et al. Epithelial cell secretions from the human female reproductive tract inhibit sexually transmitted pathogens and *Candida albicans* but not *Lactobacillus*. Mucosal Immunol 2011;4(3):335–42.
8. Wira CR, Patel MV, Ghosh M, et al. Innate immunity in the human female reproductive tract: endocrine regulation of endogenous antimicrobial protection against HIV and other sexually transmitted infections. Am J Reprod Immunol 2011;65(3):196–211.
9. Wira CR, Veronese F. Mucosal immunity in the male and female reproductive tract and prevention of HIV transmission. Am J Reprod Immunol 2011;65(3):182–5.
10. Coleman KD, Ghosh M, Crist SG, et al. Modulation of hepatocyte growth factor secretion in human female reproductive tract stromal fibroblasts by poly (I:C) and estradiol. Am J Reprod Immunol 2012;67(1):44–53.
11. Fahey JV, Bodwell JE, Hickey DK, et al. New approaches to making the microenvironment of the female reproductive tract hostile to HIV. Am J Reprod Immunol 2011;65(3):334–43.
12. Hickey DK, Patel MV, Fahey JV, et al. Innate and adaptive immunity at mucosal surfaces of the female reproductive tract: stratification and integration of immune protection against the transmission of sexually transmitted infections. J Reprod Immunol 2011;88(2):185–94.
13. Opal SM, van der Poll T. Endothelial barrier dysfunction in septic shock. J Intern Med 2015;277(3):277–93.
14. Ehrman R, Wira C, Lomax A, et al. Etomidate use in severe sepsis and septic shock patients does not contribute to mortality. Intern Emerg Med 2011;6(3):253–7.
15. Kalil AC, Opal SM. Sepsis in the severely immunocompromised patient. Curr Infect Dis Rep 2015;17(6):487.
16. Khaddaj MR, Mathew JC, Kendrick DJ, et al. The vascular endothelium: a regulator of arterial tone and interface for the immune system. Crit Rev Clin Lab Sci 2017;54(7–8):458–70.
17. Kumar A, Haery C, Parrillo JE. Myocardial dysfunction in septic shock: part I. Clinical manifestation of cardiovascular dysfunction. J Cardiothorac Vasc Anesth 2001;15(3):364–76.
18. Kumar A, Krieger A, Symeoneides S, et al. Myocardial dysfunction in septic shock: part II. Role of cytokines and nitric oxide. J Cardiothorac Vasc Anesth 2001;15(4):485–511.
19. Elenkov IJ, Chrousos GP, Wilder RL. Neuroendocrine regulation of IL-12 and TNF-alpha/IL-10 balance: clinical implications. Ann N Y Acad Sci 2000;917:94–105.
20. Elenkov IJ, Wilder RL, Chrousos GP, et al. The sympathetic nerve: an integrative interface between two supersystems—the brain and the immune system. Pharmacol Rev 2000;52(4):595–638.
21. Benias PC, Wells RG, Sackey-Aboagye B, et al. Author correction: structure and distribution of an unrecognized interstitium in human tissues. Sci Rep 2018;8(1):7610.
22. Benias PC, Wells RG, Sackey-Aboagye B, et al. Structure and distribution of an unrecognized interstitium in human tissues. Sci Rep 2018;8(1):4947.
23. Weyand CM, Goronzy JJ. Ageing of the immune system: mechanisms and therapeutic targets. Ann Am Thorac Soc 2016;13(5):S422–8.

CHAPTER 16

Acute inflammation

ZERINA TOMKINS, BAPPSC (MED LAB SCI), BAPPSC (HONS), MNSC (NURS), PHD, GRAD CERT (UNIVERSITY EDUCATION)

KEY POINTS/LEARNING OUTCOMES

1. Define inflammation and classifications of inflammation.
2. Distinguish between different causes of inflammation.
3. Explain the vascular and cellular events of a typical acute inflammatory response.
4. Link the type of injury with the acute inflammatory response.
5. Discuss how the inflammation process occurs in different body systems.

KEY DEFINITIONS

- **Acute inflammation:** a coordinated response by vascularised tissue to neutralise an injury and return the injured tissue to homeostasis.
- **Phagocytosis:** the process of engulfing or ingesting foreign particles by specialised cells, collectively called phagocytes.
- **First line of defence:** the first barrier that an injurious agent encounters, such as skin epithelial cells, cilia in the lung epithelium, secretion of acid by the gastric mucosa and saliva secretion in the mouth.
- **Second line of defence:** nonspecific immune responses that are activated by the body to destroy an invading pathogen, such as the response by the innate immune system driven by neutrophils and macrophages using phagocytosis.
- **Third line of defence:** a well-defined immune response driven by the adaptive immune system through B-cells (humoral immunity) and T-cells (cell-mediated immunity) with resolution of inflammation as the ultimate outcome.

ONLINE RESOURCES/SUGGESTED READINGS

- **Acute inflammation: educational 3D animation** available at www.youtube.com/watch?v=1SvEdg94qUA
- **Pericarditis: overview** available at www.youtube.com/watch?v=lJrXD9bJII8
- **What is croup?** available at www.youtube.com/watch?v=gxvtY2hUzWw
- **Types and causes of meningitis and meningococcal disease** available at www.meningitis.com.au/meningitis/types-of-meningitis

---

INTRODUCTION

When a harmful or injurious stimulus causes damage to the body, a range of short-term defensive responses are activated, aimed at containing tissue damage, preventing further damage and ultimately repairing the affected tissue. Collectively, these defensive responses are termed **inflammation**.

The extent of the inflammatory response reflects the nature of the injury. If an injury is small, a small-scale response is initiated, such as that mediated by biochemical, mechanical and physical barriers that constitute the innate immune response. An example of this is a skin abrasion: damage to the uppermost part of the skin, the epidermis, results in temporary loss of skin structural integrity and changes in skin pH in the injured area, which facilitates the entry of bacterial pathogens into deeper skin layers. More substantial injuries, such as a deep arm wound where the skin and underlying muscle are both damaged, may evoke a more complex inflammatory response that interlaces innate and adaptive immunity and tissue repair mechanisms aimed at sealing the wound gap. Occasionally, the extent of an injury is so significant that a systemic (whole-body) response is required. This can be observed in trauma-related injuries that involve simultaneous damage to more than one body system. For example, following a motor-vehicle accident a person may present with a fractured bone, torn muscles, broken skin, a ruptured spleen and head concussion. Inflammation takes place simultaneously at all these sites, with chemical mediators of inflammation released into the bloodstream, thus activating a systemic response. The aim is still the same: to contain the extent of the injury and to activate the repair processes.

Each organ in the body has an ability to activate the inflammatory response upon injury, with the response being reflective of the tissue composition and function. Despite this, the overall mechanisms of activation, progression and suppression of inflammation are similar and a predictable series of events occurs. Under healthy conditions, inflammation is a homeostatic event aimed at returning the injured environment back to homeostasis.

STRUCTURE AND FUNCTION OF INFLAMMATION

Inflammation is the reaction of vascularised tissue to injurious stimuli. The aim of inflammation is to repair and heal the injured area. This complex reaction is initiated by the signals generated through chemicals released during damage to tissue cells and structures such as blood vessels, lymphatic vessels and neurons. These signals initiate processes that enable vascular (blood and lymphatic) and cellular components (leucocytes and plasma proteins) to interact in an orchestrated and self-limiting manner to eliminate the injurious stimuli (such as bacteria or virus) and remove dead tissue to restore full tissue function (provided the nature of injury allows for that) (Fig. 16.1). Although inflammation most often resolves on its own, occasionally the inflammatory process can cause injury if it is inappropriately triggered or poorly controlled, causing varying degrees of damage, and even death, to otherwise healthy tissue. Examples include an extreme inflammatory response during an allergic reaction that leads to anaphylactic shock, or a debilitating autoimmune disease such as rheumatoid arthritis. In some cases, where inflammation persists over a prolonged period without being resolved, chronic

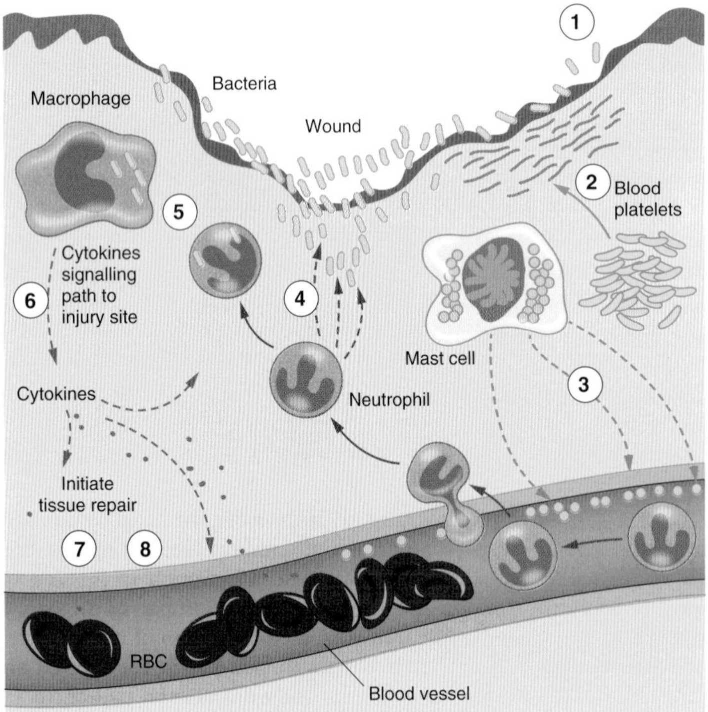

1. Bacteria and other pathogens enter the wound

2. Platelets arriving from blood release blood-clotting proteins at wound site

3. Mast cells secrete factors, such as histamine, that mediate vasodilation and vascular constriction. Increased delivery of blood, plasma and cells to injured area occurs

4. Neutrophils secrete factors that kill and degrade pathogens

5. Neutrophils and macrophages remove pathogens by phagocytosis

6. Macrophages secrete cytokines that attract immune system cells to the site of injury and activate cells involved in tissue repair

7. Inflammatory response continues until the foreign material is eliminated and the wound is repaired

8. Adaptive immune system is also activated during this process

FIGURE 16.1 **Acute inflammatory response.**

inflammation develops. Tissue injury associated with persistent low-grade production of pro-inflammatory molecules can lead to the development of chronic diseases such as diabetes, chronic kidney disease and stress-associated sleep disorders.[1]

Causes of inflammation

Damage to the body can occur **externally**, for example skin damage inflicted by scratching a hand, or **internally**, where a buildup of toxic cell metabolic products causes tissue damage. Factors that can cause injury and trigger inflammation include infectious agents, chemical and physical agents, immunological reactions, genetic abnormalities, nutritional imbalances, age-related changes and reduction in oxygen supply to cells (Fig. 16.2).

Infectious agents that may induce inflammation include bacteria and their toxins, viruses, fungi and their toxins, protozoa and prions. Note that inflammation does not necessarily mean that infection is present, but the presence of an infection will cause inflammation. **Chemical agents** that induce inflammation include tobacco, alcohol, poisons and reactive oxygen species (also known as oxygen free radicals) and substances such as cocaine, heroin and opioids. **Physical agents** include

noise, vibration, mechanical injury, radiation and extreme environmental temperature. For example, exposure to high temperatures or electricity may result in cellular protein denaturation and intracellular coagulation, a process where a cellular substance changes from a liquid to a semi-solid or solid state. Exposure to extremely low temperatures, **hypothermia**, leads to the formation of ice crystals inside cells, resulting in fragmentation of cell structure and changes in cell permeability that can lead to cell death. Similarly, **mechanical injury**, such as a knife cut, can lead to instant cell death at the wound site. Force-induced blunt trauma, for example where a cell membrane is ruptured, also results in cell death.

Immunological reactions that lead to inflammation include allergic reactions and a buildup of autoimmune cells resulting in autoimmune disease. Acute inflammation can also be triggered by **pro-inflammatory permeability mediators** made by cells such as vasoactive amines (histamine and serotonin), complement molecules (C3a and C5a, which circulate in the blood), bradykinin (also a major pain inducer), leukotrienes (produced by leucocytes), platelet-activating factor (produced by endothelial cells and leucocytes) and cytokines including interleukin-1 (IL-1) and tumour necrosis factor-alpha

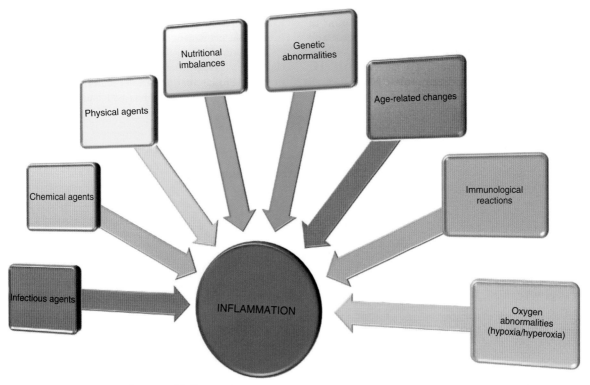

FIGURE 16.2 **Causes of inflammation.**

(TNF-α) produced by macrophages and other inflammatory cells.[2]

Genetic abnormalities resulting in inborn errors of metabolism or the presence of deformed cellular elements due to genetic mutations, such as deformed red blood cells in sickle cell anaemia and thalassaemia, also lead to inflammation. **Nutritional imbalances** are present globally but people in developed nations are disproportionately affected as they are particularly vulnerable to food insecurity, especially children. Examples of nutritional imbalances that affect the body's capacity to eliminate cell injury and inflammation include iron deficiency anaemia, iodine deficiency-induced hypothyroidism, fluoride deficiency-induced tooth decay, vitamin D deficiency-induced abnormal bone development and zinc deficiency-induced impaired healing and decreased immune defence capacity. Obesity is another example of nutrient imbalance; it is characterised by insulin resistance and altered glucose metabolism. Adipocytes from an obese individual produce pro-inflammatory molecules, such as TNF-α, IL-6 and the hormones leptin, adiponectin and resistin. As such, obesity is thought to be a pro-inflammatory condition as increased levels of these molecules are associated with increased adiposity and increased risk of developing metabolic diseases such as type 2 diabetes.[3]

Age-related changes lead to an accumulation of sub-lethal injuries so that in time, through wear and tear, tissue becomes damaged and leads to chronic injury. A simple example is deterioration of knee cartilage over time. Another more complex example is age-related cell senescence: in this case, cells stop proliferating and start to produce pro-inflammatory molecules, known as pro-inflammatory secretomes. Ageing is also associated with loss of cytokine balance between pro-inflammatory and anti-inflammatory modulators and decreasing control over immune responses.[4]

Absence of sufficient oxygen supply to the tissues is another example of injury that causes inflammation. **Hypoxia**, low oxygen levels in the blood, and **ischaemia**, low levels of oxygen in the tissues, arise either through damage to the lungs that obstructs the transport of atmospheric oxygen into the bloodstream or through obstruction of blood vessels that results in partial or complete loss of blood supply to the tissue. Similarly, too much oxygen (**hyperoxia** or **oxygen toxicity**) has serious impacts on the developing vasculature in pre-term and full-term neonates and can lead to blindness or acute respiratory distress syndrome.[5]

At any given time, more than one stimulus may be the cause of acute inflammation.

Types of inflammation

The human body encounters many physiological stresses that can lead to injury and deals with injurious stimuli as it is constantly adapting to changes in the internal (body) and external environment. These injuries can be reversible or irreversible. If an injury is **reversible**, the body has the capacity to repair the injured part. If an injury is **irreversible**, permanent damage and loss of function occur.

Based on the **duration** (time), inflammation can be classified as **acute inflammation** (less than six months) or **chronic inflammation** (greater than six months) (Fig. 16.3). Chronic inflammation is associated with ongoing

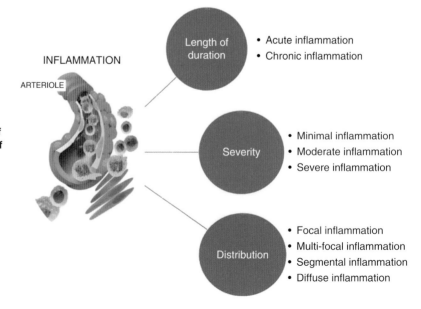

FIGURE 16.3 **Classification of inflammation based on length of duration, severity and distribution.**

INFLAMMATION

ARTERIOLE

Length of duration
- Acute inflammation
- Chronic inflammation

Severity
- Minimal inflammation
- Moderate inflammation
- Severe inflammation

Distribution
- Focal inflammation
- Multi-focal inflammation
- Segmental inflammation
- Diffuse inflammation

and greater tissue destruction, increased presence of lymphocytes and macrophages, persistent low-level proliferation of blood vessels, and ongoing deposition and remodelling of connective tissue. As mentioned earlier, changes induced by chronic inflammation increase the risk of chronic disease and contribute to age-related changes.

Inflammation can be further classified in terms of **severity** (how bad) and distribution (how widespread, pattern and changes in distribution over time) and **type of exudate** produced. The severity of inflammation can be classed as minimal, mild, moderate or severe. **Minimal inflammation** is characterised by little to no tissue destruction with a small degree of cellular exudate and is generally hardly visible, if at all. **Mild inflammation** and **moderate inflammation** are terms used interchangeably to describe a spectrum of tissue damage that is easily visible due to underlying tissue changes. **Severe inflammation** is characterised by considerable tissue damage and extensive vascular and cellular reactions that are obvious to an observer.

From a distribution perspective, inflammation may be **focal** (single location), **multi-focal** (more than one location), **locally extensive**, **segmental** or **diffuse**. **Locally extensive inflammation** is characterised by progression of focal inflammation to the surrounding tissue. **Segmental inflammation** refers primarily to intestinal lesions where inflammation is present lengthwise and interspersed among relatively normal interstitial tissue. **Diffuse inflammation** refers to inflammation present throughout an organ or system of organs.

Signs and symptoms of inflammation

For some systems, like the integumentary system, most signs and symptoms of inflammation are visible, but for others such as the cardiac and respiratory systems it is not possible to see the acute inflammation process so inflammation is identified through blood tests for markers of inflammation. In general, the symptoms of inflammation can be observed in the form of **five cardinal signs: heat, redness, swelling, pain and loss of function** (such as immobility) (Fig. 16.4). Signs of inflammation are due to underlying biological hallmark tissue responses that can be grouped as vascular cell responses, leucocyte/immune system responses or connective tissue cellular responses that form under the influence of cellular chemicals released at the time of injury. These chemicals are collectively known as **chemical mediators of inflammation**. The following section examines the role of these individual components.

Biological hallmarks of inflammation

Following acute tissue injury, cellular damage triggers the acute inflammatory response in the injured area.

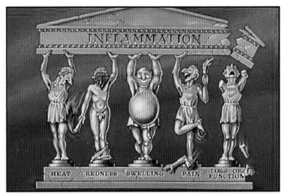

FIGURE 16.4 Five cardinal signs of inflammation.
(*Source:* Nature Reviews Immunology, 2, 787–795; © 2002 Macmillan Publishers Ltd.)

The response develops rapidly and, depending on the extent of the injury, may last hours or days with neutrophils and macrophages mediating the vascular and leucocyte responses. Although different organs have subtly different responses to injury (e.g. skin abrasion healing process versus a fractured bone), there are several fundamental common sequences of overlapping events that acute inflammatory reactions share. These events involve **vascular** and **cellular changes** (Fig. 16.5) that result in the following:

1. **dilation of small vessels** (microvasculature), such as capillaries, resulting in increased blood flow to the injured area
2. **increased permeability of the microvasculature**, which facilitates plasma protein and leucocyte movement into the injured tissue
3. **activation of the immune response** within the population of leucocytes that have emigrated from the microvasculature to the injured area, as well as leucocytes residing locally in the tissue.

This activation process is needed to eliminate the harmful agent through the innate and adaptive immune responses.

Vascular changes during inflammation. Injury is a sudden shock to the body. With respect to blood vessels, an injury either severs a vessel or causes an impact similar to bruising. If a vessel is not severed (Fig. 16.5) and blood flow is preserved within the vessel lumen, the blood vessels react to the injury by constricting the pre-capillary sphincter following release of **endothelin** from damaged endothelial cells lining the vessel lumen. Endothelin is a peptide that has both local and systemic effects.[6] This rapid and short-lived response is soon

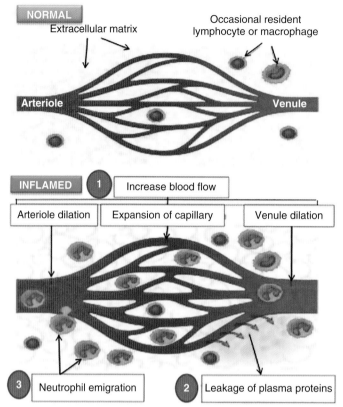

FIGURE 16.5 **Vascular changes in acute inflammation.** (*Source:* Kumar V, Abbas A, Aster JC. Robbins and Cotran pathologic basis of disease, 10 ed. St Louis: Elsevier; 2018.)

followed by relaxation of the same pre-capillary sphincter. Vasodilation follows once soluble factors are released by the injured endothelial cells, such as nitric oxide and damaged mast cells, for example histamine. Histamine acts on the vascular smooth muscle cells surrounding arterioles, capillaries and postcapillary venules to increase vessel diameter. Mast cells also synthesise **serotonin**, causing endothelial cell contraction, thus facilitating the movement of inflammatory cells across the endothelium.[2] The action of loosening cell junctions leads to vessel **hyperpermeability** and maximises the leakage of plasma proteins and migration of leucocytes and red blood cells from the blood vessel to the injured area.

Increased vessel diameter and fluid extravasation lead to slower blood flow. A secondary effect arising from the combination of increased vasodilation (increased vessel diameter), increased permeability and decreased fluid content in the vessel lumen is the slowing or stasis of blood flow. This increases blood viscosity due to the increased presence of erythrocytes and loss of laminar

flow in the capillaries, further slowing down leucocytes and thus enabling them to continue to adhere to vascular endothelial cells and migrate to injured tissue.

Stasis or **vascular congestion** is clinically evident as **erythema (redness)** and brings **warmth** to the affected area. Blood stasis induces changes on the endothelial cell surface that further enables the migration of leucocytes from the circulation into the injured area. As capillaries and postcapillary venules become hyperpermeable and allow extravasation (movement) of plasma proteins and leucocytes from blood into the injured area, local tissue oedema occurs and this becomes visible as tissue **swelling**. This important process in tissue repair delivers many proteins and nutrients such as glucose needed by the cells to perform their function during the inflammation process.

If the blood vessel is severed so that endothelial cell necrosis and detachment from the blood vessel wall occur, blood flows into the injured tissue and the clotting system will be activated to stop the bleeding.

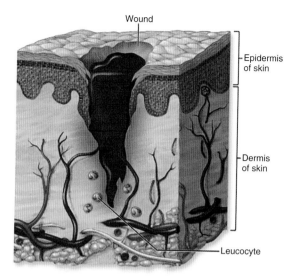

FIGURE 16.6 **Bleeding of severed blood vessels into the wound.** (*Source:* Prentice WE, Quillen, WS, Underwood, F. Therapeutic modalities in rehabilitation, 4 ed. McGraw-Hill.)

The damaged vascular endothelial cells will expose glycoproteins on their surface to capture platelets from the blood with the aim of forming a blood clot at the severed end and thus stopping the bleeding (Fig. 16.6). Leucocytes caught in the blood clot play a different role than when a vessel is not severed, simply because leucocytes are trapped in the clot and have limited potential to migrate in response to chemical mediators of inflammation.

Depending on the type of inflammation, sometimes blood vessels proliferate to cope with the requirements of healing. This process is called **angiogenesis** (Fig. 16.7). Lymphatic vessels also participate in inflammation and repair of the injured tissue. These vessels tend to increase their capacity to remove the excess fluid and help drain oedema. As cell debris, leucocytes and invading microbes enter lymphatic vessels, they carry these to lymph nodes where additional immune responses can be activated (to manage microbes) or to the central blood circulation (as a way of managing the removal of cell debris).[7] Lymphatic vessels also proliferate during inflammation and regress once they are no longer needed, as do excess angiogenic vessels.[8]

Leucocyte responses during inflammation. Leucocytes are comprised of neutrophils, monocytes, T- and B-cells, eosinophils and basophils; 40–60% of leucocytes are neutrophils. In injured tissue, leucocytes are required to facilitate elimination of injurious stimuli and cellular debris. The entire process can be summarised in three steps:

1. leucocyte **marginalisation**, where leucocytes slow down and roll on the endothelial cell lining of a postcapillary venule
2. leucocyte activation and **adhesion** to the activated endothelial cell lining
3. transmigration or **extravasation** of leucocytes across the endothelium in postcapillary venules, blood vessel basement membrane and vascular smooth muscle cells.

As blood flow stagnates in the lumen of the blood vessels in the injured area, the concentration of leucocytes

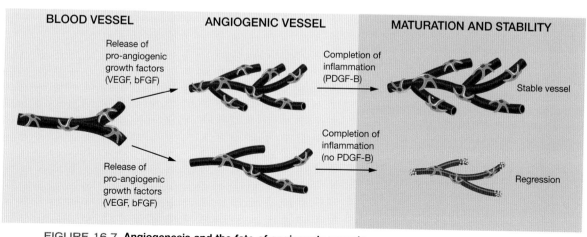

FIGURE 16.7 **Angiogenesis and the fate of angiogenic vessels.**

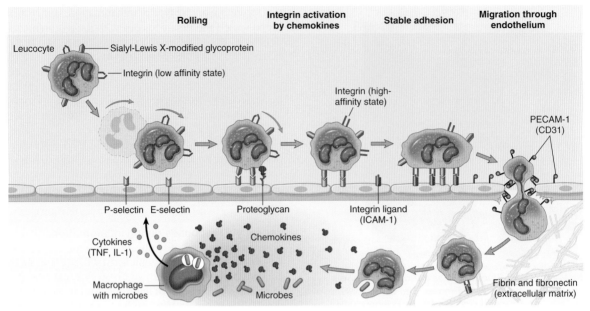

FIGURE 16.8 **Leucocyte migration through endothelial vessel.** (*Source:* Kumar V, Abbas A, Aster JC. Robbins and Cotran pathologic basis of disease, 9 ed. St Louis: Elsevier; 2015.)

increases at the site. The crowding results in leucocytes being pushed to the sides of the vessel wall, becoming **marginalised**. As leucocyte marginalisation (Fig. 16.8) takes place, leucocytes (mainly neutrophils) extravasate and accrue at the site of injury. **Extravasation** is a process of movement of leucocytes from the vessel lumen at the postcapillary venule level to extravascular tissue. Chemotactic agents released by either leucocytes or the injured tissue cells participate in these processes. For example, under the influence of TNF-α, which is a cytokine released by macrophages in the injured area, endothelial cells express cellular adhesion molecules such as P-selectin and E-selectin. The leucocytes in circulation recognise P-selectin and temporarily bind to these molecules with very weak attachments. Leucocytes are further influenced by soluble chemical mediators released by the injured tissue and they start to express activated cell receptors called **integrins**. Through interactions of selectins and integrins, leucocytes can engage with the activated endothelium. Integrins interact with **intercellular adhesion molecule-1 (ICAM-1)**, a molecule expressed on the endothelial cell surface so that firm adhesion is formed and leucocyte emigration and movement towards chemical mediators of inflammation (**chemotaxis**) can occur. Chemical mediators also induce leucocyte cytoskeletal reorganisation, which enables neutrophils to change their shape and develop

intermediate filaments, or pseudopodia, to squeeze through connective tissue and in the direction of the chemokine concentration gradient.[2,9] On the endothelial cell side, this process is mediated by the cell junction molecule **platelet endothelial cell adhesion molecule-1 (PECAM-1)**. This same adaptation enables neutrophils to migrate through the endothelial cell wall. Similar processes are involved in recruiting natural killer cells to the site of damage.

Once within the extravascular space, neutrophils continue to respond to and migrate along the chemokine concentration gradient (which is highest at the injury site) by migrating across the extracellular matrix, such as that of fibrin and fibronectin (Fig. 16.8) and towards the injured tissue, a process known as **chemotaxis**.[10] This is also evident clinically in increased neutrophil counts in blood samples as IL-1 and IL-6 (pro-inflammatory chemical mediators secreted by macrophages and natural killer cells) stimulate bone marrow to produce more neutrophils to help aid the repair process.[2] If the inflammation process is extensive or injury involves significant bleeding, the newly formed neutrophils may be relatively immature in their development. Thus, a blood test may reveal the presence of large numbers of precursor neutrophils commonly referred to as **band forms**.

Once neutrophils reach their destination, their aim is to destroy the invading pathogens or chemicals/matter

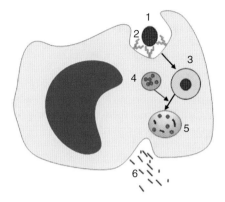

1. Bacterium
2. Phagocyte receptors/ingestion of pathogen
3. Phagosome
4. Lysosome
5. Phagolysosome (fusion of lysosome and phagosome)
6. Exocytosis of soluble debris

A

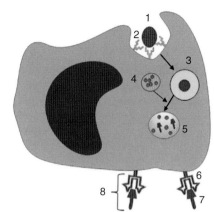

1. Bacterium
2. Phagocyte receptors/ingestion of pathogen
3. Phagosome
4. Lysosome
5. Phagolysosome (fusion of lysosome and phagosome)
6. MHC Class II molecule
7. Particle of bacteria
8. Antigen presentation

B

FIGURE 16.9 **Phagocytosis during inflammation has two major roles. A** Destruction of the pathogen. **B** Presentation of the ingested pathogen to the adaptive immune system.

that may be inducing injury. This is done through **phagocytosis** (Fig. 16.9), an active cellular process whereby neutrophils and macrophages engulf, kill and remove the injurious stimuli. Tissue macrophages are derived from monocytes that arrive into the tissue from blood circulation and are not considered to be circulating cells. Their role is to provide constant surveillance and to remove any immediate threat. To destroy or neutralise injurious stimuli, cells first must recognise the foreign matter and differentiate it from 'self'. Chapter 15 described how neutrophils and macrophages can destroy microbes that have been opsonised (tagged) with certain complement molecules such as C3b. In addition, expression of MHC Class II molecules assists in recognising 'self' molecules. Without opsonisation and MHC II molecules it would not be possible to distinguish between injurious stimuli and 'self'.

Once recognised as foreign, leucocytes engulf the injurious substance by extending their pseudopodia around the object to form a **phagolysosome** (Fig. 16.9). Leucocytes then release lysosomal contents in what is known as a **respiratory burst.**[11] This process is characterised by the production of **reactive oxygen**

species which are bactericidal. Occasionally, this process may also cause localised tissue damage when lysosomal enzymes are released into the surrounding tissue either by accident or through cell death. Pus, which is often present in a wound, arises from the by-products of inflammation such as dead phagocytes, damaged and dead tissue cells, dead bacteria, damaged and dying inflammatory cells and degradation products of the fibrin-rich exudate from damaged vessels. When too many immune cells are activated in one place and they produce too many cytokines in their attempt to combat the injurious stimuli, a **cytokine storm**, also known as a **cytokine cascade** or **hypercytokinaemia**, can develop. This may occur in waves and may be seen in patients spiking temperatures on a random basis when they are not well; it can also lead to a potentially fatal reaction when cytokines are released in massive concentrations.

Tissue response. As blood vessels constrict then vasodilate to allow increased blood flow to the area, the tissue itself forms responses. Connective tissue mast cells release histamine and tissue macrophages secrete pro-inflammatory chemokines. Tissue fibroblasts become activated and transform into **myofibroblasts**, cells that are capable of synthesising and releasing various types of collagen molecules. Collagen is deposited to repair the tissue around the same time as the inflammation process takes place.[12] The aim of this response is to either restore original tissue structure and function (**regeneration**) or **repair** tissue by replacing defective tissue with a connective tissue **scar** (Fig. 16.10). In the latter case, the tissue structure will be different and incomplete and may lead to loss of function. Both processes are dependent on cell types present in the tissue, chemical mediators regulating inflammation and growth factors and factors regulating cell signalling needed for cell proliferation, apoptosis and cell function.

Cells able to participate in regeneration constantly proliferate throughout their life. Examples include cells of the epidermis, the epithelial cells lining intestinal mucosa, bone marrow haematopoietic stem cells and resident tissue stem cells. Here cell regeneration results in replacement of lost cells with cells of the same lineage. Other cells, under normal circumstances, do not divide but can re-enter the cell proliferation cycle if needed. These cells have a very low turnover rate when compared with skin cells or gut epithelial cells.

Connective tissue cells express a variety of cell adhesion surface receptors such as integrins, cadherins and selectins, which permit them to interact with the **extracellular matrix** and **basement membrane matrix** to orientate themselves in the three-dimensional environment of our tissues. Direct contact between cells causes contact inhibition (i.e. the cells 'know' to stop dividing). If they do not, they will grow on top of each other and form tumours. Each interaction activates a different set of signalling pathways that the cell interprets in a specific way and acts according to that signal to play its part in the healing process.

Stem cells also play a role in tissue repair. A stem cell, which can be of embryonic or adult origin, is a cell that can self-renew and give rise to many different

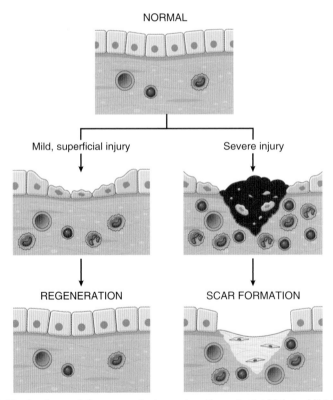

FIGURE 16.10 **Mechanisms of tissue repair depend on the extent of injury.** Mild injury results in tissue repair. Severe injury results in tissue scarring. (*Source:* Kumar V, Abbas A, Aster JC. Robbins and Cotran pathologic basis of disease, 9 ed. St Louis: Elsevier; 2015.)

lineages. Embryonic stem cells are derived from the inner cell mass of blastocysts, a layer that later forms the embryo. Embryonic stem cells are **pluripotent** (i.e. they can give rise to any tissue). Once an embryonic stem cell commits to a certain cell lineage it becomes a **progenitor cell** and can only give rise to that type of tissue. **Adult stem cells**, also referred to as **somatic (body) stem cells**, are less pluripotent than embryonic stem cells. This is because they tend to already be somewhat committed to a specific tissue pathway. **Induced pluripotent stem cells** are a relatively recent addition to the stem cell repertoire and they are a result of laboratory-driven reprogramming of adult cells to pluripotent stem cells which display the properties of embryonic stem cells.

Failure to regenerate seems to be due to loss of signalling that cells require to direct their cell function. For example, destruction of the extracellular matrix, particularly the basement membrane, may result in loss of cell orientation and significant proliferation of cells that compose part of an organ. These cells then synthesise the fibrotic tissue, preventing formation of the original tissue architecture. If tissue cannot regenerate in response to injury, a **repair** will be initiated. For regeneration and repair to occur, the acute inflammation process should be almost complete. Repair is characterised by three major overlapping and integrated events: **connective tissue deposition**, **angiogenesis** and **tissue remodelling**.

In response to injury, endothelial cells respond to growth factors present in the injured tissue. Some growth factors, such as the family of vascular endothelial growth factors (VEGF), induce endothelial cells to proliferate and form a vascular sprout (Fig. 16.7).[12] This can be imagined as the formation of a new tree branch from a sprout in a tree trunk in spring time. As part of forming the new vessel, endothelial cells degrade the surrounding matrix, which includes the basement membrane and the surrounding extracellular matrix. Guided by the chemokine gradient of pro-angiogenic factors, endothelial cells divide and migrate in the direction of the chemokine gradient. Endothelial cell migration is enabled by recognition of certain cell adhesion sites on the extracellular matrix that comprises the fibrin clot.[12] As it does so, it changes the oxygen gradient. Notably, **hypoxia** is a major stimulus for the development of new blood vessels, thus vascularised organs experiencing constant hypoxia due to injury are likely to have increased vascularisation associated with that site, which is another common characteristic of chronic inflammation.[13] Increased nutrient and oxygen supply to the injured area are needed to meet cellular metabolic demands associated with the repair process. As endothelial cells migrate as sprouts or tubes, they also form a lumen to conduct blood. Concurrently, these sprouts release growth factors of their own, which helps stabilisation of the newly built vessel, and the vessel is thought to undergo a 'maturation' process. The endothelial cells lining these vessels start to develop their normal function, such as endocrine, exocrine, cell adhesion, clotting and cell transport functions.[12]

These newly developed vessels are leaky due to pro-inflammatory chemokine gradients as well as their own immaturity. This means that plasma fibronectin and fibrinogen will leak into the extravascular space. Fibronectin and fibrinogen form a fibrin matrix that acts as a scaffold for resident fibroblasts, which are now activated (these cells are known as myofibroblasts). Myofibroblasts initially synthesise collagen type III but later as the newly deposited matrix is remodelled, type I collagen becomes the predominant form.[12] This is a sign of scar tissue with better tensile strength, which is needed if the repair is to be effective. As the tissue is repaired, the need for all the extra vessels and cells present in the repairing tissue eases. Subsequently, cells that make up the blood vessels and connective tissue start to die through programmed cell death (**apoptosis**). This leads to a reduction in cell mass and an increased role for macrophages to clean up the cell debris. The final scar tends to be avascular and acellular.[8,13]

Systemic effects of acute inflammation

During acute inflammation, additional events are triggered in the body that signal inflammation is in progress (Fig. 16.11). Chemical mediators released at the site of injury enter the blood circulation. This enables them to reach other targets in the body and initiate a systemic effect, termed the **acute phase response**. This phase consists of the following clinical changes: fever, production of acute phase proteins such as C-reactive protein (CRP), leucocytosis, increased pulse rate, increased blood pressure, decreased sweating, shivering (rigor), chills, loss of appetite (anorexia), drowsiness (somnolence) and a general feeling of discomfort (malaise). Severe infection may lead to very high concentrations of chemical mediators in the blood that can induce changes in the body that together culminate in septic shock.

Fever, which is an elevated body temperature, is induced by substances called **pyrogens**. Substances classed as pyrogens can be either **endogenous** (formed within the body) or **exogenous** (introduced into the body, for example by viruses or bacteria). In normal physiological circumstances, body temperature regulation involves communication between the autonomic nervous, endocrine and musculoskeletal systems. The

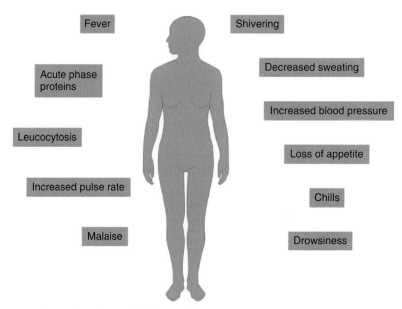

FIGURE 16.11 **Systemic effects of inflammation.**

temperature-controlling system is in the hypothalamus. The anterior hypothalamus mediates temperature decreases, while the posterior hypothalamus mediates temperature increases. The hypothalamus feedback detectors receive their information from peripheral temperature receptors distributed throughout the body including in the skin, spinal cord and viscera and central receptors located in the anterior hypothalamus.[14] During inflammation, fever is activated by endogenous pyrogens such as IL-1, TNF-α, interferon-α, prostaglandins and exogenous pyrogens released by viruses and bacteria (such as bacterial lipopolysaccharide), which stimulate IL-1 production. These pyrogens circulate in the plasma and encounter the hypothalamic temperature-regulating centre. An increase in body temperature is caused by prostaglandins. Furthermore, bacterial lipopolysaccharides stimulate leucocytes to release endogenous pyrogens IL-1 and TNF-α, which increase production of prostaglandins by hypothalamic vascular and perivascular cells. In the hypothalamus, prostaglandins stimulate the production of neurotransmitters that reset the temperature set point at a higher level.[14] These neurotransmitters cause peripheral vasoconstriction and decreased heat dissipation. The trapped heat is clinically evident as fever. It is also proposed that IL-1 enters the brain in regions where the blood–brain barrier is incomplete, such as pre-optic area, to 'reset' the set temperature point. In humans, the set temperature point is approximately 37°C.

With an increased set temperature point, muscles must work harder to produce more heat by converting food into mechanical energy, leading to shivering. Chills are also likely to be a result of responding to an increased set temperature. However, this varies diurnally, decreasing to a minimum during sleep. Fever has several advantages. It is thought that phagocytosis may be more effective at higher temperatures and some bacteria have difficulty surviving at temperatures above 37°C. With decreased pyrogen concentrations, the set temperature point returns to homeostatic levels, although vasodilation occurs followed by sweating, which aids the release of trapped heat. Release of acute phase proteins such as CRP and fibrinogen, which are made in the liver in response to increased concentrations of IL-6 and IL-1 and released into blood, can be used clinically to monitor the progress of inflammation.

An increase in leucocyte numbers (**leucocytosis**) is reflective of the body's attempts to neutralise the injury. Blood tests can clearly show an increase in neutrophil numbers in the circulation, which is referred to as **neutrophilia**. The increase is due to neutrophils having a very short life span (12–36 hours) hence requiring continuous replacement. Neutrophils recruited from the bone marrow in response to IL-1 and TNF-α secretion are of a more immature form and these immature cells are known as band cells. In pathology reports these are described as the presence of increased 'band forms' or a 'left shift' in white cell counts, indicating a release of immature neutrophils into the circulation, often due to infection but associated with the inflammatory response. The physiological basis of other signs of inflammation such as anorexia, somnolence and malaise are poorly understood.

Resolution of acute inflammation

The healing process is intended to return the injured tissue back to homeostatic balance. This outcome is referred to as **resolution** (Fig. 16.12). Typically, resolution can be complete, or result in **fibrosis** or failure to heal, which leads to chronic inflammation. **Complete resolution** refers to a return to a state that is near identical to the original homeostatic state. In other words, the tissue heals with no consequences to health. Healing by fibrosis is usually associated with extensive tissue damage and it leads to the formation of fibrotic tissue or scar (Fig. 16.13) as the affected tissue cannot regenerate.

Progression to chronic inflammation occurs when acute inflammation does not end and instead persists due to the presence of the injurious stimuli. Addressing chronic inflammation is beyond the scope of this chapter, but it is important to note that prolonged acute inflammation can lead to chronic inflammation, which can have a major effect on the person's quality of life.

At any given stage during wound healing things may go wrong. This is particularly true for patients who are malnourished or who do not receive adequate care. Furthermore, some people are genetically predisposed to complications related to scarring. In parenchymal organs such as the liver, kidneys and lungs, it is possible that persistent injury can lead to **pathological fibrosis**, loss of tissue function and, in severe cases, organ failure. Overall, the abnormalities associated with tissue repair include progression to chronic inflammation, incomplete scar formation, disproportionate formation of the connective tissue and/or blood vessels and formation of

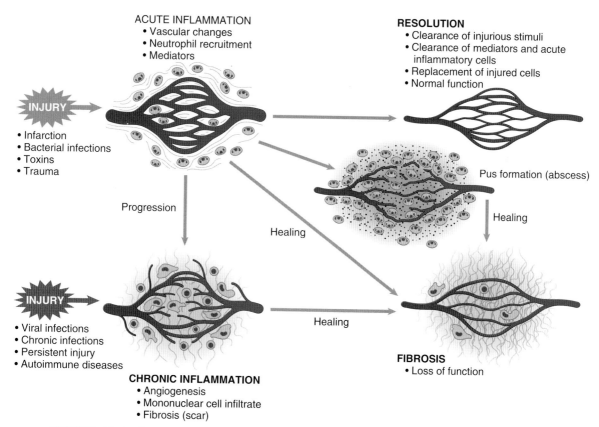

FIGURE 16.12 **Outcomes of inflammation.** (*Source:* Kumar V, Abbas A, Aster JC. Robbins and Cotran pathologic basis of disease, 9 ed. St Louis: Elsevier; 2015.)

NORMAL

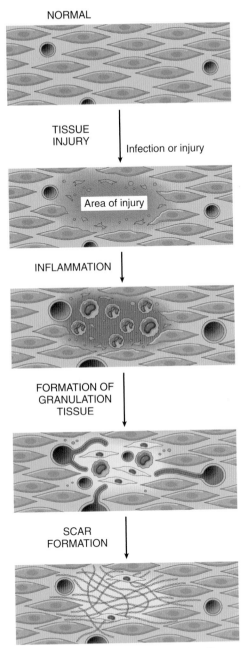

TISSUE
INJURY

Infection or injury

Area of injury

INFLAMMATION

FORMATION OF
GRANULATION
TISSUE

SCAR
FORMATION

FIGURE 16.13 **Repair by scar formation.** (*Source:* Kumar V, Abbas A, Aster JC. Robbins and Cotran pathologic basis of disease, 9 ed. St Louis: Elsevier; 2015.)

contractures. **Wound breakdown** (dehiscence) and **ulceration** can occur where the deposition of granulation tissue is inadequate. If too much collagenous tissue is deposited, a raised scar develops, known as a **hypertrophic scar**. A **keloid scar**, also due to excessive connective tissue deposition, outgrows the boundaries of the original wound and does not regress.

INTEGRATION OF ACUTE INFLAMMATION WITH OTHER BODY SYSTEMS

The following section covers the most common acute inflammatory states that affect each body system and that can resolve with prompt treatment. Many are frequently encountered in community settings.

Integumentary system

The healing process can be observed when assessing cuts and bruises, surgical wounds or red swollen skin in the event of a skin-specific fungal infection. The skin is also an easy way to identify if someone has a fever, a sign of a systemic inflammatory response. When considered in the context of wound size and nature, skin wound healing may occur by first or second intention healing (Fig. 16.14). An example of **first intention healing** is a surgical wound where the wound edges are closely approximated by sutures (they are very near to each other). The outcome is minimal scarring. In **second intention healing** the wound edges are far apart, the tissue must contract to close the wound gap and more prominent scarring is evident. Both processes share common healing mechanisms guided by principles of tissue repair through regeneration and scar formation.

Healing by first intention is characterised by surgically made close alignment of the wound edges where the area for repair and the distance the endothelial and connective tissue cells need to travel is small. This is a way of limiting the extent of injury. Following surgical incision, blood vessels are severed and the coagulation cascade is activated to form a fibrin-rich thrombus and seal the wound gap. This prevents further blood loss and seals the bleeding vessels.[12] On the surface, the clot will polymerise to form a dry scab or eschar. Underneath the eschar, the fibrin matrix contains trapped leucocytes and platelets, which release pro-inflammatory cytokines, growth factors and chemokines. Fibrin becomes a provisional matrix which fibroblasts and endothelial cells move and migrate to invade the injured area in response to the cytokine gradient. Pro-angiogenic growth factors, secreted by the trapped leucocytes, resident fibroblasts and injured endothelial cells, induce new

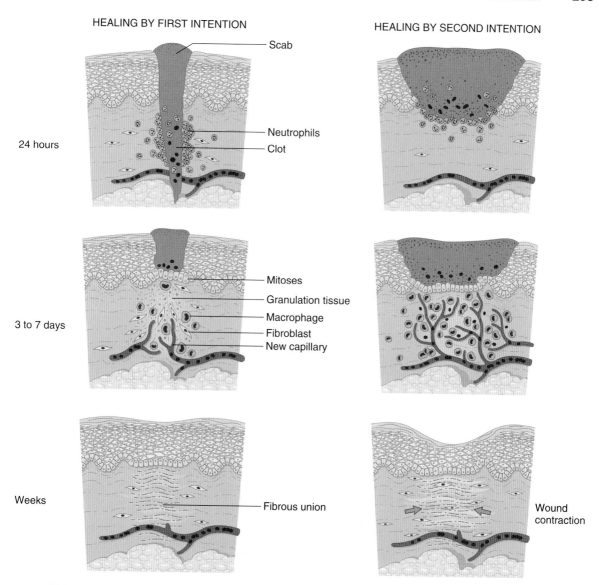

HEALING BY FIRST INTENTION

HEALING BY SECOND INTENTION

Scab

24 hours

Neutrophils
Clot

3 to 7 days

Mitoses
Granulation tissue
Macrophage
Fibroblast
New capillary

Weeks

Fibrous union

Wound contraction

FIGURE 16.14 **Healing by first and second intention in skin tissue.** (*Source:* Kumar V, Abbas A, Aster JC. Robbins and Cotran pathologic basis of disease, 9 ed. St Louis: Elsevier; 2015.)

vessel growth (both lymphatic and vascular), increase permeability and subsequent oedema.

The first angiogenic sprouts start to appear within 72 hours of injury (Fig. 16.12). Hyperpermeable vessels enable migration of neutrophils and other leucocytes into the damaged area. Neutrophils release proteolytic enzymes that cleave the fibrin clot. At the edge of the damaged epidermis, keratinocytes start to secrete epidermal growth factor, which stimulates further keratinocyte division. As keratinocytes migrate underneath the clot

along the dermis, they deposit basement membrane. Eventually the two keratinocyte migrating fronts meet beneath the eschar to form a continuous epithelial layer that closes the wound and forms a barrier to further pathogen invasion.

At around the same time, fibroblasts are activated and start to deposit type III collagen. The endothelial cells, keratinocytes and fibroblasts proliferate simultaneously at the periphery of the wound gap and start to invade the fibrin matrix. At around 72 hours post injury, blood monocytes will have become tissue macrophages and together with the resident macrophage population they commence clearing extracellular debris, fibrin and other foreign material. Macrophages secrete growth factors that drive angiogenesis, vessel interconnections and extracellular matrix deposition.[12]

As repair progresses, granulation tissue—a highly vascular newly developed tissue—continues to form and fills in the wound space, while fibrin clot is gradually degraded by tissue macrophages and myofibroblasts. Remodelling of granulation tissue commences through matrix metalloproteinases, enzymes that predominantly degrade different types of matrix molecules including collagen. The keratinocyte layer thins out as it returns to its normal thickness and position. During this time, local fibroblasts continue to synthesise collagen but they also start to replace collagen type III with a more durable collagen type I. At the same time, they contract the wound to reduce the total scarring area and improve scar tensile strength. Leucocytes apoptose, oedema is reduced and the vasculature regresses, also through apoptosis.[12]

Wounds that are not surgically closed undergo a similar process, except that the response tends to be magnified. This is because larger defects require more granulation tissue to form and seal the wound. Keratinocyte migration is slower and occurs after the granulation tissue has already formed. A bigger avascular scar may eventuate. This type of healing is more prone to the development of secondary inflammation and complications related to scar formation, such as pathological fibrosis or wound contracture.

Burns are another common type of injury to the skin. They can be caused by thermal injury, electricity, chemicals, friction or radiation. In thermal burns, the local inflammatory response involves vasodilation and increased vascular permeability. The degree of oedema is dependent on the amount of tissue damage, with greater damage leading to more extensive oedema. Fluid and electrolyte losses may be influenced by the volume and type of fluid replacement, while aggressive fluid replacement (especially with crystalloids) in the presence of airway burns can promote rapid development of compromising airway obstruction secondary to oedema. Healing will depend on the extent or thickness of the burn. A small burn will have a limited acute response, whereas a deep burn will involve scar formation. As skin integrity is lost, a major effort is directed at preventing wound infection. Major burns can be complicated by **contracture**, meaning that instead of developing elastic tissue as part of the healing process, the scar tissue is comprised of inelastic tissue. As this tissue remodels it contracts even further, thus limiting movement of the skin or the limb it is related to. Contractures, as complications of burns healing gone wrong, can also occur in ligaments, muscles and tendons.

Wound exudate observed during acute inflammation can be classified as **serous** (protein-rich clear fluid exudate), **catarrh** (hypersecretion of mucus), **fibrinosis** (polymerised extravascular fibrinogen) and **suppurative** or **purulent** (formation of pus). In sub-acute inflammation lymphocytic exudate can also be observed, characterised by nearly pure leucocyte infiltration in the tissue, whereas in chronic inflammation granulomatous exudate is present (characterised by macrophage infiltration).

Musculoskeletal system

Bone fractures heal by forming **bone callus** at the site of fracture (Fig. 16.15). When a bone is fractured, blood pours into the injured area to form a clot. This is known as a **fracture haematoma** and its role is to act as a provisional scaffold for migration of cells and a source of growth factors released by the haematopoietic cells trapped in the haematoma. These growth factors induce the migration and proliferation of osteoblasts, fibroblasts and mesenchymal cells, which form a type of granulation tissue around each fracture end, thus forming a bridge between the separated ends.[15]

In the first week of injury, the granulation tissue gives rise to islands of **cartilaginous procallus**, also known as **soft callus**, to anchor the broken ends together. Within two to three weeks, through a process known as **endochondral ossification**, the soft callus is slowly converted to a hard bony framework to further stabilise the connection between the separated ends. Between four to 16 weeks, the callus is remodelled so that the cartilaginous structure converts to calcified bone matrix and the bone is shaped to return towards the near-normal shape and function, including clear separation of the medullary cavity from the compact bone (Fig. 16.15).[15]

The most important factors that influence bone healing include blood supply, mechanical stability, the location of the injury and bone loss due to age-associated changes or the extent of trauma to the bone. Patient diet also has an impact on the quality of formed bone; for example, nutritional deficiencies in calcium and vitamin D or loss of capacity to absorb calcium through procedures such as gastric bypass. Medication prescribed, such as bisphosphonates, also affects a patient's capacity to generate good-quality bone.[16]

Nervous system

The structure of the brain and spinal cord has been covered in Chapter 7. For the purposes of this section it

Fracture types

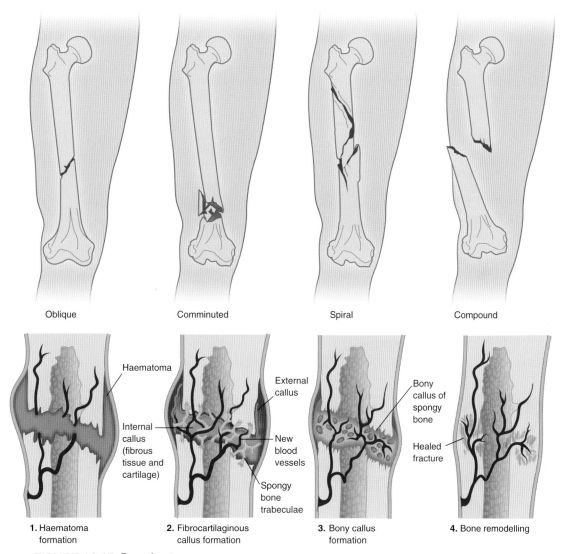

Oblique | Comminuted | Spiral | Compound

Haematoma

Internal callus (fibrous tissue and cartilage)

External callus

New blood vessels

Spongy bone trabeculae

Bony callus of spongy bone

Healed fracture

1. Haematoma formation

2. Fibrocartilaginous callus formation

3. Bony callus formation

4. Bone remodelling

FIGURE 16.15 **Bone fracture.**

is important to be aware of two specific structures: the meninges and the blood–brain barrier. The **meninges** are comprised of three layers: the pia mater, arachnoid mater and dura mater. The **pia mater** is the innermost highly vascularised membrane adhering to the brain surface, the **arachnoid mater** is a delicate richly vascularised membrane and the **dura mater** is the tough fibrous outermost membrane. The pia mater and arachnoid mater are separated by the subarachnoid space which contains **cerebrospinal fluid (CSF)**. The **blood–brain**

barrier is a specialised structure that shields the brain from harmful blood-borne substances and pathogens. It is composed of a continuous layer of capillary endothelial cells joined by tight endothelial cell junctions, astrocyte end feet encasing the capillary and pericytes that are embedded in the basement membrane. The basement membrane is unique as it is synthesised by both astrocytes and endothelial cells. The brain is separated from leucocytes in the blood by the blood–brain barrier. It has its own specialised immune cells that help mediate neuroinflammation and associated repair. These cells are glial cells and astrocytes. **Neuroinflammation** is a term commonly used to describe acute inflammation of the nervous system. The most commonly known states of inflammation affecting the nervous system are stroke and meningitis.

Meningitis is inflammation of the membranes surrounding the brain and spinal cord, the meninges, the subarachnoid space, ventricular space and CSF (Fig. 16.16). It can be either bacterial- or viral-induced. In terms of bacterial infection, the most common causes are meningococcal bacteria, pneumococcal bacteria, tuberculosis, Group B streptococcus and *Escherichia coli*.[17] Early symptoms include a runny nose, irritation, sensitivity to bright light, fever, confusion, neck stiffness and possibly seizures. These occur in advance of non-blanching petechial or purpuric rash, which arises from bleeding into the skin or mucosa. Initially, the rash is

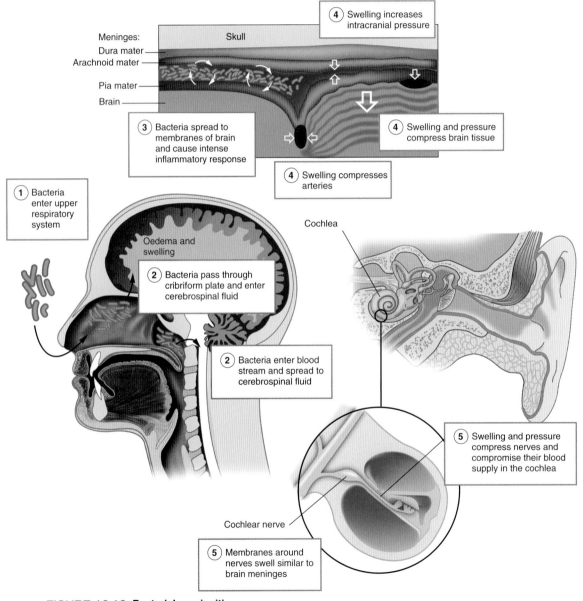

FIGURE 16.16 **Bacterial meningitis.**

about 1–2 mm in size; as meningitis progresses, it can progress to gangrene and may lead to amputation of the affected body part. Seizures can also develop.

When bacteria are present in the blood, they enter the meninges through the **choroid plexus**, a site of CSF formation and where the blood–brain barrier is weakest. Alternatively, bacteria may enter from the nasal cavity, which is in direct contact with the meninges. The response of the immune system to the invading bacteria is what leads to the subsequent signs and symptoms of this condition. Namely, after recognising the bacterial cell components, astrocytes and neuroglia, which have an immune role in the brain, respond by releasing chemokines that recruit lymphocytes to the site of infection. This leads to increased permeability of the blood–brain barrier, leading to **cerebral oedema**, which results in increased cerebral pressure. **Interstitial oedema** also occurs, characterised by swelling of the meninges. Blood vessels become inflamed and this restricts blood flow and leads to cytotoxic oedema. Collectively, this leads to an increase in **intracranial pressure**, further compressing the brain and vascular structures and thus compromising blood flow and impairing delivery of oxygen and nutrients to the brain, leading to cell death in the brain and associated structures.[18]

Vaccination is the most effective protection against bacterial meningitis, but vaccines have not been developed for all types of bacteria. As there is the potential for a pregnant mother who is a carrier of Group B streptococcus to pass on the bacteria to her newborn, thus increasing the risk of bacterial meningitis in the newborn, in Australia all pregnant women are screened or tested for Group B streptococcus. If positive, antibiotics are administered during labour to prevent passing the bacteria to the newborn.

Viral infection of the meninges can be caused by mumps virus, herpes simplex virus (which causes chickenpox), varicella zoster virus (which causes shingles), measles virus, influenza virus or other less well-known viruses such as the family of non-polio enteroviruses. Although milder than bacterial meningitis, this condition can still pose life-threatening complications in vulnerable populations and requires urgent attention. Children under the age of five and people with a weakened immune system are at greater risk of developing viral meningitis than the rest of the population.

Special senses: hearing, balance and vision

Ear infections (Fig. 16.17), scientifically known as **otitis media**, are more common in children and may be due

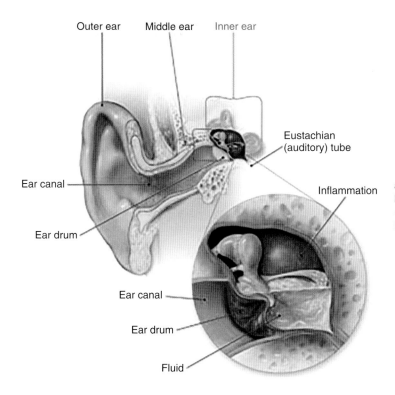

FIGURE 16.17 Ear infection and associated inflammation and fluid buildup. (*Source:* www.cdc.gov/antibiotic-use/community/for-patients/common-illnesses/ear-infection.html)

to viral infections such as those associated with the common cold or bacterial infections of the respiratory system. This is because the eustachian tubes, small passageways that connect the throat to the middle ear, are shorter and more level in children compared with adults. Furthermore, children have a weaker immune system and their adenoids may trap bacteria from the mouth and nose that can then travel to the eustachian tubes and middle ear.[19]

Ear infections can be grouped into acute otitis media, otitis media with effusion and chronic otitis media with effusion. **Acute otitis media** is characterised by parts of the middle ear being infected and swollen with fluid trapped behind the eardrum. **Otitis media with effusion** occurs when, after the ear infection has passed, fluid stays trapped behind the eardrum. This may temporarily affect hearing. In **chronic otitis media with effusion**, the infection has passed but fluid accumulated behind the ear either remains in the middle ear or repeatedly occurs. This may affect the child's hearing and language development as sound transmission between the eardrum and cochlear nerve is affected.

Signs and symptoms of an ear infection include tugging, constantly rubbing or pulling on ears, general irritability, fluid draining from the ear, and problems with balance and hearing. In children who experience otitis media with effusion, if a hearing test is done, mild hearing loss may be recorded; this result will be followed up three months later to determine whether the fluid has drained or intervention such as grommets is required to drain the fluid.

Conjunctivitis is inflammation of the conjunctiva, a clear membrane that covers part of the front surface of the eye and inner surface of the eyelid (Fig. 16.18). This condition is common in children, particularly if a child attends childcare, as it is highly contagious. It can be either viral or bacterial, with the child remaining infectious as long as there is discharge from the eye. Conjunctivitis can also be caused by an allergic reaction such as that seen in hay fever. Evidence of conjunctivitis includes a red or pink eye/s, itchiness of the eye/s, redness behind the eyelid/s, swelling of the affected eyelid, tears or yellow discharge from the eyes that dries when the child sleeps, leading to crusting.

Cardiovascular system

Inflammation of the myocardium is termed **myocarditis**. The cause of myocarditis can be either infectious or non-infectious and it can affect anyone. Most cases are caused by viruses that originate from something as simple as the common cold, herpes or influenza viruses. Bacterial infection of the myocardium is usually blood-borne but

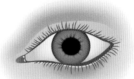

Normal eye
In a healthy eye, the sclera is essentially white with only a few small blood vessels visible. There is an adequate tear film, with no significant discharge or watering.

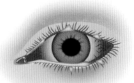

Bacterial conjunctivitis
A red eye with a sticky yellow/green discharge. Eyelids may be stuck together upon waking. Can affect one or both eyes. Usually spread by direct contact only.

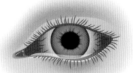

Viral conjunctivitis
The type of conjunctivitis most commonly associated with the term 'pink eye'. Appearance: red, itchy, watery eye. Can affect one or both eyes. Highly contagious.

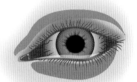

Allergic conjunctivitis
Very similar in appearance to viral conjunctivitis, but accompanied by nasal congestion, sneezing, eyelid swelling and sensitivity to light. Both eyes are affected. Not contagious

FIGURE 16.18 Conjunctivitis.

can also come from bacterial tonsillitis and scarlet fever. Fungal infections of the myocardium are usually seen in immunocompromised individuals such as those with AIDS or on chemotherapy. Non-infectious causes are attributed to immune system dysfunction, such as rheumatoid disease.

Inflammation of the pericardium is called **pericarditis**. Inflammation of these two layered membranes surrounding the heart can lead to restrictions in heart movement during impulse conduction (heartbeat), thus it is important to treat it early. Treatment will be driven by the cause of pericarditis. **Vasculitis** is a term used to describe inflammation of the blood vessels. It can be chronic or acute. Associated swelling, weakening of the vessel walls and scarring of the vessel may impact blood flow, which may lead to organ and tissue damage.

Lymphatic system

The lymphatic system is composed of the lymphatic vessels and lymphoid organs, which include the tonsils, spleen, thymus and lymph nodes. The role of the lymphatic system is in tissue fluid balance, immunity and transport of chylomicrons from the gastrointestinal system to systemic blood circulation. When bacteria invade the lymphatic vessels, this leads to inflammation of the lymphatic vessels, termed as **lymphangitis**.

Characteristics of lymphangitis include red streaks radiating from the site of infection towards the nearest lymph node when part of skin infection. Other causes of inflammation of lymphatic vessels include metastasis of tumours such as breast cancer, lung cancer and prostate cancer. Bacterial lymphangitis spreads quickly and can lead to cellulitis, a generalised skin infection, and, if not treated in time, to sepsis, a body-wide infection.

Respiratory system

Inflammation of the respiratory system can be due to infections or disease processes. With respect to infections, these can be grouped into **upper respiratory tract infections** and **lower respiratory tract infections**. Examples of upper respiratory tract infections include the common cold, sinusitis, laryngitis (inflammation of the voice box) and epiglottitis (inflammation of the epiglottis). In children, **croup**, a viral infection of the trachea, larynx and bronchi, may become life-threatening due to oedema-induced obstruction of the airway (Fig. 16.19A). Lower respiratory infections include bronchitis, bronchiolitis and pneumonia.

While the pathogenesis of these conditions is beyond the scope of this book, it is important to note that in terms of acute inflammation of the upper respiratory tract, infectious organisms predominantly gain access to the respiratory tract by inhalation of droplets containing infectious particles. The infectious particles invade the **first line of defence**, which is comprised of epithelial cells lining the respiratory tract and the secretions made by those cells. Once broken, the subsequent tissue damage induced by the infectious particles activates the **second line of defence**. This may be visible in the throat as redness and swelling, accompanied occasionally by haemorrhage and exudate.

With respect to the lower respiratory tract, organisms enter the lungs by inhalation or aspiration. **Aspiration** is defined as inhalation of foreign matter such as a piece of food or a drink while drawing in a breath, thus permitting access to the lungs. Similar to upper respiratory tract infection, the virus and bacteria pass the first line of defence, which is the respiratory tract epithelial cell lining, and infect the underlying cells.

Bronchitis and bronchiolitis are infections of the bronchi and bronchioles, respectively. **Bronchiolitis** is a viral infection in infants caused predominantly by respiratory syncytial virus. Copious secretions are produced; infants cough frequently with deepening cough, and an increased respiratory rate is common, as are retractions of the chest wall, nasal flaring and grunting. As infant airways are easily obstructed, medical attention should be obtained as early as possible.

Pneumonia is inflammation of the lung alveoli where the alveolar space can be filled with fluid or pus, causing coughing with phlegm (Fig. 16.19B). It can be caused by infectious particles such as bacteria, viruses or fungi. As secretions exist in the alveolar space, the capacity of the alveoli to participate in effective oxygen exchange becomes impaired. Young children and the elderly are at higher risk of developing pneumonia.

Gastrointestinal system

Both food poisoning and alcohol poisoning are afflictions most people are likely to have either experienced

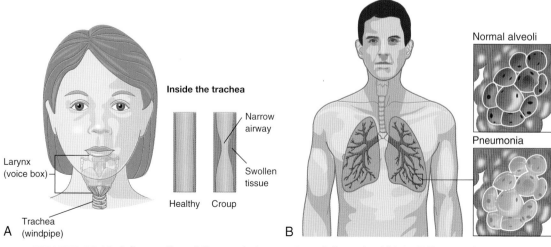

FIGURE 16.19 **Inflammation of the respiratory system. A** Croup in children. **B** Pneumonia.

firsthand or witnessed in others. Food poisoning is predominantly associated with bacterial contamination, bacterial toxins or chemical substances. It may result in diarrhoea, nausea, vomiting and abdominal cramping. Note that if food poisoning is due to toxins, the responding mechanism is not that of an infection but rather that of managing toxin neutralisation. In the gut, the first line of defence is the epithelial cells lining the gut and the symbiotic bacteria living in the gut. Damage to the epithelial cell lining will initiate the second and third line of the acute inflammatory response. The effect of enterotoxins on the secretory mechanism of the gut mucosa leads to the formation of large watery stools. Vomiting is another part of the first line of defence in the acute inflammatory response, also in response to bacterial toxins. How toxins cause diarrhoea and vomiting is a topic of research.

Alcohol-induced intoxication is a common presentation to hospital emergency departments. Alcohol affects all parts of the gastrointestinal system, including the gut mucosa, liver and pancreas. In a healthy adult, alcohol is metabolised by the liver to the compound acetaldehyde by the enzyme alcohol dehydrogenase (ADH). This enzyme is widely distributed throughout the body. Acetaldehyde is metabolised further to acetate by acetaldehyde dehydrogenase (ALDH), which is found in liver mitochondria. Acetate is used as fuel by the muscles to produce acetyl-coenzyme A (acetyl-CoA) using the enzyme acetyl-CoA synthetase.[20] Acetyl-CoA is used in the citric acid cycle, which releases stored energy in cells dependent on oxygen for survival. Although certain concentrations of alcohol can be metabolised, excessive intake leads to physical and psychological impairment. In the early stages of alcohol-related liver disease, the liver appears to preferentially metabolise alcohol over lipids.[20] This leads to the intracellular accumulation of fat particles within the liver, thus the name alcoholic fatty liver (alcoholic hepatosteatosis). It is a mild condition and may be asymptomatic; unlike later stages of alcoholic liver disease, it is reversible if alcohol intake is stopped. Chronic abuse of alcohol can lead to alcoholic liver disease and liver failure.

As alcohol is a central nervous system depressant, large consumption of alcohol can lead to depression of the respiratory centre and loss of capacity to maintain a patent airway. An intoxicated person can become unconscious and if they vomit while unconscious, they may aspirate and choke on their vomit. Ethanol also inhibits gluconeogenesis, thus causing hypoglycaemia, and may cause lactic acidosis, ketoacidosis and acute kidney failure. Alcohol also causes pancreatic acinar cell injury that generates an inflammatory response, although the mechanism is not clear. To date, it is proposed that pancreatic injury, clinically known as **acute pancreatitis**, and subsequent inflammation are in response to the accumulation of toxic acetaldehyde through oxidation of alcohol to acetaldehyde via ADH by the acinar cells, inhibition of blood flow to the pancreas, increased production of digestive enzymes by pancreatic acinar cells following alcohol consumption and an increase in pancreatic cell necrosis.[21]

Urinary system

Nephritis is acute inflammation of the kidneys. There are three types of nephritis, affecting three distinct areas in the kidneys. **Interstitial nephritis** affects the interstitial space between the kidney tubules. It is usually due to an allergic reaction to an antibiotic or medication. **Pyelonephritis** is caused by an infection, mostly due to *Escherichia coli*—bacteria that happily live in your intestine but when they reach your bladder via the urethra to the kidneys cause an infection. Other causes include medical procedures such as cystoscopy or surgery on components of the urinary system, and kidney stones.

Glomerulonephritis is inflammation of the kidney glomerulus. Glomerular injury can arise from hypoxia, immunological diseases, infections, toxins and some prescribed medications and may be associated with chronic diseases such as diabetes mellitus. Acute glomerulonephritis is most often associated with a streptococcal infection where the injury is due to streptococcal antigen-antibody complexes depositing in the glomerular basement membrane. This causes activation of the complement pathways and release of inflammatory mediators, which cause endothelial and epithelial cell damage in the glomerulus.

Failure to treat nephritis can lead to acute kidney failure, a life-threatening condition.

Reproductive system

Vaginitis is inflammation of the vagina, the muscular canal that connects the cervix to the outside of the body in females (Fig. 16.20). In adults, it is usually due to an infection such as *Candida albicans* (a fungus), a bacterial infection or trichomoniasis. It can also be a consequence of some antibiotic treatments, as antibiotics do not differentiate between pathogenic and non-pathogenic bacteria and therefore disrupt the vaginal bacterial flora. Inflammation is evident as redness and swelling of the labia majora and labia minora and perineal area. Discharge may be present and passing urine can be painful. Reduced oestrogen levels after menopause can also cause vaginitis. In children, the

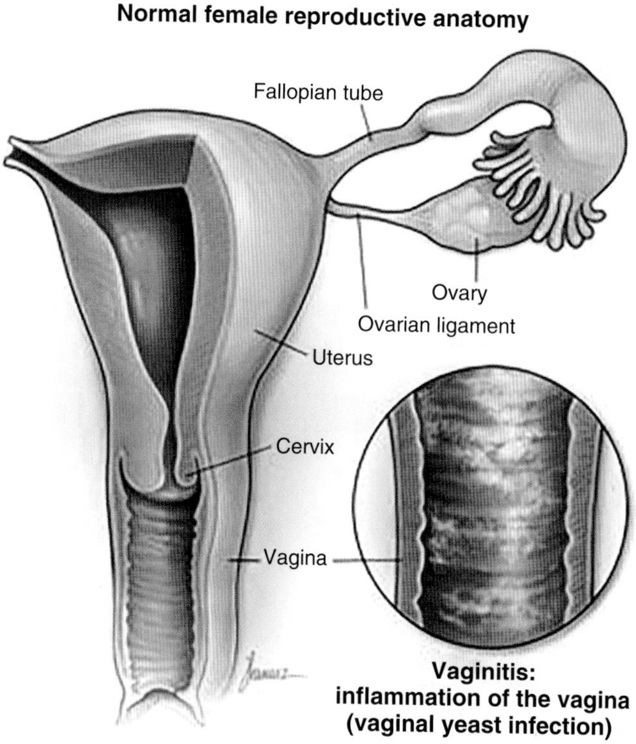

Normal female reproductive anatomy

FIGURE 16.20 Vaginitis. (*Source:* https://my.clevelandclinic.org/health/diseases/9131-vaginitis)

condition is often seen during toilet training if the child is not dried after passing urine. Threadworms may also cause vaginitis in children. Inflammation of the glans penis and foreskin in children is called **balanitis** and is characterised by minor redness and soreness of the tip of the foreskin. **Pelvic inflammatory disease** refers to inflammation processes affecting the uterus, ovaries, fallopian tubes and cervix due to infection. Causes are usually attributed to sexually transmitted infections such as gonorrhoea or chlamydia.

AGE-RELATED CHANGES

During early gestation the fetus has the ability to heal skin wounds without forming scars. As the fetus grows this capacity is lost and by the time the fetus is born, and subject to wound size and depth, this capacity is mostly lost, with bigger wounds leaving scars behind.[22] Due to skin composition changes in older adults such as collagen deposition and the strength of newly formed scars, older people have a higher risk of wound break-down and complications of wound healing.[23]

The ageing process is associated with loss of cellular capacity to divide (senescence) and reduced capacity to effectively respond to causes of inflammation. Through gradual reduction in cell repair mechanisms and reduced ability to effectively degrade cellular waste by autophagy, the body starts to accumulate damaged molecules such as DNA and protein. This may contribute to the ageing process as well as increasing a person's risk of developing chronic conditions characterised by an accumulation of defective cellular structures. Ageing is also associated with an increased risk of infections, increased susceptibility to sepsis, an increase in pro-inflammatory prostaglandins and upregulation of pro-inflammatory mediators. The prolonged presence of a pro-inflammatory state also leads to the development of chronic inflammation and associated chronic diseases.[4] Older individuals are also at risk of altered haemostasis regulation, leading to an increased risk of thrombotic complications during critical illness.[24] It is proposed that by understanding and regulating age-related processes it may be possible to delay the development of chronic diseases.[4]

CONCLUSION

Acute inflammation is an orchestrated sequence of events that involves vascular, immune and tissue responses that collectively aim to return injured tissue back to a near-normal state through repair and remodelling processes.

Such homeostatic balance ensures the continuity of tissue structure and function. The body's capacity to heal reduces as we age so that older adults have a higher risk of experiencing inflammatory conditions and have an increased risk of thrombosis and wound dehiscence.

CASE STUDY 16.1

Sahara went on a five-day ski trip to Mount Hotham with her friends but unfortunately she forgot to pack her ski boots. Her friends had no spare boots to loan her and she was not keen to buy new ski boots so she wore her leather boots instead. As her boots were not waterproof, by the second day of the trip Sahara's feet were soaking wet. On the fourth day Sahara started to experience shortness of breath when climbing the stairs. This worsened over the next day as she also developed a sore throat, fever, cough and a mild wheeze. Once back home, she went to her doctor who told her that she had acute bronchitis.

Q1. Fever is a manifestation of:
   a. upregulation of connective tissue deposition.
   b. systemic effect of inflammation.
   c. angiogenesis.
   d. localised inflammatory response.

Q2. Mild wheezing in Sahara's case is likely to be due to:
   a. oversecretion of sputum, which restricts air flow.
   b. swelling of the bronchi, which restricts air flow.
   c. alveolar inflammation, which restricts air flow.
   d. sinusitis, which restricts air flow.

Q3. Which of the following molecules is/are associated with resetting the hypothalamic set temperature point?
   a. Endogenous pyrogens
   b. Exogenous pyrogens
   c. C-reactive protein
   d. Both a and b are correct

Q4. Considering that Sahara was diagnosed with acute bronchitis, suggest what changes you would expect to be present in her lung bronchi as part of the acute inflammatory response.

Q5. As this is acute rather than chronic bronchitis, suggest what the likely outcome will be if Sahara takes good care of herself.

CASE STUDY 16.2

Nellie is an 89-year-old retiree. Last week she had a procedure to remove a mole from above her left eyebrow that the doctor thought might be skin cancer. The doctor stitched the wound and placed a dressing over it, telling Nellie to come back for a checkup in a week's time. At the checkup the dressing was wet; when it was removed, the wound seemed to have opened on the end closer to the eyebrow and it was oozing yellow cloudy pus.

Q1. Age-related changes are associated with impaired wound healing.
   a. True
   b. False

Q2. Resolution is a process of:
   a. formation of new blood vessels.
   b. deposition of collagen tissue.
   c. leucocyte diapedesis.
   d. return of injured tissue to near homeostatic balance.

Q3. Healing by first intention refers to:
   a. healing of large open wounds.
   b. polymerisation of the fibrin matrix.
   c. surgically-made close alignment of wound edges.
   d. activation of the systemic inflammatory response.

Q4. Suggest why the ageing process may contribute to Nellie's wound not closing completely.

Q5. Explain how the pus might have formed in Nellie's case and the reason why it is oozing.

CASE STUDY 16.3

Banjo, a geology student, went on a two-week field trip with his classmates to New Zealand. During the day, the students were busy mapping the geology of New Zealand but in the evening they let their hair down and enjoyed a drink or two. One evening, Banjo, who was not much of a drinker, decided to try to keep up with his more seasoned mates and drank more alcohol than ever before. At around 4 am he woke up feeling very unwell, nauseated and experiencing severe abdominal pain. His roommates helped him to the toilet where he vomited. As he vomited eight times in the space of an hour and seemed unlikely to stop, one of his mates called for an ambulance. Banjo was taken to hospital where he was diagnosed with acute pancreatitis.

Q1. Inflammation can be caused by:

a. infectious agents such as viruses and bacteria.

b. physical agents such as vibration and noise.

c. overconsumption of alcohol.

d. all of the above.

Q2. With respect to duration, inflammation can be:

a. acute or chronic.

b. multifocal.

c. segmental.

d. diffuse.

Q3. Inflammation of any tissue involves the following processes:

a. tissue-specific vascular, leucocyte and tissue-related responses aimed at repair.

b. overgrowth of scar tissue to ensure healing is complete.

c. uncontrolled blood vessel growth in the injured area.

d. the formation of new tissue structure different to original tissue.

Q4. Suggest why alcohol might have caused acute pancreatitis.

Q5. What could be a consequence of acute pancreatitis if untreated?

CASE STUDY 16.4

Sydney, a four-year-old boy, was admitted to the local hospital due to heightened light sensitivity, fever, vomiting and headache. On admission, he was increasingly confused and drowsy. A provisional diagnosis of meningitis was made. To investigate a cause, blood tests and imaging were ordered, and cerebrospinal fluid was collected for microbiology tests to see whether viral or bacterial infection could be detected.

Q1. Meningitis is a term used to describe:

a. inflammation of the blood–brain barrier.

b. inflammation of the hypothalamus.

c. inflammation of the meninges.

d. inflammation of the myocardium.

Q2. Young children are at higher risk of developing meningitis because of:

a. a less developed immune system.

b. a less developed blood–brain barrier.

c. both a and b are correct.

d. all children being carriers of Group B streptococcus.

Q3. Non-blanching rash is an early sign of meningitis.

a. True

b. False

Q4. Discuss how acute inflammation might be affecting the brain in Sydney's case.

Q5. If meningitis is not effectively treated, what might be the sequelae of this infection?

REFERENCES

1. Pahwa R, Jialal I. Chronic inflammation. Treasure Island, FL: StatPearls; 2019.

2. Abdulkhaleq LA, Assi MA, Abdullah R, et al. The crucial roles of inflammatory mediators in inflammation: a review. Vet World 2018;11(5):627–35.

3. Makki K, Froguel P, Wolowczuk I. Adipose tissue in obesity-related inflammation and insulin resistance: cells, cytokines, and chemokines. ISRN Inflamm 2013;139239.

4. Rea IM, Gibson DS, McGilligan V, et al. Age and age-related diseases: role of inflammation triggers and cytokines. Front Immunol 2018;9:586.

5. Perrone S, Bracciali C, Di Virgilio N, et al. Oxygen use in neonatal care: a two-edged sword. Front Pediatr 2016;4:143.

6. Tani K, Ogushi F, Shimizu T, et al. Protease-induced leukocyte chemotaxis and activation: roles in host defense and inflammation. J Med Invest 2001;48(3–4):133–41.

7. Lokmic Z. Utilizing lymphatic cell markers to visualize human lymphatic abnormalities. J Biophotonics 2018; 11(8):e201700117.

8. Lokmic Z, Darby IA, Thompson EW, et al. Time course analysis of hypoxia, granulation tissue and blood vessel growth, and remodeling in healing rat cutaneous incisional primary intention wounds. Wound Repair Regen 2006;14(3):277–88.

9. Hamidzadeh K, Christensen SM, Dalby E, et al. Macrophages and the recovery from acute and chronic inflammation. Annu Rev Physiol 2017;79:567–92.

10. Sarris M, Sixt M. Navigating in tissue mazes: chemoattractant interpretation in complex environments. Curr Opin Cell Biol 2015;36:93–102.

11. Gordon S. Phagocytosis: an immunobiologic process. Immunity 2016;44(3):463–75.

12. Gonzalez AC, Costa TF, Andrade ZA, et al. Wound healing: a literature review. An Bras Dermatol 2016;91(5): 614–20.

13. Lokmic Z, Musyoka J, Hewitson TD, et al. Hypoxia and hypoxia signaling in tissue repair and fibrosis. Int Rev Cell Mol Biol 2012;296:139–85.

14. Zhao ZD, Yang WZ, Gao C, et al. A hypothalamic circuit that controls body temperature. Proc Natl Acad Sci USA 2017;114(8):2042–7.

15. Loi F, Cordova LA, Pajarinen J, et al. Inflammation, fracture and bone repair. Bone 2016;86:119–30.

16. Bedogni A, Blandamura S, Lokmic Z, et al. Bisphosphonate-associated jawbone osteonecrosis: a correlation between imaging techniques and histopathology. Oral Surg Oral Med Oral Pathol Oral Radiol Endod 2008;105(3):358–64.

17. Oordt-Speets AM, Bolijn R, van Hoorn RC, et al. Global etiology of bacterial meningitis: a systematic review and meta-analysis. PLoS ONE 2018;13(6):e0198772.

18. Koedel U, Klein M, Pfister HW. New understandings on the pathophysiology of bacterial meningitis. Curr Opin Infect Dis 2010;23(3):217–23.

19. Yiengprugsawan V, Hogan A. Ear infection and its associated risk factors, comorbidity, and health service use in Australian children. Int J Pediatr 2013;2013:963132.

20. Manzo-Avalos S, Saavedra-Molina A. Cellular and mitochondrial effects of alcohol consumption. Int J Environ Res Public Health 2010;7(12):4281–304.

21. Chowdhury P, Gupta P. Pathophysiology of alcoholic pancreatitis: an overview. World J Gastroenterol 2006; 12(46):7421–7.

22. Larson BJ, Longaker MT, Lorenz HP. Scarless fetal wound healing: a basic science review. Plast Reconstr Surg 2010; 126(4):1172–80.

23. Sgonc R, Gruber J. Age-related aspects of cutaneous wound healing: a mini-review. Gerontology 2013;59(2):159–64.

24. Kale SS, Yende S. Effects of aging on inflammation and hemostasis through the continuum of critical illness. Aging Dis 2011;2(6):501–11.

CHAPTER 17

Respiratory system

NICK BRIDGE, MASTER OF HEALTH EDUCATION • ZERINA TOMKINS, BAPPSC (MED LAB SCI), BAPPSC (HONS), MNSC (NURS), PHD, GRAD CERT (UNIVERSITY EDUCATION)

KEY POINTS/LEARNING OUTCOMES

1. Identify the general functions of the respiratory system and describe the functions of each component of the system, including age-related changes.
2. Explain how inspiration and expiration are accomplished and how these processes are regulated.
3. Describe the structure and function of the respiratory membrane and the importance of partial pressure in the diffusion of gases.
4. Explain how blood transports oxygen and carbon dioxide.
5. Describe the interactions between the respiratory, cardiovascular, endocrine and nervous systems in the normal regulation of respiratory function, transport of oxygen and removal of carbon dioxide.

KEY DEFINITIONS

- **Anatomical dead space:** the sum of volume of air trapped in the conducting portions of the respiratory tract (from the trachea to the terminal bronchi) that conduct air to the respiratory bronchioles and alveoli but do not participate in the process of gas exchange.
- **Minute ventilation:** the volume of gas inhaled or exhaled per minute.
- **pH:** an abbreviation for a phrase meaning 'the power of hydrogen'; it is used to mean the relative hydrogen ion (H^+) concentration of a solution. The more H^+ dissolved in a solution, the more acidic it is. On a scale of 0 to 14, 7 is neutral while 0 is highly acidic. The normal pH of blood is 7.4.
- **Partial pressure:** Dalton's law states that in a mixture of non-reacting gases the total pressure exerted is equal to the sum of the partial pressures of the individual gases; i.e. total pressure $(P_T) = P_1 + P_2 + P_3 + \dots + P_n$.
- **Tidal volume:** the volume of gas inhaled or exhaled in a single breath during regular (normal) breathing.
- **Ventilation perfusion match (V/Q):** optimal gas exchange that occurs when regions of lung are ventilated (V) in proportion to their perfusion (Q)—that is, V and Q are matched.

ONLINE RESOURCES/SUGGESTED READINGS

- **Human Respiratory System Best Resources** available at www.onlinenursingprograms.net/resources/respiratory.html
- **Advanced respiratory system physiology** available at www.khanacademy.org/science/health-and-medicine/respiratory-system
- **Anatomy of a child's lung** available at www.pedilung.com/pediatric-lung-diseases-disorders/anatomy-of-a-childs-lung/
- **Effects of ageing on the respiratory system** available at www.msdmanuals.com/en-au/home/lung-and-airway-disorders/biology-of-the-lungs-and-airways/effects-of-aging-on-the-respiratory-system
- **Ageing changes in the lungs** available at https://medlineplus.gov/ency/article/004011.htm

INTRODUCTION

To survive, we are dependent on our ability to absorb oxygen from air and remove carbon dioxide produced during cellular metabolism. The specialised organs and structures of the respiratory system facilitate the movement of gases from the environment to blood and from blood to the environment. By its very nature, the interface between the environment and the respiratory system requires these tissues to possess characteristics that support this activity and reduce the possibility of injury or infection. The functions of the respiratory system include maintenance of acid–base balance in the body and production of speech (phonation), but the primary function is gas transfer and exchange, specifically oxygen and carbon dioxide. For gas transfer to occur, we need to breathe or ventilate the units of lung tissue known as alveoli.

In this chapter we review some of the essential anatomy and physiology of the respiratory system and discuss the integration of the respiratory function and physiology with other body systems such as the cardiovascular system. A thorough knowledge of the structure and normal function of the respiratory system underpins an understanding of the signs and symptoms indicative of conditions of respiratory distress and disease.

THE STRUCTURE AND FUNCTION OF THE RESPIRATORY SYSTEM

The human respiratory system is comprised of specific functional components whose role is to facilitate either air movement—ventilation—or gas exchange—respiration. The respiratory system is divided into the upper and lower respiratory tracts. The **upper respiratory tract** (Fig. 17.1), consisting of the nasal cavity, nasopharynx, oropharynx, laryngopharynx and larynx, is concerned with facilitating the conduction of air in and out of the **lower respiratory tract** (the lungs and associated structures). These tissue components have structures that maintain airway patency and filter and humidify inhaled gases.

Breathing can be oral (through the mouth) or nasal. **Nasal breathing** offers improved filtration and humidification of inhaled air particles. Within the nasal cavity, **olfactory sensors** in the nose detect potentially harmful gases and the hairs called **vibrissae** filter large particles. The **nasal septum** and **turbinates**, collectively known as the **vestibule** (Fig. 17.2), have a large mucosal surface area and blood flow. Vestibular tissue is lined with **pseudostratified ciliated columnar epithelium**, which is rich in goblet cells (Fig. 17.3), sebaceous glands and sweat glands—these provide humidification and add heat and moisture to inhaled gases. Collectively, the structures aid the upper respiratory tract to moisten inhaled air but

also filter and trap inhaled particulate matter in the viscous mucus. The epithelial cilia move in a wavelike motion, which has the effect of moving secretions upwards from the lower respiratory tract. The cellular epithelial features of the upper and lower respiratory tracts help protect us from infection, but the delicate structures can be damaged by noxious gases and toxins, such as tobacco smoke.

With nasal breathing, the turbinates generate turbulent airflow, which maximises the humidification process. Turbulence also increases airflow resistance. In circumstances requiring higher **minute ventilation** (the respiratory rate per minute multiplied by the **tidal volume** in litres), such as with exercise, mouth breathing is preferred. Neonates, however, preferentially nose breathe and hence nasal congestion can have a significant impact on airflow resistance and the effort, or work, of breathing, even at rest.

The cilia and mucus secretion structures in the upper respiratory tract support or protect activities related to breathing by providing a mechanism not only for humidification but also to transport and remove trapped particulate matter out of the respiratory tract. In addition, the presence of lymphoid tissue in the form of the pharyngeal, palatine and lingual tonsils provides a first line of defence against ingested or inhaled foreign pathogens. This tonsillar tissue forms part of the lymphatic defence system. As soon as germs enter through the mouth or nose and encounter the lymphoid tonsils, the immune system is activated. The location of the tonsils is ideal in terms of assisting immune function. Recent evidence suggests that there is an increased long-term risk of respiratory, allergic and infectious diseases if the tonsils and adenoids are removed in childhood,[1] which highlights the interaction between this component of the immune and respiratory systems.

The **pharynx**, more commonly known as the throat, is a passageway that serves both the digestive and respiratory systems. Air enters and leaves the lower respiratory tract via the pharynx through the nose or mouth. Given that this is a common passageway for air, food and drink, several specific muscles are activated on eating and drinking. These muscles, which include the genioglossus and levator veli palatini, comprise the **soft palate** (Fig. 17.2), located posterior to the bony hard palate. During swallowing they contract to elevate and close off the nasopharynx, which prevents nasal reflux. The soft palate plays an important role in speech to produce certain sounds. It also prevents pharyngeal collapse during negative-pressure ventilation (spontaneous breathing) and sleep.[2] Problems with soft palate muscle function may cause snoring and obstructive sleep apnoea.

The **larynx** is important for airway protection and speech. It is composed of cartilaginous and muscular

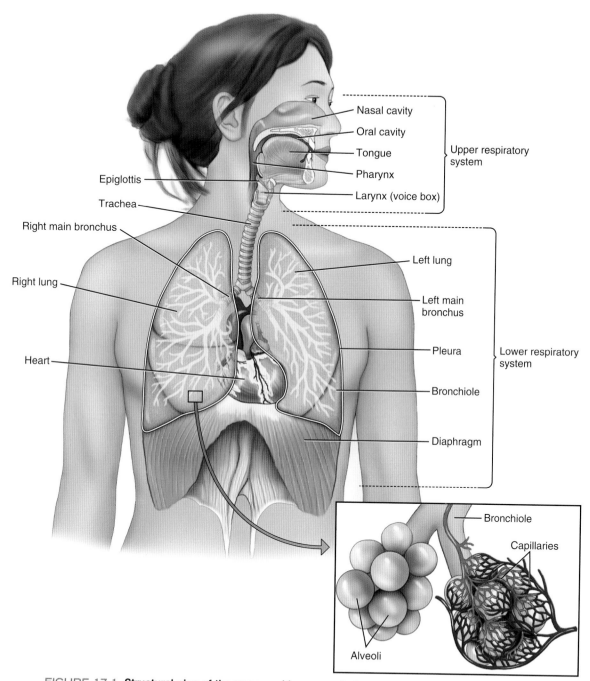

FIGURE 17.1 **Structural plan of the upper and lower respiratory tracts.** (*Source:* Van Meter KC, Hubert RJ. Microbiology for the healthcare professional, 2 ed. Elsevier; 2016.)

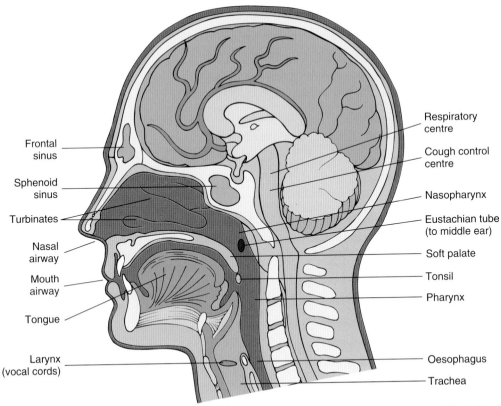

FIGURE 17.2 **Upper respiratory tract.** (*Source:* Willihnganz MJ, Gurevitz SL, Clayton BD. Clayton's basic pharmacology for nurses, 18 ed. Elsevier; 2019.)

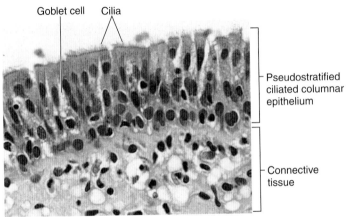

FIGURE 17.3 **Respiratory mucosa.** (*Source:* Patton KT, Thibodeau GA, editors. Anatomy and physiology, 9 ed. London: Elsevier Health Sciences; 2015.)

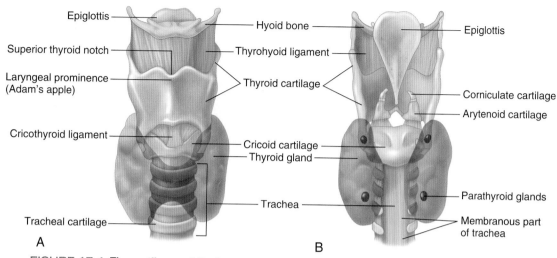

FIGURE 17.4 **The cartilages of the larynx. A** Anterior view. **B** Posterior view. (*Source:* Patton KT, Thibodeau GA. Mosby's handbook of anatomy & physiology, 2 ed. Elsevier; 2014.)

structures to provide support to the conducting airway and prevent closure during breathing. It also contains the 'voice box', more specifically the vocal cords (Fig. 17.2). Perhaps one of the most important structures of the larynx is the **epiglottis**, which is fundamental

to airway protection. The epiglottis is a flexible elastic cartilage (Fig. 17.4) covered with mucous membrane that lies posteriorly to the tongue and is attached to the entrance to the larynx (Fig. 17.5). This anatomical position enables the epiglottis to act as a 'trapdoor'

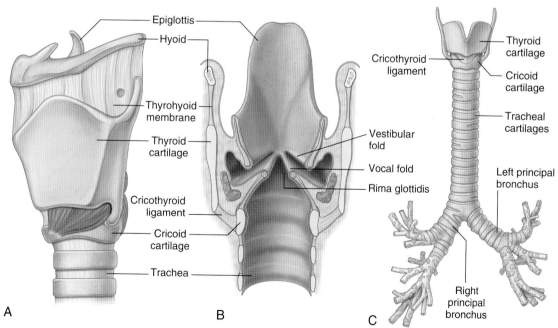

FIGURE 17.5 **The larynx. A** Components of the larynx. **B** Coronal section through the larynx viewed posteriorly showing the position of the vestibular and vocal cords. **C** Anterior aspect of the trachea and principal bronchi. (*Source:* Soames R, Palastanga N. Anatomy and human movement: structure and function, 7 ed. Elsevier; 2019.)

during swallowing to prevent the entry of food and drink into the airway and direct it posteriorly into the oesophagus. The vocal cords and the opening between them, collectively known as the **glottis**, while obviously used in phonation and speech, also have the capacity to seal off the respiratory tract, which is known as effort closure, and allow the performance of the Valsalva manoeuvre and cough. The **Valsalva manoeuvre** and cough involve the generation of an increase in intrathoracic pressure against a closed glottis, which adds to the protective role of this portion of the upper respiratory tract.

The actions of the muscles that comprise the glottis and the larynx have a specific role in inspiration and expiration and are controlled by the tenth cranial nerve, the vagus nerve. The glottis within the larynx is a relatively narrow portion of the airway. The narrower the airway, the more resistance there is to airflow and the more effort is required to breathe. During **inspiration**, the cricoarytenoid muscles abduct the vocal cords to reduce resistance to airflow; during expiration, the thyroarytenoid muscles adduct the vocal cords and increase resistance during expiration. This provides a form of positive intrapulmonary pressure known as intrinsic **positive end-expiratory pressure (PEEP)**. PEEP assists in maintaining opening and inflation of small airways and the alveoli at the end of expiration, which maximises the exchange of oxygen (O_2) and carbon dioxide (CO_2) and reduces the effort required to breathe. The larynx and the point at which the trachea bifurcates (known as the carina) are one of the most sensitive regions of the conducting airways. When chemical, inflammatory or mechanical irritation of nerve endings occurs here, this induces the cough reflex, forcing any particles of foreign matter lodged here out of the respiratory tree through sudden contraction of the diaphragm and intercostal muscles. The interaction between the nervous system and the actions of the small laryngeal muscles, combined with the larger skeletal muscles of respiration, results in the ability to cough, clear and protect the airway.

Below the larynx is the **trachea**, which is the first portion of the lower respiratory tract and **tracheobronchial tree** (Fig. 17.6). The tracheobronchial tree is divided into two zones—the conducting zone and the respiratory zone—based on whether they contain alveoli and can therefore participate in gas exchange. The conducting zone does not contain alveoli and forms a continuous passageway for the movement of air in and out. It is composed of cartilaginous rings and smooth muscle which maintain opening and have the ability to dilate and constrict in response to nervous system

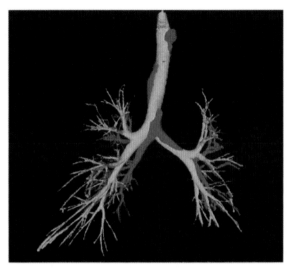

FIGURE 17.6 **The tracheobronchial tree.** Inspiratory and expiratory chest CT scan. Tracheobronchial tree on full inspiration in grey and on end-exhalation from tidal volume in blue. (*Source:* Chen A, Pastis N, Furukawa B, Silvestri GA. The effect of respiratory motion on pulmonary nodule location during electromagnetic navigation bronchoscopy. Chest 2015;147(5):1275–81.)

inputs. Bronchial smooth muscle constriction is caused by parasympathetic nervous system stimulation and leads to excess mucus production. Inflammation and allergic reactions also induce this response. Conversely, bronchial dilation occurs in response to sympathetic stimulation.

The upper portion of the trachea is also lined with ciliated pseudostratified columnar epithelium which supports immunity and lung protection by preventing pathogens from entering the lower respiratory tract. The ciliated mucous tissue acts as an escalator, wafting inhaled trapped foreign particles upwards to the pharynx where they can be swallowed or expectorated. Further down the tracheobronchial tree, the **ciliated pseudostratified columnar epithelium** of the bronchi eventually transitions to simple cuboidal epithelium, then squamous epithelium. This transition to thinner epithelium is important because the thickness of the respiratory membrane directly affects the ability of oxygen and carbon dioxide to move from air to blood and vice versa within alveoli in the respiratory zone. This structure also leads to lower airflow resistance, as inhaled and exhaled air travels in and out of smaller and smaller bronchioles that lead to the alveoli. There is no cartilage in the bronchioles, so they are held open by the volume of air in the lungs. In a healthy person, when lung volume decreases, such as in the supine position or when sitting, these smaller airways become narrowed or collapse, leading to changes in the ability of air to flow in and out of the alveoli. Air flow in the conducting zone during inspiration is fast and turbulent, but as it moves through the distal bronchioles it slows and becomes less turbulent due to the lowered resistance.

The low airflow resistance means the muscle work and energy required to move air in and out of the very small conducting airways during breathing is minimal in normal healthy lungs. Exchange of oxygen or carbon dioxide does not occur in the conducting zone. Instead, this space is filled with air on inspiration and expiration and is therefore known as **anatomical dead space.** As the bronchial tree divides into smaller and smaller bronchioles, they become alveolar ducts which end in alveolar sacs composed of many alveoli surrounded by a fine mesh of capillaries (Fig. 17.7). This is the interface where gas exchange occurs. There are millions of alveoli in our lungs: in adults the surface area for gas exchange is estimated to be almost the size of a tennis court. The proximity of the pulmonary capillaries to the alveoli facilitates gas exchange.

The alveoli and pulmonary capillaries are separated by a thin membrane known as the respiratory membrane across which gas transfer can occur (Fig. 17.8). The alveolar and pulmonary capillary walls are only a single cell layer thick. Each alveolar sac structure is surrounded by multiple pulmonary capillaries, with the two structures separated by the thin **respiratory membrane.** This membrane facilitates maximum exposure of deoxygenated blood to the air in each alveolus. This is known as **ventilation perfusion matching (V/Q),** which is essential if gas exchange is to occur efficiently and at a rate that meets the body's metabolic demand for oxygen and removal of carbon dioxide.

The pulmonary blood vessels that surround each alveolus can reflexively constrict in response to **hypoxia,** a response known as **hypoxic pulmonary vasoconstriction (HPV)** that is unique to the pulmonary circulation. In hypoxia, which is low partial pressure of inspired oxygen (PO_2), the reflex contraction of vascular smooth muscle in the pulmonary circulation diverts blood away from alveoli that are poorly ventilated towards alveoli that are better ventilated.[3] Hence, deoxygenated blood is 'shunted'

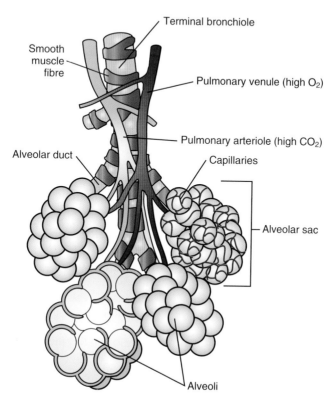

FIGURE 17.7 **The terminal bronchioles and alveoli.** (*Source:* Colville T, Bassert JM, Clinical anatomy and physiology for veterinary technicians, 3 ed. Elsevier; 2016.)

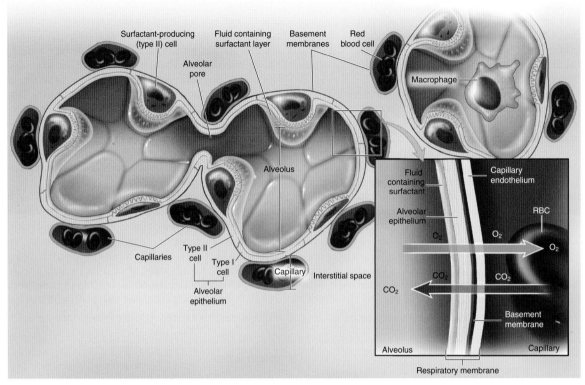

FIGURE 17.8 Gas exchange between the alveoli and pulmonary capillaries. (*Source:* Patton KT, Thibodeau GA, editors. Anatomy and physiology, 9 ed. London: Elsevier Health Sciences; 2015.)

towards alveoli that have a higher PO_2, improving the matching of ventilation to perfusion, and improve the uptake of oxygen by haemoglobin in red blood cells. This is opposite to the normal response to hypoxia of the systemic vasculature, which typically vasodilates in response to low PO_2 to increase blood flow to the area to alleviate hypoxia. It is worth noting at this stage that lungs also require oxygen for function and that oxygen supply is delivered by the bronchial artery.

Each alveolus is composed mainly of **thin squamous epithelial cells (type I pneumocytes)** and to a lesser extent **type II pneumocytes**, which produce a substance known as surfactant. Surfactant reduces the surface tension of fluid, which is the propensity of water molecules to attract each other, so that the alveoli don't collapse and close. If we didn't have surfactant, each exhalation would result in alveolar collapse, and each inhalation would require significant effort to reinflate the collapsed alveoli. This is not dissimilar to trying to inflate a balloon: initially it is very difficult, but as the balloon fills with some air, it gets easier to inflate.

Another specialised cell in the alveoli is the **alveolar macrophage** (Fig. 17.8). This immune cell ingests and removes inhaled pathogens and prevents them from causing injury or infection in the alveoli. Because we breathe air, our lungs are always exposed to the external environment, including microorganisms, so the presence of immune cells at the interface between the body and the environment is vital in the early activation of an immune response to an injurious or pathogenic invader.

Breathing

How we breathe is controlled by highly regulated and integrated processes involving the nervous, cardiovascular, musculoskeletal and respiratory systems. Understanding the structure of the respiratory system is fundamental in understanding the physiology of respiration. Respiration is a term that refers to both the movement and exchange of gases in the lungs—**external respiration**—and the exchange of gases in the tissues and cells—**internal respiration** and **cellular respiration**, respectively (Fig. 17.9).

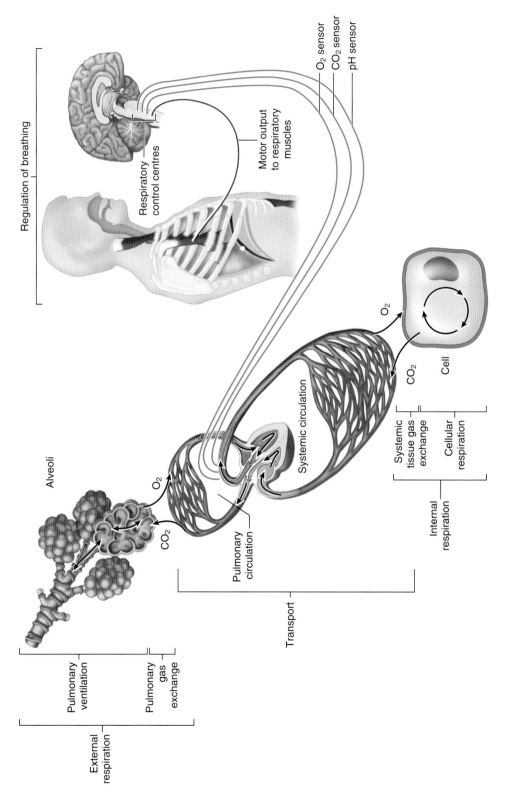

Regulation of breathing

Respiratory control centres

Motor output to respiratory muscles

O_2 sensor
CO_2 sensor
pH sensor

Alveoli

O_2

CO_2

Pulmonary circulation

Systemic circulation

O_2

CO_2

Cell

Systemic tissue gas exchange

Cellular respiration

Internal respiration

Transport

Pulmonary ventilation

Pulmonary gas exchange

External respiration

FIGURE 17.9 Regulation of breathing and the physiology of respiration. (*Source*: Patton KT, Thibodeau GA, editors. Anatomy and physiology; 9 ed. London: Elsevier Health Sciences; 2015.)

The integrated work of the nervous, cardiovascular, haematological and respiratory systems is vital to the uptake and delivery of oxygen to the tissues and cells, to the transport and removal of the by-product of aerobic respiration (carbon dioxide) and to maintain the balance and control of the pH of blood and body fluids. With normal cellular function and human metabolism, small alterations in blood pH are normal, but if the blood pH becomes too acidic (known as **acidaemia**) or too basic (known as **alkalaemia**), it affects the enzymatic activities in the cell, which then negatively affects cellular and organ function. Through its interactions with special sensory neurons in the nervous system, the respiratory system can directly alter the blood pH by changing the rate and depth of breathing.

Control of breathing

Movement of air in and out of the lungs is controlled by several factors. These include nervous system inputs, which are activated by special sensory neurons located in the carotid artery and the aorta. The neurons, which form part of the parasympathetic division of the autonomic nervous system, extend from the brain stem directly to the inner surface of these two arteries. The nerve fibres concerned are the glossopharyngeal and vagus nerves, which are known as cranial nerves because they extend directly from the brain rather than from the spinal cord. The carotid and aortic sensory nerve endings, or carotid and aortic bodies, are very sensitive to changes in blood pH and levels of carbon dioxide and oxygen in the blood. If the blood pH falls, blood becomes more acidic; if blood carbon dioxide rises, the sensory nerves will be activated, causing an increase in nerve impulse transmission to the muscles of the respiratory system. This feedback mechanism means that as our metabolic rate increases, so too does the level of aerobic activity in the cells to generate more energy to meet cellular activity. The net effect of this increase in metabolic activity and aerobic metabolism is the production of more carbon dioxide and the lowering of pH. The neurons sense this rise in carbon dioxide and lowering in pH, which initiates a rise in respiratory muscle activity to increase the rate of removal of excess carbon dioxide and return the pH to normal.

The oxygen cascade

Our cells depend on receiving an adequate supply of oxygen because it is only when oxygen is present in cells that the maximum amount of adenosine triphosphate (ATP) can be produced in the mitochondria. If oxygen becomes unavailable, the production of ATP from oxidative phosphorylation stops. Oxidative phosphorylation is a process of aerobic metabolism that generates energy through a series of chemical reactions in the inner membrane of mitochondria to create ATP and during carbohydrate breakdown produces almost 90% of the ATP required for cells to function. A deficiency in oxygen quickly leads to inadequate ATP production to meet the homeostatic requirements of cells and results in the increased production of lactic acid via anaerobic glycolysis (the production of ATP from glucose in the absence of oxygen). The **oxygen cascade** describes the transfer of oxygen from the air to the mitochondria in the cells. Oxygen delivery to the systemic tissues relies on the passive movement of gas along decreasing partial pressure gradients, where at each step in the cascade (Fig. 17.10) the partial pressure of oxygen (PO_2) falls. The important point to remember here is that oxygen is important for normal cellular function and it is partial pressure that determines the rate and extent of gas transfer (Fig. 17.11).

Carbon dioxide transport

Blood pH is determined by the amount of H^+ in solution; the more carbon dioxide we produce or retain, the more the following equation moves to the right. This is expressed by the chemical equation $CO_2 + H_2O \Leftrightarrow H_2CO_3 \Leftrightarrow H^+ + HCO_3^-$. The equation moves from left to right in tissue cells because as we use oxygen to produce energy, this produces carbon dioxide as a by-product. When carbon dioxide is transported to the lungs dissolved in blood and bound to haemoglobin, then exposed to ventilated alveoli, the equation moves from right to left because carbon dioxide leaves the red blood cells and enters the alveoli where it can be exhaled. In the alveoli the oxygen from air then binds to the haemoglobin molecule.

When carbon dioxide is produced in the tissues, it diffuses from the tissues into the red blood cells, where it mostly dissociates to form hydrogen ions (H^+) and bicarbonate ions (HCO_3^-). Red blood cell haemoglobin molecules transport most carbon dioxide in the form of HCO_3^- (Fig. 17.12); carbon dioxide is carried to the lungs where it is exhaled either:

- dissolved as HCO_3^- ions in plasma
- dissolved as CO_2 in plasma
- bound to haemoglobin molecules as carbamino-haemoglobin (haemoglobin CO_2) and haemoglobin.

In normal physiology, it is the use of oxygen in aerobic respiration to produce energy (in the form of ATP) that leads to the by-product of carbon dioxide, which is responsible for 'driving' ventilation, the movement of air in and out of the lungs.

Dry atmospheric gas	• Air is comprised mostly of 79% nitrogen and 21% oxygen • Atmospheric partial pressure of oxygen is a function of the barometric pressure of air • At sea level, the barometric pressure of air is 760 mmHg; therefore the partial pressure of oxygen at sea level is equal to 21% of 760 = 159 mmHg
Humidified tracheal gas	• As we breathe in, air is heated and moisturised, which means water vapour is added which reduces the total partial pressure of inspired oxygen • Water vapour has a partial pressure of almost 50 mmHg
Alveolar gas	• By the time the air breathed in at sea level reaches the alveolus, the partial pressure of oxygen has fallen to between 100 and 105 mmHg
Arterial blood	• Oxygen diffuses from the alveolus into the pulmonary capillary blood leading to a normal arterial PO_2 of 80–100 mmHg
Systemic cells Mitochondria	• Depending on metabolic demand, the PO_2 in the cells is between 20 and 40 mmHg • In the mitochondria, oxygen is continually used in the process of aerobic cellular respiration • The PO_2 here is typically between 5 and 20 mmHg, so oxygen readily diffuses down along this pressure gradient from the arterial blood into the cells
Venous blood	• The result is a decrease in PO_2 in arterial blood from 80–100 mmHg to a PO_2 of approximately 40 mmHg where, when it returns to the lungs, the partial pressure rises again due to the higher PO_2 in the alveoli

FIGURE 17.10 **The steps of the oxygen cascade.**

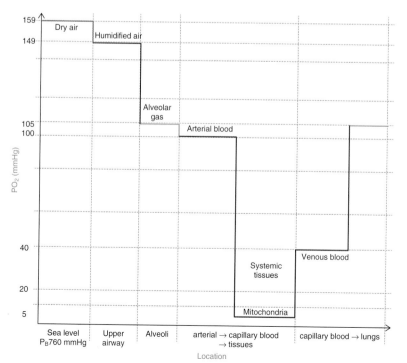

FIGURE 17.11 **The oxygen cascade.** As oxygenated blood travels through the systemic circulation where the tissue PO_2 is low, oxygen diffuses along this partial pressure gradient into the cells. (*Source:* Adapted from Lambertz M, Hsia C, Schmitz A, Lambertz M, Perry S, Maina J. Evolution of air breathing: oxygen homeostasis and the transitions from water to land and sky. Comprehensive Physiol 3(2):849–915.)

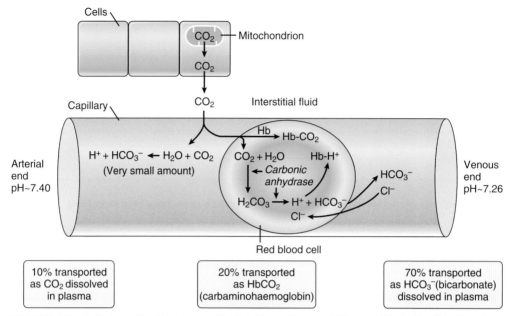

FIGURE 17.12 Carbon dioxide transport in the blood. (*Source:* O'Connell TX, Pedigo RA, Blair TE. Crush step 1: the ultimate USMLE step 1 review, 2 ed. Elsevier; 2018.)

In the haematological system, haemoglobin molecules within red blood cells have specific properties that promote the uptake of oxygen in the lungs, transporting and releasing oxygen to the tissues. The ability to bind to and release oxygen is represented by the oxyhaemoglobin dissociation curve, which demonstrates that as PO_2 rises, haemoglobin develops a higher affinity to bind with it; and as PO_2 falls, so too does the affinity of haemoglobin to bond to oxygen (Figs 17.13 and 17.14). The characteristics of haemoglobin molecules

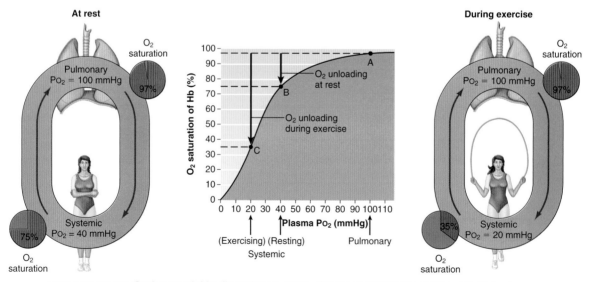

FIGURE 17.13 Oxyhaemoglobin dissociation curve. (*Source:* Adapted from Patton KT, Thibodeau GA, editors. Anatomy and physiology, 9 ed. London: Elsevier Health Sciences; 2015.)

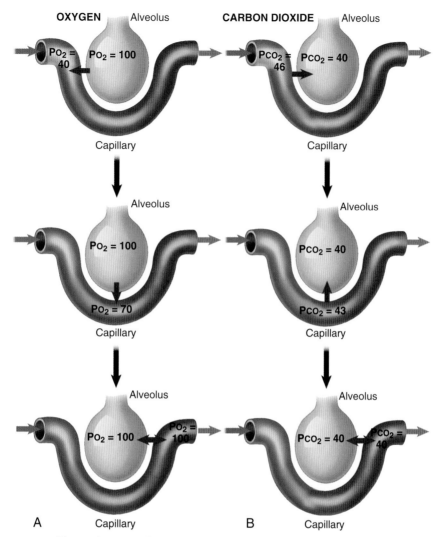

FIGURE 17.14 The exchange and partial pressure changes of oxygen and carbon dioxide between the lungs and systemic tissues. (*Source:* Adapted from Patton KT, Thibodeau GA, editors. Anatomy and physiology, 7 ed. London: Elsevier Health Sciences; 2010.)

are such that the sigmoid shape of the oxyhaemoglobin dissociation curve offers several physiological advantages. The plateau between points B and A in Fig. 17.13 means that the amount of oxygen in the blood remains high even if the partial pressure falls, and the steep section below point B demonstrates that a large amount of oxygen can still be delivered to the tissues with only a small drop in PO_2. This means that when there is an increase in oxygen demand, such as when exercising, the rate of oxygen delivery to the systemic tissues can still

be maintained because the pressure gradient between the capillary blood and the systemic tissues is steep, as illustrated in Fig. 17.13.

The movement of air

What causes air to enter and leave the lungs? The right and left lungs are surrounded by a dual-layered serous membrane called the pleura. The outer membrane (**parietal pleura**) attaches to the inner surface of the thoracic cage, while the inner membrane (**visceral pleura**)

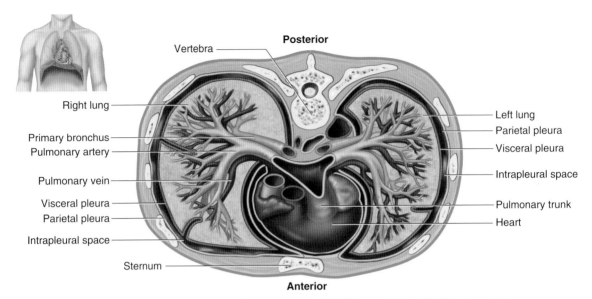

FIGURE 17.15 **The lungs and pleura (transverse section).** (*Source:* Patton KT, Thibodeau GA, editors. Anatomy and physiology, 9 ed. London: Elsevier Health Sciences; 2015.)

encloses the lung tissue itself (Fig. 17.15). Between these two layers is serous fluid, a lubricant, that decreases the friction each time the lungs expand and contract. Contraction and relaxation of the muscles of respiration cause several important changes to pressures in the intrathoracic cavity. The structure of the thoracic cavity with the ribs and sternum anteriorly, the spine posteriorly and the diaphragm inferiorly creates and surrounds a space that expands and contracts with the movement of respiratory muscles.

Inspiration

During **inspiration**, the diaphragm—which is enervated by phrenic nerves from C3, C4 and C5—and the external intercostal muscles contract. When this occurs, the diaphragm pushes the intra-abdominal contents down, increasing the thoracic volume and generating a negative intra-pleural and intrathoracic pressure. The external intercostals, enervated by intercostal nerves from the same spinal level, pull the ribs upwards and outwards, which increases the thoracic volume, creating a negative pressure. Provided the diaphragm is intact, reduced functional ability of the external intercostals does not have a dramatic effect on inspiration. In hyperventilation, there are additional, or accessory, muscles to assist in the movement of the thoracic cage. Accessory muscles include the sternocleidomastoid and the scalene, which elevate the sternum and the first two

ribs, respectively. When the external intercostal muscles and the diaphragm contract, the increase in thoracic volume causes a decreased air pressure within the lungs (**intrapulmonary pressure**). The fall in intrapulmonary pressure below atmospheric pressure creates a gradient, causing air to flow into the lungs along this gradient.

Expiration

For **expiration** to occur the respiratory muscles must relax and the rib cage return to its resting position, which decreases the volume of the thoracic cage, causing a rise in intrapulmonary pressure above atmospheric pressure, and air flows out along the pressure gradient. During quiet breathing, the elastic recoil of the lungs and thoracic tissues means that expiration is a passive process requiring little energy. However, expiration becomes an active process when ventilation requirements are high, such as during exercise or an increased metabolic rate. In this situation the abdominal wall muscles (rectus abdominis, internal oblique, external oblique and transversus abdominis) contract and force the diaphragm up by raising intra-abdominal pressure. In addition, the internal intercostals contract, pulling the ribs downwards and inwards, further decreasing thoracic volume. The movement of the thoracic cage and respiratory muscles creates negative and positive pressure changes with respect to atmospheric pressure and this is why ventilation of the

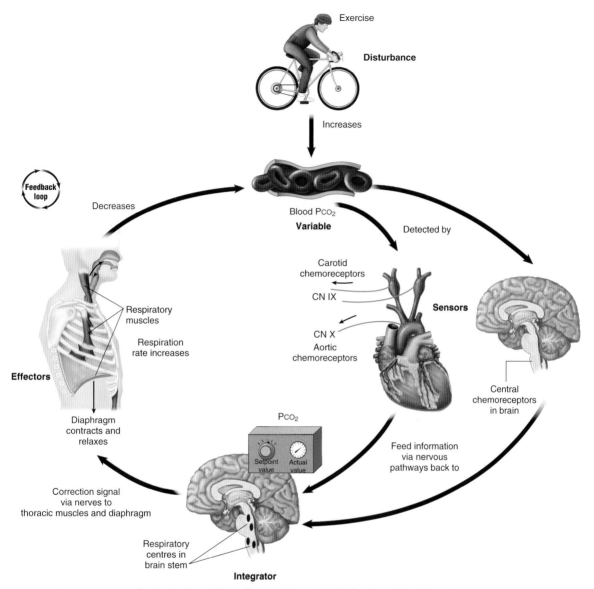

FIGURE 17.16 **Control of breathing.** (*Source:* Patton KT, Thibodeau GA, editors. Anatomy and physiology, 9 ed. London: Elsevier Health Sciences; 2015.)

alveoli occurs, hence the uptake of oxygen and removal of carbon dioxide from the blood.

When chemoreceptors are stimulated by low pH, elevated carbon dioxide levels or low oxygen levels, they initiate activation of the respiratory muscles to generate the changes in intrapulmonary pressure that result in ventilation. This interaction between the nervous, respiratory and musculoskeletal systems in effect assists in

oxygen uptake by the red blood cells and regulates blood pH levels. However, as shown in Fig. 17.16 it is not only the levels of oxygen and carbon dioxide or the blood pH that influences ventilation. The cortex and the limbic system as well as receptors in skeletal muscle also influence the activities of the respiratory muscles via the respiratory control centre located in the brain stem, specifically in the pons and the medulla. This is why in highly emotional states or during periods of increased skeletal muscle activity, the respiratory rate can rise. The cortical and limbic influences can stimulate increased sympathetic nervous system output (Fig. 17.17),[4] resulting in the release of hormones from the adrenal medulla (adrenaline [epinephrine] in particular) that act to increase not only the respiratory rate but also the heart rate, resulting in increased cardiac output and therefore increased transport of oxygen to the tissues and transport of carbon dioxide for removal. Adrenaline (epinephrine)

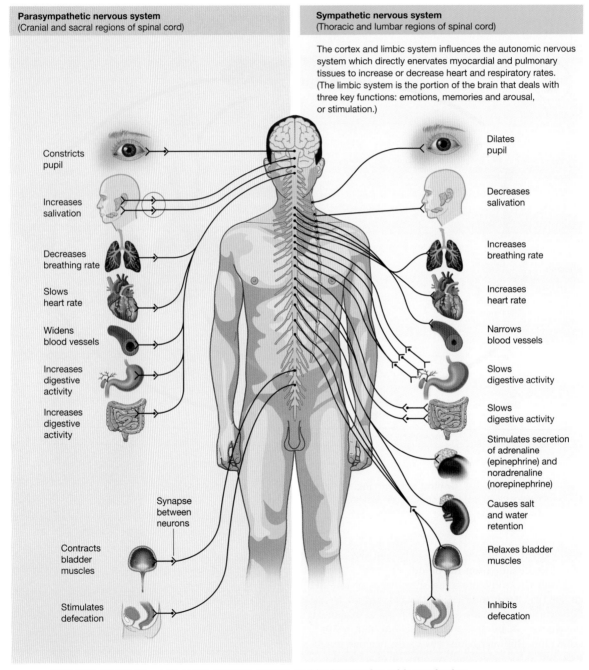

Parasympathetic nervous system
(Cranial and sacral regions of spinal cord)

Constricts pupil

Increases salivation

Decreases breathing rate

Slows heart rate

Widens blood vessels

Increases digestive activity

Increases digestive activity

Synapse between neurons

Contracts bladder muscles

Stimulates defecation

Sympathetic nervous system
(Thoracic and lumbar regions of spinal cord)

The cortex and limbic system influences the autonomic nervous system which directly enervates myocardial and pulmonary tissues to increase or decrease heart and respiratory rates. (The limbic system is the portion of the brain that deals with three key functions: emotions, memories and arousal, or stimulation.)

Dilates pupil

Decreases salivation

Increases breathing rate

Increases heart rate

Narrows blood vessels

Slows digestive activity

Slows digestive activity

Stimulates secretion of adrenaline (epinephrine) and noradrenaline (norepinephrine)

Causes salt and water retention

Relaxes bladder muscles

Inhibits defecation

FIGURE 17.17 **The autonomic nervous system and its integration with respiration.**

also increases the diameter of the bronchioles by relaxing bronchial smooth muscle, which reduces the resistance to airflow associated with higher respiratory rates.

The nervous system is integrated with the respiratory system through a number of sensory inputs that include chemoreceptors located centrally in the brain stem and peripherally in the aortic arch and carotid bodies. There are also pulmonary stretch receptors, mechanoreceptors, which reduce the respiratory rate by initiating the Hering–Breuer reflex via the vagus nerve. Mechanoreceptors are also located in the joints, tendons and muscles of the chest wall. Within the alveoli are receptors known as juxta-pulmonary capillary receptors, or J receptors, which respond to increased interstitial fluid that may occur in conditions such as heart failure, infection or asthma, or in allergic responses. These sensors respond to chemicals released by immune cells such as mast cells and leucocytes when an inflammatory response is activated.

The lungs also have a role in the regulation of blood pressure. Breathing, or pulmonary ventilation, occurs due to the contraction and relaxation of the muscles of respiration. During inspiration, the negative intrathoracic pressure that facilitates the inward flow of air also promotes the venous flow of blood from the peripheries to the central circulation and back to the heart. In this way, breathing promotes venous return and assists with the filling of the right atria and ventricle prior to contraction. This is similar in effect to the action of the lower limb skeletal muscles when they contract and promote venous flow back towards the heart through a 'muscle pump' action.

In addition, located within the endothelial cells of the pulmonary capillaries is **angiotensin converting enzyme (ACE)**, which is responsible for the conversion of angiotensin I to angiotensin II, a potent vasoconstrictor and hormone that stimulates the release of aldosterone to increase sodium and water retention by the kidneys. In this way, the lungs interact with the endocrine system (Fig. 17.18). When renal perfusion is reduced, this stimulates the renal release of renin, which triggers the cascade of reactions that result in the production of

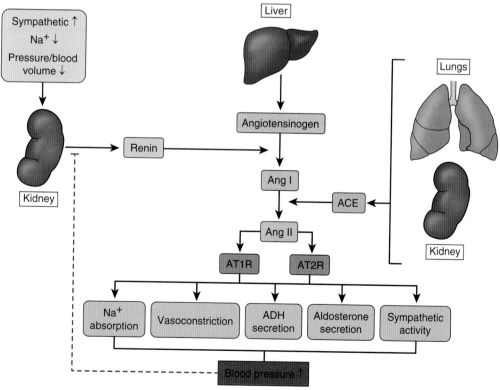

FIGURE 17.18 **The role of the lungs in the renin-angiotensin-aldosterone system (RAAS) for regulating aldosterone secretion.** (*Source:* Sidawy AN, Perler BA. Rutherford's vascular surgery and endovascular therapy, 9 ed. Elsevier; 2019.)

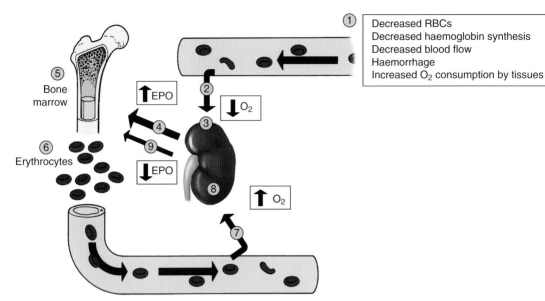

FIGURE 17.19 **Hypoxia and erythropoietin.** Decreased arterial oxygen levels (1) result in decreased tissue oxygen (hypoxia) (2) that stimulates the kidneys (3) to increase production of erythropoietin (4). Erythropoietin is carried to the bone marrow (5) and binds to erythropoietin receptors on precursor red blood cells (proerythroblasts), resulting in increased red cell production and maturation and expansion of the erythrocyte population (6). The increased release of red cells into the circulation frequently corrects the hypoxia in the tissues (7). Perception of normal oxygen levels (8) by the kidneys causes diminished production of erythropoietin (negative feedback) (9) and return to normal levels of erythrocyte production. (*Source:* Huether K, McCance S. Pathophysiology: the biologic basis for disease in adults and children, 7 ed. St Louis: Elsevier; 2015.)

angiotensin I. When angiotensin I circulates in the blood to the lungs, it is converted by ACE to angiotensin II.

Another area where respiratory system function directly interacts with the endocrine system is in the production of erythropoietin (EPO). Lack of oxygen (hypoxia) is a stimulus for the synthesis of EPO, primarily in the kidneys. If oxygen levels decrease, the kidneys detect and release increasing amounts of EPO, which stimulates red bone marrow to accelerate its production of reticulocytes (immature red blood cells). The oxygen capacity of the blood increases with the enhanced erythropoiesis. There are extra-renal sites (such as the liver, brain and skin) that also contribute to the control of renal EPO synthesis but in particular the kidneys respond to hypoxia in a negative feedback loop (Fig. 17.19). With an increase in red blood cells, the oxygen-carrying capacity of the blood increases and oxygen delivery to tissues increases, which leads to a reduction in EPO production and consequently less red bone marrow stimulation for red blood cell production.[5] The concept map in Fig. 17.20 summarises the stimulatory and inhibitory influences on breathing.

INTEGRATION OF THE RESPIRATORY SYSTEM WITH OTHER BODY SYSTEMS

All body cells and tissues depend on adequate supply of oxygen and efficient removal of carbon dioxide, but the extent to which cells depend on oxygen differs. For example, cartilage and chondrocytes require a very low amount of oxygen; in contrast, cells that make up the heart and brain can survive only minutes without oxygen. Without intact structure and function of the respiratory system to uptake and transport oxygen and carbon dioxide, cardiovascular and nervous system function would be significantly impaired.

Integumentary system

Adequate perfusion with oxygen via blood circulation results in adequate nourishment of the skin. This large organ is highly vascularised and reflects whether oxygen is perfusing well to the tissue peripheries. For example, in the absence of adequate oxygen perfusion due to impaired lung function, skin often appears cyanotic or blue. In contrast, increased delivery of oxygenated blood, such as during inflammation, is evident as red, flushed

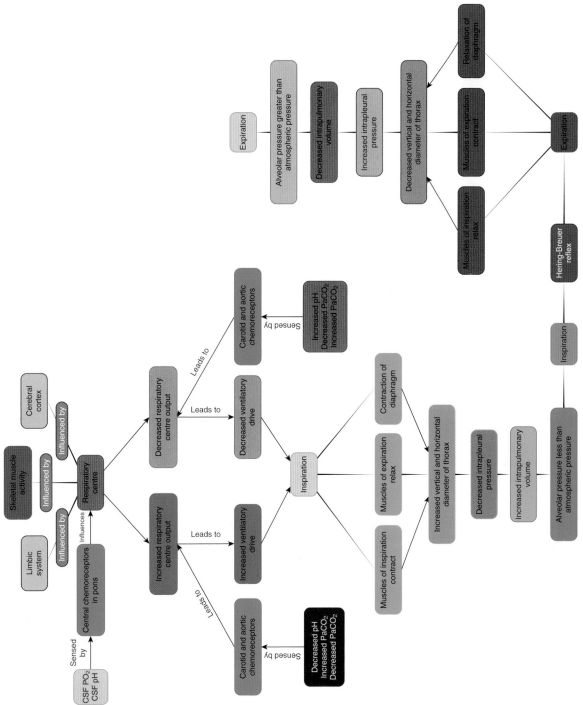

FIGURE 17.20 **Concept map depicting the stimulation and inhibition of ventilation.**

skin. Pollutant air particles, including tobacco,[6] that a person breathes in are significantly correlated to extrinsic (visible) signs of skin ageing, such as pigment spots and wrinkles.

Musculoskeletal system

Our ability to sit, walk, run and stretch depends on effective communication between muscles, bones and the nervous system and the delivery of adequate oxygen and nutrient supplies to the tissues needed to coordinate these functions. As demonstrated earlier, oxygen supply is heavily dependent on a functional respiratory system. Thus, any disease affecting the transport of oxygen from the air into the body (such as diseases affecting the surface area in the lungs needed for adequate air exchange) will automatically impact on the delivery of oxygen to the rest of the body, including the muscles.

Nervous system

Neuronal cells in the brain require a high level of oxygen and nutrients to function effectively and cannot survive long without oxygen supply. If oxygen delivery decreases, such as during transient constrictions of the blood vessels in the brain, the affected individual will display clear signs of confusion. In cases of chronic respiratory diseases that affect the delivery of oxygen from the air into the tissues, there will be a degree of adjustment to these changes, but control of nervous system function will ensure that the brain receives adequate oxygen supplies.

Cardiovascular system

As noted above, the cardiovascular system collaborates closely with the respiratory system to deliver oxygen to cells and remove carbon dioxide. Thus the functionality of the respiratory system has a direct impact on the function of the structural components of the cardiovascular system. For example, cardiac cells (cardiomyocytes) have a high metabolic demand and use oxygen through aerobic metabolism to facilitate heart contraction following electrical stimulation received from the sinoatrial node. Reduced oxygen supply—through vascular obstruction or loss of function at the respiratory membrane site—means that cardiomyocytes experience cellular stress and therefore cannot effectively react to the electrical impulse. Furthermore, prolonged deprivation of oxygen quickly results in cardiomyocyte death and loss of function. In the most severe case, deprivation of oxygen to the self-paced cells of the sinoatrial node would lead to the person's death as there is no ability to generate an impulse. Blood vessels, like all tissues, need oxygen to live and function. What is not commonly known is that blood vessels have their own blood supply through a network of small vessels known as the vasa vasorum. Similar to other tissues, obstruction of the vasa vasorum will lead to death of the vessel it supplies and therefore loss of function of that vessel.

Endocrine system

The endocrine system can be thought of as a regulator and the integrator of physiological functions needed to maintain homeostasis, thus ensuring internal adaptations to changes that occur in the body or the external environment, such as a change in temperature. This regulation is delivered through complex networks regulated by hormones, the chemical substances released by endocrine glands and organs. Hormones have a high potency and simultaneously act on a range of bodily functions; this effect is mediated by a tightly defined set of negative and positive feedback loops that span several body systems (Chapter 10). Endocrine glands are heavily vascularised. This should not be surprising considering they predominantly exert their effects via hormones released into the blood circulation. This vascularisation also serves the oxygen and nutritional needs of endocrine glands and the removal of metabolic waste. Subsequently, if oxygen delivery is impaired, this will affect the capacity of the endocrine structures to perform their functions. What is also worth mentioning is that components of the endocrine system can affect how oxygen is consumed, thus indirectly affecting the demand on the respiratory system. For example, thyroxine, a hormone secreted into the bloodstream by the thyroid gland, stimulates oxidative metabolism in cells and increases oxygen consumption and heat production of most tissues.

Blood and haemostasis

Earlier it was described that the kidneys can sense a low amount of oxygen in the blood and produce erythropoietin in response. This hormone acts on the haematopoietic stem cells in bone marrow to induce commitment to the red blood cell lineage and stimulate increased production of red blood cells that then pick up whatever oxygen may be available at the respiratory membrane site and deliver it at the tissue level. Little is known of the effect of oxygen on platelets and overall activity of the coagulation system to form a thrombus. However, very old data examining animals exposed to high levels of oxygen suggest that exposure to too much oxygen decreased coagulation ability. No information was identified on the effect of low oxygen levels on white blood cell production and the function of these cells in immunity. However, it is thought that tissue hypoxia experienced during wound injury stimulates release of some immune cell mediators (cytokines) that then participate in the cascade aimed at resolving tissue injury.

Lymphatic system

Lymphatic vessels collect tissue fluid that is thought to contain low levels of oxygen. To date there is no evidence that any part of the lymphatic system contains the equivalent of vasa vasorum in either humans or animals. Therefore, the effect of impaired respiratory function in terms of oxygen delivery and carbon dioxide uptake on the lymphatic system is yet to be delineated.

Gastrointestinal system

The gastrointestinal and respiratory systems share some common structures. These include the mouth, oropharynx, laryngopharynx and epiglottis. While it may seem that the two systems are disparate, they function together in several ways. The digestive tract requires peristalsis—muscular contractions—to break up food and move it along the intestine. Smooth muscle requires oxygen to perform this function. Oxygen is also required by other cells in the gastrointestinal tract to perform the chemical reactions needed to break down complex carbohydrates, fats and proteins. Similarly, the gastrointestinal system provides energy derived from digested food to respiratory muscle cells (such as those of the diaphragm and intercostal muscles) and other cell populations within the respiratory system so that breathing can take place.

Urinary system

The links between the urinary and respiratory systems are multifaceted. For example, the respiratory system is responsible for oxygen delivery to and the removal of metabolic waste from the cells that constitute the organs of these systems. Furthermore, in addition to regulating the secretion of EPO in the presence of hypoxia, these systems play a crucial role in maintaining blood pH as described above in the section on breathing. Effective communication between the systems is regulated by the endocrine system through secretion of hormones such as aldosterone and ACE that regulate kidney filtration and therefore urine excretion by the urinary system.

Reproductive system

The reproductive system is composed of primary and secondary reproductive organs that have the same dependency on oxygen as any other vascularised tissue.

However, what is different is that the female reproductive system is responsible for the development of a fetus. As the fetus grows (Chapter 22), anatomical and physiological changes occur in the respiratory system to meet the increasing oxygen and metabolic demands of the mother, the placenta and the growing fetus. As the pregnant uterus grows and changes shape, it pushes the diaphragm above its usual position. The chest cavity adapts by increasing the transverse diameter of the chest, which results in a decreased thoracic cavity. The lungs adjust to this new space and modify breathing function to meet demand. Pregnancy-related hormonal changes, such as the release of progesterone and relaxin, assist these changes by softening lung cartilaginous joints, which permits increased flexibility of the chest wall and expansion of the chest outwards. Progesterone modifies bronchial and tracheal airway resistance, the result being reduced work of breathing. Significantly, during pregnancy progesterone enhances sensitivity to carbon dioxide in the respiratory centre and lowers the threshold for carbon dioxide levels, which may contribute to the pregnant woman's feelings of shortness of breath.

AGE-RELATED CHANGES

When a baby is born prematurely, its lungs are unable to produce lung surfactant, which provides surface tension and maintains the lung alveoli open. This leads to an inability to expand the lungs and breathe in oxygen and exhale carbon dioxide. Medical intervention is needed to help these babies to survive. Babies born after 30 weeks of gestation have a capacity to produce lung surfactant. Premature babies are also at risk of ceasing to breathe. This is known as apnoea of prematurity. Those born before 28 weeks of gestation have an almost 100% risk of apnoea, whereas those born after 34 weeks are much less likely to develop it.[7]

At birth, the newborn's lungs can expand and inhale and exhale air just as an adult does. However, structural differences exist. For example, the ribs in infants and young children are positioned more horizontally than in older children and adults. Rib cartilage in children is also more elastic and flexible, while the intercostal muscles are not developed to their full capacity. As infants and young children have larger heads than adults, this can cause their necks to flex and partially obstruct the airways.[8] The internal diameter of children's airways tends to increase in size as they get older but the airways are more prone to obstruction due to their high elasticity. Infants also have a high respiratory rate which decreases as they get older to match that of adults by the time they reach adolescence (12–20 breaths per minute).

As adults age, there are changes in the structure and function of the intercostal muscles, ribs, spine and lungs. Muscles become weaker, which impacts on how the diaphragm expands, while bones become thinner and tend to change shape. Changes in muscles also impact airway structures, resulting in structures more prone to collapsing, while the alveoli tend to change shape and become less efficient at air exchange.[9] Nerves innervating the lungs and that trigger the cough reflex can also become less sensitive, leading to reduced capacity to expel germs and pollutants. The breathing centre also declines in function, which may affect how oxygen and carbon dioxide are exchanged. Smoking and lack of exercise accelerate age-related changes in the lungs, while smoking also increases the risk of developing respiratory diseases and lung cancer.

CONCLUSION

The respiratory system is intimately connected with and regulated by complex interactions between the involuntary or autonomic nervous system, via special sensors within the blood vessels, the brain and skeletal muscles, and the voluntary nervous system via cortical and limbic structures. Normal control of breathing is highly regulated, not only to ensure adequate uptake of oxygen from the air but also to help maintain the normal pH of blood and body fluids. In circumstances where the homeostatic balance of oxygen and carbon dioxide shifts, numerous cardiovascular, nervous and endocrine responses are stimulated to induce smooth muscle, vasomotor and ventilatory responses that act to increase the diameter of the airways and the rate and depth of ventilation, as well as to maximise the matching of perfusion to the ventilation of the alveoli. The respiratory system, not unlike the gastrointestinal and integumentary systems, is continuously exposed to environmental threats such as airborne toxins, viruses and bacteria, so it is not surprising that within the complex structure of this system there are elements of the first lines of immune defence to protect and prevent injury and loss of homeostasis. After all, the ability to breathe, to take up oxygen from the air, is fundamental to the very survival of every cell and system in our body.

CASE STUDY 17.1

Every year, many tourists fly into Lukla in Nepal from Kathmandu on their way to Everest Base Camp. Lukla sits at an altitude of 2860 metres. At this altitude there is 72% of the oxygen available at sea level, which with normal lung function means a PO_2 in the arterial blood of 57 mmHg. By the time trekkers have reached Everest Base Camp they will have climbed to 5380 metres where there is only 53% of the oxygen normally available at sea level,[10] meaning the blood oxygen level will have fallen to 45 mmHg. Many trekkers experience difficulties in breathing at this altitude.

Q1. Transport of oxygen from the air into the bloodstream occurs through:

    a. lung alveolar capillaries.

    b. carotid artery.

    c. coronary sinus.

    d. phrenic nerve.

Q2. Diffusion of oxygen from the air into the bloodstream is due to:

    a. decrease in blood pH.

    b. increase in blood pH.

    c. increased permeability of bronchial epithelial cells.

    d. difference in the partial pressure of oxygen between the air and the bloodstream.

Q3. Oxygen is transported by red blood cells through the bloodstream predominantly:

    a. bound to albumin.

    b. bound to haemoglobin molecules to form oxyhaemoglobin.

    c. bound to bicarbonate ions.

    d. as free oxygen molecules.

Q4. Explain how the respiratory system of a trekker arriving in Lukla to commence a trek to Everest Base Camp will respond in this environment.

Q5. What responses could be expected from the cardiovascular, nervous and endocrine systems?

CASE STUDY 17.2

The lungs of a baby are normally considered to have matured by week 36 of gestation. One of the problems faced by babies who are born prematurely is that the cells in the alveoli that produce surfactant are also immature.

Q1. The cells in the alveoli that produce surfactant are:
   a. type II alveolar cells.
   b. endothelial cells.
   c. macrophages.
   d. red blood cells.

Q2. Which anatomical structure protects a baby's lungs from damage from external forces?
   a. The ribs and their associated joint and muscles
   b. Trachea

   c. Alveoli
   d. Nasopharynx

Q3. Expansion of the ribcage outwards and inwards is aided by:
   a. cartilage joints that connect the ribs to the sternum and spinal cord.
   b. alveolar sacs.
   c. bronchi.
   d. bronchioles.

Q4. Explain the location and role of surfactant in breathing.

Q5. Explain how a lack of surfactant affects the breathing of a baby born prematurely.

CASE STUDY 17.3

Some people say 'relax, take a deep breath' as a way to reduce stress or anxiety or help someone to calm down. For thousands of years Buddhist and Hindu traditions have used yogic techniques of breathing in meditation to influence physiological and emotional regulation.

Q1. The parasympathetic innervation of lungs and viscera comes from the:
   a. phrenic nerve.
   b. facial nerve.
   c. vagus nerve.
   d. cardiac nerve.

Q2. The space between the visceral and parietal membranes is called the:
   a. thoracic cavity.
   b. pleural cavity.

   c. bronchus.
   d. sternum.

Q3. The major blood vessel that supplies the respiratory system with oxygenated blood is the:
   a. pulmonary artery.
   b. pulmonary vein.
   c. alveolar capillaries.
   d. bronchial artery.

Q4. What is the relationship between voluntary control of breathing and the sympathetic and parasympathetic nervous systems?

Q5. How might voluntary regulation of breathing rate and depth affect heart rate, blood pressure and blood glucose levels?

CASE STUDY 17.4

After winning a 1500-metre swimming race, a young athlete emerges from the pool to be interviewed by waiting journalists. When asked to describe her experience of the race, she is visibly breathless, tachypnoeic and only able to speak in words rather than full sentences, and shows active use of the accessory muscles of respiration.

Q1. Which of the following does not constitute gas–blood barrier?
   a. White blood cell membrane
   b. Alveolar capillary endothelium
   c. Alveolar epithelium
   d. Alveolar endothelial–epithelial membrane

Continued

CASE STUDY 17.4—cont'd

Q2. The space in the lungs where oxygen and carbon dioxide do not participate in gas exchange is known as the:

a. alveolar dead space.

b. epithelial dead space.

c. bronchial dead space.

d. anatomical dead space.

Q3. During inspiration, the external intercostal muscles:

a. relax.

b. contract.

c. do not participate in inspiration.

d. both contract and relax.

Q4. Explain the physiological respiratory response to strenuous exercise and homeostatic control of respiration in this situation.

Q5. Why does the heart rate increase in response to exercise?

REFERENCES

1. Byars SG, Stearns SC, Boomsma JJ. Association of long-term risk of respiratory, allergic, and infectious diseases with removal of adenoids and tonsils in childhood. JAMA Otolaryngol Head Neck Surg 2018;144(7):594–603.

2. Patton K, Thibodeau G. Ventilation. In: Patton KT, Thibodeau GA, editors. Anatomy and physiology, 9 ed. London: Elsevier Health Sciences; 2015.

3. Lumb AB, Slinger P. Hypoxic pulmonary vasoconstriction: physiology and anesthetic implications. Anesthesiology 2015;122(4):932–46. doi:10.1097/ALN.0000000000000569.

4. Murray AJ, Horscroft JA. Mitochondrial function at extreme high altitude. J Physiol 2016;594(5):1137–49.

5. Jelkmann W. Regulation of erythropoietin production. J Physiol 2011;589(6):1251–8. doi:10.1113/jphysiol.2010.195057.

6. Vierkötter A, Schikowski T, Ranft U, et al. Airborne particle exposure and extrinsic skin aging. J Invest Dermatol 2010;130(12):2719–26.

7. Colin AA, McEvoy C, Castile RG. Respiratory morbidity and lung function in preterm infants of 32 to 36 weeks' gestational age. Pediatrics 2010;126(1):115–28.

8. www.pedilung.com/pediatric-lung-diseases-disorders/anatomy-of-a-childs-lung.

9. Thannickal VJ, Murthy M, Balch WE, et al. Blue Journal Conference: aging and susceptibility to lung disease. Am J Respir Crit Care Med 2015;191(3):261–9.

10. Marshall J, Raynor M. Myles textbook for midwives, 16 ed. Sydney: Churchill Livingstone Elsevier; 2014.

CHAPTER 18

Gastrointestinal system

WEI HENG ON, MBCHB • YEONG JER LIM, MBCHB • KIRYU YAP, BMEDSC, MBBS

KEY POINTS/LEARNING OUTCOMES

1. Describe the structure and function of the gastrointestinal tract.
2. Describe the passage of food through the gastrointestinal tract and its regulation.
3. Link the process and regulation of food digestion and absorption.
4. Discuss the structure and function of the liver and pancreas.
5. Integrate the gastrointestinal system with other systems in the body.

KEY DEFINITIONS

- **Digestion:** the mechanical, enzymatic and chemical breakdown of food to nutritional by-products that can be absorbed into the bloodstream and transported to target organs.
- **Gastrointestinal (GI) tract:** also known as the digestive tract or alimentary canal, the organ system involved in the ingestion and breakdown of food, the absorption and regulation of energy and nutrients, and the expulsion of waste as faeces.
- **Mucosa:** the membranous lining of the gastrointestinal tract consisting of an epithelial layer that secretes lubricating mucus, an underlying connective tissue layer and a layer of smooth muscle.
- **Peristalsis:** involuntary coordinated wave-like movements that propel food along the gastrointestinal tract.

ONLINE RESOURCES/SUGGESTED READINGS

- **Digestive system I: the upper gastrointestinal tract** available at https://study.com/academy/lesson/digestive-system-i-the-upper-gastrointestinal-tract.html
- **Digestive system II: the lower gastrointestinal tract** available at https://study.com/academy/lesson/digestive-system-ii-the-lower-gastrointestinal-tract.html
- **Gastrointestinal system** (clinical reviews, translational and basic science research studies related to the gastrointestinal system) available at www.nature.com/subjects/gastrointestinal-system
- **General motility disorders: diarrhoea and constipation** available at https://study.com/academy/lesson/general-motility-disorders-diarrhea-and-constipation.html
- **Digestive system** available at www.healthdirect.gov.au/digestive-system

INTRODUCTION

The gastrointestinal (GI) tract is a contiguous muscular tube extending from the mouth to the anus and is responsible for the transport, digestion, absorption and expulsion of ingested food.[1] It primarily functions to absorb nutrients essential for life. This is facilitated by digestive enzymes secreted by organs of the gastrointestinal system, the effective movement of ingested food through the gastrointestinal tract and the large total intestinal surface area for absorption of nutrients—thought to be up to 260–300 m^2, comparable to the size of a tennis court. The GI system also functions to protect the body by removing harmful infectious organisms, materials and allergens, facilitated by the well-developed innate and adaptive immune responses present throughout the gastrointestinal mucosa and in GI organs

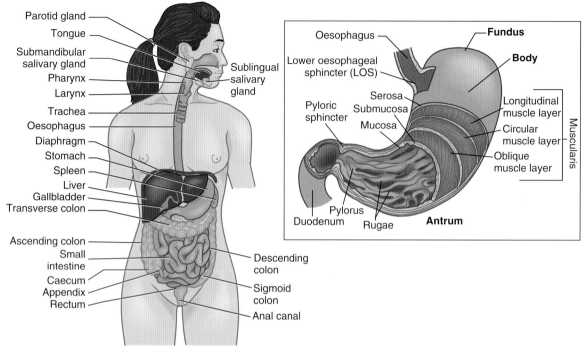

FIGURE 18.1 Organs of the gastrointestinal system. (*Source:* Lewis S, Bucher L, Heitkemper M. Lewis's medical-surgical nursing: assessment and management of clinical problems, 3 SE ed. Elsevier India; 2018.)

like the liver. Furthermore, the gut (in particular, the large intestine) hosts a range of microorganisms that have a symbiotic (beneficial) relationship with the host and are involved in the metabolism of toxins, absorption of nutrients, maintenance of intestinal wall health and regulation of immunity. This chapter reviews the anatomy and physiology of the major organs of the GI system (Fig. 18.1), which includes the mouth, tongue and salivary glands, oesophagus, stomach, small intestine, liver, pancreas, large intestine and rectum. We also integrate the GI system with the other body systems and demonstrate its role in day-to-day activities.

STRUCTURE AND FUNCTION OF THE GASTROINTESTINAL TRACT
Oral cavity
The oral cavity is the opening where food enters the GI system. It commences with the **lips** that bound its opening anteriorly, **cheeks** on both sides forming its lateral walls, the **hard palate** forming its roof anteriorly and the **soft palate** posteriorly, and the **tongue** as its floor (Fig. 18.2). It is lined by a moist mucous membrane traditionally divided into lining, masticatory and specialised mucosa.

The mucosa acts as a barrier against contaminants and microorganisms attempting to enter surrounding tissues. The mucosa lines most of the oral cavity including the soft palate, ventral (underside) surface of the tongue, floor of the mouth and internal surface of the lips and cheeks. The masticatory mucosa lines areas of the oral cavity that are exposed to masticatory forces such as the hard palate and gingiva (gums). It is firmly bound onto overlying teeth or bones and is keratinised to withstand high masticatory forces. Lastly the specialised mucosa is found in the dorsum (upper surface) of the tongue and contains taste receptors (or taste buds) that allow us to taste and enjoy the food we eat.

Tongue
When you put food in your mouth and chew (masticate), the food is moved around your mouth by the motion of your tongue. This richly vascularised and innervated muscular organ aids the crushing of food against the hard palate and the processing of food towards a state where it can be swallowed. At the back of your tongue are the lingual tonsils, which play a role in the immune system. The tongue's upper surface (dorsum) is covered in small projections called papillae, which house taste

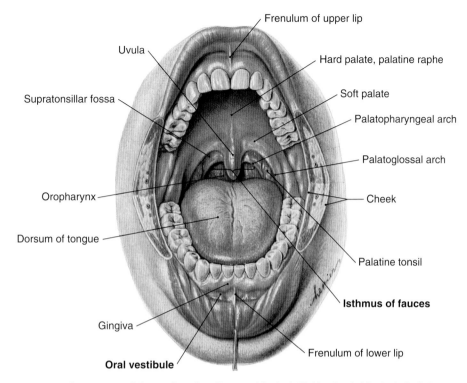

Frenulum of upper lip

Uvula

Hard palate, palatine raphe

Supratonsillar fossa

Soft palate

Palatopharyngeal arch

Palatoglossal arch

Oropharynx

Cheek

Dorsum of tongue

Palatine tonsil

Isthmus of fauces

Gingiva

Frenulum of lower lip

Oral vestibule

FIGURE 18.2 **Structures of the oral cavity.** (*Source:* Klonisch T, Hombach-Klonisch S. Sobotta: clinical atlas of human anatomy. Elsevier; 2019.)

buds. Based on their structure, the papillae are divided into four different types: fungiform papillae, circumvallate papillae, foliate papillae and filiform papillae. In the past it was believed that different parts of the tongue sensed different tastes but scientists have shown that this is not the case and that all tastes can be detected on all parts of the tongue.

Taste buds house **chemoreceptors** or **gustatory cells** whose surface is covered by tiny hair-like projections known as **cilia** or **gustatory hairs.** Gustatory cells are surrounded by supporting cells that comprise the epithelial cell capsule. Gustatory hairs have direct contact with the external environment (the mouth cavity) through taste pores. This means that they are constantly exposed to saliva. Chemoreceptors sense different types of chemicals (tastants) dissolved in saliva as you chew food and generate action potentials which are translated into nerve signals by afferent nerves and conducted to the brain via cranial nerves VII (supplying two-thirds of the tongue), IX (supplying the posterior one-third of the tongue) and X (which extends from the pharynx to the back of the tongue) where they are interpreted to help recognise tastes. Overall, a healthy person has the ability to detect different tastes due to a combination of five primary taste sensations: salty, sour, bitter, sweet and umami.

Salivary glands

Saliva is secreted into the oral cavity by three major salivary glands: **parotid**, **submandibular** and **sublingual** (Fig. 18.3). Acinar cells within salivary glands produce and secrete saliva through salivary ducts into the oral cavity, averaging 1–1.5 L daily in healthy adults. Saliva consists of a variety of salts and minerals with important proteins and enzymes that complement its functions to lubricate the mouth, protect against foreign microorganisms, maintain appropriate pH, initiate digestion of starches and lipids, and facilitate the taste of food.[2]

Lingual and palatine tonsils

Tonsils are part of the lymphatic system and are located at the posterior end of the oral cavity. The palatine tonsil is located at the end of the uvula, while the lingual tonsil is located near the base of the tongue. Both tonsils are part of the adaptive immune response, which enables the body to recognise foreign microorganisms and form a targeted response against them.

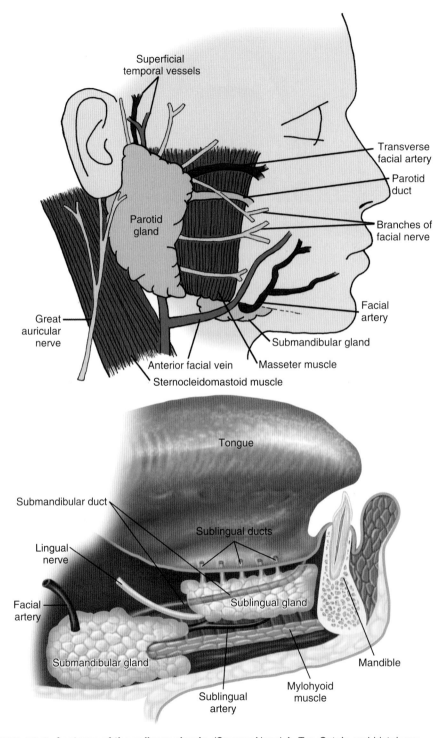

FIGURE 18.3 Anatomy of the salivary glands. (*Source:* Nanci A. Ten Cate's oral histology: development, structure, and function, 9 ed. Elsevier; 2018.)

Pharynx and the mechanism of swallowing

Once food has been ingested into the oral cavity, it is mixed with saliva and physically broken down. The **mastication** process grinds food into smaller components while the tongue mixes and aids lubrication of food. The **swallowing** process starts when the tongue voluntarily collects the oral contents and pushes it posteriorly into the pharynx. This is followed by an involuntary response controlled by cranial nerves from the brain, which leads to simultaneous contraction of the pharyngeal muscle, inhibition of breathing and closure of the glottis (entrance to the larynx/trachea) with a flap of tissue called the epiglottis, which allows food to enter the oesophagus via the upper oesophageal sphincter (Fig. 18.4). Failure of this regulation (which may inadvertently occur when one talks while eating and swallowing) will lead to a cough reflex to expel any solids or liquids that may have travelled down the trachea instead of the oesophagus.

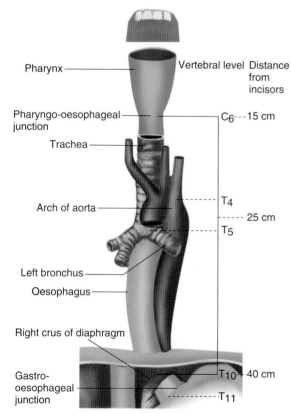

Pharynx		
Pharyngo-oesophageal junction	C6	15 cm
Trachea		
Arch of aorta	T4	25 cm
	T5	
Left bronchus		
Oesophagus		
Right crus of diaphragm		
Gastro-oesophageal junction	T10	40 cm
	T11	

Vertebral level   Distance from incisors

FIGURE 18.4 The oesophagus and associated structures. (*Source:* Dhingra PL, Shruti Dhingra S. Diseases of ear, nose and throat: head and neck surgery, 7 ed. Elsevier India; 2018.)

Oesophagus

The **oesophagus** is a muscular tube that is approximately 25 cm long in adults connecting the pharynx to the stomach. Upon swallowing, food travels through the upper oesophageal sphincter into the oesophagus, which extends from the neck through the thoracic cavity and diaphragm into the stomach.

Microanatomy of the oesophagus

From the oesophagus, all organs along the GI tract contain several layers (see Fig. 18.8 later in the chapter). This is not dissimilar to other luminal structures in the body but there are several unique features to complement the function of the GI tract. The **mucosa**, the innermost luminal layer, contains three layers. The **epithelium** abuts the luminal contents and acts as a protective layer against repeated mechanical injury during food movement and peristalsis (intestinal movement). The underlying loose connective tissue known as the **lamina propria** is further surrounded by a layer of smooth muscle, the **muscularis mucosae**, which separates the mucosa from the submucosal layer.

Underneath the mucosa lies the **submucosa**, a loose connective tissue layer that loosely attaches the mucosa to the muscularis externa and mainly contains larger blood vessels and nerves. In the submucosa of the oesophagus and duodenum, mucous glands secrete lubricating mucus.

Surrounding the submucosa is the **muscularis externa**, a thick muscular layer within the oesophagus wall that is responsible for the peristaltic movement of food. It consists of an inner circular layer and outer longitudinal layer of smooth muscle for most of the GI tract.

The outer surface of the oesophagus is lined by a protective membrane called the **serosa**, which contains an epithelial layer known as the mesothelium, which secretes lubricating serous fluid, and connective tissue, which contains blood vessels and nerves.

Propulsion of food along the oesophagus

Movement of food along the oesophagus, and indeed the whole GI tract (oesophagus to large intestine), is facilitated by the mechanism of **peristalsis**, which provides rhythmic contractile movements. The peristaltic process starts when stretch of the gut wall triggers an involuntary contraction behind the food bolus, pushing it forward; this in turn stretches the next segment of the gut wall, leading to a wave of contractions directing the food towards the rectum. This movement is aided by gravity when the person is sitting upright. In the oesophagus, peristalsis starts once food enters via the upper oesophageal junction and is pushed to the end of the oesophagus, where it passes through the lower oesophageal sphincter before entering the stomach. Both oesophageal sphincters are constantly under contraction until stimulated to relax by nerve transmissions, and they prevent unintended entry of substances into the oesophagus, such as gastric juices that are highly acidic and harmful to the oesophageal mucosa. This is in contrast to the rest of the oesophageal mucosa, which is in a resting state at baseline until stimulated by stretch receptors to contract.

Stomach

The **stomach** is a roughly J-shaped organ located in the left side of the upper abdominal cavity, lying immediately below the diaphragm, and is partially covered by the liver on its right. It has two orifices: the cardiac orifice connects the oesophagus to the stomach (regulated by the lower oesophageal sphincter) and the pylorus connects the stomach to the duodenum (regulated by the pyloric sphincter). The stomach is divided into several areas. The cardiac region surrounds the cardiac orifice and is named due to its proximity to the heart. The fundus is the top part of the stomach lateral to the cardiac region, the pylorus is the terminal part of the stomach that connects into the duodenum and the body is all other areas between the fundus and the pylorus (Fig. 18.5). Towards the liver is the lesser curvature of the stomach that connects to the lesser

omentum and on its other side is the greater curvature of the stomach that connects to the greater omentum.

Microanatomy of the stomach

The gastric mucosal epithelium consists of a single layer of columnar cells that secrete a layer of alkaline mucus that protects the gastric walls from the digestive effects of gastric juices. Within the epithelium there are gastric pits that lead into blind gastric glands, which are responsible for the production and secretion of gastric juices and consist of parietal cells and chief cells interspersed between mucosal columnar cells. **Parietal cells** secrete hydrochloric acid, a strong acid leading to a pH of 2–3 within the stomach, which provides a suitable environment for the breakdown of protein (termed proteolysis) and works as an innate protection against ingested microorganisms. These cells also secrete intrinsic factor, which is an important glycoprotein necessary for the absorption of vitamin B12. **Chief cells** secrete pepsinogen, which differentiates into pepsin in the stomach leading to the initiation of proteolysis, and lipase, which initiates lipid digestion.

The stomach has an oblique muscular layer in addition to the longitudinal and circular muscle layers of the muscularis externa. This enables a churning and mixing motion that further helps in the breakdown and mixing of food with enzymes. This combination of

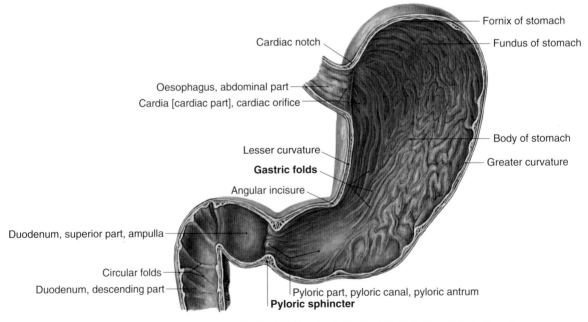

FIGURE 18.5 **The stomach.** (*Source:* Klonisch T, Hombach-Klonisch S. Sobotta: clinical atlas of human anatomy. Elsevier; 2019.)

movements is not required elsewhere in the GI tract and hence is present only in the gastric wall.

Regulation of gastric juices

Due to the corrosive nature of gastric juices, robust regulation of secretion is necessary to prevent breakdown of the stomach's mucosal wall. Gastric secretion is stimulated by three mechanisms: the hormone gastrin released by G-cells found in the pyloric antrum; histamine released by entero-chromaffin-like cells (ECLs) interspersed in gastric glands; and enteric nerve endings found in the fundus. These three mechanisms are synergistic. At a resting state before food is encountered, gastric juices are inhibited by the hormone somatostatin, released by delta cells found in the stomach. When food is seen, smelled, tasted or even thought of, the enteric nerve endings are stimulated, resulting in small releases of gastric juices. This is the cephalic phase response to a meal (see later). When food is ingested, the presence of protein in the stomach and the stretch of its mucous membrane further amplifies the enteric nerve endings and stimulates gastrin secretion, which causes histamine release. Working together these mechanisms lead to the release of copious amounts of gastric juices to process and digest the food. The reduction in acidity when food enters the stomach also leads to inhibition of somatostatin secretion, and this reduces its inhibitory effect on gastric juices. Once food exits the stomach, somatostatin

is released again, leading to the inhibition of further gastric juice release. After food is processed in the stomach it enters through the pylorus into the small intestine, and at this stage it has a heavy cream-like appearance and is known as **chyme**.

Small intestine

The small intestine is the longest portion of the GI tract measuring on average 5 m in adults. It connects the pyloric sphincter in the stomach to the large intestine through the ileocaecal valve. It functions as a major digestive organ where nearly all nutrients are digested and absorbed. There are three subdivisions in the small intestine: the duodenum, accounting for approximately 5% of the total small intestine; the jejunum, accounting for almost 40%; and the ileum, which accounts for almost 60%.

The **duodenum** is the shortest and widest portion of the small intestine and forms an elongated C shape that accommodates the head of the pancreas. It is penetrated by the hepatopancreatic ampulla (known also as the ampulla of Vater or major duodenal papilla) and the accessory pancreatic duct that allows secretion of bile and pancreatic enzymes into the GI tract. The duodenum (Fig. 18.6) transitions into the next section of the small intestine via the duodenojejunal junction. This then continues as the **jejunum**, which contains a rich blood supply to allow for most of the absorption

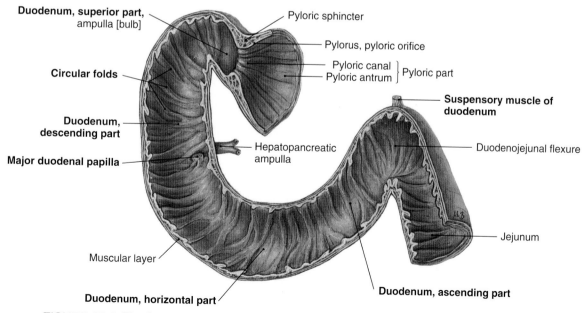

FIGURE 18.6 The duodenum. (*Source:* Klonisch T, Hombach-Klonisch S. Sobotta: clinical atlas of human anatomy. Elsevier; 2019.)

of nutrients and fluids, then gradually transitions to the ileum with no clear border. The **ileum** has the smallest diameter, has a thinner wall compared with the jejunum and has less pronounced circular folds. The jejunum and the ileum lie in the central and lower part of the abdominal cavity bordered by the large intestine.

On the anterior front, the small intestine is covered by the greater omentum (Fig. 18.7), which hangs down like an apron from the stomach as a loose fold of serous membrane (**peritoneum**). All intra-abdominal organs are lined by folds of peritoneum that attach the organs to the abdominal wall, produce lubricating serous fluid that enables gliding motion of visceral organs against each other, contain fat that provides soft intra-abdominal cushioning and contain lymph nodes, lymphatic vessels and immune cells that play a role in GI immunity. These folds of peritoneum were traditionally thought to be fragmented and associated individually with each visceral organ, but in fact are now known to be one continuous structure classified as a new abdominal organ in itself, the **mesentery**.[3]

Microanatomy of the small intestine

The presence of a large mucosal surface area enables effective digestion and absorption of food in the small intestine. On the inner surface of the intestinal walls lie deep mucosal and submucosal folds called circular folds or valves of Kerckring; within these folds lie finger-like structures known as villi that project 0.5–1.5 mm into the lumen (Fig. 18.8). The mucosal cells that line each villus contain even smaller finger-like structures known as microvilli. Cumulatively, this hierarchy of folds leads

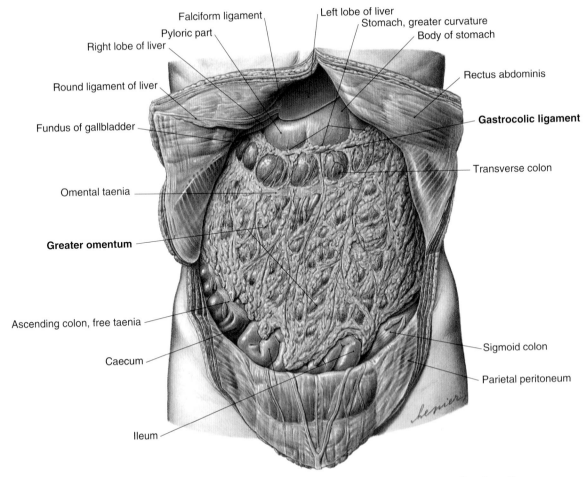

FIGURE 18.7 **The greater omentum, overlying the viscera like an apron descending from the lower border of the stomach.** (*Source:* Klonisch T, Hombach-Klonisch S. Sobotta: clinical atlas of human anatomy. Elsevier; 2019.)

to a total mucosal surface area that is 400–500 times more than what it would be if the inner surface of the small intestine consisted of a flat mucosal surface.

Another unique feature of the small intestinal wall is the presence of aggregates of lymphoid cells called Peyer's patches within the submucosa. These are present mostly in the ileum and function to develop an immune response against potentially harmful microorganisms found in undigested food residue.

Transition of food through the small intestine

In addition to peristaltic movement that occurs in all lumens of the GI tract, the movement of chyme through the small intestine involves segmental contractions and

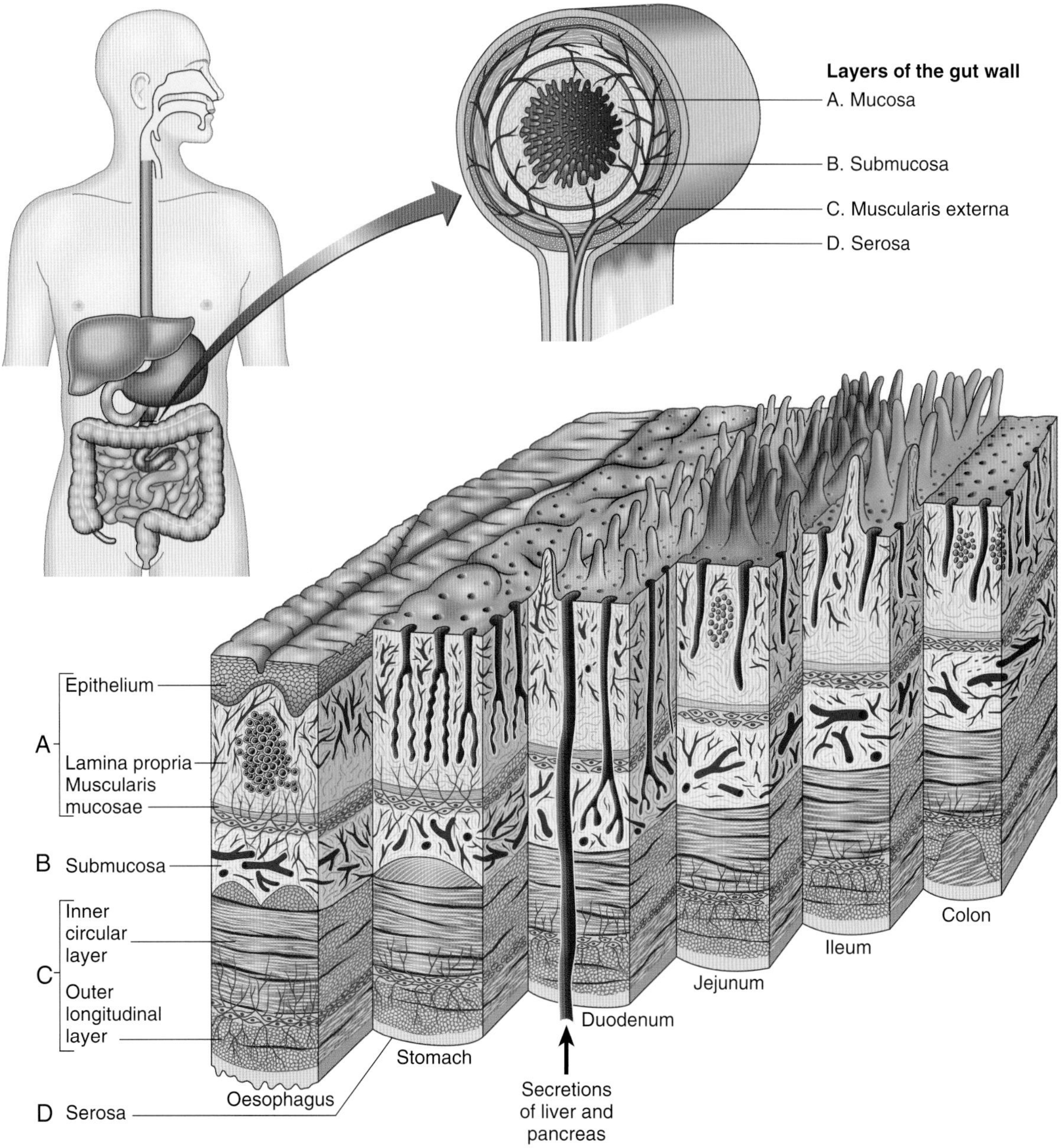

Layers of the gut wall
A. Mucosa
B. Submucosa
C. Muscularis externa
D. Serosa

A { Epithelium
Lamina propria
Muscularis mucosae

B Submucosa

C { Inner circular layer
Outer longitudinal layer

D Serosa

Oesophagus
Stomach
Duodenum
Secretions of liver and pancreas
Jejunum
Ileum
Colon

FIGURE 18.8 **Microanatomy of the wall of the gastrointestinal tract.** (*Source:* Standring S. Gray's anatomy, 41 ed. New York: Elsevier; 2016.)

tonic contractions. In segmental contractions chyme is mixed backwards and forwards, while in tonic contractions a segment of the bowel is isolated for a period. These two mechanisms aid in regulating and slowing gut transit time to maximise mucosal contact with chyme, which is another feature of the small intestine that results in the efficient absorption of food nutrients. When food residue reaches the end of the ileum, it enters the large intestine regulated by the ileocaecal valve.

Digestion of nutrients in the small intestine

Once chyme enters the small intestine, it is mixed with intestinal juices, pancreatic juices and bile, which are responsible for the digestion of most of its nutrients. Intestinal juices are produced by intestinal cells and are present at the microvilli. Although the main function remains to line and protect the mucosa, intestinal juices contain several important enzymes that aid in the final breakdown of carbohydrates and protein. Pancreatic juices also contain numerous enzymes that play a role in the digestion of most nutrients, including proteins, carbohydrates, triglycerides and cholesterol. Pancreatic juices are produced and released from alveolar glands in the pancreas (described later). In contrast to gastric secretions, pancreatic juices are alkaline and neutralise the previously acidic chyme, raising pH to approximately 6–7, which facilitates enzymatic activity. Bile is produced in the liver, stored in the gallbladder and secreted into the small intestine mixed with pancreatic juices (described later). Triglycerides are broken down by pancreatic lipase into fatty acids and glycerol, which associate together with bile salts and phospholipids to form small microscopic cylindrical and spherical structures called micelles. Through their incorporation in micelles, fatty acids, monoglycerides, cholesterol and fat-soluble vitamins, which are poorly soluble in water, can be transported towards the intestinal wall where they are absorbed.

Regulation of digestive secretions

Digestive secretions in the intestine are regulated by the actions of hormones and the enteric nervous system. Cholecystokinin (CCK) is a hormone produced mainly by I-cells in the small intestine but is also produced elsewhere such as in the brain and in the nerves around the body. It is secreted in response to the contact of chyme with the intestinal mucosa, and works by stimulating the secretion of pancreatic juices, gallbladder contraction and relaxation of the hepatopancreatic sphincter that ultimately leads to the release of digestive enzymes into the duodenum. Secretin is the second important hormone produced by S-cells in the small intestine, in response to contact of acidic chyme with the intestinal mucosa. It amplifies

the actions of CCK and further increases the alkalinity of pancreatic juices. It also decreases gastric juices and leads to contraction of the pyloric sphincter, allowing a phased and controlled transit of food residue from the stomach to the duodenum. This results in neutralisation of the acidic chyme as it transits in the small intestine.

The enteric nervous system is a vast and complex pathway containing about 100 million neurons—similar to the total number of neurons found in the whole spinal tract itself! It independently regulates intestinal motility and enzyme secretion in response to changes in the intestinal environment. Because of its complexity and independence from the central nervous system, it is often called the 'second brain' in the body.

Pancreas

The **pancreas** is an important accessory digestive organ that connects to the duodenum. It is creamy pink in colour and is divided into head, neck, body, tail and uncinate process (Fig. 18.9). Its head rests within the

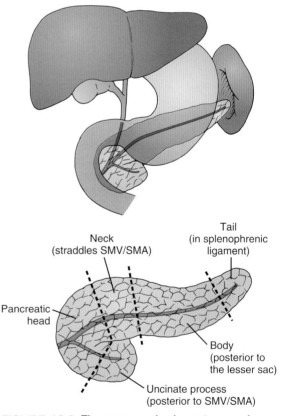

FIGURE 18.9 **The pancreas: basic anatomy and microstructure.** (*Source:* Roth CG, Deshmukh S. Fundamentals of body MRI, 2 ed. Elsevier; 2017.)

C-loop of the duodenum and extends horizontally to form a flattened tongue-like tissue pointing towards the spleen. The pancreas has two main functions: to produce exocrine digestive enzymes that are released into the pancreatic duct and endocrine hormones released into the bloodstream. Exocrine function is covered in this chapter while endocrine function was discussed in Chapter 10.

Microanatomy of the pancreas

The main pancreatic duct extends within the pancreas where it branches out and ultimately leads to an acinar gland, which consists mostly of acinar cells responsible for the production of pancreatic juices. When stimulated, these acinar glands secrete pancreatic juices consisting of numerous enzymes as described above. The juices flow into the main pancreatic duct and are released into the small intestine through the ampulla of Vater, which is the same point where the common bile duct releases bile from the gallbladder.

Liver

The **liver** is an accessory digestive organ and the largest organ in the abdomen. It occupies the right upper quadrant of the abdomen and lies below the diaphragm where it is moulded to the lower surface of the right hemidiaphragm, causing it to have a wedged appearance. It is suspended by the falciform ligament, which arises near or at the umbilicus and continues on to the front of the liver extending to the lower surface of the diaphragm, where it becomes the left and right coronary ligaments. Anatomically it is divided into four lobes: left, right, caudate and quadrate.

The liver has a rich blood supply and is unique in that it receives blood from two sources: the hepatic artery, which contributes 25–30% of blood supply; and the portal vein, which contributes the remaining 70–75% but can rise to 90% after a heavy meal (Fig. 18.10). The portal vein delivers all absorbed nutrients to be metabolised in the liver. It receives nutrition-rich blood from the superior mesenteric vein, splenic vein and gastric

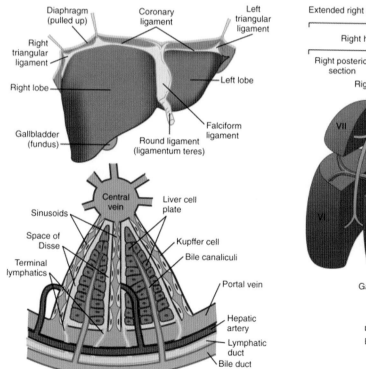

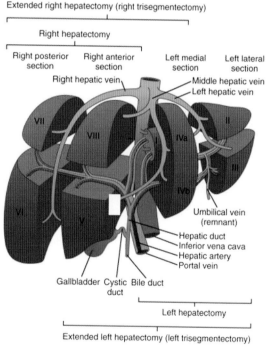

FIGURE 18.10 **The liver: basic anatomy and microstructure.** (*Source:* Ducheyne P. Comprehensive biomaterials II. Elsevier; 2017.)

veins, which in turn receive blood from all veins draining from digestive organs like the small and large intestine. These veins that eventually drain into the portal vein from the digestive organs are collectively called the **portal venous system**. As the portal vein enters the liver it is further divided into smaller branches and is ultimately mixed with the hepatic arterial blood into a capillary system within the liver called the hepatic sinusoids, which eventually drain back into the systemic circulation via the hepatic vein.

Microanatomy of the liver and its functions

The microscopic structure of the liver goes hand in hand with its function. It is worth mentioning that the liver has many other functions not covered in this chapter, such as in metabolism and storage of nutrients, synthesis of important glycoproteins and coagulation factors, and production of vitamin A, as well as playing a role in immunity. In fact, the liver is estimated to have approximately 500 different functions in the body.[4] In this chapter we focus on its role in processing absorbed digestive products and acting as a gatekeeper between blood from the GI tract and the systemic circulation (the rest of the body); and its role in the synthesis and circulation of bile.

Role of the liver as a filtrating and detoxifying organ

Blood enters the liver through the portal vein and hepatic artery, which eventually converges into a series of sinusoids. These sinusoids lie adjacent to the main parenchymal cells in the liver (hepatocytes) and then drain into a central vein that eventually converges with other central veins into a large hepatic vein. The sinusoids are unique in their morphology, with fenestrated endothelium (containing pores) and patchy basement membrane, which enables the formation of 'sieves' that allow the transit of large proteins like albumin and intraportal nutrients that can be metabolised by hepatocytes. In addition, the liver filters and protects the body from potentially harmful substances by two mechanisms. First, Kupffer cells (resident macrophages in the sinusoids) phagocytose and remove substances and microorganisms that may pass from the intestine. Second, each hepatocyte is equipped with numerous enzymes that inactivate potentially harmful substances such as toxins and xenobiotics and process their excretion through the gut as bile or through the kidneys as urine. You may be interested to know that alcohol is mainly metabolised in the liver where the enzyme alcohol dehydrogenase oxidises alcohol to acetaldehyde. Subsequently, the enzyme aldehyde dehydrogenase oxidises acetaldehyde to acetate. Acetate is transported outside the liver to other tissues where it is further metabolised and excreted.

Role of the liver in the production of bile

Hepatocytes that line bile ducts or canaliculi are responsible for the production of bile. Bile contains bile acids, phosphatidylcholine and cholesterol as its major components in a ratio of 10:3:1, respectively. It functions not only to solubilise lipid to enable its digestion and absorption, but also as a mechanism for excretion of waste products like conjugated bilirubin (described later) and a variety of other metabolites. When bile is released into the small intestine, it facilitates lipid digestion. The majority of used/unused bile is then reabsorbed by the gut and transported back to the liver. This pathway is termed the enterohepatic circulation. As a result, only a small fraction of total bile needs to be produced daily (approximately 10% per day) to replace what little is lost in the gut.

Following its formation in the bile canaliculi, bile drains into biliary ductules and ducts lined by cells called cholangiocytes. These bile ducts eventually drain into the right and left hepatic ducts, which combine to form the common hepatic duct. The common hepatic duct is then joined by the cystic duct arising from the gallbladder into the common bile duct, which opens into the ampulla of Vater, regulated by the sphincter of Oddi (Fig. 18.11). When the sphincter of Oddi is closed (i.e. when no food is ingested), bile flows through the cystic duct into the gallbladder and is stored until required. When food is ingested, hormones such as CCK and secretin and stimulation of the enteric nervous system result in increased bile production, gallbladder contraction and relaxation of the ampulla of Vater to enable secretion of bile and pancreatic juices.

Large intestine

The large intestine is about 1–1.5 m long and is the most distal segment of the GI tract (Fig. 18.12). It starts at the caecum, which lies in the right lower quadrant of the abdomen. It is connected to the ileum (through the ileocaecal valve) and to the vermiform appendix, which is a blind finger-like pouch extending off the caecum. It then extends upwards into the ascending colon and makes a turn to the left near the liver (hence this turn is called the hepatic flexure) and travels horizontally as the transverse colon. It then turns again, this time downwards upon reaching near the spleen (hence it is termed the splenic flexure), and extends downwards as the descending colon on the left of the abdomen. Upon reaching the pelvis, it makes a horizontal

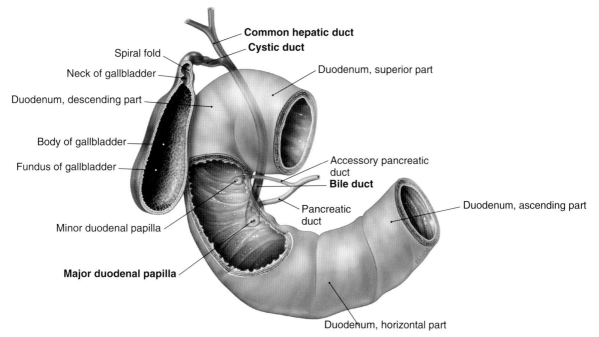

FIGURE 18.11 **Association of the gallbladder and duct transporting bile, and the pancreatic duct transporting pancreatic juice.** (*Source:* Klonisch T, Hombach-Klonisch S. Sobotta: clinical atlas of human anatomy. Elsevier; 2019.)

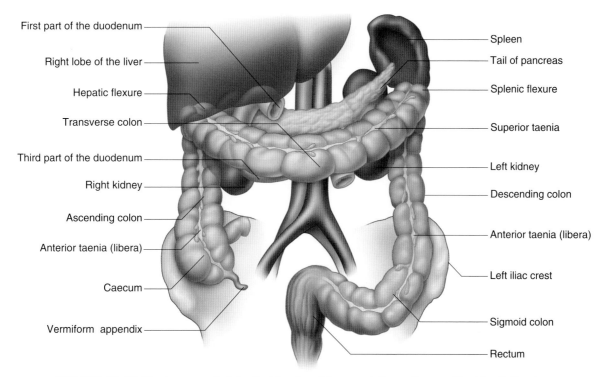

FIGURE 18.12 **The lower gastrointestinal tract and its associations.** (*Source:* Standring S. Gray's anatomy, 41 ed. New York: Elsevier; 2016.)

'S' shape to become the sigmoid colon and continues as the rectum. The distal end of the rectum curves forwards before it curves backwards at an angle as the rectum.

The large intestine differs from the small intestine in several aspects. It is larger in diameter and mostly anchored in position in the intra-abdominal cavity. It also has three separate bands of muscles known as taeniae that run parallel to each other at 120° intervals throughout the large intestine. In between these taeniae the bowel wall forms small outpouching sacs known as haustra, which give the bowel its typical segmented appearance.

Microanatomy of the large intestine

Microscopically the large intestinal mucosa is characterised by crypts of Lieberkuhn, which predominantly consist of goblet cells that secrete mucin to aid the passage of faeces. The large intestine also contains its own biological ecosystem consisting of trillions of commensal microbes, which enjoy a symbiotic relationship with the host. For example, commensal bacteria metabolise residual undigested food into products and nutrients that can be absorbed into the bloodstream and compete with invading pathogens to limit their colonisation of the gut. In turn, they thrive on the nutrition available in the gut.

Movement of undigested food residue

Undigested food residue in the colon is moved by peristaltic and segmental contractions, similar to the small intestine. Additionally, in a third type of contraction unique to the large intestine, known as mass action contraction, there is simultaneous contraction of smooth muscle over a large area. Movement and contractions are almost completely regulated involuntarily by the enteric nervous system, in contrast to the small intestine, where there is synergistic regulation by hormones. As food residue travels through the large intestine, sodium, water and other minerals are absorbed. To enable efficient absorption of water and electrolytes, the food residue advances slowly once in the large intestine, taking an average of 12 hours to travel from the caecum to the sigmoid colon. Once it reaches the rectum, its distension triggers the defecation reflex (described later).

Anal canal and anus

The anal canal is the final portion of the GI tract measuring approximately 4 cm in length. Food residue (referred to as faeces) is expunged from the rectum through the anal canal and past the anus (Fig. 18.13). Two muscular rings wrap around the anal canal: the internal anal

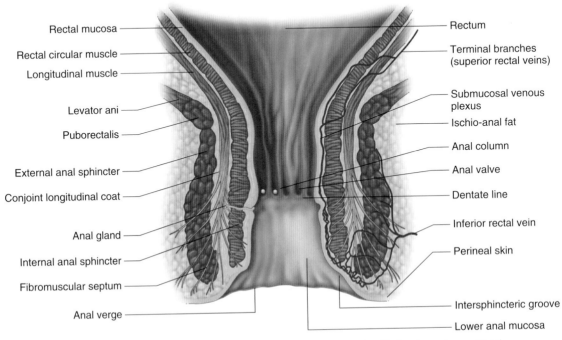

FIGURE 18.13 **The rectum, anal canal and anus.** (*Source:* Standring S. Gray's anatomy, 41 ed. New York: Elsevier; 2016.)

sphincter and the external anal sphincter. These muscles, alongside the pelvic floor muscles (levator ani and coccygeus), play an integral part in the defecation process (described later). The inferior part of the anal canal is lined by squamous epithelium and opens out to form the anus, while the superior part is lined by columnar epithelium, similar to the rectum.

Mechanism of defecation

The process of defecation begins even before the defecation urge occurs. It comprises an orchestrated series of sensorimotor pathways involving the central, peripheral and enteral nervous systems. Ingestion of food triggers the gastrocolic reflex, which is mediated by gut hormones and stretch receptors in the stomach. This reflex is responsible for large colonic motor contractions and it is the increase in colonic motility and propulsion of gut contents towards the anus that represents the start of the process of defecation.

The rectum is generally empty: when faeces enter the rectum this triggers the stretch receptors, which initiate the defecation reflex. Signalling via the parasympathetic pathways of the sacral portion of the spinal cord reaches the brain and triggers the defecatory urge. The anal canal is instrumental in maintaining continence and this is controlled by two muscles: the internal anal sphincter (under involuntary control) and the external anal sphincter (under voluntary control). The pelvic floor muscles also help maintain continence by being in a state of continuous contraction at rest, and this is mediated by the lower and sacral portion of the spinal cord. Filling of the rectum causes relaxation of the internal anal sphincter, but the act of defecation can be delayed by voluntary contraction of the external anal sphincter as well as the pelvic floor muscles, which is paramount if the timing of defecation is inconvenient.

The process of defecation is initiated by the simultaneous actions of the aforementioned gatekeepers of continence. Effectively, the anal sphincters and pelvic floor muscles relax and intrarectal pressure is elevated. Straining may be required using the Valsalva manoeuvre, which increases intra-abdominal pressure. Following successful defecation, everything returns to the resting state.

INTEGRATION OF THE GASTROINTESTINAL SYSTEM WITH OTHER BODY SYSTEMS

Homeostasis is a complex evolutionary mechanism that enables the human body to compensate for variations in its natural state. It is perhaps most evident from our understanding of the GI system, which is incredibly elaborate, consisting of various organs with multiple functions. The ultimate role of the GI system is to digest food, absorb nutrients and eliminate waste in the form of faeces. To achieve its role, coordinated interactions must take place between the GI system and various other body systems, most importantly the nervous, endocrine and musculoskeletal systems.

Nervous system

The gut–brain axis refers to bidirectional communication between the central nervous system and the enteric nervous system, linking processes such as cognition and emotion with digestion and defecation. These interactions also involve crosstalk between the endocrine system (via the hypothalamic-pituitary-adrenal axis) and the immune system.

A good example of this interplay is the mechanism of hunger and satiety. The state of hunger is triggered by a combination of factors: (1) the vagus nerve detecting an empty stomach, (2) high circulating levels of the hormone ghrelin which is produced by the stomach and (3) low blood sugar levels. These factors are relayed to the hunger centres in the hypothalamus and brain stem, inducing the feeling of hunger, which is processed by the cerebral cortex.

Ingestion of food triggers stretch receptors located in the stomach and this leads to the feeling of 'fullness' as stomach capacity is reached. The stretching of stomach receptors also stops the secretion of ghrelin. The introduction of food into the digestive tract triggers the release of gut hormones such as leptin, cholecystokinin and peptide YY. These hormones act on the hypothalamus in the brain to suppress appetite and to trigger the secretion of digestive enzymes. Peristaltic movements progress the food through the digestive tract and digestive enzymes and intestinal secretions break down the solid food into liquid, which is absorbed via the intestinal mucosa. As time passes, the stretch receptors within the digestive tract detect the relative 'emptiness' in the stomach, secretion of ghrelin increases, the feeling of hunger recurs and the whole cycle repeats. However, this hunger–satiety circuit is not a simple one-way path, but is influenced by other factors such as emotional cues including anxiety and the brain's pleasure centre (which derives satisfaction from a good meal), sensory inputs such as smell and vision, and nutrient balance.[5]

Endocrine system

The liver produces albumin, a major carrier protein in the blood which binds to many hormones such as steroid and lipophilic hormones that would otherwise be difficult to dissolve in blood. Another major integration between the endocrine and GI systems occurs in the pancreas, where secretion of the endocrine hormones insulin and glucagon regulates energy balance. Somatostatin is another hormone produced in the stomach's pyloric antrum, duodenum and pancreatic islet, and acts to inhibit GI activity by suppressing the secretion of GI hormones (e.g. gastrin, cholecystokinin) and reducing gastric motility and pancreatic activity. Somatostatin also acts on the anterior pituitary gland to inhibit its release of hormones.

During the body's fight or flight response, activation of the sympathetic nervous system, inhibition of the parasympathetic nervous system and the secretion of cortisol and adrenaline (epinephrine) from the adrenal gland lead to changes in the GI system. This includes inhibition of GI motility and secretions; constriction of the gastro-oesophageal, pyloric and anal sphincters; and reduced blood flow within the GI tract. This allows redirection of blood and energy resources to organs vital for the fight and flight response, such as the heart, lungs and skeletal muscles.

Integumentary system

Allergic conditions such as eczema and food allergies can manifest in the skin as pruritus (itching) and rashes. This has been linked in part to defective intestinal barrier function, where increased permeability can lead to leakage of potential allergens into the bloodstream, triggering an immune response.[6] Liver disease can lead to decreased excretion of bile breakdown products (bilirubin), which can circulate in the blood and become deposited in the skin to give patients a yellow hue, a condition known as jaundice. In many cases, bilirubin and bile salts under the skin can cause pruritus.

Skeletal system, joints and bone

The GI system's role in the absorption and regulation of calcium, magnesium and vitamin D is essential for maintaining bone and joint health. Skeletal muscles store energy in the form of glycogen, which is stored in cells in response to the hormone insulin produced by the pancreas. During periods of exercise (and the fight or flight response), glycogen is converted to glucose and used for energy; this occurs in response to the hormone glucagon, which is also released from the pancreas.

Cardiovascular system

The GI system is dependent on the cardiovascular system to distribute energy and nutrients, and to receive endocrine hormones that affect its activity. Inorganic minerals essential for electrical activity in the heart and to make

blood include sodium, potassium, magnesium, phosphate and iron.

Lymphatic system

Lymphatic vessels and lymph nodes throughout the GI system are required for transport as well as immune regulation. In the small intestine, each villus contains a lymphatic structure called lacteals, which transports digested lipids and drains into mesenteric and coeliac lymph nodes. These subsequently drain into abdominal lymph trunks and the thoracic duct, which transports lipids back into the bloodstream.

Immune system

The GI system is a major point of entry for a large range of pathogenic microorganisms, and as such lymphoid tissues are embedded throughout the tract. These include the tonsils in the pharynx, as well as throughout the GI mucosa scattered on the luminal surface as intraepithelial or lamina propria lymphocytes or embedded in the mucosa/submucosa as lymphoid follicles, such as Peyer's patches found in the small intestine.

Additionally, the GI tract is host to a large community of microorganisms, particularly in the small and large intestines—this is initially established prior to birth through the mother's own microbiota (community of microorganisms). From birth, the GI microbiota gradually diversifies through oral contact with microorganisms present in the environment, such as during passage through the birth canal and feeding. These microorganisms remain relatively stable after the age of 3–5 years but can be altered through events such as infection by a pathogenic (harmful) microorganism not usually present in the GI tract, through the administration of antibiotics, or by choice of diet and lifestyle.[7] The intestinal microbiota maintains a symbiotic relationship with the host whereby it obtains its nutrition from passing food, and in turn the microorganisms help maintain the mucosal surface; compete with harmful foreign microorganisms to decrease their chances of settling in the gut, causing an infection; assist with the breakdown and excretion of bile acids; and regulate the immune system. Disruption of the gut microbiota can cause changes in the immune system, leading to inflammatory diseases such as food allergies and inflammatory bowel disease.[8]

Respiratory system

The GI system works with the respiratory system to supply the essential components required by cells to produce energy and maintain cellular processes: glucose and oxygen. Additionally, the two systems are in close physical proximity, particularly in the pharynx where passage of food is kept out of the larynx and trachea by the epiglottis, instead passing into the oesophagus.

Urinary system

Metabolic and xenobiotic by-products that have been absorbed and processed in the GI system are often excreted via the urinary system. Additionally, the GI system works with the urinary system to regulate sodium levels in the body, and this 'gastrointestinal-renal axis' is involved in the regulation of blood pressure by mediating sodium levels.[9] For example, vasoactive intestinal peptide (VIP) produced in the small intestine works on the proximal tubules of the kidney nephrons to increase excretion of sodium and potassium, whereas insulin and C-peptide released by the pancreas promote sodium retention in the body.

Reproductive system

Nutrition and immune regulation by the GI system (and its associated microorganisms) are important for fertility, and the major reproductive hormones testosterone, oestrogen and progesterone are all metabolised in the liver. During pregnancy, major physiological alterations occur including hormonal changes and a shift in metabolism to an anabolic state to support the growing fetus. Decreased intestinal motility allows for maximal absorption of important nutrition to support both the mother and the fetus. Concurrently, increased appetite, nausea, bloating and constipation are all examples of symptoms that occur due to hormonal changes and interactions between the GI and reproductive systems. Key nutrients essential for pregnancy, such as folate and iron, are absorbed and regulated by the GI system.

AGE-RELATED CHANGES

The GI system is not immune to age-related effects. Babies do not have any voluntary control over defecation, but young children learn to voluntarily control this process during toilet training, which usually occurs anywhere from 18 months of age onwards.[10] This control remains with us for life, unless a medical condition impairs it. Diet changes significantly in the first two years of life,

from being breastfed/formula-fed to eating a large variety of foods. What is eaten affects stool consistency, colour and smell.

As we age we may lose teeth, which impacts mastication.[11] Age-related loss of teeth is due to loss of bone in the jaw. Taste buds become less sensitive, food becomes less tasty and appetite decreases. There is also loss of smooth muscle tone in the oesophagus and intestinal tract, which impacts on peristalsis, and relaxation of the oesophageal sphincter may lead to increases in indigestion-related issues. The stomach lining thins out and fewer digestive enzymes and less hydrochloric acid are secreted, which affects both digestion and immune function (remember that hydrochloric acid constitutes part of the innate immune response as it destroys bacteria ingested with food). Intestinal smooth muscle atrophies, which leads to slowing down of peristaltic motion and loss of small intestine tonicity, negatively impacting on the gut's ability to expand.[11,12] This results in loss of surface area needed for food absorption. Similar events occur in the large intestine, but here intestinal atrophy leads to thinning of the intestinal wall and an increased risk of developing diverticulitis.[13] Production of digestive enzymes by GI structures also decreases with age, affecting the capacity to optimally digest and therefore absorb food components, which may lead to malnutrition (see Chapter 19). Constipation (hardening of the stools), faecal incontinence (due to loss of bowel control) and haemorrhoids (swollen blood vessels in the anorectal region that can rupture during straining when a person is constipated) are also more common in the older population.[12,13]

CONCLUSION

The ultimate role of the GI system is to digest food, absorb nutrients and eliminate waste in the form of faeces. It works in harmony with other body systems and with commensal bacteria residing within the GI tract. In fact, imbalance or disruption of intestinal flora has been implicated as a potential cause of GI diseases. This chapter has described GI anatomy, regulation of food transit together with digestion and absorption, the metabolic functions of the liver and the digestive function of the pancreas.

CASE STUDY 18.1

After a long morning in the lecture hall, John felt hungry and made his way to the cafeteria. He indulged in a meal of fish and chips followed by chocolate cake. He satisfied his hunger pangs and felt that his stomach was full. Contented, he felt ready to face a full afternoon of lectures.

Q1. Which structures in the tongue are responsible for John's ability to feel the deliciousness of a chocolate cake?

    a. Supporting epithelial cells

    b. Gustatory cells

    c. Palatine tonsil

    d. Uvula

Q2. When John places a piece of cake in his mouth, the chemoreceptors in his taste buds will be able to detect the sweet sensation because:

    a. there is a specific receptor for chocolate in his gustatory cells.

    b. there is a specific receptor for sweet taste located at the tip of his tongue.

    c. as John masticates, the chocolate cake will be crushed by his tongue and coated in saliva,

which will enable the chemicals found in the cake to bind to his taste bud receptors.

    d. there is a receptor located at the palatine tonsil that detects sweet flavours.

Q3. John can differentiate between the taste associated with fish and chips and chocolate cake because:

    a. chemical receptor stimulation leads to generation of an action potential, which is then carried to the brain via cranial nerves where it is interpreted correctly.

    b. each area of the tongue has specific receptors for fish taste, chips taste and chocolate taste.

    c. each taste bud is specific for only one type of stimulant—for example, salty, sweet, sour, bitter and umami.

    d. John knows the difference as he eats fish and chips every day and he has trained his brain to remember this taste.

Q4. How does John know when he is hungry and when he is full?

Q5. Describe the passage of food through John's GI tract.

CASE STUDY 18.2

Sam spent his morning at an outdoor food festival and enjoyed a variety of food and drinks. He started to feel the urge to defecate but did not feel comfortable using the portable toilets at the festival so he decided to walk home, a 15-minute journey, as he felt that he could 'keep it in'. Once at home, he felt relaxed about defecating in a familiar environment and did so successfully.

Q1. Which part of the intestinal system is responsible for bowel elimination?

    a. Duodenum

    b. Jejunum

    c. Rectum

    d. Ileum

Q2. With respect to the GI system, as a person ages which of the following conditions is likely to be increasingly experienced?

    a. Diarrhoea

    b. Constipation

    c. Improved appetite

    d. Better teeth and gum health

Q3. Sam is capable of exerting voluntary control of defecation because:

    a. the defecation reflex can be controlled from birth.

    b. it is an automatic process that occurs from around 18 months of age.

    c. it is a learned skill that children develop as they are toilet-trained.

    d. defecation cannot occur without voluntary control.

Q4. Explain how the ingestion of food leads to an urge to defecate.

Q5. How does Sam's choice of food affect defecation?

CASE STUDY 18.3

Chen finished her exams and decided to celebrate by going to the pub with her friends. She drank two pints of lager and started to feel flushed. Her friends commented that she looked very red. Not long afterwards, she had the urge to urinate. As the night went on, she found herself making multiple trips to the toilet to empty her bladder.

Q1. The liver has the following functions:

   a. bile production, metabolism and detoxification.

   b. production of urine.

   c. production of vitamin C.

   d. formation of new white blood cells.

Q2. How does the pancreas support GI function?

   a. Secreting carbohydrates that regulate cell metabolism

   b. Digesting dietary fibre

   c. Controlling the function of the duodenum

   d. Releasing digestive enzymes that help break down ingested food

Q3. Which vessel supplies the majority of blood to the liver?

   a. Hepatic artery

   b. Portal vein

   c. Mesenteric artery

   d. Inferior vena cava

   e. Hepatic vein

Q4. Describe the metabolism of alcohol.

Q5. Explain why Chen feels the urge to urinate after drinking alcohol.

CASE STUDY 18.4

Liam met up with his family at his grandmother's house for a Sunday roast lunch, which is a family tradition. Busy catching up with his relatives and talking with his mouth full, Liam suddenly choked and had a coughing fit. This was settled with a good thumping of the chest and sips of water.

Q1. Which cell secretes hydrochloric acid in the stomach to maintain its pH?

   a. Goblet cells

   b. Cholangiocytes

   c. Enterocytes

   d. Parietal cells

   e. Chief cells

Q2. What type of epithelium lines the oesophagus?

   a. Stratified squamous epithelium

   b. Cuboidal epithelium

   c. Columnar epithelium

   d. Squamous epithelium

   e. Transitional epithelium

Q3. Which anatomical structure prevents food from entering the respiratory tract during swallowing?

   a. Tongue

   b. Palatine tonsil

   c. Epiglottis

   d. Lingual tonsil

Q4. Explain why food does not normally enter the respiratory tract via the trachea.

Q5. After passing into the oesophagus, how is food entry into the stomach regulated?

REFERENCES

1. Patton KT, Thibodeau GA. Anatomy and physiology, 9 ed. London: Elsevier; 2015.

2. Humphrey SP, Williamson RT. A review of saliva: normal composition, flow, and function. J Prosthet Dent 2001; 85(2):162–9.

3. Coffey JC, O'Leary DP. The mesentery: structure, function, and role in disease. Lancet Gastroenterol Hepatol 2016;1(3):238–47.

4. Sanyal AJ, Boyer TD, Lindor KD, et al, editors. Zakim and Boyer's hepatology. 7th ed. Philadelphia: Elsevier; 2018.

5. Panduro A, Rivera-Iniguez I, Sepulveda-Villegas M, et al. Genes, emotions and gut microbiota: the next frontier for the gastroenterologist. World J Gastroenterol 2017;23(17): 3030–42.

6. Konig J, Wells J, Cani PD, et al. Human intestinal barrier function in health and disease. Clin Transl Gastroenterol 2016;7(10):e196.

7. Rodriguez JM, Murphy K, Stanton C, et al. The composition of the gut microbiota throughout life, with an emphasis on early life. Microb Ecol Health Dis 2015;26:26050.

8. Hooper LV, Littman DR, Macpherson AJ. Interactions between the microbiota and the immune system. Science 2012;336(6086):1268–73.

9. Yang J, Jose PA, Zeng C. Gastrointestinal-renal axis: role in the regulation of blood pressure. J Am Heart Assoc 2017; 6(3):e005536.

10. Sreedharan R, Mehta DI. Gastrointestinal tract. Pediatrics 2004;113:1044–50.

11. Rémond D, Shahar DR, Gille D, et al. Understanding the gastrointestinal tract of the elderly to develop dietary solutions that prevent malnutrition. Oncotarget 2015; 6(16):13858–98.

12. Saffrey JM. Aging of the mammalian gastrointestinal tract: a complex organ system. Age (Dordr) 2014;35:1019–32.

13. Greenwood-Van Meerveld B, Johnson AC, Grundy D. Gastrointestinal physiology and function. In: Greenwood-Van Meerveld B, editor. Gastrointestinal pharmacology. New York: Springer; 2017.

CHAPTER 19

Nutrition and metabolism

ERIN LAING, BNUTDIET (HONS)

KEY POINTS/LEARNING OUTCOMES

1. Define metabolism and key macro- and micronutrients.
2. Describe the role of each nutrient in metabolism.
3. Discuss how the body receives and uses energy from food.
4. Explain the concept of energy balance.
5. Link the interaction between metabolism and body systems.

KEY DEFINITIONS

- **Anabolism:** the formation of substances from nutrients.
- **Basal metabolic rate (BMR):** the body's resting rate of energy expenditure or output.
- **Catabolism:** breakdown of nutrients for energy.
- **Excretion:** removal of a substance from the body.
- **Osmosis:** movement of water from an area of high concentration to an area of low concentration.

ONLINE RESOURCES/SUGGESTED READINGS

- **Australian Dietary Guidelines** available at eatforhealth.gov.au
- **Metabolism** available at www.betterhealth.vic.gov.au/health/conditionsandtreatments/metabolism
- **Nutrient reference values for Australia and New Zealand** available at www.nrv.gov.au/nutrients
- **Nutrition Education Materials Online (NEMO)** available at www.health.qld.gov.au/nutrition
- **Basics of metabolism** available at www.youtube.com/watch?v=wQ1QGZ6gJ8w

INTRODUCTION

Nutrients are substances generally sourced from foods that are required by the body for energy, growth, repair and maintenance of body functions. After food has been ingested, its nutrients are processed by the gastrointestinal (GI) tract and broken down into smaller substances. Some nutrients are considered essential, meaning that they must be sourced from food and cannot be synthesised by the body. The primary role of nutrients is to provide the building blocks for efficient functioning and body maintenance.[1] Nutrients are divided into six categories: carbohydrates, proteins, fats (lipids), vitamins, minerals and water. **Macronutrients** (carbohydrates, proteins and fats) are required in large quantities and comprise most of what we ingest from our diet.

Micronutrients are vitamins and minerals we require but in much smaller amounts.

Metabolism refers to the use of nutrients from food to make energy and products for body functions. The process of metabolism includes catabolism and anabolism (Fig. 19.1). **Catabolism** is the breaking down of food into smaller particles that are then used to release energy. **Anabolism** is the process of synthesis or formation of substances such as cell membranes, bone or

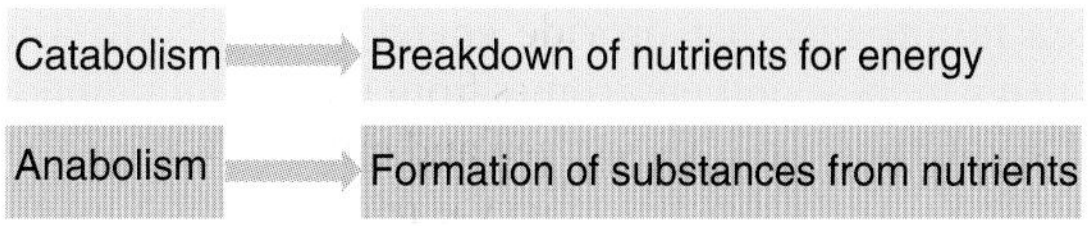

Catabolism ⟹ Breakdown of nutrients for energy

Anabolism ⟹ Formation of substances from nutrients

FIGURE 19.1 **Catabolism and anabolism.**

muscle. While most nutrients ingested are used for catabolism or anabolism, excess nutrients will either be stored by the body or end up as by-products of metabolism that are excreted from the body. These by-products can also be thought of as metabolic waste and this waste is excreted through the lungs, kidneys or large intestine. The lungs excrete metabolic waste in the form of carbon dioxide and water; the kidneys filter the blood and aid in excretion of urea (a by-product of protein catabolism), excess water and salts; and during digestion the intestine absorbs broken down nutrients for use by cells, and any unused nutrients, including fibre and excess water, are excreted in faeces. The body's resting metabolic rate, or **basal metabolic rate (BMR)**, is the amount of energy required for essential bodily functions at rest, such as maintenance of body structures (bone, muscles and organs), synthesis of new cells and structures, and functioning of vital organs. Movement, exercise and illness increase the body's need for energy and use of nutrients to provide this energy.

It is essential to consume a balanced diet from a range of food sources to ensure adequate ingestion of nutrients. Carbohydrates are the preferred source of energy and easiest for the body to process through catabolism, but proteins and fats are also used for energy during normal metabolism and can be used preferentially in the absence of carbohydrates. Excess nutrients are stored in different forms—for example, excess glucose is stored as **glycogen** in the liver; and excess protein and fat are often converted and stored as **adipose tissue** (fat).[1] Glycogen and adipose tissue can be broken down for energy, particularly when the body has not ingested adequate nutrients, such as in a state of starvation or continuous exercise. Conversely, if excess nutrients are ingested, the body will increase its storage of them, usually through conversion to adipose tissue, leading to weight gain and obesity. Hence, a balance between energy input through food and energy output through exercise is important.

STRUCTURE AND FUNCTION

Foods usually contain a mixture of nutrients but are categorised depending on the predominant nutrient—for example, bread is categorised as a carbohydrate but it also contains water, protein and some vitamins and minerals.[1] Carbohydrates, proteins and fats are the key macronutrients that provide energy to the body. The energy in these nutrients comes from the chemical bonds that combine hydrogen, oxygen and carbon.[1] When these nutrients are catabolised, energy is released and available for use by cells. Energy released from food is measured

in kilojoules or calories. In Australia, the most common terminology used is kilojoules (kJ). One calorie is equal to 4.2 kilojoules (Fig. 19.2). The key macronutrients result in different energy outputs after catabolism and can therefore be thought of as having different energy content. Carbohydrates and proteins have the same energy per gram of weight, whereas fats have double the energy per gram weight and are therefore a more energy-dense nutrient (Table 19.1).

1 calorie = 4.2 kilojoules

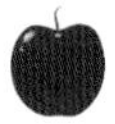

For example, an apple contains 52 calories or 218 kilojoules

FIGURE 19.2 **Measuring energy: calories and kilojoules.**

TABLE 19.1 Energy content of macronutrients	
Energy content (kJ) per 1 gram of weight	
Carbohydrates	17 kJ
Protein	17 kJ
Fat	37 kJ
Alcohol	29 kJ

Carbohydrates

There are two types of **carbohydrates**: simple carbohydrates or sugars; and complex carbohydrates, which include starch and some fibres. Simple carbohydrates are found in foods such as fruit, milk, table sugar (white or brown) and honey. Fruit and honey contain a sugar substance called fructose, while milk and dairy products contain the sugar substance lactose. Complex carbohydrates are found in cereals, grains, pasta, rice, fruit and vegetables. Fruit is an example of a food that contains both simple and complex carbohydrates, due to its combination of fructose, complex carbohydrate and fibre. When digested in the GI tract, food containing carbohydrate is broken down into glucose, the simplest form of carbohydrate and an essential form of energy for the brain, muscles and organs. The process of glucose breakdown is known as **glycolysis**. Glycolysis results in the production of **adenosine triphosphate (ATP)**, which transports energy within cells for metabolism.[2] Any glucose not required for ATP production is converted by the liver, through a process known as glycogenesis, and stored as glycogen.[2] Fibre is commonly found in carbohydrates but it is not broken down by the digestive system and therefore provides little energy. Instead, dietary fibre benefits the body by assisting with nutrient transit and water absorption in the GI tract and is useful to prevent constipation.

Proteins

Proteins are a source of energy and building blocks in the structure of muscles and bones (through collagen production), hormone and enzyme synthesis, the immune system and cell membranes.[1] Proteins are made up of links of amino acids in various combinations. Ingested proteins are broken down into amino acids, absorbed by the small intestine and circulated for use by the body. The liver plays a key role in the breakdown of proteins to amino acids and releases enzymes to assist in this process. Amino acids are primarily used for protein synthesis and are a source of energy when glucose stores are low. The process of converting amino acids to glucose is known as **gluconeogenesis**, which refers to the synthesis of glucose from a non-carbohydrate source.[2] There are 21 amino acids required to create the proteins essential for body functions. Some amino acids are formed or synthesised by the body, while others must be sourced from food and so are considered to be essential amino acids. There are nine essential amino acids: histidine, isoleucine, leucine, lysine, methionine, phenylalanine, threonine, tryptophan and valine. These essential amino acids can be ingested from various plant and animal sources including meat, chicken, fish, some dairy products, grains, some legumes, nuts and seeds. A varied intake of different plant and animal protein sources is the best way to ensure consumption of all essential amino acids. If excess protein is consumed, it is broken down into amino acids and then converted to storage forms of carbohydrate (glycogen) or fat (adipose tissue), or excreted by the kidneys as urea.

Fats

Fats or **lipids** are an essential nutrient for our bodies when taken in moderation, but excess consumption leads to obesity as fat contains the most energy per gram of weight. Fat plays a vital role in organ protection (organs are cushioned by surrounding fat cells), temperature regulation (the fat layer under the skin acts as insulation) and assisting in the transport of fat-soluble vitamins (A, D, E and K).[1] Fats can be grouped into three types—triglycerides, phospholipids and sterols—and can be ingested from both plant and animal sources.[1] The majority of fat metabolised (90%) is in the form of triglycerides, as this is the most common form of fat in animal and plant sources.[2] During digestion, fat is mixed with bile and pancreatic enzyme lipase, which aids in the breakdown of fat to glycerol, fatty acids and monoglycerides (a glycerol molecule joined to a fatty acid). Some fatty acids and glycerol are transported to the liver where they are used to produce energy and heat.[1] Like amino acids, glycerol can be converted to glucose and used for energy through gluconeogenesis.[2] Essential fatty acids (EFAs) must be consumed through diet and cannot be made by the body. They have an important role in cell membrane and nerve tissue production, and in the synthesis of prostaglandins which aid regulation of blood pressure, blood clotting, gastric acid secretions and muscle function.[1] Excess fatty acids are stored as adipose tissue (i.e. fat cells). Adipose tissue can be broken down and used as an energy source when glucose is not available.

Animal sources of fat include meat (beef, chicken, pork, lamb), fish, egg yolks and dairy products. Plant sources include nuts, avocado and plant oils (canola oil, olive oil). Animal products tend to contain saturated fatty acids, which are solid at room temperature and when eaten in excess can contribute to cholesterol production and heart disease risk. Most plant products contain unsaturated fatty acids, which are liquid at room temperature. Unsaturated fatty acids oppose the function of saturated fatty acids by aiding in cholesterol excretion, in turn lowering cholesterol and triglyceride levels. A small number of plant sources contain saturated fatty acids, including coconut oil, palm oil and peanuts. Fish and fish oils contain two types of unsaturated fatty acid—omega-3 and omega-6—which have a role in blood clotting and inflammation. Regular consumption of these unsaturated fatty acids may reduce the risk of clotting and cardiovascular disease.[3] While fats are essential for the body, they should be consumed in moderation due to their high energy content, with a focus on unsaturated rather than saturated fats.

Vitamins

Vitamins are essential for function and have various roles in the body including in the formation and function of blood, bone and teeth, and energy metabolism.[1] Vitamins are grouped into two categories, water-soluble and fat-soluble, which refers to the substance in which they dissolve and are transported throughout the body. The different vitamins, their food sources and function are listed in Table 19.2.

Vitamins are ingested through food and absorbed in the small intestine, where they then move into the bloodstream and are transported throughout the body. However, some vitamins are partially synthesised by the body, including vitamins D and K, and biotin.[1] Some

TABLE 19.2
Vitamins

	Food source	Function
WATER-SOLUBLE VITAMINS		
Vitamin B1 (thiamine)	Pork, wholegrains, legumes, seeds, nuts	Coenzyme for energy metabolism; muscle and nerve function
Vitamin B2 (riboflavin)	Dairy products, meat, fish, chicken, eggs, dark leafy greens, wholegrains, fortified cereals	Coenzyme for energy metabolism
Vitamin B3 (niacin)	Meat, chicken, fish, legumes, fortified cereals, milk	Cofactor for enzymes involved in energy metabolism; aids in glycolysis
Vitamin B5 (pantothenic acid)	Most foods, wholegrain cereals, legumes, meat, fish, chicken	Synthesis of red blood cells; energy metabolism
Vitamin B6 (pyridoxine)	Wholegrains and cereals, legumes, chicken, fish, pork, eggs	Synthesis of haemoglobin
Vitamin B7 (biotin)	Most foods, liver, kidney, peanut butter, egg yolk, yeast	Metabolism of macronutrients
Vitamin B9 (folate)	Fortified cereals, bread, pasta, flour, legumes	Aids in metabolism of amino acids, red blood cells and DNA
Vitamin B12	Meat, fish, chicken, eggs, dairy products	Transport/storage of folate for blood cell formation and function
Vitamin C	Citrus fruits, red and green capsicum, strawberries, tomato, potato, green leafy vegetables	Growth and repair of tissues; synthesis of proteins; wound healing
FAT-SOLUBLE VITAMINS		
Vitamin A	Full-cream milk, butter, liver, egg yolks, fatty fish	Bone growth; epithelial cell maintenance; gene expression regulation
Vitamin D	Butter, egg yolk, fatty fish, liver; consumption of calcium and vitamin D through milk aids in absorption	Bone mineralisation
Vitamin E	Vegetable oils, margarine, wholegrains, seeds, nuts, green leafy vegetables	Antioxidant; reduces damage by free radicals
Vitamin K	Dark-green leafy vegetables	Aids in synthesis of blood clotting factors; protein formation

Source: Grodner M, Escott-Stump S. Nutritional foundations and clinical applications: a nursing approach, 6 ed. St Louis: Mosby; 2016.

vitamins require other factors for optimal function. Vitamin D is a good example, as ultraviolet exposure from sunlight is required to activate its synthesis in the body. Therefore, people with fair skin and/or low sun exposure are at risk of vitamin D deficiency.

Fat-soluble vitamins require bile to be released from the gallbladder to assist their absorption. Bile is a substance produced by the liver and stored in the gallbladder. In combination with lipase enzymes released from the pancreas, bile has an essential role in the absorption of fat and fat-soluble vitamins. If lipases and bile are not available in the small intestine, which may occur due to surgery or illness, the person is at risk of fat malabsorption and subsequent fat-soluble vitamin deficiency. While vitamins are required by the body in only small amounts, it is essential to consume them through diet, and a balanced diet from a wide range of different foods will ensure ingestion of all vitamins. Fresh fruit and vegetables are good sources of vitamins, as are meat, fish, chicken, eggs, dairy products and wholegrains.

It is possible to consume more vitamins than the body requires for essential functions, particularly if taking vitamin supplements in addition to dietary sources.

Water-soluble vitamins are not generally stored and instead are excreted through the kidneys in urine. This means that there is a low risk of toxicity, as any excess is generally removed by the body. Water-soluble vitamins therefore need to be consumed on a daily basis to ensure adequate levels in the body.[1] Fat-soluble vitamins do not have the same efficient excretion process and fatty tissues in the body can retain fat-soluble vitamins.[1] They are therefore at greater risk of toxicity when consumed in excess. For this reason, fat-soluble vitamins are not recommended to be taken in a supplement form unless a deficiency is observed.

If vitamins are not adequately consumed in the diet there is a risk of deficiency. Mild vitamin deficiency may not cause any symptoms initially, but severe deficiency can lead to illness. Take niacin (vitamin B3) for example, which is essential for the synthesis of the amino acid tryptophan and works as a coenzyme in energy metabolism. Niacin deficiency can lead to the condition pellagra, which is characterised by symptoms of dermatitis (skin pigmentation and inflammation), dementia (confusion and anxiety) and diarrhoea. Most vitamins are required in small amounts for essential body functions and therefore there is a low risk of deficiency if a balanced diet is consumed. In Australia vitamin deficiencies are generally rare among the general population, but people with illness, restricted diets and altered GI function are at greater risk of vitamin deficiencies.

Minerals

Minerals have several functions in the body including contributing to the structure of teeth and the skeleton, assisting muscle and nerve function, acting as cofactors for enzymes, and helping to maintain the acid–base balance of body fluids.[1] **Acid–base balance** refers to the degree of acidity or alkalinity of the blood, as indicated by a pH level. Acidity occurs when there is a higher level of acid products in the blood, while alkalinity occurs when there are reduced levels of acid products in the blood. The pH level can be between 0 (strongly acidic) and 14 (strongly alkaline) but the body attempts to keep the blood pH level close to 7.4 to allow for optimal function.

There are 16 essential minerals required by the body and these are often categorised into major and trace minerals depending on the quantity required. A list of major and trace minerals is provided in Table 19.3. Major minerals are required in the diet on a daily basis in amounts of 100 mg or higher. Trace minerals are also required daily but in amounts of 20 mg or less.[1] Minerals are sourced through various foods, and both plant and animal foods are good sources of minerals, including

TABLE 19.3 Minerals	
Major minerals	**Trace minerals**
Calcium	Chromium
Chloride	Copper
Magnesium	Fluoride
Phosphorus	Iodine
Potassium	Iron
Sodium	Manganese
Sulfur	Molybdenum
	Selenium
	Zinc

beef, chicken, eggs, fish, fruit, vegetables, legumes, wholegrains and dairy products. Minerals obtained from animal sources are traditionally easier for the body to absorb, because many plant products have substances called binders that cause the minerals to bind to plant fibre structures, making it harder for them to be digested and absorbed from food.[1] Minerals are inorganic substances and therefore are not metabolised by the body. Instead they are used to assist metabolic processes as cofactors. Table 19.4 summarises the functions of some of the key minerals.

Water and electrolytes

Water comprises approximately 50–60% of total body weight and has many important roles in the body. It assists in regulation of body temperature through blood vessel dilation and sweating, and acts as a lubricant assisting in swallowing, eye function (tears), spinal cord cushioning and basic cellular function.[4] Water is also a significant component of blood, which transports nutrients and oxygen around the body for use by tissues and cells, as well as waste products for excretion. Water has an integral role in metabolism, including the use of ATP for energy, and is often a by-product of catabolism.[4] **Electrolytes** are minerals that carry an electrical charge or ions when dissolved in water. They can be classified into positively and negatively charged ions, known as cations and anions. Sodium (Na^+), potassium (K^+), chloride (Cl^-), phosphorus (PO_4^{3-}) and magnesium (Mg^{2+}) are the key electrolytes.

Water and electrolytes exist in intracellular fluid (within the cell), interstitial fluid (between the cells) and extracellular fluids (interstitial fluid and all other fluids outside cells).[4] To maintain fluid balance, hormones control the movement of electrolytes within and outside cells. The concentration of electrolytes within cells is also controlled by the movement of water through the process

TABLE 19.4
The function of minerals

Mineral	Function
Calcium	Structure of bones; aids in central nervous system; muscle contraction; blood clotting; blood pressure regulation
Chloride	Maintains fluid balance inside and outside cells; component of stomach acid
Fluoride	Tooth and bone formation
Iodine	Aids in regulation of growth and development
Iron	Transport and use of oxygen
Phosphorus	Structure of bones and teeth; aids in energy transfer during metabolism; composition of genetic material; acid–base balance
Potassium	Maintains fluid levels within cells; nerve and muscle function
Sodium	Body fluid and blood pressure regulation; nerve function
Sulfur	Structure of proteins; acid–base balance
Zinc	Enzyme function; immune system regulation; carbohydrate metabolism through hormone regulation

Source: Grodner M, Escott-Stump S. Nutritional foundations and clinical applications: a nursing approach, 6 ed. St Louis: Mosby; 2016.

of osmosis. **Osmosis** is the movement of water from an area of high concentration to an area of low concentration through a selective permeable membrane.[4] To function normally the body must be able to maintain levels of electrolytes within narrow limits.[4] The concentration of electrolytes in blood and cells will impact on osmosis and the movement of water in the body. For example, if there is a high concentration of sodium in blood, water will move from cells into the blood, increasing the blood volume and lowering the concentration of sodium. Ingestion of water and electrolytes plays an important role in osmosis and the regulation of blood volume. Excessive consumption of sodium chloride (i.e. salt) over time can increase a person's blood volume and risk of high blood pressure.[5,6]

Each day water is excreted through air, sweat, urine and the GI tract as part of normal metabolism. Approximately 2.5% of the body's total water is excreted through these processes every day.[4] Water is an essential component of the diet in order to maintain life and body function. General water consumption recommendations for adults are at least 2 litres per day, sometimes more. Water can be consumed through a variety of fluids including juice and milk and is contained in many foods in smaller amounts. Some fruits contain a high amount of water (up to 95%).[4]

Balancing nutrient intake

A balanced diet is essential for good health. Our bodies need a combination of different nutrients to ensure adequate energy and building blocks for growth and cell function. Dietary guidelines direct the optimal intake of macronutrients and food types to ensure the body is receiving adequate nutrients for normal function. Our diet should contain approximately 45–60% carbohydrates, 10–35% protein and 20–35% fat. A variety of foods will then ensure ingestion of all the essential micronutrients, vitamins and minerals. The Australian Dietary Guidelines divide food into five main groups: vegetables (including legumes), fruit, grains (includes cereals, bread, pasta, oats, noodles, quinoa, barley), lean meats (including poultry and fish) and dairy (milk, yoghurt, cheese and/or alternatives).[7] The recommended daily intake of each food group is highlighted in Table 19.5. In order to obtain all the nutrients required for general health and metabolism, a range of food groups should be consumed—for example, over a week it is ideal to consume red meat, chicken and/or fish, at least five different types of fruit and vegetables, and different grains such as cereals, pasta and bread.

Energy balance

Energy balance is the measure of energy input in relation to energy output. Energy input is determined by the quantity and type of food we consume, which can be affected by our appetite, food preferences and social factors. Energy output is determined by many factors including metabolism of nutrients for synthesis and growth, production of heat for thermoregulation, and the activity of our muscles (Fig. 19.3).

The energy released from the catabolism of nutrients is used for essential processes such as muscle and organ function, cell synthesis and repair. The amount of energy required by the body for these essential functions while at rest is the BMR. Like energy derived from food, BMR is often measured in kilojoules. BMR is affected by a person's age, sex, hormone function and genetics.[2] A person's BMR also increases as their muscle mass increases, due to the energy required to work and maintain increased

TABLE 19.5
Recommended food groups and serving sizes

Food group	Serving size	Example	Total serves recommended (per day)
Fruit	350 kJ	1 apple	2
Vegetables	100–350 kJ	½ cup cooked vegetables 1 cup leafy vegetables	5
Grains	500 kJ	1 slice bread ½ cup porridge	4–6
Lean meat	500–600 kJ	65 g cooked red meat 100 g cooked fish 80 g cooked chicken 2 eggs	1–2
Dairy	500–600 kJ	1 cup milk 40 g hard cheese ¾ cup yoghurt	2–3

Source: National Health and Medical Research Council. Australian guide to healthy eating, 2017. Available from: www.eatforhealth.gov.au/guidelines/australian-guide-healthy-eating, on 30 August 2018.

muscle function. Someone who exercises regularly will have a higher muscle mass and therefore a higher BMR. The higher the BMR, the higher the rate and efficiency of nutrient metabolism. The requirement for nutrients increases as energy use by the body increases. BMR is a measurement of the energy required for essential functions, but other factors increase energy use and output such as movement, exercise, illness and inflammation, which in turn increase the occurrence of and requirement for catabolism and anabolism.

Exercise increases energy use due to the work of muscles and organs during activity. Energy is required to fuel muscle contractions during exercise and this energy is in the chemical form of ATP. ATP is produced by glycolysis. As exercise increases the use of ATP, the requirement for glucose increases. While glucose is a preferred source of energy for muscles during activity, the body also metabolises fat and protein for essential metabolic functions and during exercise. At most times of the day, including at rest, macronutrients are metabolised,

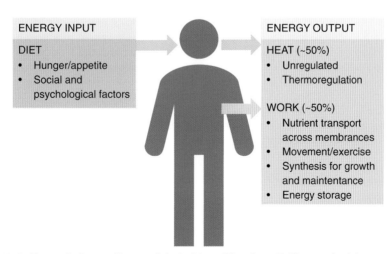

FIGURE 19.3 **Energy balance.** (Source: Adapted from Silverthorn D. Human physiology: an integrated approach, 7 int ed. San Francisco: Pearson; 2015.)

but not at the same rate or efficiency. Fat can be used by muscles for energy when catabolised into fatty acids or converted to glucose through gluconeogenesis. However, this process is much slower than glycolysis and therefore used to a lesser degree. Stored fat in adipose tissue is often used during exercise once glycogen (storage form of carbohydrate) is depleted. The liver is able to store only a small amount of glycogen at any one time, and therefore if the body's requirement for energy exceeds input or ingestion of carbohydrates, glycogen stores will be depleted.

When the body is in a fed state and there are adequate nutrients available for metabolism, the body will preferentially use the nutrients and preserve glycogen and adipose tissue. However, if the body is in a fasted state and nutrients are no longer available in the blood, the body will initiate catabolism of stored nutrients. However, this process is more complex and inefficient, and therefore the body will only use this pathway when glucose is not available.[2] The process of ATP production from fatty acids is known as ketosis and results in the by-product ketones.[2] Ketosis indicates the predominant catabolism of fatty acids and is most common in reduced consumption of carbohydrates and increased consumption of proteins and fats. In the short term, ketosis may not be harmful but long term there can be negative side effects. Ketones can be harmful by lowering the body's pH and increasing the risk of metabolic acidosis.[2] Long-term ketosis can also lead to dehydration, electrolyte loss and kidney impairment. If the body's requirement for energy is greater than the energy consumed, then energy stored as glycogen and adipose tissue will be broken down. Those trying to lose weight should aim to consume a balanced diet but overall less energy than their body requires, measured by the amount of macronutrients consumed. Those trying to gain weight should aim to consume more energy through nutrients than their body is metabolising due to BMR, activity and/or illness.

During illness or inflammation the body requires more energy to fuel cell repair and heightened immune function. People suffering from illness are often at risk of losing weight due to raised metabolism and increased energy expenditure, leading to catabolism of adipose tissue and muscle.

Cellular respiration: conversion of nutrients to energy

Cellular respiration involves the oxidation of nutrients to create energy in two forms: heat and ATP. ATP is the chemical form of energy used in metabolism. The process of cellular respiration requires oxygen and as a result is also referred to as **aerobic respiration**. The process of aerobic respiration begins with glycolysis, the catabolism of glucose, and is followed by chemical reactions known as the citric acid cycle (or Krebs cycle) and oxidative phosphorylation.[8] Glycolysis results in the production of pyruvic acid and 2 ATP molecules.[8] Pyruvic acid is converted to acetyl-CoA, which enters the citric acid cycle to produce water (H_2O), 2 ATP molecules and carbon dioxide (CO_2) as its by-product.[8] The CO_2 is expelled through the blood and respiratory system. Oxidative phosphorylation occurs within the cell mitochondria and produces 34 ATP molecules using a process known as electron transport.[8,9] ATP is also used to facilitate the same process that produces it. Glycolysis and the citric acid cycle both require 2 ATP molecules to function, but the total net gain of ATP through the completion of aerobic respiration is 38 ATP molecules.[8] Oxygen is essential for aerobic respiration. In the setting of low oxygen, such as during prolonged exercise, the body undergoes anaerobic respiration, producing lactic acid as its by-product. Anaerobic respiration cannot produce as much ATP as aerobic respiration and is considered less efficient.[8]

INTEGRATION OF NUTRITION AND METABOLISM WITH OTHER BODY SYSTEMS

The nutrients in the food we eat play a role in the function and processes of many body systems and through metabolism provide energy and building blocks for vital organs, muscles, the nervous system, the immune system and bone. For example, calcium and vitamin D have an important role in the structure of the skeletal system; muscle contraction occurs due to the energy made available by catabolism of carbohydrates and proteins; the endocrine system produces hormones that aid in metabolism; and the kidneys play a vital role in the filtering and excretion of excess nutrients and by-products of metabolism. The GI tract has a vital connection to the metabolism of food, as it is the system that digests food, leading to the breakdown of nutrients, which are then available for metabolism.

Gastrointestinal system

The process of digestion begins as soon as food enters the mouth, comes into contact with saliva and is chewed by the teeth. As food moves down the GI tract it is broken down into smaller nutrient particles that are then used for metabolism. Each section of the GI tract has a different role in the digestion and absorption of nutrients. When nutrients enter the small intestine, they are absorbed through the intestinal wall into the blood and circulated throughout the body. The majority of nutrient absorption occurs in the small intestine, but different sections of the small intestine are responsible for absorption of various macronutrients, vitamins and minerals. When food reaches the large intestine, it is mostly remaining electrolytes and water that are absorbed. The availability of nutrients for metabolism is dependent on the function of the GI tract: if it is altered, nutrients may not be broken down and absorbed appropriately, impacting on their availability for metabolism.

Respiratory system

The respiratory system plays an important role in the excretion of substances left over after metabolism. By-products of metabolism—CO_2 and water—are transported in the blood to the lungs, where they are expelled through air.

Urinary system

The kidneys filter blood and excrete waste products in urine. By-products of metabolism—including urea and creatinine (by-products of protein catabolism), water, excess water-soluble vitamins, minerals and electrolytes— pass through the kidneys and are filtered into urine for excretion. The concentration of vitamins and minerals in urine depends on their balance in the body; their concentration in urine will be higher when they are in excess or the person is ill.

Endocrine system

Various hormones within the endocrine system play a vital role in the metabolism of nutrients and how we ingest nutrients through hunger regulation. Hormones such as insulin, glucagon, amylin, adipokines, adrenaline (epinephrine), cortisol and growth hormone assist the control of glucose, lipid and amino acid metabolism. Hormones can facilitate nutrient catabolism and conversion or stimulate the use of stored nutrients. Take insulin and glucagon, for example, hormones with a key role in the metabolism of carbohydrates. During carbohydrate metabolism, insulin stimulates uptake of glucose by muscles and adipose tissue and prompts the storage of excess glucose as glycogen in the liver; glucagon has the effect of breaking down glycogen and adipose tissue to glucose and fatty acids, respectively, which are then used for energy when the body is in a fasted state.

AGE-RELATED CHANGES

Age is one of the main drivers influencing changes in how the body metabolises food to produce energy. A baby starts life by consuming enough breast milk or baby formula to meet their metabolic needs and provide all essential nutrients. Although it is difficult to define the precise nutritional needs of each infant, overall infants need enough energy to meet many physiological changes such as growth, capacity to develop fine and gross motor skills, and to increase mental capacity. This energy need is affected by the infant's body size and composition at birth and, as the infant grows, the infant's physical activity, genetic factors, growth rate and any illnesses experienced. For breastfeeding the mother needs to be well-nourished and maintain a high-quality diet, as her own diet will affect what is delivered in the breastmilk to her infant.

By 6 months of age, the infant has almost doubled their birth weight and as their mouth, tongue, teeth and GI system start to mature, they will be ready to taste different types of food and learn to recognise food taste and texture. Metabolic needs expand as the toddler grows rapidly, both physically and cognitively. This is also the age where toddlers start to experiment with food and proactively decide what they will and will not eat. By the age of 2 to 4 years, parents may experience significant concerns about whether their child is getting enough nutrition to grow and develop appropriately, as children continue to favour some foods over others.

Older people start to lose their capacity to smell and taste different foods due to age-related loss of associated receptors and neuronal pathways. Age-related diseases may also impact on the capacity to process food in the GI system. Gastric emptying slows down and loss of muscle mass means that there is a reduction in BMR and therefore a reduction in appetite.[10] Malnutrition in the elderly is complex but for the purpose of this chapter it is valuable that you are aware that malnutrition in this group tends to be driven by factors other than food availability. These factors can be broadly grouped as cognitive, psychological and social. For example, cognitive factors may include conditions such as Alzheimer's disease or mental health conditions such as depression; and social factors may include isolation, low income or grief at losing a loved one. Malnutrition in the elderly is associated with poor health outcomes and an accurate assessment of the person's nutritional status must be considered as part of a patient's health assessment.

CONCLUSION

Nutrients are essential for our bodies to maintain growth, function and provide energy. Macronutrients (carbohydrates, proteins and fats) are responsible for providing the building blocks for energy production, tissue growth and repair. While all macronutrients are used for energy metabolism in varying degrees, carbohydrates are the preferred source through the process of glycolysis, particularly for vital organs such as the heart and brain. Proteins and fats are commonly used for the synthesis of tissues and maintenance of essential functions such as temperature regulation and transport of vitamins. Micronutrients provide coenzymes that aid in energy metabolism, as well as substances that assist in the synthesis of tissues such as bone, blood and nerves.

Each macro- or micronutrient has an important role but is most effective when ingested in combination with other nutrients, as each makes a unique contribution to the function of the body. Daily intake of a range of foods and nutrients will ensure adequate nutrition for homeostasis, growth and activity. Energy balance is achieved when the input of nutrients through food matches the output of energy from resting metabolic processes, exercise and events of illness and inflammation. Energy imbalance occurs when the body's energy input is altered, due to a change in food intake or improper digestion and absorption of nutrients in the GI tract; or when the body's energy output exceeds the nutrients available for energy production, such as during intense and prolonged exercise or increased catabolism due to illness. An understanding of the nutrient content of food and the resulting metabolism of nutrients will help ensure that individuals provide their body with the appropriate elements for good health.

CASE STUDY 19.1

Anna is a 27-year-old woman who has been training for a marathon; in recent weeks she has been running 15–20 kilometres three times per week. Before each run Anna drinks at least 2 litres of water and has a small snack, either a banana or yoghurt, so she has energy but does not feel too full before running. After 8 weeks of training Anna is surprised that her body weight is the same: she thought she might have lost weight after running frequently for the past few weeks.

Q1. Which of the following nutrients will be metabolised while Anna is running?

    a. Carbohydrate

    b. Protein

    c. Protein and fat

    d. Carbohydrate, protein and fat

Q2. Carbohydrate is stored in the body as:

    a. glucose.

    b. glycogen.

    c. ATP.

    d. fibre.

Q3. Which of the following affects basal metabolic rate?

    a. Height

    b. Age

    c. Diet

    d. Sleep

Q4. Consider the primary nutrient that is being metabolised during Anna's run and explain whether this nutrient will be depleted at the end of each run.

Q5. Think about why Anna's body weight has remained the same. What changes to Anna's body may have occurred after she has been running this distance frequently for 8 weeks?

CASE STUDY 19.2

Sally has been talking to her friends about the best way to follow a healthy diet. One friend suggested that a diet high in protein and low in carbohydrate would be the best and might even help Sally to lose some weight. Sally decided to try this diet and stopped eating fruit, grains, cereals and starchy vegetables such as potato and corn, increasing her intake of meat, eggs and dairy. Sally followed this diet for a month but found she was often hungry and more tired during the day.

Q1. How many daily serves of fruit are recommended as per the *Australian Guide to Healthy Eating*?

    a. 4–5

    b. 2

    c. 1

    d. 0–2

CASE STUDY 19.2—cont'd

Q2. What nutrients are contained in a glass of full-cream milk?

   a. Fat

   b. Fat and protein

   c. Carbohydrate

   d. Carbohydrate, fat and protein

Q3. Vitamin B12 can be found in various foods; which of the following is not a dietary source of vitamin B12?

   a. Red meat

   b. Fish

   c. Cereal

   d. Dairy

Q4. What essential nutrients is Sally missing in her new diet and what is the function of these nutrients?

Q5. Explain why Sally is feeling more tired than previously and how metabolism may have changed in her body.

CASE STUDY 19.3

Rob is worried about his diet and whether he is getting all the nutrients his body needs. He tries to eat a range of foods each day including a serving of meat, at least 4–5 serves of grains, 1–2 pieces of fruit and 4–5 servings of vegetables, but to guarantee that he is getting enough, he decides to start taking vitamin supplements. After a visit to the pharmacy Rob purchases a multivitamin and vitamin C tablets. He starts taking these on a daily basis but after a few days he notices that his urine is bright yellow, and even after drinking more water the colour does not change.

Q1. Would 4–5 serves of vegetables per day be considered adequate according to the *Australian Guide to Healthy Eating*?

   a. No

   b. 5 serves is the recommended amount

   c. It depends what vegetables are included

   d. At least 4 is adequate

Q2. Which of the following foods contains vitamin C?

   a. Fish

   b. Cereal

   c. Yoghurt

   d. Tomato

Q3. Which of the following vitamins is considered fat-soluble, meaning it is stored and transported in the body by fat tissue?

   a. Vitamin C

   b. Vitamin B12

   c. Vitamin E

   d. Folate

Q4. Explain whether Rob is at risk of consuming vitamins in excess based on the information provided.

Q5. Explain why Rob's urine is bright yellow and what might be contributing to this.

CASE STUDY 19.4

Greg, a 67-year-old male, visited his GP for a check-up and had his blood pressure measured. His GP told Greg that his blood pressure was high and asked him whether anyone else in his family had high blood pressure as well as about his diet, particularly how much salt he consumed. Greg explained that he adds salt to most of his food because he likes the taste and has been doing this for years.

Q1. Which of the following is commonly found in salt and salt products?

   a. Vitamin B6

   b. Chloride

   c. Phosphorus

   d. Sodium

Continued

CASE STUDY 19.4—cont'd

Q2. Which sentence best describes the process of osmosis?

   a. The movement of water from an area of low concentration to an area of high concentration

   b. The movement of water from an area of high concentration to an area of low concentration

   c. The movement of water between areas of similar concentration

   d. The movement of sodium from an area of high concentration to an area of low concentration

Q3. Sodium is an electrolyte; which of the following is also an electrolyte?

   a. Magnesium

   b. Folate

   c. Vitamin C

   d. Water

Q4. Explain why a high intake of salt would lead to increased blood pressure.

Q5. How would the body manage a high salt intake from the diet? Think about the role of both the GI tract and the kidneys.

REFERENCES

1. Grodner M, Escott-Stump S. Nutritional foundations and clinical applications: a nursing approach, 6 ed. St Louis: Mosby; 2016.

2. Silverthorn D. Human physiology: an integrated approach, 7 ed. San Francisco: Pearson; 2015.

3. Nettlejohn JA, Brouwer IA, Geleijnse JM, et al. Saturated fat consumption and risk of coronary heart disease and ischemic stroke: a science update. Ann Nutr Metab 2017;70(1):26–33.

4. Peate I, Nair M. Fundamentals of anatomy and physiology: for nursing and healthcare students, 2 ed. Wiley-Blackwell; 2016.

5. Intersalt Cooperative Research Group. Intersalt: an international study of electrolyte excretion and blood pressure. Results for 24h urinary sodium and potassium excretion. BMJ 1988;297:319–28.

6. Ha SK. Dietary salt intake and hypertension. Electrol Blood Press 2014;12(1):7–18.

7. National Health and Medical Research Council. Australian guide to healthy eating; 2017. Available from: www.eatforhealth.gov.au/guidelines/australian-guide -healthy-eating, on 30 August 2018.

8. Waugh A. The digestive system. In: Waugh A, Grant A, editors. Ross and Wilson anatomy and physiology in health and illness, 13 ed. Elsevier; 2018.

9. McCance K. Cellular biology. In: Huether S, McCance K, editors. Understanding pathophysiology, 6 ed. St Louis: Elsevier; 2017.

10. Leslie W, Hankey C. Aging, nutritional status and health. Healthcare 2015;3(3):648–58.

CHAPTER 20

Urinary system

JED MONTAYRE, RN, PHD • RACHEL MACDIARMID, RN, BSC, MHSC, DHSC •
ELISSA M MCDONALD, PHD • PADMAPRIYA SARAVANAKUMAR, RN, PHD

KEY POINTS/LEARNING OUTCOMES

1. Describe the anatomy and physiology of the urinary system.
2. Link the structure of the nephron with its function of glomerular filtration.
3. Discuss the normal physiological process of urine formation and the homeostatic role of the kidneys.
4. Link the physiological changes in urine formation and the physiological responses to maintain fluid and electrolyte balance.
5. Discuss the process of micturition relating to the structure and function of the urinary system.

KEY DEFINITIONS

- **Acid–base balance:** in terms of renal function, this refers to a homeostatic process whereby in order to maintain a stable pH level in blood plasma, the kidneys reabsorb bicarbonate ions and excrete hydrogen ions in urine.
- **Glomerular filtration rate (GFR):** the rate of fluid (blood) movement passing through the glomerulus to the capsular space in one minute.
- **Micturition:** also referred to as voiding or urination, the process that regulates the release of urine from the bladder, via the urethra.
- **Renal perfusion:** also known as renal blood flow, refers to the volume of blood delivered to the kidneys; in an adult, 25% of cardiac output goes to the kidneys.
- **Urine formation:** the production of waste end-product (urine) from the kidneys' filtration of blood. There are three main steps in urine formation: glomerular filtration, reabsorption and secretion.

ONLINE RESOURCES/SUGGESTED READINGS

- **Urinary system** available at www.innerbody.com/image/urinov.html
- **Urinary system** available at www.kenhub.com/en/library/anatomy/urinary-system
- **Kidneys** available at www.kenhub.com/en/library/anatomy/kidneys
- **Teach me anatomy: the kidneys** available at https://teachmeanatomy.info/abdomen/viscera/kidney
- **Teach me anatomy: the urinary bladder** available at https://teachmeanatomy.info/pelvis/viscera/bladder

INTRODUCTION

The functions performed by the urinary system, also known as the renal system, can be considered as routine (i.e. production and excretion of urine), protective (i.e. elimination of toxins, reactive to blood pressure changes) or balancing (i.e. pH control in the blood and subsequently the urine, and electrolyte reabsorption during formation of urine). The term 'renal' simply denotes something that relates to or involves the kidneys. Clinically, urinary system functions are carefully considered in the context of age-related and developmental characteristics when prescribing medications, as medication dosages and their effectiveness are heavily dependent on renal function. The urinary system has an incredible capacity to cope with adversity; for example, when a diseased kidney is removed, the body can still function effectively with only one kidney.

This chapter examines the structure and function of the urinary system and how different components of the system complement each other to maintain homeostatic balance through maintenance of acid–base balance in the blood, elimination of metabolic waste products and tight control of blood electrolyte balance. To function effectively, the kidneys—the masters of these processes—are heavily dependent on adequate blood perfusion, which is partially dictated by blood volume, a concept also explored in this chapter.

STRUCTURE AND FUNCTION OF THE URINARY SYSTEM
Macro anatomy
The urinary system consists of the kidneys and the urinary tract, which is composed of the ureters, bladder and urethra. Collectively, these structures facilitate the principal function of excretion of waste products and regulate the biochemical composition of blood.

Kidneys
The **kidneys** are bean-shaped organs with an average size of 11 cm × 7 cm × 3 cm (about the size of a clenched fist). They are located at a position referred to as retroperitoneal, meaning at the back of the peritoneum and against the abdominal wall (Fig. 20.1). The upper part of each kidney is protected by the 12th rib (also known as a floating rib). The right kidney is positioned slightly lower than the left. Located posteriorly and cushioned with adipose tissue, the kidneys are vulnerable to trauma and infection. However, the internal kidney structures are well-protected by connective tissues covering its surface.

The kidneys have layers that serve as a protective barrier separating them from other organs and secure their position to the abdominal wall. These three layers are the renal capsule, adipose capsule and renal fascia. The **renal capsule** is the surface covering of the

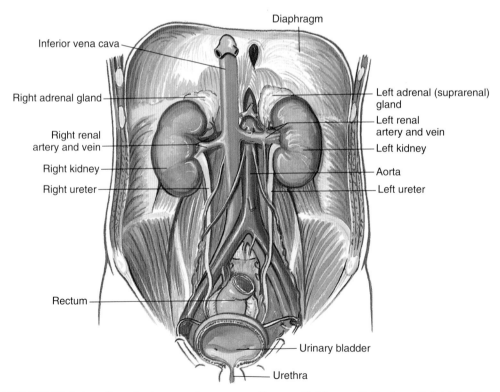

FIGURE 20.1 **Location of urinary system organs.** (*Source:* Christensen B, Kockrow E. Adult health nursing, 6 ed. Elsevier; 2010.)

kidneys. It is thin but tough and fibrous. It serves as a barrier against trauma and infection. Outside the renal capsule is the **adipose capsule**, a mass of fatty tissue that acts as a shock absorber and protects the kidneys from physical trauma. The outermost layer is the **renal fascia** which anchors the kidneys to the abdominal wall.

A coronal view of the kidney (Fig. 20.2) demonstrates the renal cortex (outermost region), renal medulla (interior region) and renal pyramids (extensions of the medulla forming triangular structures). In between each renal pyramid are extended cortical tissues referred to as **renal columns**. Each pyramid has a pointed base called a papilla, which has openings that drain urine through a cuplike structure known as the **calyx**. Minor calyces directly drain the papilla, which join and form the bigger calyces known as major calyces, which empty towards the renal pelvis.

The kidneys are generously supplied with blood vessels, hardly surprising when you consider that their function is to control the composition of blood. The two kidneys receive 25% of cardiac output (i.e. about 1200 mL of blood per minute). Fig. 20.3 illustrates the flow of blood from the abdominal aorta through the renal artery to the arterioles and back to the venous circulation (inferior vena cava) through the renal veins.

Ureters

The **ureters** are tubular structures originating from the renal pelvis, which means they drain urine from the kidneys to the urinary bladder. The ureters have unique anatomical features such as the oblique (diagonal) attachment of the end part of the tube towards the bladder floor creating a 'valve junction' regulating urine flow (slows the urine drain) to a full bladder and preventing backflow (Fig. 20.4). You might wonder whether urine flow from the ureters is influenced by gravity, or what happens when a person is lying flat? Overall, urine flow within the ureters is facilitated by ureteral peristalsis, a propelling movement due to muscular contraction. Even when lying flat, the ureters can propel urine because of their middle muscular layer with a unique stretchable lining that facilitates peristalsis.

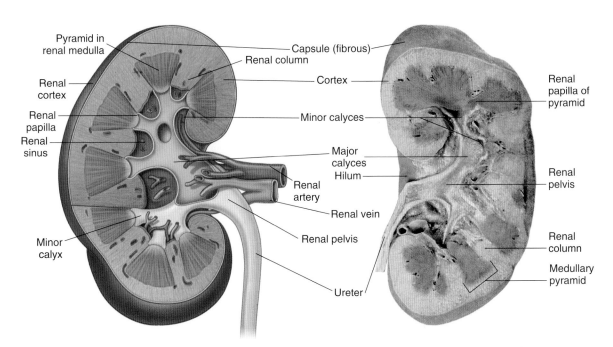

FIGURE 20.2 **Internal structure of the kidney.** (*Source:* Craft JA, Gordon CJ, Huether SE, McCance KL, Brashers VL, Rote NS. Understanding pathophysiology, 3 ed. Sydney: Elsevier; 2019.)

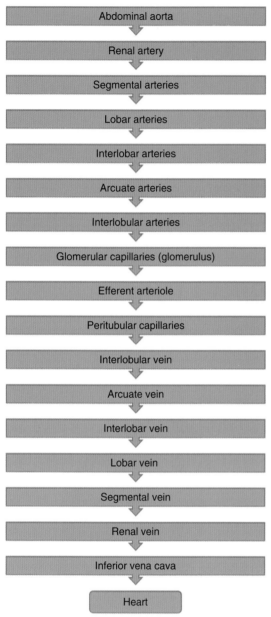

FIGURE 20.3 **Renal blood flow.** (*Source:* Patton KT, Thibodeau. The human body in health and disease, 6 ed. St Louis: Mosby; 2014.)

Bladder

The **bladder** stores urine before excreting it out of the body. Its internal muscular layer, the **detrusor muscle**, aids in moving urine towards the urethra (Fig. 20.5). The bladder can hold 300–400 mL of urine before the person starts to feel discomfort and a need to urinate. This urine-holding capacity is due to the presence of stretchable folds (rugae) in the bladder, which allow bladder expansion and distension. In females, the bladder is located anterior and slightly superior to the vagina and directly in front of the uterus. In males, the bladder is located on top of the prostate. The location of the urinary bladder in females structurally accommodates the reproductive organ changes that occur during pregnancy. These changes include enlargement of the uterus, which can increase external pressure on bladder function by limiting its capacity to expand, thus leading to more frequent urination. For males, an increase in the size of the prostate will exert pressure on the bladder and can obstruct urine flow. Collectively, these changes negatively affect urine storage and urine excretion from the bladder.

Urethra

The **urethra** is a tubular structure that originates from the bladder floor, a triangle-shaped area known as the trigone (Fig. 20.5), and extends to the urinary meatus (urethral opening) where urine is removed from the body into the external environment. In males, the urethra passes through the penis and has a dual function: to allow passage of urine and to enable the ejaculation of semen from the male reproductive tract. The male urethra is divided into functional sections named according to the adjacent organs it passes through. It extends a long way from the bladder floor and passes through the prostate gland, where it joins the ejaculatory ducts within the interior of the prostate gland (prostatic urethra), then exits the prostrate and passes through the bulbourethral gland (membranous urethra), extending down the penis (penile urethra) to the base of the urinary meatus. The female urethra is at the back of the symphysis pubis and in front of the vagina, and is much shorter than the male urethra. The close proximity of the urinary meatus to the anal opening in females is considered to be one of the reasons why females are more likely to experience urinary tract infections (UTIs) than males.

Micro anatomy
Nephron

Examination of a longitudinally sliced kidney with the naked eye shows light and dark pigmented regions, the

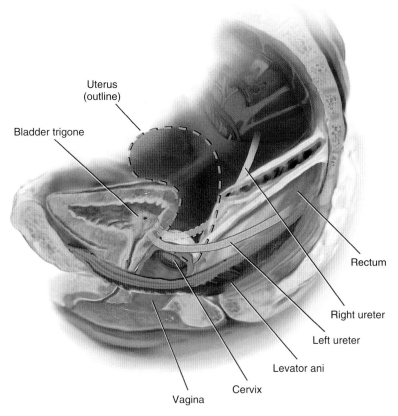

Uterus (outline)

Bladder trigone

Rectum

Right ureter

Left ureter

Levator ani

Cervix

Vagina

FIGURE 20.4 Ureter-bladder junction. Sagittal view of the ureters and urinary bladder shown in relation to the vagina (green) and uterus (dark pink). (*Source:* Baggish MS, Karram MM. Atlas of pelvic anatomy and gynecologic surgery, 4 ed. Elsevier; 2016.)

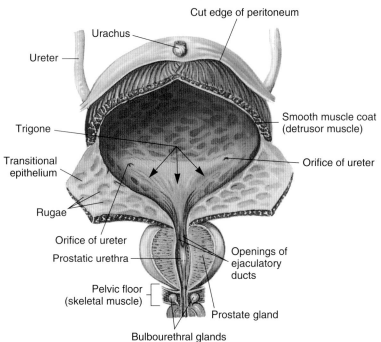

Cut edge of peritoneum

Urachus

Ureter

Trigone

Transitional epithelium

Rugae

Orifice of ureter

Prostatic urethra

Pelvic floor (skeletal muscle)

Smooth muscle coat (detrusor muscle)

Orifice of ureter

Openings of ejaculatory ducts

Prostate gland

Bulbourethral glands

FIGURE 20.5 Structure of the urinary bladder in the male. (*Source:* Monahan F, Green CJ, Marek JF, Sands JK. Phipps' medical-surgical nursing: health and illness perspectives, 8 ed. Mosby; 2006.)

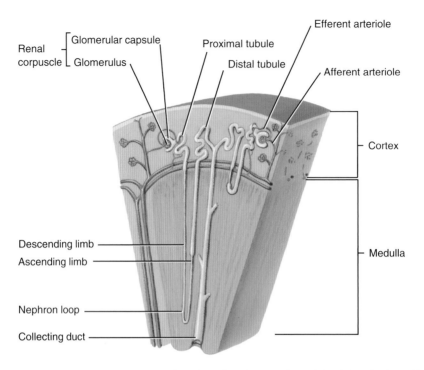

FIGURE 20.6 **Nephron.** (*Source:* Shiland BJ. Medical assistant: urinary, blood, lymphatic and immune systems with laboratory procedures. Elsevier; 2005.)

cortex and **medulla** (Fig. 20.6). The patch-like appearance is due to the arrangement of the 'functional units' of the kidney, the **nephrons**. There are approximately one million nephrons in each kidney. Nephrons are referred to as 'functional units' because it is here that the filtration of blood takes place and urine production occurs. In terms of cell regeneration, it is thought that nephrons have an extremely limited capacity to renew.[1]

There are two types of nephrons, named after their anatomical location within the kidneys. The majority of nephrons are located in the renal cortex and hence are called cortical nephrons; those originating close to the cortex and within the renal medulla are called juxtamedullary nephrons (*juxta* means 'close to'). Nephron distribution within the kidneys gives rise to the dark and light shades of colour seen in the renal layers from a coronal view.

At a microscopic level, the nephron structure is described as a tuft of blood vessels (capillaries) extending towards a tubular path (Fig. 20.7). The vascular tuft is protected by a double-walled cup comprised of inner and outer epithelial cell walls. Because of the unique association between the epithelial structures of the nephron and nephron capillaries, each nephron is able to both filter blood and facilitate reabsorption of electrolytes sensitive to changes of body fluid composition.

There are two major parts to the nephron: the renal corpuscle and the renal tubule. Each structure has a unique role in blood filtration, reabsorption of biochemicals needed by the body and secretion of urine.

Renal corpuscle. The **renal corpuscle** is the blood-filtering part of the nephron and it is formed from the tuft of blood capillaries, commonly known as the **glomerulus**, and the glomerular capsular space where the glomerulus is found. This capsule is known as Bowman's capsule or glomerular capsule. The capillary network of the glomerulus has a unique structure of large pores (fenestrae) not covered by a diaphragm that permits passage of water, ions and small molecules into the glomerular capsular space, thus enabling blood filtration to occur within the nephrons of a healthy kidney. Blood enters the glomerulus through the afferent arteriole and exits through the efferent arteriole. Bowman's capsule facilitates the filtration process within the renal corpuscle by providing the intimate layer covering the glomerular capillaries called the visceral wall, which separates filtered blood and the space where the glomerular filtrate (soon

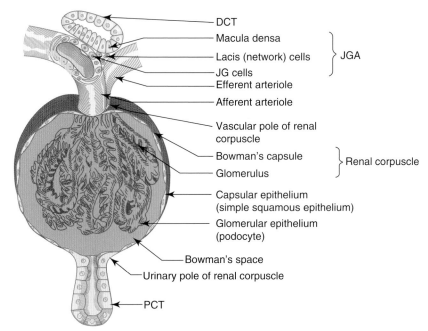

DCT
Macula densa
Lacis (network) cells ⎫
⎬ JGA
JG cells
Efferent arteriole
Afferent arteriole
Vascular pole of renal corpuscle
Bowman's capsule ⎫
⎬ Renal corpuscle
Glomerulus
Capsular epithelium (simple squamous epithelium)
Glomerular epithelium (podocyte)
Bowman's space
Urinary pole of renal corpuscle
PCT

FIGURE 20.7 **Structure of the renal corpuscle.** (*Source:* Gunasegaran JP. Textbook of histology: a practical guide, 2 ed. Elsevier; 2010.)

to be urine) enters before it travels to the renal tubules. The layers of Bowman's capsule and the pores within the lining of the glomerular endothelium are collectively referred to as the filtration barrier.

Renal tubule. The **renal tubule** extends out from Bowman's capsule and is subdivided into four segments: the proximal convoluted tubule, loop of Henle, distal convoluted tubule and collecting ducts. The first segment of the renal tubule originating from Bowman's capsule is the **proximal** (nearest) **convoluted** (winding) **tubule (PCT)**. The filtrate passes through the parietal wall of Bowman's capsule and enters the proximal convoluted tubule, which has brush-like structures on its cell lining, called microvilli, that increase the surface area, facilitating its absorptive function. The next tube segment is the nephron loop, also known as the **loop of Henle**. The loop has two sub-segments: the descending loop and the ascending loop. The epithelial cell lining of the nephron loop changes as the loop reaches the ascending loop, leading to a thicker segment. The structural difference in terms of wall thickness is important to the permeability and transport functions of water molecules, urea and electrolytes. The descending limb allows easy diffusion of water and waste products like urea while the ascending limb limits diffusion of molecules and

performs a selective reabsorption function. This nephron loop extends to the **distal convoluted tubule (DCT)**. This tubule has a similar cell lining to the PCT, although the cells are thinner and have no absorptive function. The **collecting ducts** are at the end of the renal tubules and receive the filtrate from nephrons. These ducts contain epithelial cells with microvilli, which control the reabsorption of water and maintain electrolyte balance, particularly of sodium. The collecting ducts aggregate towards renal calyces and drain the remaining filtrate (now urine) towards the renal pelvis.

Nephron capillary network

To understand the process of urine production and the kidneys' role in regulating fluid composition, it is important to know how the nephron capillary networks are structurally designed. Probably the most unusual feature of blood flow in the kidneys is the fact that two capillary networks exist in series. The two networks are the glomerular capillaries (glomerulus) and the peritubular capillaries.

An important feature of blood flow to the kidneys that contributes to the high rate of filtration is the relatively high blood pressure in each nephron's glomerulus. This arises because the glomerular efferent arteriole is narrower than the afferent arteriole, leading to increased peripheral resistance to blood flow, which is evident as a naturally high-pressure environment. This can be easily imagined if you consider what occurs when water moves from a pipe with a wider spout to a hose with a narrower spout and observe the pressure at which water flows (i.e. wider spout, lower pressure; narrower hose, greater pressure of flow).

In the rest of the body blood would flow from an arteriole through a capillary network then be drained into a venule, but within the renal circulation the pathway is not the same. In the glomerulus, blood flows from the efferent arteriole into a specialised capillary network, the peritubular capillaries (Fig. 20.8). The efferent arteriole leaves the glomerular capillary tuft and branches into the peritubular capillaries which supply the tubule. Peritubular capillaries (*peri* means around) facilitate two important processes: reabsorption of water and electrolytes from the filtrate to the systemic circulation; and secretion of excess/unneeded substances to maintain homeostasis such as the acid–base balance.

Physiological process of urine formation

Urine is formed as a result of three processes that take place in the nephrons: glomerular filtration, tubular reabsorption and tubular secretion (Fig. 20.9). When urine is formed it consists of water, sodium, chloride, magnesium, sulfates, phosphates, bicarbonates, uric acid, ammonium ions, creatinine and urobilinogen, a by-product of bilirubin breakdown.

Glomerular filtration

Filtration is the first step in urine formation. This process captures mechanisms responsible for the movement of water and small solutes from the blood passing through the glomerular capillaries into the glomerular capsule to form filtrate, which is a precursor urine. The glomerulus is an efficient filter and fluid moves across a permeable membrane with a large surface area. It is estimated that in the healthy adult kidney 180 L of filtrate is formed per day. Fluid movement is caused by the relationship between glomerular hydrostatic pressure, blood colloid

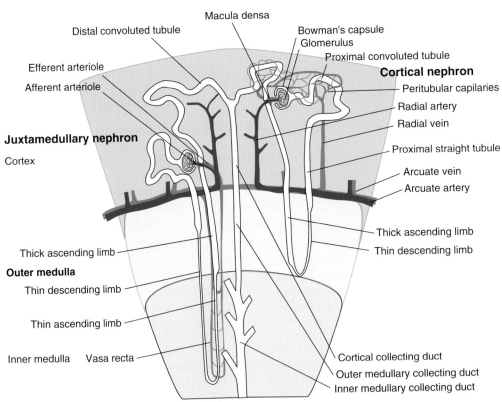

FIGURE 20.8 Blood supply to the nephron. Two general kinds of nephrons are shown: a juxtamedullary nephron and a cortical nephron. Blood supply is partially shown, with most capillaries omitted. (*Source:* Feher J. Quantitative human physiology: an introduction. 2 ed. Elsevier; 2017.)

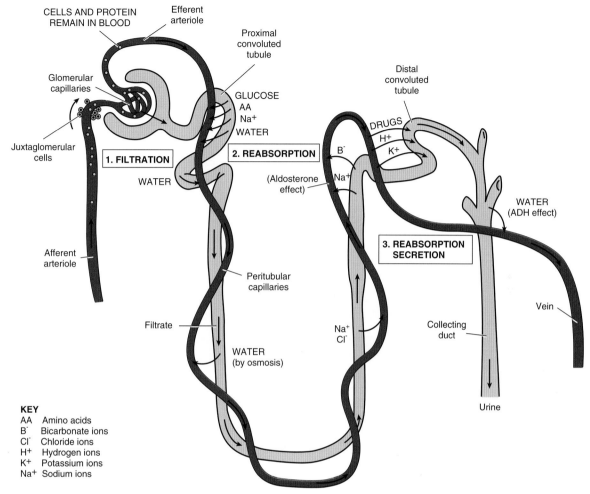

CELLS AND PROTEIN
REMAIN IN BLOOD

Efferent
arteriole

Proximal
convoluted
tubule

Glomerular
capillaries

Distal
convoluted
tubule

GLUCOSE
AA
Na⁺
WATER

DRUGS

H⁺

K⁺

Juxtaglomerular
cells

1. FILTRATION

2. REABSORPTION

B⁻

WATER

(Aldosterone
effect)

Na⁺

WATER
(ADH effect)

Afferent
arteriole

**3. REABSORPTION
SECRETION**

Peritubular
capillaries

Vein

Filtrate

Na⁺
Cl⁻

Collecting
duct

WATER
(by osmosis)

Urine

KEY
AA   Amino acids
B⁻   Bicarbonate ions
Cl⁻ Chloride ions
H⁺   Hydrogen ions
K⁺   Potassium ions
Na⁺ Sodium ions

FIGURE 20.9 **Overview of urine formation.** (*Source:* Hubert RJ, Van Meter KC. Gould's pathophysiology for the health professions, 6 ed. Elsevier; 2018.)

osmotic pressure and capsular hydrostatic pressure (Fig. 20.10).

Glomerular hydrostatic pressure is a force that moves water and solutes into the glomerular space. It is equivalent to the blood pressure of the afferent arteriole in the glomerulus. It is influenced by systemic blood pressure and the resistance of the glomerular capillaries. The resistance of the glomerular capillaries is due to the smaller diameter of the efferent arteriole (this arteriole leaves the glomerulus). Hydrostatic pressure causes the movement of water and solutes from the plasma into the filtrate.

Blood colloid osmotic pressure is a form of osmotic pressure exerted by proteins, predominantly albumin, present in the blood plasma. An increase in the number

of plasma proteins increases the osmotic pressure. The effect of blood colloid osmotic pressure is to draw water out of filtrate and into the plasma.

Capsular hydrostatic pressure opposes glomerular hydrostatic pressure. Basically, it is a force exerted against the filtration membrane in Bowman's capsule and the end result is to force water and solutes from the filtrate back into the plasma. It is through this process that the body preserves these important blood components.

Another important concept in renal anatomy and physiology is that of the **glomerular filtration rate (GFR)**. Clinically, you will see this parameter reported when a patient's renal function is assessed. The GFR is the amount of filtrate the kidneys produce each minute. The rate at which plasma is filtered is estimated to be

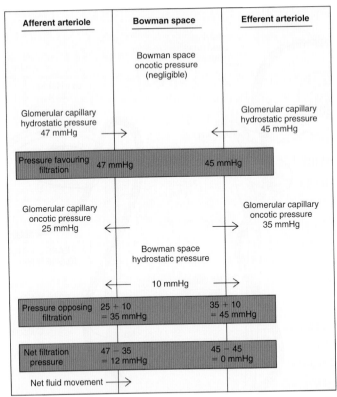

FIGURE 20.10 **Pressure affecting glomerular filtration.** Angiotensin II increases filtration pressure by (1) increasing pressure in the afferent arteriole (secondary to increasing systemic arterial pressure) and (2) constricting the efferent arteriole, thereby generating back-pressure in the glomerulus. (*Source:* McCance K, Huether S. Pathophysiology: the biologic basis for disease in adults and children, 8 ed. Elsevier; 2019.)

125 mL per minute in a healthy adult. There are two levels of control of the GFR. One occurs within the kidneys and is therefore referred to as a locally controlled process that constitutes renal autoregulation. The other occurs through collaboration of the endocrine, renal and vascular systems and is thus known as central regulation. Renal autoregulation involves a response to a change in blood pressure or constriction and dilation of arterioles in an attempt to maintain normal GFR. Central regulation involves the action of hormones such as renin, aldosterone, anti-diuretic hormone (ADH) and atrial natriuretic peptide (ANP) to maintain the normal GFR when renal autoregulation is insufficient (Fig. 20.10).[3,4]

Tubular reabsorption

Reabsorption, the second step in urine formation, involves the removal of water and solutes from the filtrate and their return into the blood. Most of the reabsorbed solutes are fundamental to homeostasis. While reabsorption occurs along the entire length of the tubule, most reabsorption takes place in the PCT (Fig. 20.9).

The processes of reabsorption and secretion in the kidneys involve a combination of diffusion, osmosis, channel-mediated diffusion and carrier-mediated transport. Diffusion is the passive movement of a substance from an area of high concentration to an area of low concentration across a semi-permeable membrane. Osmosis describes the movement of water across a semi-permeable membrane. In the kidneys, water moves from the tubule fluid into the peritubular fluid through water channels known as aquaporins. In channel-mediated diffusion, molecules diffuse across the membrane through channels. These channels are like tunnels and are very selective about the molecules they accept for transport across the membrane. In carrier-mediated transport, proteins bind to specific ions and carry them across the membrane. Active transport uses ATP as energy and can work against the concentration gradient to move sodium, potassium and chloride ions out of the tubular fluid. Each cycle of the pump carries sodium, potassium and two chloride ions into the tubular cell. Potassium ions diffuse back into the tubules and the end result is that sodium and chloride enter the peritubular fluid.

Reabsorption and secretion in the PCT. The PCT is involved in both reabsorption and secretion (Fig. 20.9). The PCT has five functions: (1) reabsorption of organic nutrients; (2) active reabsorption of ions; (3) reabsorption of water; (4) passive reabsorption of ions; and (5) secretion. Organic nutrients are reabsorbed through facilitated transport and active transport known as co-transport. Co-transport involves a carrier molecule that binds two molecules, such as sodium and glucose. Both molecules use different mechanisms to move. For example, sodium moves down a concentration gradient from an area of high concentration to an area of low concentration, but glucose requires no energy because it is 'riding the coattails' of sodium.[4] Normally, all the

glucose that was filtered out initially in the glomerulus returns to the blood using this mechanism, so there is only a very small amount of glucose in urine. However, this is limited by the number of co-transporters available. Ions such as sodium (Na^+), potassium (K^+) and bicarbonate (HCO_3^-), plus magnesium phosphate and sulphate, are reabsorbed by active transport. Notably, bicarbonate is important in maintaining blood pH homeostasis (see the following section on acid–base balance). Water moves by osmosis out of the tubular fluid and into the peritubular fluid. Passive reabsorption of urea, chloride ions and lipid-soluble ions takes place by diffusion into the peritubular fluid (Fig. 20.11). Secretion involves the transport of solutes (such as hydrogen, ammonium ions, creatinine, some drugs and toxins) from the peritubular fluid into the lumen of the renal tubule.[4]

Reabsorption in the DCT. Sodium is reabsorbed by active transport in the DCT similarly to the PCT. Cells in the DCT walls are mostly impermeable to water so

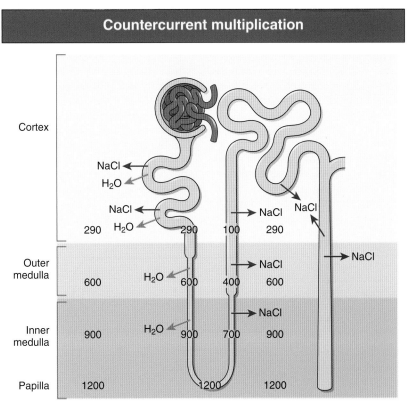

FIGURE 20.11 **Production of hypertonic urine.** (*Source:* Feehally J, Floege J, Tonelli M, Johnson RJ. Comprehensive clinical nephrology, 6 ed. Elsevier; 2019.)

water does not follow sodium. This means that the solute concentration in the tubule fluid increases.[4] Two hormones (aldosterone and ADH) influence fluid balance in the DCT. Aldosterone influences reabsorption of sodium and water in the DCT, while ADH influences water reabsorption from the collecting ducts, thus preventing excessive water loss (Fig. 20.9). Only 15–20% of the initial filtrate volume ends up reaching the DCT. Both secretion and reabsorption happen in the DCT. Sodium ions are reabsorbed as an exchange for potassium ions. If the pH decreases, hydrogen ions (H⁺) are exchanged with sodium ions.

Tubular secretion

Tubular **secretion** is the third step in urine formation and involves the movement of solutes from the peritubular capillaries into the tubular filtrate. Potassium, ammonia and other waste products are secreted from the peritubular capillaries into the distal tubules (Fig. 20.12). This process involves active transport. Potassium ions and hydrogen ions are actively transported out of the blood into the tubule fluid in exchange for sodium ions.

Composition of urine

The normal composition of urine is water and waste products. Because urine production is a direct reflection of kidney function, it is important to recognise normal and abnormal urine contents and composition. Table 20.1 presents the normal and abnormal composition of urine.

Acid–base balance

The acid–base composition of the extracellular and intracellular environments needs to be regulated constantly to achieve homeostasis. A narrow pH range of 7.35–7.45 ensures optimal functioning of the body at the cellular level. For example, normal pH ensures the ability of mitochondria to produce energy, helps enzymes to function optimally and is crucial for cell membrane excitability.[5] Three main systems are involved in correcting the pH when there is an imbalance in the acid and base composition of blood: the chemical buffers, respiratory system and urinary system. The kidneys play a major role particularly in correcting the metabolic component of the acid–base balance. To achieve this balance, the kidneys perform several processes simultaneously: secretion of hydrogen ions, reabsorption of bicarbonate ions and excretion of excess hydrogen ions by buffering with ammonium and phosphate.

For simplicity, let us look at two main processes: bicarbonate reabsorption and hydrogen ion excretion. By controlling bicarbonate reabsorption and hydrogen ion excretion, the pH of the blood plasma is kept within normal limits. For example, if blood is too acidic, more hydrogen ions are excreted; if blood is too basic, fewer hydrogen ions are excreted. The excretion of hydrogen ions is determined by the concentration of hydrogen ions (pH), bicarbonate and the partial pressure of CO_2 (pCO₂). This relationship is described by the Henderson-Hasselbalch equation:[6]

$$pH = 6.1 + \log \frac{HCO_3^-}{0.03 \times pCO_2}$$

where HCO_3^- is in milliequivalents per litre and pCO₂ is in millimetres of mercury.

The acid–base regulatory processes happen at different locations in the nephron. As the filtrate leaves the glomerulus, it first enters through the PCT. Most of the bicarbonate that is filtered at the glomerulus is reabsorbed at the PCT. The bicarbonate combines with hydrogen ions that are secreted by the tubular cells, forming carbonic acid. The enzyme carbonic anhydrase acts on this carbonic acid ($H_2CO_3^-$), which then dissociates into

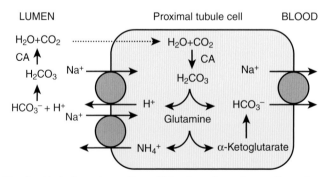

FIGURE 20.12 **Proximal tubule reabsorption of bicarbonate and secretion of ammonium.** (*Source:* Martin RJ. Fanaroff and Martin's neonatal-perinatal medicine, 10 ed. Philadelphia, NJ: Saunders; 2015.)

TABLE 20.1
Characteristics of urine

	Normal characteristics	Abnormal characteristics

Colour and clarity	Normal urine should be clear; colour varies with specific gravity
	Dilute urine: transparent straw colour
	Concentrated urine: deep yellow amber
	(Occasionally, normal urine may be cloudy because of high dietary levels of fat or phosphate)
	
	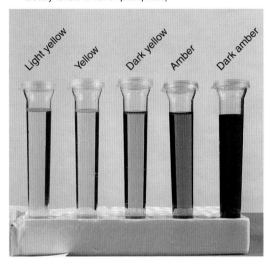
		Abnormally coloured urine may result from (1) pathological conditions; (2) certain foods; and (3) numerous drugs:
		1. Pathological conditions (examples):
		  Kidney cancer (haemorrhage—red (red blood cells [RBCs])
		  Bile duct obstruction (gallstone)—orange/yellow (bilirubin)
		  Pseudomonas infection—green (bacterial toxins)
		2. Foods (examples):
		  Beets—red
		  Rhubarb—brown
		  Carrots—dark yellow
		3. Drugs (examples):
		  Pyridium (urinary tract analgesic)—orange
		  Dilantin (anticonvulsant)—pink/red brown
		  Dyrenium (diuretic)—pale blue
		Cloudy urine may result from (examples):
		1. Bacteria—active infection of urinary system organs
		2. Blood cells
		  RBCs—haemorrhage from kidney cancer
		  WBCs—pus from urinary tract infection (UTI)
		3. Casts—various types of tubelike clumps (blood cell, epithelial, hyaline, waxy, etc.) that form in diseased renal tubes
		4. Proteinuria—protein—usually albumin—in urine
		5. Crystals—usually uric acid or phosphate/calcium oxalate in concentrated urine

Compounds	Mineral ions (for example, Na^+, Cl^-, K^+) Nitrogenous wastes: creatine, urea, uric acid Urine pigment: urochrome (product of bilirubin metabolism)	Ketones—generally acetone Protein—generally albumin Glucose Crystals—generally uric acid and phosphate or calcium oxalate Pigments—abnormal levels of bilirubin metabolites
Odour	Slight aromatic Some foods produce a characteristic odour (asparagus) Ammonia-like odour on standing may result from decomposition in stored urine	Strong, sweet, fruity (acetone) odour—uncontrolled diabetes mellitus Foul odour—urinary tract infections (UTIs) Musty odour—phenylketonuria Maple syrup odour—congenital defect in protein metabolism
pH	4.6–8.0 (average 6.0) Towards low normal: some foods (meat and cranberries) and drugs (chlorothiazide diuretics) Towards high normal: some foods (citrus fruits, dairy products) and drugs (bicarbonate antacids)	High in alkalosis (kidneys compensate by excreting excess base) Low in acidosis (kidneys compensate by excreting excess H^+)
Specific gravity	Adult: 1.005–1.030 (usually, 1.010–1.025) Elderly: values decrease with age Newborn: 1.001–1.020	Above normal limits: glycosuria, proteinuria, dehydration, high solute load (may result in precipitation of solutes and kidney stone formation) Below normal limits: chronic renal diseases (inability to concentrate urine), overhydration

Light yellow Yellow Dark yellow Amber Dark amber

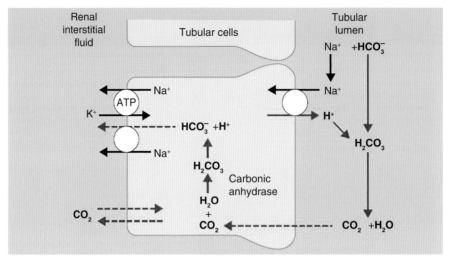

FIGURE 20.13 **Bicarbonate reabsorption.** (*Source:* McTavish AD, Sharma M-P. Renal physiology: acid–base balance. Anaesth Intensive Care Med 2018;19(5):233–8.)

carbon dioxide and water. This process is shown in the following equation:

$$HCO_3^- + H^+ \leftrightarrow H_2CO_3 \leftrightarrow H_2O + CO_2$$

Water remains in the filtrate that passes through the lumen, when carbon dioxide enters the tubular cell by diffusion, where the reverse of the same process happens: cellular carbonic anhydrase aids the combination of carbon dioxide and water. The resulting carbonic acid dissociates, forming hydrogen and bicarbonate ions (Fig. 20.13). The hydrogen ion is exchanged for sodium and

excreted via active transport into the filtrate in the lumen. The bicarbonate ion is moved across the basolateral membrane of the tubular cell along with the sodium ion. When the filtrate passes through the DCT, bicarbonate is again reabsorbed. In the PCT cell, there is another process that helps to get rid of hydrogen ions, through ammonium formation. This is via glutamine (an amino acid) that breaks down into ammonia and bicarbonate ions. While bicarbonate is moved into the bloodstream, the intracellular ammonia combines with hydrogen ions to form ammonium (Fig. 20.14). The ammonium is exchanged for sodium and moved into

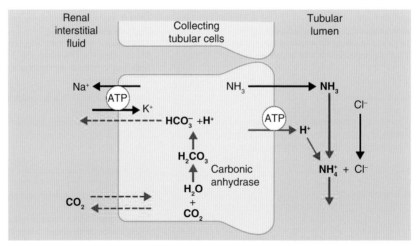

FIGURE 20.14 **Hydrogen ion excretion.** (*Source:* McTavish AD, Sharma M-P. Renal physiology: acid–base balance. Anaesth Intensive Care Med 2018;19(5):233–8.)

the filtrate. This then combines with chloride in urine, forming ammonium chloride (NH_4Cl). In the filtrate, there is another buffer, phosphate (formed from dissociation of sodium hydrogen phosphate in the developing urine), which binds with the excreted hydrogen ions to form di-hydrogen phosphate ions ($H_2PO_4^-$):[7]

$$HPO_4^{-2} + H^+ \leftrightarrow H_2PO_4^-$$

Blood volume and blood pressure regulation

The kidneys participate in the regulation of blood volume and pressure, through a process initiated by a group of hormones that constitute the **renin-angiotensin-aldosterone system (RAAS)**.[3,4] Note that earlier we discussed how this same system regulates the GFR.

Juxtaglomerular cells are cells that are receptive to signals generated by detecting low blood pressure, sympathetic stimulation and secretion of adenosine (by macula densa cells in response to increased GFR). In response to these signals, juxtaglomerular cells release the enzyme **renin** into the bloodstream.[2] Renin then reaches the liver, where it interacts with the protein **angiotensinogen** and converts it into **angiotensin I**, which then circulates in the blood. Endothelial cells, particularly those that line the lungs, contain the enzyme **angiotensin converting enzyme** (ACE). ACE converts angiotensin I to **angiotensin II**.[2,3] This molecule causes systemic vasoconstriction, meaning that all blood vessels in the body decrease their vessel lumen, thus increasing resistance to blood flow. Angiotensin II also binds to the angiotensin receptors in the afferent and efferent arterioles in the nephrons, leading to vasoconstriction of these vessels, which impacts on renal blood flow and the GFR. At the proximal tubule, it causes increased sodium ion reabsorption, which is followed by osmotic movement of water. Angiotensin II also stimulates the production of **antidiuretic hormone (ADH)**. ADH increases water reabsorption from the distal tubule[2] and the collecting ducts to conserve blood volume. This process results in increasing the blood pressure. Lastly, the RAAS also responds by another chain of events that is set off by angiotensin II. Angiotensin II stimulates the adrenal gland to secrete **aldosterone**. Aldosterone has an effect on the filtration function of the kidneys so that it conserves blood volume through increased function of the sodium-potassium ion pumps in the distal tubule and the collecting ducts. This enables movement of sodium ions into the blood in exchange for potassium ions. Movement of sodium into the blood changes the concentration gradient and hence is followed by the osmotic movement of water, which increases the blood volume and pressure. Angiotensin II also stimulates the release of adrenaline (epinephrine) and noradrenaline (norepinephrine), which enhance the vasoconstriction that assists in the regulation of blood pressure and maintenance of the GFR.[2]

Micturition

Micturition—also known as voiding the bladder, passing urine or urinating—is the release of urine collected from the kidneys and stored in the bladder via the urethra (Fig. 20.15). This is usually under conscious (voluntary) control from the age of two to three years. The process of micturition is under the control of autonomic and somatic nervous system innervation to the detrusor muscle of the bladder and the internal and external urethral sphincters.

An important distinction needs to be made between the different muscle types within the urinary system, as this dictates function and control. The detrusor muscle, which comprises the greater proportion of the bladder, is composed of smooth muscle. Smooth muscle is involuntary, non-striated muscle that lines hollow internal organs. This muscle type enables contraction of the bladder. Within the bladder, the detrusor muscle fibres are oriented in three directions to retain its structural integrity when it stretches.[4] As the internal urethral sphincter is a thickened extension of the detrusor muscle, it is under the control of the autonomic nervous system (parasympathetic and sympathetic nervous systems) and

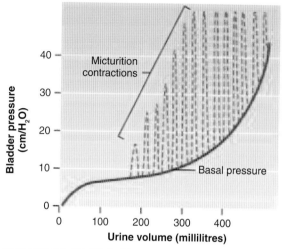

FIGURE 20.15 **Micturition reflex.** (*Source:* Patton KT, Thibodeau GA. Anatomy and physiology, 10 ed. St Louis, MI: Elsevier; 2019.)

TABLE 20.2
Musculature and innervation of the internal and external urethral sphincters

	Internal urethral sphincter	External urethral sphincter
Muscle type	Smooth	Skeletal
Control	Involuntary	Voluntary
Prevent micturition	Sympathetic nervous system	Somatic nervous system: pudendal nerve
Initiate conscious micturition	Parasympathetic nervous system	Somatic nervous system: pudendal nerve
Involuntary micturition (babies and infants)	Parasympathetic nervous system	Parasympathetic nervous system

therefore is not controlled consciously. In contrast to this, skeletal muscles are striated voluntary muscles that are attached to bone via tendons and enable body movement. The external urethral sphincter is composed of skeletal muscle and is under the control of the somatic nervous system via the pudendal nerve. This difference in muscle types is what provides the ability to control when micturition occurs (Table 20.2).

Storage of urine in the bladder
Storage of urine in the bladder is controlled by both the autonomic and somatic nervous systems. Sympathetic stimulation via the **hypogastric nerve** causes contraction of the internal urethral sphincter and inhibits contraction of the detrusor muscle. Stimulation of the sympathetic nervous system inhibits micturition. As the detrusor muscle in the bladder relaxes, it can accommodate an increasing amount of urine produced by the kidneys. The internal urethral sphincter contracts to enable the bladder to retain the urine it has collected. The external urethral sphincter is constantly stimulated by the pudendal nerve in the somatic nervous system to enable it to remain contracted and prevent micturition (Fig. 20.16).

The micturition reflex
The micturition reflex is under the control of the autonomic and somatic nervous systems. Parasympathetic

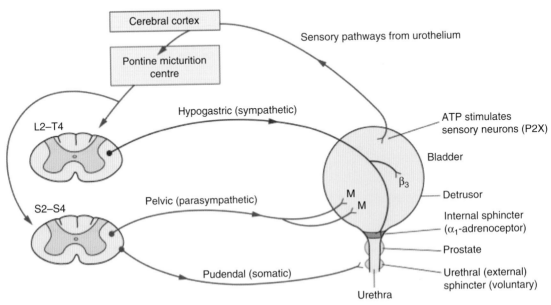

FIGURE 20.16 Aspects of the bladder/prostate structures and the innervation involved in the micturition reflex. (*Source:* Waller DG, Sampson T. Medical pharmacology and therapeutics. Elsevier Health Sciences; 2017.)

control of micturition[8] originates in the micturition centre located in the pons of the brain. Parasympathetic nerves from this centre travel down the spinal cord to the splanchnic nerves in the sacral area and innervate the detrusor muscle in the bladder and the internal urethral sphincter via the pelvic nerve. Parasympathetic nerves stimulate contraction of the detrusor muscle once the volume of urine reaches approximately 200 mL, as illustrated in Fig. 20.15. Stretch receptors in the bladder wall are stimulated by distension of the bladder, sending signals to the micturition centre in the pons, which then relays signals down the spinal cord to the splanchnic nerves.[2] Stimulation of these nerves causes the detrusor muscle to contract and the internal urethral sphincter to relax, enabling micturition to occur. This sequence of events enables urine to be expelled from the bladder via the urethra. The parasympathetic division stimulates micturition.

Urinary control also involves coordination of the levator ani muscle, the thoracic diaphragm and the abdominal musculature. Neuronal links between the spine and the cerebral cortex are not firmly established until approximately two years of age, therefore toilet training before this time may not be physiologically possible. By learning to use these systems of control, children can double their bladder capacity between the ages of two and four and a half years. A larger bladder capacity, along with firmly established neuronal control, enables children to control urine storage overnight.

Conscious awareness of bladder fullness can override signals from the micturition centre, although it can take up to one minute before the detrusor muscle contractions subside and the immediacy of the urge passes. During conscious suppression of micturition, the bladder keeps filling and the urge to urinate becomes stronger. Micturition usually occurs before the volume of urine reaches 400 mL in the bladder, although the bladder can stretch to accommodate up to 800–1000 mL of urine. However, there is a tipping point where conscious control is overridden by the parasympathetic nervous system and micturition occurs involuntarily. After micturition, approximately 10 mL of urine is left in the bladder and the storage reflex (sympathetic nervous system) is activated to begin the process of urine collection again.

The pudendal nerve is able to contract the external urethral sphincter voluntarily to control the timing of micturition.[2] Urinary continence is dependent on the descending spinal pathways inhibiting parasympathetic stimulation to the bladder and stimulating the pudendal nerve (somatic nervous system) supplying the external urethral sphincter.[8]

INTEGRATION OF THE URINARY SYSTEM WITH OTHER BODY SYSTEMS

Integumentary system

When a person sweats a lot, either through excessive exercise or due to the high temperature of the environment, water is lost through the skin. This loss affects the blood volume and will be detected by the kidneys. The response will be to initiate compensatory mechanisms to adjust to that water loss. Another link between the urinary system and the skin is vitamin D synthesis. As mentioned in Chapter 3, a precursor of vitamin D is formed in skin cells. This precursor form is transported to the kidneys where is its converted into the active form of vitamin D, which then impacts on bone health.

Skeletal system

As the active form of vitamin D is synthesised by the kidneys, the kidneys' ability to do so directly impacts on blood levels of calcium ions, which are needed for bone remodelling, a process that involves both bone growth and bone repair.

Muscular system

Muscle contraction is heavily dependent on the tight control of blood calcium, sodium and potassium ion levels. Concentration of sodium and potassium ions is regulated by the kidneys through the GFR, whereas concentration of calcium ions is indirectly regulated through kidney-driven vitamin D synthesis. We have already noted that contraction of renal tubules depends on the contraction of smooth muscle cells, while kidney protection from external trauma is provided by the skeletal muscles of the ribs at the back of the body. The bladder's capacity to expand to accommodate increased urine volume and the ureter's capacity to excrete urine are also dependent on muscular cells.

Nervous system

Similar to the muscular system, conduction in the cells of the nervous system is heavily dependent on the levels of sodium, potassium and calcium ions, blood levels of which are dependent on effective kidney function. Furthermore, the kidneys, via the RAAS, communicate with the nervous system to regulate systemic blood pressure as previously described. In this case, it is important to note that renin release can also be stimulated by sympathetic nerve activation via beta$_1$ adrenoceptors.[2] Angiotensin II also stimulates the thirst centre in the brain and facilitates the noradrenaline (norepinephrine) release while inhibiting noradrenaline (norepinephrine) uptake, which enhances the sympathetic adrenergic effects.

When the bladder is full, signals are sent to the autonomic nervous system, which controls the muscles that permit bladder stretch but also the muscles in the ureter to release and constrict during voluntary expulsion of urine, as discussed above.

Endocrine system

Kidney function is heavily regulated by the endocrine system. The kidneys have an endocrine-like role as they convert the inactive form of vitamin D to the active form in collaboration with parathyroid hormone (PTH), which is secreted by the parathyroid gland. In this case PTH acts on the PCT to enable the final conversion of the inactive form of vitamin D to the active form. PTH also prevents reabsorption of phosphate ions, leading to loss of phosphate ions in the urine. This is an important step as excess phosphate ions in the circulation would lead to the formation of calcium phosphate molecules, which would decrease the available calcium ions in the blood.

The hormones renin, angiotensin and aldosterone and their role in the regulation of kidney function with respect to urine formation, blood pressure and peripheral vascular resistance are discussed in detail earlier above. The cardiac hormone ANO, which is secreted from the heart's atria in response to stretching of the atrial walls, directly impacts the process by increasing sodium excretion in an attempt to decrease blood pressure.

Blood

The kidneys secrete the hormone erythropoietin, which leads to the formation of new blood cells (Chapter 11).

Cardiovascular system

Earlier it was explained that systemic blood pressure can be regulated through the RAAS and that the kidneys' juxtaglomerular apparatus has a fundamental role in detecting changes in systemic blood pressure by sensing changes that occur as blood transitions from afferent to efferent arterioles.[2] Furthermore, the kidneys help maintain the chemical composition of the blood, including electrolyte balance and pH. This filtered blood is what the cardiovascular system delivers to cells and thus enables appropriate function of those cells. In response to excessive stretching of the atrial cardiac muscle and therefore the atrial wall, the cardiac hormone ANP is secreted to force a reduction in blood pressure by directly impacting on the GFR.

Lymphatic system

Very little is known about the human lymphatic system. In normal kidneys, the lymphatics are reported to be located in the interstitium around the lobular and arcuate arteries and veins but seldom present around glomerular arteries or between tubules in the cortex or in the medulla.[9] Studies that examine the role of lymphatics in kidney health—including lymph transport, participation in the regulation of blood pressure, transport of antigens and white blood cells and participation in the immune defences of the kidneys—are lacking.

Respiratory system

The link between the respiratory and urinary systems is best observed in acid–base regulation with respect to pH maintenance. As you are aware, the lungs are responsible for ensuring that blood is oxygenated and carbon dioxide is effectively removed from the blood. If excess carbon dioxide needs to be removed from the blood in order to adjust pH to the reference range, for example, the lungs will increase the work of breathing to exhale more carbon dioxide.

In addition, it is in the lung capillary endothelial cells that ACE converts angiotensin I to angiotensin II to enable regulation of blood pressure. As some water is lost through expiration, the kidneys compensate for this through renal autoregulation to adjust to the small loss of water from the blood.

Reproductive system

In males, part of the urinary system is shared with the reproductive system, as the penis serves as a common passage for both urine and semen. In contrast, the female ureter is separate from the vagina and the birth canal.

Pregnancy

Growth of a new human being inside the uterus places an extraordinary demand on all body systems. With respect to the kidneys, in order to meet the demands of the pregnant body, the GFR increases 50% with a decrease in serum creatinine, urea and uric acid values. The thresholds for thirst and antidiuretic hormone secretion are depressed, while blood pressure decreases approximately 10 mmHg by the second trimester, even though there is an increase in intravascular volume of 30–50%. The kidneys increase in length and volume, and physiological changes resembling those associated with urine buildup in the kidneys (hydronephrosis) are reported in up to 80% of pregnant women.[10]

AGE-RELATED CHANGES

Changes that affect micturition occur across the lifespan (Table 20.3). Overall, they involve changes in renal blood flow, changes in vascular resistance due to cardiovascular diseases and gradual destruction of nephron structures. As we age, the bladder also shrinks in size and frequency

TABLE 20.3
Age-related changes to micturition across the life span

Age	Urine volume	Conscious control	Physiological changes	Functional changes
Premature babies–6 months post full-term	400 mL/day (~20 voids per day)	Classic micturition reflex	As kidneys continue to develop until 40 weeks gestation, urine of premature babies contains stem cells that have been proven to protect other cells from damage, and repair and restore aged or damaged adult kidney tissue.[11]	
6–12 months		Conscious awareness developing	Increased ability to inhibit micturition unconsciously as brain matures and changes in functional capacity of the bladder occur. Neural maturation of frontal and parietal lobes.	
~15 months		Conscious awareness	Child learning to identify, contract and relax pelvic muscles including striated urethral muscles.	Most toddlers know when they have passed urine.
~1.5 years		Conscious control developing		
~2 years		Conscious control possible	Direct control of detrusor muscle occurs	Can temporarily postpone micturition and hold urine for up to 2 hours.
~4 years		Nocturnal control developing	Cortical inhibitory control achieved	Bedwetting may occur in 10–15% of children older than 4 years.
~6 years				Ability to initiate urination even when bladder has not given a full signal.
Adolescence–adulthood	1500 mL/day	Full control	Main issues are urinary tract infections and sexually transmitted infections.	
Older adult		More prone to incontinence and retention	Increased collagen content of bladder wall makes bladder less elastic. Urethra can become impeded via bladder/vaginal prolapse in women or enlarged prostate in men.	Bladder capacity is decreased to ~250 mL resulting in increased frequency of micturition during day and night.

in urination increases, including during the night (known as nocturia).

CONCLUSION

The urinary system is fundamental to homeostasis in conjunction with other body systems. Renal function is highly sensitive to the amount of blood that reaches both kidneys. With adequate renal perfusion, the kidneys balance fluids and chemicals within the blood, by reabsorbing useful substances into the bloodstream and excreting excess metabolic products in urine. Through these mechanisms, the body maintains internal stability in terms of fluid volume regulation, concentration of electrolytes in the blood and elimination of harmful toxins. The urinary system also contributes to and participates in compensatory responses to systemic changes such as low blood pressure by releasing hormones capable of initiating a cascade of corrective actions; one example is the RAAS. The organs of the urinary system work together to carry out the main system functions, at the same time protecting the kidneys from injury and infections.

CASE STUDY 20.1

Sandra is 65 years old and is not fond of drinking 'plain' water as she considers it to be tasteless. Instead, she drinks fizzy and flavoured drinks. She also eats very salty foods. During the last heatwave, when the temperature outside reached 40° Celsius and Sandra went to a local park with her friends, she ran out of her flavoured drink and chose not to drink water, even though she felt very thirsty. On going to the toilet, she noticed that her urine was dark-brown with a very strong offensive smell. She told her friend who insisted that Sandra drink two glasses of plain water straight away.

1. All of the following except which one are primary functions of the urinary system?

   a. Urine formation

   b. Detoxification of medications

   c. Excretion of wastes

   d. Regulation of blood and fluid composition

2. In which situation will the kidneys perform a homeostatic and protective function?

   a. When the person is not eating enough carbohydrates

   b. When the person is sweating a lot

   c. When the person's blood pressure drops

   d. When the person's heart rate increases

3. Which of the following is an example of form and function relationships within the urinary system?

   a. Microvilli in renal tubules: tubular absorption

   b. Renal capsule: urine formation

   c. Efferent arteriole: renal perfusion

   d. Renal medulla: BP regulation

4. How would drinking two glasses of water help Sandra's body to maintain normal urine specific gravity?

5. Discuss how Sandra's refusal to drink plain water impacts on overall kidney function.

CASE STUDY 20.2

Marisa is a 59-year-old office worker. She went to see her GP as she had been feeling more tired lately. While taking Marisa's health history the GP asked Marisa whether she had noticed an increase in urine output, and Marisa realised that she had been passing urine more often. The GP requested a urine test. A large amount of glucose was found in her urine.

Q1. A person drinks 240 mL of water 6–8 times per day. The kidneys react to this change by:

   a. producing aldosterone.

   b. secreting renin.

   c. increasing urine output.

   d. secreting erythropoietin.

Q2. What is the normal GFR?

   a. 125 mL/day

   b. 100 mL/minute

   c. 500 mL/minute

   d. 125 mL/minute

Q3. Glucose is not normally found in urine because it:

   a. does not pass through the walls.

   b. is kept in the blood by oncotic pressure.

   c. is reabsorbed by tubular cells.

   d. is removed before it reaches the kidneys.

Q4. Outline the three major processes in the formation of urine.

Q5. How does glucose end up in urine?

CASE STUDY 20.3

Rob, a 72-year-old businessman, suffered food poisoning after eating at a new restaurant. He had been vomiting for three days and was feeling unwell, but his wife became worried when she saw him getting confused and took him to the nearest hospital. On assessment, the emergency department nurse noted that Rob was experiencing bradypnoea (a low respiratory rate of 10 breaths per minute) and high blood pressure (160/100 mmHg).

1. Which of the following triggers from Rob's condition could have activated the RAAS?

   a. Bradypnoea

   b. High blood pressure

   c. Dehydration

   d. Overhydration

CASE STUDY 20.3—cont'd

2. Reabsorption of most nutrients, water and electrolytes takes place in which part of the nephron?
   a. Proximal convoluted tubule
   b. Distal convoluted tubule
   c. Henle's loop
   d. Collecting ducts

3. Which of the following laboratory tests would indicate damage to the kidneys because of hypertension?
   a. Coagulation panel
   b. Serum aldosterone
   c. Complete blood count
   d. Urinalysis

4. Discuss the acid–base imbalance that Rob is experiencing and the initial compensatory actions that take place in the kidneys.

5. Discuss why Rob is experiencing bradypnoea.

CASE STUDY 20.4

Jo is trying to toilet-train her two-year-old daughter, Amy, without much success. Amy tells her that she needs to pass urine, but wets herself before she makes it to the toilet. Jo asks you, the nurse at the Well Child Clinic, to explain why Amy can recognise the feeling of having to pass urine but is unable to hold on for any length of time yet.

1. Involuntary parasympathetic stimulation of the bladder leads to:
   a. relaxation of the detrusor muscle and the external urethral sphincter.
   b. contraction of the detrusor muscle and relaxation of the internal urethral sphincter.
   c. relaxation of the internal and external urethral sphincters.
   d. contraction of the detrusor and internal urethral sphincters.

2. Micturition occurs when the _____ contracts.
   a. detrusor muscle
   b. internal urethral sphincter
   c. external urethral sphincter
   d. all of the above

3. Babies and infants are unable to voluntarily control micturition as they need signals from which nerve to override the parasympathetic nervous system signals from the bladder and control their external urethral sphincter?
   a. Pelvic nerve
   b. Parasympathetic nerve
   c. Pudendal nerve
   d. Hypogastric nerve

4. Discuss how Amy's age affects the development of conscious control of micturition.

5. Describe how micturition is controlled by the nervous system.

REFERENCES

1. Thomasova D, Anders HJ. Cell cycle control in the kidney. Nephrol Dial Transpl 2014;30(10):1622–30.
2. Patton KT, Thibodeau GA. Urinary system. In: Patton KT, Thibodeau GA, editors. Anatomy and physiology, 9 ed. London: Elsevier Health Sciences; 2015.
3. Ferrão FM, Lara LS, Lowe J. Renin-angiotensin system in the kidney: what is new? World J Nephrol 2014;3(3):64–76.
4. Patton KT, Thibodeau GA. Urinary system. In: Patton KT, Thibodeau GA, editors. Anatomy and physiology, 10 ed. London: Elsevier Health Sciences; 2019.
5. McTavish AD, Sharma M-P. Renal physiology: acid–base balance. Anaesth Intens Care Med 2018;19(5):233–8.
6. Hamm LL, Nakhoul N, Hering-Smith KS. Acid-base homeostasis. Clin J Am Soc Nephrol 2015;10(12):2232–42.
7. Atherton JC. Role of the kidney in acid-base balance. Anaesth Intens Care Med 2015;16(6):275–7. doi: doi.org/10.1016/j.mpaic.2015.03.002.
8. Sugaya K, Nishijima S, Miyazato M, et al. Central nervous control of micturition and urine storage. J Smooth Muscle Res 2005;41(3):117–32.
9. Ishikawa Y, Akasaka Y, Kiguchi H, et al. The human renal lymphatics under normal and pathological conditions. Histopathol 2006;49(3):265–73.
10. Cheung KL, Lafayette RA. Renal physiology of pregnancy. Adv Chronic Kidney Dis 2013;20(3):209–14.
11. Arcolino FO, Zia S, Held K, et al. Urine of preterm neonates as a novel source of kidney progenitor cells. J Am Soc Nephrol 2016;27(9):2762–70.

CHAPTER 21

Reproductive system

ANGELA FRASER, MBBS, MPHTM, FACEM

KEY POINTS/LEARNING OUTCOMES

1. Describe the anatomy and overall functions of the male and female reproductive systems.
2. Describe the process of sperm production in males; describe the processes of egg production, ovulation and the menstrual cycle in females.
3. Understand the processes of the male and female sexual acts.
4. Understand the hormones involved in the development and maintenance of the male and female reproductive systems.
5. Understand how the functions of the male and female reproductive systems integrate with other body systems.

KEY DEFINITIONS

- **Gamete:** a mature reproductive cell able to combine with a gamete of the opposite sex to produce a fertilised egg; sperm or spermatozoa in males, and egg, ovum or oocyte in females.
- **Gametogenesis:** the process by which gametes are made by the gonads; in males the specific term is *spermatogenesis* and in females it is *oogenesis*.
- **Gonad:** a reproductive gland that produces gametes; testis or testicle (testes or testicles) in males and ovary (ovaries) in females.
- **Gonadotropin:** a hormone produced by the anterior pituitary gland in the brain that acts on the gonads, stimulating them to produce gametes and, in females, regulating the menstrual cycle; follicle-stimulating hormone (FSH) and luteinising hormone (LH) are gonadotropins.
- **Sex hormone:** a chemical messenger produced by the gonads; for example, testosterone, oestradiol and progesterone.

ONLINE RESOURCES/SUGGESTED READINGS

- **Reproductive system introduction** available at www.khanacademy.org/science/health-and-medicine/human-anatomy-and-physiology#reproductive-system-introduction
- **Reproductive system organs** available at www.kenhub.com/en/videos/organs-of-reproductive-system
- **Endocrinology of male reproduction** available at www.endotext.org/section/male
- **Endocrinology of female reproduction** available at www.endotext.org/section/female
- **The female reproductive tract** available at https://teachmeanatomy.info/pelvis/female-reproductive-tract/
- **Why do human testicles hang like that?** available at https://blogs.scientificamerican.com/bering-in-mind/why-do-human-testicles-hang-like-that/

INTRODUCTION

The reproductive system has one simple aim: procreation for the survival of the species. Even before birth, as a tiny embryo growing inside our mother, we are programmed to produce sex hormones and to develop the sexual organs required for reproduction. Once sexual maturity is reached at the completion of puberty, we are physically ready to continue the cycle of life.

The male and female reproductive systems can be thought of as having three main functions:
1. the production of gametes (sperm or eggs)
2. the act of sexual intercourse (bringing together the gametes so that fertilisation can occur)

3. the production and regulation of sex hormones (chemical messengers essential for the development, function and homeostasis of the reproductive system).

Anatomically, each reproductive system comprises:

- two gonads (testes or ovaries, in which gametes and most sex hormones are produced)
- a reproductive tract (a series of tubes and ducts designed to permit the passage of gametes from the gonads, so that fertilisation can occur)
- accessory glands (which provide lubrication and nourishment to help the gametes pass through the reproductive tract).

In this chapter we discuss the male and female reproductive systems, using case studies to highlight key concepts of how homeostasis is maintained in these systems. Pregnancy, childbirth and breastfeeding, three other important functions of the female reproductive system, are discussed in Chapter 22.

STRUCTURE AND FUNCTION
Male reproductive system

The male reproductive system (Fig. 21.1A) comprises a pair of testes, epididymides, vasa deferentia, seminal vesicles, ejaculatory ducts and bulbourethral glands, together with a single prostate gland, urethra and penis. The **urethra** is shared by both the urinary and the reproductive systems in that both urine and semen traverse it during urination and ejaculation, respectively. The **testes** sit outside the abdomen, in the **scrotum** (Fig. 21.1B), and together contain nearly one kilometre of tiny coiled tubes called **seminiferous tubules**. The seminiferous tubules are arranged in such a way to give each testis the appearance of a mandarin segment. These tubules converge to join at the upper aspect of each testis before connecting to the **epididymis**, which in turn connects to a muscular tube known as the **vas deferens**. Each vas deferens passes up into the abdomen, looping backwards and downwards under the bladder,

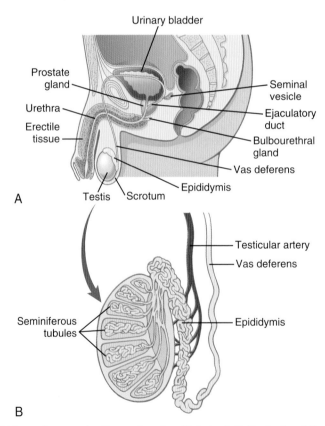

A

B

FIGURE 21.1 **A The male reproductive system (sagittal view). B Contents of the hemiscrotum.**
(*Source:* Modified from Hall JE. Guyton and Hall textbook of medical physiology, 13 ed. Saunders; 2015.)

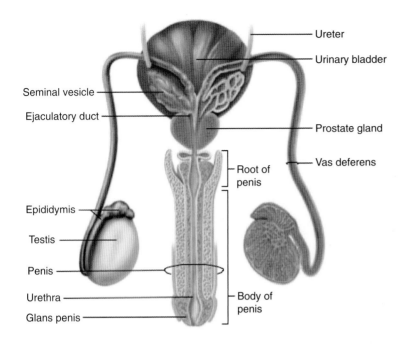

Ureter

Urinary bladder

Seminal vesicle

Ejaculatory duct

Prostate gland

FIGURE 21.2 **The male reproductive system (coronal view).** (*Source:* Modified from www.slideshare.net/1957Hamlet/chapter-22-reproductive-system-8713222.)

Vas deferens

Root of penis

Epididymis

Testis

Penis

Urethra

Glans penis

Body of penis

where it is joined by a **seminal vesicle** before entering the prostate gland to form an **ejaculatory duct**. The **bulbourethral gland**, which is found beneath the prostate gland, adds fluid to the semen during ejaculation. The two ejaculatory ducts empty into the single urethra, which passes the bulbourethral glands as it continues through to the tip of the **penis** (Fig. 21.2).

The three main functions of the male reproductive system are the production of **sperm (spermatogenesis)**, sexual intercourse, and the production and regulation of the male sex hormone **testosterone**.

Spermatogenesis

Spermatogenesis begins at puberty, at an average age of 13 years, and occurs throughout most of adult life, decreasing with advancing age. It takes places within the seminiferous tubules of the testes in response to stimulation by **gonadotropic hormones** released from the anterior pituitary gland. Precursor sperm cells, lying dormant within the seminiferous tubules since embryonic development, multiply by mitosis and differentiate in response to these hormones. Some then go on to multiply by meiosis, resulting in the production of immature sperm cells containing just one copy of each chromosome (half the genetic material of the male). It takes approximately 74 days for a precursor sperm cell to get to this point.[1] Sperm then take a few days to travel through the epididymis, where they mature and learn to swim. They wait for up to several months, most of

them in the epididymis and some in the lower portion of the vas deferens, surrounded by a nourishing and sedating fluid, until they are propelled forwards during ejaculation.[1,2] Up to 120 million sperm are produced each day.[1]

Normal spermatogenesis requires a testicular temperature about 2° Celcius below that of the intra-abdominal core temperature.[2] Below this, testicular function decreases. Above this temperature, testicular tubular cells degenerate, resulting in inefficient or inhibited spermatogenesis, and existing sperm die prematurely due to excessive activation. The human body has a clever way of keeping the testes cool: the scrotum. The **scrotum** is a skin-covered pouch that sits behind the penis. Once testicular descent has occurred (usually during the last month of gestation) the testes remain within the scrotum for the remainder of the male's life. Although more vulnerable to injury in this location, it allows regulation of testicular temperature for optimal spermatogenesis. Just beneath the skin of the scrotum lies a muscle called the **dartos muscle** (Fig. 21.3). It involuntarily contracts in response to cold, wrinkling the scrotal skin and reducing the surface area of the scrotum through which heat can be lost. In warmer conditions the muscle relaxes and the scrotal skin smooths out as its surface area increases, allowing more heat to be lost from the skin. Another muscle, the **cremaster muscle**, runs from the lower abdomen down into the scrotum where it envelops each testis. This muscle involuntarily

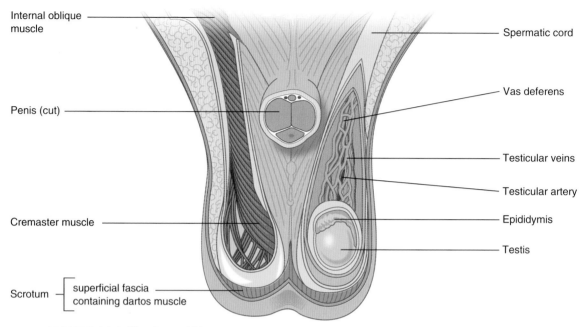

Internal oblique muscle

Penis (cut)

Cremaster muscle

Scrotum —⎰ superficial fascia
           ⎱ containing dartos muscle

Spermatic cord

Vas deferens

Testicular veins

Testicular artery

Epididymis

Testis

FIGURE 21.3 **Muscles and blood vessels of the scrotum.**

contracts in response to cold, elevating the testes and holding them close to the body to keep them warm. In response to warmth, the cremaster muscle relaxes, letting the testes fall back down into the scrotum (further away from the abdomen) where they can cool down. Additionally, the scrotal skin contains multiple sweat glands, which contribute to testicular cooling.

Additional thermoregulation occurs through the cardiovascular system. The first mechanism is counter-current heat exchange. The **testicular artery**, branching from the abdomen to each testis, and the **testicular vein**, running from each testis to the abdomen, form a plexus of blood vessels (Fig. 21.3). Heat is transferred from the warmer arterial blood (from the abdomen) to the cooler venous blood (from the testes), cooling the arterial blood as it travels towards the testes. This process becomes less effective as ambient (and therefore testicular) temperature increases. The second mechanism is regulation of blood flow to the peripheries. In response to environmental cold, peripheral vasoconstriction occurs within the skin, including that of the genitals. This reduces blood flow to the less critically important parts of the body (such as the fingers, face and genitals) while diverting blood to central organs (such as the brain, heart and lungs) in order to conserve heat and life-sustaining functions. Constriction of blood vessels results in smaller tissue volume. For example, a person's rings will become looser

on their fingers in the cold, when their fingers have shrunk due to decreased blood volume in their vessels. The opposite happens in warmer weather: blood vessels dilate, increasing the tissue volume of the fingers, making the rings tighter. The same process happens within the external genitalia: an increase in ambient temperature causes increased blood volume and increased tissue size, and the opposite occurs in the cold.

A mature sperm cell comprises a head, a body and a long mobile tail (Fig. 21.4). On top of the **head** sits a cap-like structure called an **acrosome**; it contains enzymes capable of breaking down the wall of an egg so that fertilisation can occur. The **tail**, or **flagellum**, is long and mobile and it propels the sperm forwards in a liquid medium by its forwards and backwards motion.

Male sexual act

Sexual intercourse is the act of transferring sperm from the male reproductive tract into the female reproductive tract, with the aim of fertilising an egg. There are four main stages of the male sexual act: **arousal**, erection, emission and ejaculation, and resolution. **Erection** of the penis is the first effect of sexual arousal, which may be physical or psychological, or a combination of both. Arteries in the penis dilate, causing an influx of blood. These enlarged arteries compress the veins, impairing venous outflow from the penis, resulting in a net increase

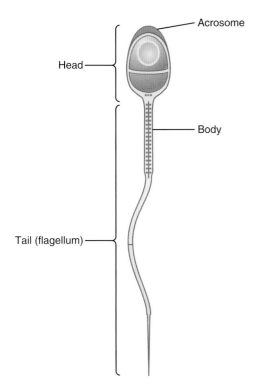

FIGURE 21.4 **Structure of a sperm cell.** (*Source:* Modified from Hall JE. Guyton and Hall textbook of medical physiology, 13 ed. Saunders; 2015.)

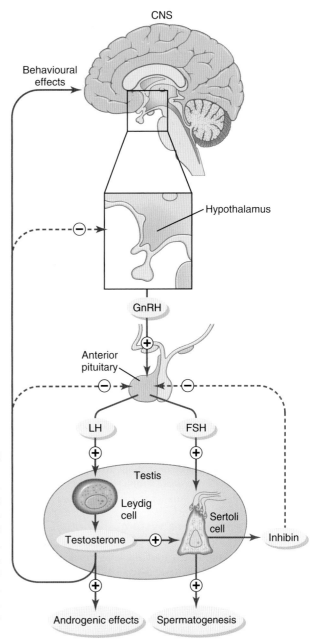

in penile blood volume. This manifests as lengthening and hardening of the penis.

Once sexual arousal intensifies, reflex centres in the lower spine signal to the reproductive tract that it is time for **emission**. In response, the vas deferens contracts, propelling sperm into the urethra where the sperm combine with fluid from the prostate gland and the seminal vesicles to form semen. Once the urethra is full of semen a signal is sent to the sacral nerves and coordinated rhythmic contractions of the internal genital organs and genital muscles result in expulsion of the semen from the end of the penis. The process of emission and **ejaculation** is known as an **orgasm**. Within one to two minutes post orgasm, sexual arousal diminishes and the erection resolves in a process known as resolution.

Hormonal control of the male reproductive system

Hormonal control of the male reproductive system depends on communication between the brain and the testes via a system known as the **hypothalamic-pituitary-testicular**

FIGURE 21.5 **Hypothalamic-pituitary-testicular axis.** (*Source:* Hall JE. Guyton and Hall textbook of medical physiology, 13 ed. Saunders; 2015.)

axis (Fig. 21.5). The hypothalamus produces a hormone called **gonadotropin-releasing hormone (GnRH)**. As its name suggests, it causes the release of gonadotropes from the adjacent anterior pituitary gland. The two gonadotropes released from the anterior pituitary are luteinising hormone (LH) and **follicle-stimulating hormone (FSH)**.

LH acts on the Leydig cells in the testes, stimulating them to make **testosterone**. Testosterone is the main male sex hormone and is responsible for masculine characteristics including genital growth, pubic and facial hair, increased muscle mass and deepening of the voice. It is also essential for sperm production. Adequate or high testosterone blood levels are sensed by both the hypothalamus and the anterior pituitary, resulting in a decrease in GnRH secretion and, as a follow-on effect, a decrease in LH and FSH secretion by the pituitary gland and an overall reduction in testosterone production to ensure optimal blood levels of the hormone.

FSH acts on Sertoli cells in the testes. Sertoli cells can be thought of as being 'sperm nannies': they support sperm production within the seminiferous tubules. Spermatogenesis is dependent on both Sertoli cell activity and adequate testosterone levels. If too many sperm are being produced, Sertoli cells produce a hormone called inhibin. Inhibin travels in the blood and feeds back to the anterior pituitary gland to tell it to secrete less FSH. This is an example of how negative feedback contributes to homeostasis.

Stress of any kind activates the release of the hormone cortisol by the adrenal glands. **Cortisol** has a negative feedback effect on the male reproductive system at two levels: the hypothalamus, to reduce the secretion of GnRH; and the anterior pituitary gland, to reduce the secretion of FSH and LH. Chronic stress can cause similar adverse effects on the male reproductive system as observed in chronic abuse of anabolic-adrenergic steroids: reduced intra-testicular testosterone production, reduced spermatogenesis and smaller testicular volume.

Female reproductive system

The female reproductive system (Fig. 21.6) comprises two ovaries and a reproductive tract, the latter being made up of the vagina, cervix, uterus and a pair of **fallopian tubes**. The **ovaries** consist of multiple bubble-like structures called **follicles** and within each follicle lies an egg. The two most important types of follicular cells are **theca** and **granulosa cells**. The ovaries are not continuous with the fallopian tubes; instead, they sit nearby within the pelvis. Once an egg is released from an ovary it is quickly swept up by special finger-like projections called **fimbriae**, present on the end of the adjacent fallopian tube. If fertilisation is to occur, it will usually do so in the fallopian tube. The inside of the fallopian tube is lined with tiny, hair-like projections called **cilia**, whose function it is to propel the egg (fertilised or otherwise) towards the uterus. The **uterus** is a muscular, upside-down-triangle-shaped

structure, the lower portion of which becomes the cervix and protrudes into the vagina. The **vagina** is a hollow structure with an opening (the introitus) between the labia majora and the labia minora, and posterior to the clitoris and urethra. Collectively, the external genitalia make up the vulva. Two small glands, called **Bartholin's glands**, sit just behind the vaginal introitus; these glands produce mucus which helps to lubricate the vagina during sexual intercourse.

Three important functions of the female reproductive system include egg production and release (oogenesis and ovulation, respectively), sexual intercourse, and the production and regulation of the female sex hormones oestradiol and progesterone. Pregnancy, childbirth and breastfeeding are discussed in Chapter 22.

Oogenesis

Oogenesis occurs during embryonic development, reaching completion by the fifth month of gestation, so that a baby girl has about one to two million eggs (oocytes) within her ovaries when she is born. By the time she reaches puberty at the average age of nine to 12 years, only about 300 000 eggs remain.[1,2] These eggs are diploid (they contain all the genetic material of the female), having not yet undergone meiosis. Each egg lies within an ovarian follicle, surrounded and nourished by a layer of specialised cells called granulosa cells. During a woman's fertile life only about 400–500 follicles will mature enough for their eggs to undergo meiosis and to then be released; the remainder degenerate and are resorbed by the body.[1]

Female sexual act

There are four stages to the female sexual act: arousal, erection and lubrication, orgasm and resolution. Sexual desire differs with sex hormone levels, increasing pre-ovulation as oestrogen levels rise. Sexual arousal results from a combination of physical and psychological stimulation, the **clitoris** being especially sensitive to physical stimulation. As in the male, the female genitals contain erectile tissue: it surrounds the vaginal opening and extends into the clitoris. **Sexual arousal** results in vasodilation within and increased blood flow to these tissues. The Bartholin's glands secrete mucus into the vaginal opening, providing most of the lubrication required for sexual intercourse.

As sexual stimulation peaks it initiates a reflex in the lower spine and orgasm results, causing the genital muscles to contract rhythmically. **Oxytocin** (a hormone released from the posterior pituitary gland, responsible for the 'loved-up' feeling) causes uterine contractions. It is thought that these contractions may assist sperm in

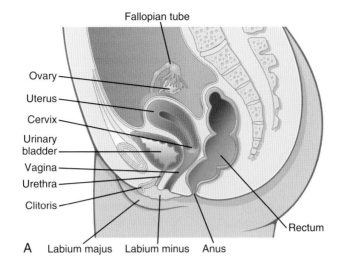

Fallopian tube

Ovary

Uterus

Cervix

Urinary bladder

Vagina

Urethra

Clitoris

Rectum

A Labium majus Labium minus Anus

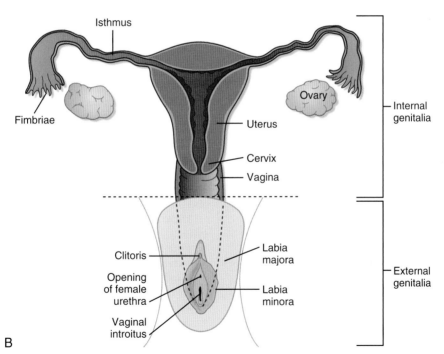

Isthmus

Ovary

Fimbriae

Uterus

Cervix

Vagina

Internal genitalia

Clitoris

Labia majora

Opening of female urethra

Labia minora

Vaginal introitus

External genitalia

B

FIGURE 21.6 **Female reproductive organs. A** Sagittal. **B** Coronal. (*Source:* **A,** Hall JE. Guyton and Hall textbook of medical physiology, 13 ed. Saunders; 2015. **B,** Modified from Koeppen B, Stanton B. Berne & Levy physiology, 6 ed. Mosby; 2009.)

travelling upwards towards the fallopian tubes in their quest to fertilise an egg. Additionally, it is thought that the cervix remains open for about 30 minutes post orgasm, facilitating sperm entry into the uterus. Post orgasm, the female experiences an intense sense of relaxation and her erectile tissue reduces in size; this is known as resolution.

Hormonal control of the female reproductive system

As in males, puberty is heralded by an increase in the release of GnRH from the hypothalamus and the subsequent secretion of LH and FSH from the anterior pituitary gland (Fig. 21.7). LH and FSH stimulate ovarian

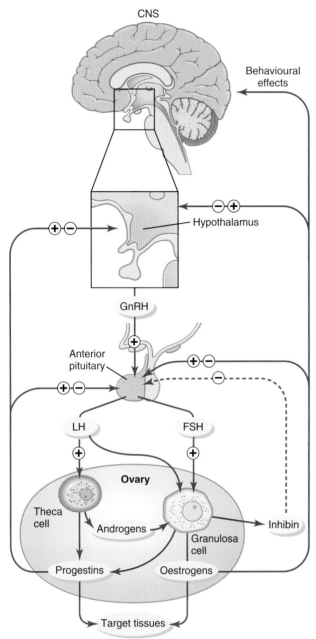

FIGURE 21.7 **Hypothalamic-pituitary-ovarian axis.**
(*Source:* Hall JE. Guyton and Hall textbook of medical
physiology, 13 ed. Saunders; 2015.)

production of progestins, androgens (male hormones)
and oestrogens from cholesterol. The major progestin is
progesterone, while the major oestrogen is oestradiol. At
puberty, oestrogen production surges about twenty-fold,
and is responsible for the development of secondary

sex characteristics including breast growth, increased
fatty deposition (especially around the buttocks and
thighs), growth and maturation of reproductive organs,
and enlargement of the external genitalia. Oestrogens
also decrease bone breakdown, resulting in a net increase
in bone density and strength. Pubic and underarm hair
growth is due to a normal increase in androgen secretion
by the female at this time. Progesterone has two main
functions: preparation of the breasts for lactation, and
preparation of the uterine lining (the endometrium) in
the second half of the menstrual cycle. The increasing
release of FSH and LH stimulates ovarian growth and
the onset of the monthly menstrual cycle. The onset
of menstruation is known as **menarche** and occurs at
an average age of 11 to 15 years. Regular menstruation
usually continues, perhaps punctuated by one or more
pregnancies, until the age of 40 to 50 years, when the
cycle becomes more irregular and, eventually, **anovula-
tory**. Cessation of the menstrual cycle (and the concurrent
decline in female sex hormones) is known as **menopause**.

The menstrual cycle

The **menstrual cycle** (Fig. 21.8) is a complex and regular
set of events resulting from the coordinated action of
the hypothalamus, anterior pituitary gland, ovaries and
endometrium. Each cycle results in ovulation of a single egg
and preparation of the endometrium for the reception of a
fertilised egg. The average length of a cycle is 28 days—day 1
being the first day of menstruation and ovulation occurring
on day 14—but cycle length can vary from 20 to 45 days.
The first half of the cycle is known as the **follicular phase**
and the second half as the **luteal phase**.

There are five major components of the menstrual
cycle:
- secretion of GnRH by the hypothalamus
- secretion of FSH and LH by the anterior pituitary
  gland
- secretion of progesterone, androgens and oestradiol by
  the theca and granulosa cells of the ovarian follicles
- development of ovarian follicles, ovulation and the
  formation and demise of the corpus luteum
- proliferation, maturation and shedding of the
  endometrium.

At the beginning of the cycle the anterior pituitary gland
and ovaries are in a relatively quiet state with FSH, LH,
oestradiol and progesterone levels all at baseline. No
longer suppressed by ovarian hormones from the luteal
stage of the previous cycle, the hypothalamus increases
its secretion of GnRH and a modest increase in anterior
pituitary secretion of FSH ensues. The FSH spike results
in the recruitment and rapid growth of up to 20 ovarian
follicles. As these selected follicles grow, they produce

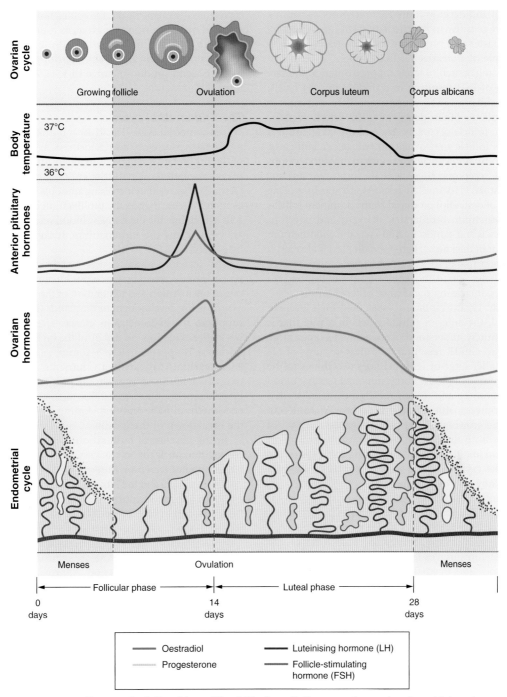

FIGURE 21.8 **Temporal relationships of the follicular, pituitary, ovarian and endometrial cycles.**

oestradiol and develop more FSH receptors, becoming even more sensitive to the circulating FSH and therefore growing faster and producing more oestradiol. This is an example of a positive feedback loop.

Increasing oestradiol levels suppress anterior pituitary secretion of FSH resulting in a decline in FSH levels; however, the most FSH-responsive follicle continues to thrive while the others degenerate. This selection of the dominant follicle occurs by day 8 of the cycle and it is from this follicle that ovulation will occur mid-cycle. As this dominant follicle continues to grow it develops more LH receptors; these will be important for the pre-ovulatory LH surge. In response to the increasing amounts of oestradiol produced by the dominant follicle, the endometrium proliferates, thickens and develops blood vessels and glands. By mid-cycle the endometrium is 3–5 mm in thickness. High oestradiol levels also result in the production of sticky, egg-white-like cervical mucus; this facilitates sperm movement from the vagina into the uterus, increasing the chance of fertilisation.

On day 12, in response to sustained high levels of oestradiol, the anterior pituitary acts in a way that is not yet entirely understood: it suddenly becomes more sensitive to GnRH, resulting in a massive surge of LH and a smaller surge of FSH. LH does two things to the follicle: oestradiol production is inhibited (so that blood levels plummet); and follicular cells are altered so that they become capable of producing progesterone. On day 14 the growing follicle pushes against the wall of the ovary from the inside, causing an outward bulge, before bursting through and releasing its egg into the abdominal cavity adjacent to the fallopian tube, in a process known as **ovulation**.

The ruptured follicle, now devoid of its egg, forms a structure called the **corpus luteum** (Latin for 'yellow body'), so-named due to its high fat content, giving it its yellow colour. Supported by basal levels of LH, the corpus luteum survives for about 14 days. It produces progesterone and, in smaller amounts, oestradiol, levels of which both peak on day 21. Progesterone results in the organisation, maturation and stabilisation of the endometrium which prepares it for implantation, while oestradiol enhances the action of progesterone on the endometrium. The corpus luteum also secretes inhibin, which, as in males, results in negative feedback to the anterior pituitary gland to suppress FSH secretion. The corpus luteum regresses from day 21, reducing the amount of progesterone, oestradiol and inhibin produced so that it is at baseline by about day 24. After this time the corpus luteum degenerates and is resorbed by the ovary.

Without oestradiol or progesterone to support it, the endometrium shears off and is expelled through the cervix into the vagina by uterine contractions. This process is called **menstruation** and averages four to seven days in length. The decline in ovarian hormones in the last few days of the cycle allows the anterior pituitary gland to once again produce a surge in FSH, leading to the start of a new cycle.

The endometrial cycle

The **endometrial cycle** (Fig. 21.9) comprises three stages: proliferative, secretory and menstrual. At the beginning of the proliferative stage, immediately after completion of menstruation, very little endometrium remains. Oestradiol, secreted in increasing amounts by the growing ovarian follicles, triggers the proliferation of endometrial cells, which line the uterus. New blood vessels and glands are formed, and the endometrium thickens to 3–5 mm by mid-cycle.

The secretory phase occurs mostly in response to progesterone secreted by the corpus luteum. Progesterone causes organisation and maturation of the endometrium, as well as the development of the glands within it. Blood supply to the endometrium increases and, about one week after ovulation, on day 21 of the cycle, endometrial thickness is approximately 5–6 mm. At this stage the endometrium is packed with nutrients with which to nourish a fertilised egg, should implantation occur. Progesterone continues to stabilise the fragile, blood-filled endometrium by promoting clotting and discouraging the breakdown of these clots.

In the absence of fertilisation, degeneration of the corpus luteum leads to the cessation of progesterone and oestradiol secretion. In response, the endometrium rapidly involutes and the blood vessels within it constrict and break down, resulting in an endometrial haemorrhage that separates the dead layer of endometrium from the underlying tissue. The uterus then contracts to allow the shed endometrium to be expelled through the cervix and out through the vagina as menstruation, more commonly known as a period. Approximately 40 mL of blood is lost in each menstrual cycle.

A proliferative phase then begins to quickly resurface the raw tissue from which the endometrium has detached; this occurs within four to seven days and corresponds with the cessation of menstruation.

INTEGRATION OF THE MALE AND FEMALE REPRODUCTIVE SYSTEMS WITH OTHER BODY SYSTEMS

Endocrine system

The development and function of the male reproductive system are entirely dependent on the endocrine system,

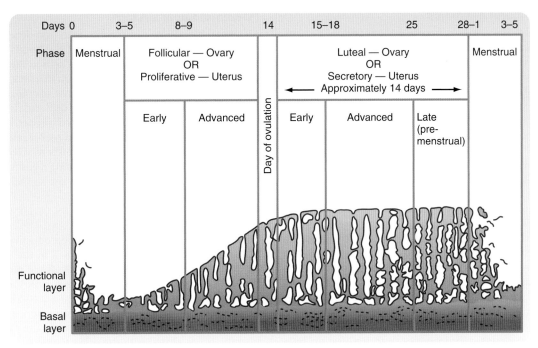

FIGURE 21.9 **Endometrial cycle.** (*Source:* Koeppen B, Stanton B. Berne & Levy physiology, 6 ed. Mosby; 2009.)

without which it would not exist. The male sex hormone testosterone, responsible for the development of male reproductive organs and secondary sexual characteristics, and integral to spermatogenesis, is produced by testicular Leydig cells in response to either placental human chorionic gonadotropin (hCG) (during gestation and infancy) or LH which, in turn, is produced in response to GnRH. FSH, also required for spermatogenesis, produced in response to GnRH. This hypothalamic-pituitary-testicular axis is regulated by negative feedback to ensure maintenance of a hormonal steady-state.

In contrast to the male testes, the female ovaries are hormonally silent during embryonic development. At puberty, oestradiol, progesterone and small amounts of androgens begin to be produced by the ovaries in response to hypothalamic and anterior pituitary activity; without these hormones there would be no secondary sex characteristics—the reproductive organs would remain child-size and the menstrual cycle would not occur. The hypothalamic-pituitary-ovarian axis is integral to the normal functioning of the female reproductive system and both negative and positive feedback occur along this axis to produce the cyclical changes necessary for fertility.

Another two hormones, ghrelin and leptin, also play an important role in the hypothalamic-pituitary-ovarian axis. **Ghrelin**, secreted by the stomach in conditions of low weight or intense exercise, acts to increase the appetite. People responding to internal ghrelin secretion ideally seek food, thereby increasing their kilojoule intake and helping to counteract the metabolic imbalance created by their physique or lifestyle. But ghrelin has another important function: suppression of GnRH secretion by the hypothalamus. In response, FSH and LH secretion from the anterior pituitary gland decreases and the effects flow on to the ovaries and endometrium, impairing or stopping ovarian and endometrial function.

Leptin, secreted by the body's fat cells, acts in the opposite way to ghrelin: it reduces appetite. Underweight individuals have fewer fat cells and therefore reduced circulating leptin. The hypothalamus detects the low leptin level and, unsurprisingly, reduces its secretion of GnRH, resulting in impairment or cessation of the function of the hypothalamic-pituitary-ovarian axis. Low leptin and high ghrelin levels present in the underweight state work to restore appetite and increase kilojoule intake. This would lead to recovery of adequate body fat stores, a decrease in ghrelin levels and an increase in leptin levels, the net effect being normalisation of hypothalamic secretion of GnRH and a return to normal ovarian and endometrial function.

Genes and genomics

In males, precursor sperm cells replicate within the seminiferous tubules to produce exact copies of themselves in a process known as **mitosis**. Following this, they undergo meiosis during which they produce immature sperm cells that each contain half the genetic material of the male, with either one X or one Y chromosome. During these processes of replication and division, existing genetic mutations are copied and new mutations may occur. If a mutation exists within the germ cells it can be transmitted to new generations—this is known as a **germ-line mutation**.

In females, precursor egg cells containing two X chromosomes replicate by mitosis within the embryonic ovaries from the sixth week of gestation. By the time they have finished replicating, by about the fifth month of gestation, there are approximately seven million precursor egg cells. They then begin meiotic division but pause in the first stage: they won't complete meiosis until a few hours before ovulation, years later. After ovulation the egg cell begins to divide again by meiosis, but again the process is paused. This second meiotic division occurs only in response to fertilisation by a sperm cell. All normal haploid eggs contain one X chromosome. As with sperm production, existing genetic mutations are copied and new mutations may occur during this process.

Cardiovascular system

The achievement and maintenance of a male erection is required for sexual intercourse and therefore reproduction. Penile arteries must be able to adequately relax to allow the influx of blood necessary for erection to occur. Arteries that are dysfunctional, damaged or narrowed due to diseases that affect blood vessels cannot dilate properly. In fact, the most common cause of impotence in males aged over 40 years is cardiovascular disease.

The testes, which essentially dangle in the scrotum on their spermatic cord, require constant blood supply to function and survive. The spermatic cord can twist, blocking blood flow to and from the testis, causing lack of oxygen and nutrients and a buildup of waste products, causing irreversible injury to and death of the testis.

During their reproductive years, women are protected from many diseases as oestrogens have a protective effect against blood vessel disease (atherosclerosis). This means that coronary artery disease, stroke and peripheral vascular disease are all less common in females of reproductive age. After menopause, males and females have an almost equal risk of cardiovascular disease.

The ovaries, like the testes, are also prone to twisting. If they do so they risk cutting off their blood supply, causing death to the ovary and impairing fertility.

Haematological system

Menstrual blood loss can contribute to iron deficiency and anaemia. Approximately 75% of the body's total iron content is found inside red blood cells in the form of haemoglobin. In its early stages iron deficiency can occur without any effect on the body's haemoglobin count, but once iron stores have been depleted haemoglobin can no longer be synthesised properly and anaemia follows. Ordinarily, once red blood cells die, after about 120 days in circulation, iron is recycled and returned to the circulation. However, during menstruation red blood cells are lost from the body and so their iron cannot be recycled.

Urinary system

The urethra is shared by the male reproductive and urinary systems so semen may be noted in the urine, particularly in the first void of the day. If the prostate gland undergoes benign or cancerous growth this can cause obstruction of the urethra. This may lead to more frequent voiding, complete bladder obstruction, kidney obstruction and kidney failure. In women, the vaginal opening is not shared with the urinary system, but the urethra and vagina are anatomically closely located.

Musculoskeletal system

The reproductive and musculoskeletal systems are influenced by some of the same hormones. For example, testosterone causes muscle growth and increased bone density. Oestrogen causes bone growth and increased bone density during the reproductive years, meaning that postmenopausal women are at risk of decreased bone density, osteoporosis and fractures.

Nervous system

Erection is dependent on parasympathetic stimulation from the sacral nerves at the base of the spine, while emission and ejaculation are sympathetic responses from the thoracolumbar nerves. These actions can occur independently of the brain, such as in the case of a spinal cord injury.

Psychological system

While erection, emission and ejaculation can occur without any input from the brain (psychological stimulation is not required for sexual intercourse), the sexual act is usually a combination of both physical and psychological stimulation. Men who find it difficult to achieve psychological arousal may have sexual dysfunction. Women also require both physical and psychological arousal in order to reach orgasm; women who have psychological difficulties may therefore be unable to do so. Stress, and the resultant increase in circulating cortisol, can suppress the hypothalamic-pituitary-testicular axis, ultimately leading to infertility in both men and women.

AGE-RELATED CHANGES

The male reproductive system undergoes changes over time, having four distinct phases: fetal, neonatal, pubertal and adult. In utero, the hormone hCG secreted by the placenta acts on the male embryo's Leydig cells in a similar manner to that of LH: it stimulates the production of testosterone. This embryonic secretion of testosterone is critical to the development of the male reproductive organs, including testicular descent. Testicles begin high up within the abdomen and, during the third trimester, descend into the scrotum where they remain for life. Without this secretion of testosterone, the testes remain intra-abdominal. If uncorrected, irreversible damage to the seminiferous tubules can occur, impairing or inhibiting the testes' ability to produce sperm. At birth, testosterone levels fall (so that males and females are born with very similar testosterone levels). Testosterone rises for the first three to six months before falling away again to very low concentrations by the age of one year. It is not yet clear why this surge in infancy occurs. At puberty, in response to a surge in gonadotropins from the anterior pituitary gland, testosterone secretion abruptly increases, reaching normal adult levels by about 17 years of age. Testosterone secretion continues throughout adulthood, progressively decreasing from the fifth decade of life. This decline correlates with a progressive reduction in sperm production.

The female reproductive system is also affected by age-related changes. Of these, the most significant is menopause, which arises due to changes in hormonal levels in the ageing female body. While menopause is considered a normal part of the ageing process and is generally experienced between the ages of 45 and 55 years, it is not an easy transition. As ovaries cease to make progesterone and oestrogen and stop producing eggs, menstruation ceases. The vaginal walls become dryer and thinner, and the external genitalia become thinner and smaller. Breast tissue also decreases in size. Concurrently, women may experience hot flushes, mood changes, headaches, insomnia and decreased sex drive and sexual responses. In the absence of protective oestrogen effects, bone density decreases, thus increasing the risk of developing osteoporosis. Furthermore, there is a loss of muscle tone in the pelvic area, which may lead to increased risk of prolapse of the vagina, uterus and/or urinary bladder.[3]

CONCLUSION

The reproductive system is perfectly purpose-built: gametes are produced in the gonads and, through the act of sexual intercourse, these gametes traverse their respective reproductive tracts to meet in the female fallopian tube so that fertilisation can occur. The development and function of the reproductive system are dependent on the production and regulation of sex hormones and the hypothalamic-pituitary-testicular/ovarian axis governs both systems. Anything that alters this complex interplay of hormones can threaten homeostasis. The male and female reproductive systems are complex yet simple: the goal is procreation, but not at the expense of human health or life.

CASE STUDY 21.1

For as long as he can remember, Jack, an 11-year-old boy, has known that it is common for males to experience 'shrinkage' when exposed to the cold. He definitely noticed it last weekend when he went swimming at the beach on a cold, wintery morning. When he jumped into the water he felt his scrotum tighten so that his testicles were pushed up higher and he was certain that everything 'down there' got a bit smaller. Of course, when he warmed up after his swim everything returned to normal, but he is curious about why this occurred.

Q1. The ideal testicular temperature for optimal sperm production is:

a. 36°C.

b. 2°C lower than normal core body temperature.

c. 2°C higher than normal core body temperature.

d. core body temperature.

e. 32°C.

Q2. The following responses occur when the male external genitalia are exposed to heat.

a. Vasoconstriction, contraction of the cremaster muscle, depression of the testes

b. Vasoconstriction, relaxation of the cremaster muscle, elevation of the testes

c. Vasodilation, relaxation of the cremaster muscle, depression of the testes

d. Vasodilation, contraction of the cremaster muscle, elevation of the testes

e. Vasodilation, relaxation of the cremaster muscle, elevation of the testes

Continued

CASE STUDY 21.1—cont'd

Q3. Testicular descent usually occurs:

a. at puberty.

b. at one year of age.

c. at seven weeks' gestation.

d. in the last month of gestation.

e. just prior to puberty.

Q4. Why is temperature regulation of the testes important, and by what mechanisms does the male reproductive system achieve this?

Q5. How does the cardiovascular system contribute to thermoregulation of the testes and penis?

CASE STUDY 21.2

Matt, a 28-year-old security guard, is a self-confessed gym junkie. He loves to lift weights and hardly misses a workout, not wanting to lose any of the strength and bulk he has developed over the years. Over the past few months he and some of his gym buddies have been using testosterone supplements to boost their training. They bought the supplements over the internet, illegally. Matt found that he could lift more and was perhaps starting to put on a bit of bulk. A few days ago, however, Matt became concerned about the unwanted side effects of this regimen after he read in a men's health magazine there was a chance it could affect his fertility and make his testicles shrink. He was quite worried about this and decided to speak to a healthcare professional about his concerns.

Q1. Thinking about the negative feedback effect of testosterone on the hypothalamic-pituitary-testicular axis, which of the following effects would testosterone supplementation have on the male reproductive system?

a. Raised inhibin levels

b. Raised sperm count

c. Increased intra-testicular testosterone

d. Reduced testicular size

e. Increased secretion of FSH and LH

Q2. Which of the following statements is *incorrect* about cortisol?

a. Chronically elevated cortisol levels can suppress the hypothalamic-pituitary-testicular axis

b. A man with chronically elevated cortisol levels would have low inhibin levels

c. Cortisol acts on the hypothalamus to increase GnRH secretion

d. Cortisol is produced by the adrenal glands in response to stress

e. Cortisol acts on the anterior pituitary gland to decrease FSH and LH secretion

Q3. What are some other important side effects of anabolic-adrenergic steroid use?

a. Male breast development

b. Acne

c. Damage to the heart muscle, impairing its ability to contract and relax

d. Aggression and violence

e. All of the above

Q4. Testosterone, or synthetic forms of it, is not uncommonly obtained illegally for the purposes of increasing strength and muscle bulk. The terms 'anabolic steroids' and 'anabolic-adrenergic steroids' refer to these kinds of supplements. Thinking about the hypothalamic-pituitary-testicular axis, what effect would the addition of extra testosterone have on the reproductive system? If Matt ceased using these supplements, how would his body respond to restore homeostasis?

Q5. How might stress-reduction techniques help Matt's reproductive system to recover after he stopped taking these testosterone supplements?

CASE STUDY 21.3

Sarah, a 20-year-old engineering student, consulted her GP because she had been feeling more tired than usual. She was otherwise well and considered herself quite healthy. She has been a vegetarian for the past year, trying to eat a wide variety of fresh healthy foods when her budget allows. Sarah reported regular periods that tended to be on the heavier side, bleeding for seven days each cycle. Sarah's GP suspected that she might be iron-deficient: her dietary intake was probably inadequate to replenish the iron lost each month during menstruation. He arranged

CASE STUDY 21.3—cont'd

a panel of blood tests, including iron levels, and was unsurprised to see that Sarah was mildly iron deficient but not yet anaemic.

Q1. What is the average volume of blood lost during each menstrual cycle?

    a. 4 mL

    b. 40 mL

    c. 400 mL

    d. 8 mL

    e. 80 mL

Q2. In relation to a normal endometrial cycle, which is true?

    a. Progesterone secretion by the developing follicles promotes proliferation of the endometrium.

    b. Oestradiol secretion by the developing follicles promotes shedding of the endometrium.

    c. Progesterone levels remain low during the secretory phase, to ensure maturation and stabilisation of the endometrium.

    d. Progesterone levels increase during the secretory phase, ensuring maturation and stabilisation of the endometrium.

    e. In response to falling levels of both progesterone and oestrogen, the endometrium begins to detach from day 21 of a 28-day cycle.

Q3. In which scenario is gastrointestinal absorption of iron increased?

    a. Drinking a cup of tea with a steak

    b. Drinking a glass of cow's milk with a steak

    c. Eating a piece of citrus fruit with a steak

    d. Drinking a glass of soy milk with a steak

    e. Drinking a cup of tea with cow's milk in it

Q4. How does the endometrium change during the menstrual cycle? Despite the physiological requirement for monthly blood loss, how does the reproductive system regulate and minimise this bleeding while ensuring it can continue to prepare the uterine lining for implantation each month?

Q5. Why are menstruating women at risk of iron deficiency? How does the body respond to reduced iron stores?

CASE STUDY 21.4

Taryn, a 26-year-old teacher and amateur triathlete, has ramped up her training over the past six months in preparation for her first big race. She has always been a healthy eater and of slim build but she has been quite strict with her diet recently and this, plus her increased training, has resulted in noticeable weight loss. A couple of her friends have mentioned that she has perhaps lost too much weight, but Taryn doesn't think so: she feels faster and fitter than ever. It wasn't until a chat with her older sister that she realised she hasn't had a period in a few months. She has been so busy with work and training that she's not really noticed; besides, it is much more convenient not having periods with all of the time spent in the pool. It took considerable convincing by her sister for Taryn to make an appointment to see her GP about it.

Q1. What is the evolutionary rationale for stress-induced cessation of the menstrual cycle?

    a. A pregnancy at this time would pose a risk to the health or perhaps life of the mother

    b. A woman does not have to worry about getting her period when she is experiencing emotional or physical stress

    c. A pregnancy at this time would be more likely to produce twins

    d. Cessation of the menstrual cycle alerts the woman to a problem

    e. Ongoing menstrual blood loss would significantly contribute to the worsening nutritional status of the woman

Q2. Which of the following is a consequence of stressors such as intense exercise and weight loss?

    a. Low ghrelin, high leptin, low GnRH, low FSH, low LH

    b. High ghrelin, low leptin, low GnRH, high FSH, high LH

    c. Low ghrelin, low leptin, high GnRH, low FSH, low LH

    d. High ghrelin, low leptin, low GnRH, low FSH, low LH

    e. High ghrelin, high leptin, low GnRH, low FSH, low LH

Continued

CASE STUDY 21.4—cont'd

Q3. Which of the following is a proven method of reducing levels of the stress hormone cortisol?
   a. Slow, diaphragmatic breathing
   b. Yoga
   c. Adequate, restful sleep
   d. Spending time with loved ones and pets
   e. All of the above

Q4. Assuming that Taryn is not pregnant and there is no underlying disease state, what is the likely mechanism for this change in her cycle? What can the reproductive system do to try to return to homeostasis?

Q5. Do any other hormones play a role in the recovery of Taryn's menstrual cycle?

REFERENCES

1. Hall JE. Guyton and Hall textbook of medical physiology. 13th ed. Philadelphia: Elsevier; 2016. p. 1021–54.
2. Koeppen BM, Stanton BA. Berne & Levy physiology, 7 ed. Philadelphia: Elsevier; 2018. p. 787–97.
3. MedlinePlus. Aging changes in the female reproductive system. Available from https://medlineplus.gov/ency/article/004016.htm.

CHAPTER 22

Pregnancy and lactation

BETHANY CARR, BMIDWIF, BCLINMIDWIF

KEY DEFINITIONS

- **Embryo:** the developing individual from fertilisation until week 8 of gestation.
- **Fetus:** the developing individual from week 9 of gestation until birth.
- **Postpartum:** the period after the baby is born when the mother recovers, the baby transitions to extrauterine life and breastfeeding is established.
- **Term (pregnancy/gestation):** the period between 37 and 42 weeks of pregnancy when the fetus is matured enough for birth; this is the expected time women will go into labour.

ONLINE RESOURCES/SUGGESTED READINGS

- **Diagnosis of pregnancy** available at www.youtube.com/watch?v=OnlHXSBv0M4&t=130s
- **Implantation** available at www.youtube.com/watch?v=1KL8HAm3uSY
- **Pregnancy physiology** available at www.youtube.com/watch?v=IKRT-boQTr0&index=2&list=PLbKSbFnKYVY2yzzd3a3WShJxjc_aAt4Vk
- **Labour** available at www.youtube.com/watch?v=Bf04LcSBpDw&list=PLbKSbFnKYVY2yzzd3a3WShJxjc_aAt4Vk&index=3
- **Breastfeeding: letdown reflex** available at www.youtube.com/watch?v=cMhgFt1xT7c

INTRODUCTION

During pregnancy a woman experiences dramatic yet normal physiological and anatomical changes, as pregnancy leads to major demands on all body systems. These changes enable the baby to be born and for the woman's body to meet the nutritional needs of her baby after birth. Although the female body undergoes visible changes to accommodate a growing fetus, pregnancy is a normal physiological state. As a future clinician, it is important to understand the 'normal' anatomical and physiological changes associated with pregnancy so that you can more easily recognise any deviations from normal. The functions of major body systems have been discussed elsewhere in this book and need to be understood before reading this chapter to facilitate a more comprehensive understanding of the changes that occur during pregnancy.

INTEGRATION OF PREGNANCY WITH OTHER BODY SYSTEMS

Reproductive system

Some of the most significant changes in a pregnant woman's body occur in her reproductive system. Chapter 21 noted that the essential organs of the female reproductive system are the ovaries, while the accessory organs include the uterus (which includes the cervix), fallopian tubes, vagina, external genitalia and mammary glands—the last of which are discussed in this chapter with regard to lactation. The reproductive organs are essential for pregnancy to begin.

Conception and implantation

During ovulation, an ovum is released into the abdominopelvic cavity then travels to the fallopian tube. This is where conception or fertilisation occurs. During intercourse, sperm cells that are released through male ejaculation swim through the female cervix and uterine cavity to the fallopian tubes. It is estimated that only 50–100 out of 250 million sperm make it to the ovum.[1] Once a sperm reaches the surface of the ovum the receptor molecules on the ovum and sperm bind together and a biochemical reaction occurs (called an acrosome reaction). The tip of the sperm head contains enzymes that break down the outer layer of the ovum, enabling the sperm to reach the surface of the ovum.[1] No other sperm can enter once the sperm and ovum have fused due to a complex mechanism whereby enzymes are released that inactivate the receptor molecules on the surface of the ovum.[1] The fertilised ovum is genetically complete and now called a **zygote**—the first cell of a new individual.[1] Although fertilisation has occurred, pregnancy has not yet begun. Pregnancy begins once implantation occurs. Development of the zygote is divided into three periods: the two weeks following fertilisation, which includes implantation into the endometrium, is the pre-embryonic period; weeks two to eight are the embryonic period; and the fetal period is from week eight until birth.[2]

After fertilisation, the zygote travels along the fallopian tube to the uterus (Fig. 22.1). Along this journey, which takes about one week, the zygote undergoes transformation and it divides (cleaves) into a **morula** (which has an inner cavity) and then into a **blastocyst**, a hollow ball containing 58 cells.[1,2] The blastocyst has two components: an inner cell mass known as an embryoblast and an outer cell mass known as the trophoblast.[2] The

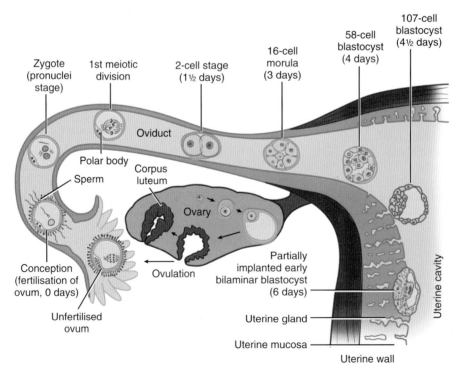

FIGURE 22.1 **Fertilisation and implantation.** (*Source:* Goljan EF. Rapid review pathology, 5 ed. Elsevier; 2019.)

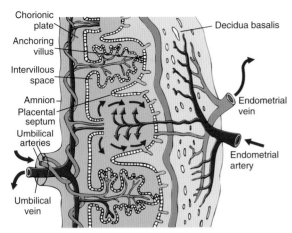

Chorionic plate
Anchoring villus
Intervillous space
Amnion
Placental septum
Umbilical arteries
Umbilical vein
Decidua basalis
Endometrial vein
Endometrial artery

FIGURE 22.2 **Placenta.** Deoxygenated blood leaves the fetus through the umbilical arteries and enters the placenta, where it is oxygenated. Oxygenated blood leaves the placenta through the umbilical vein, which enters the fetus via the umbilical cord. (*Source:* Perry SE, Lowdermilk DL, Cashion K, Rhodes Alden K, Hockenberry MJ et al. Maternal child nursing care, 6 ed. Elsevier; 2018.)

embryoblast forms the **embryo**, amnion and umbilical cord and the trophoblast forms into the placenta and chorion. The chorion and amnion are the membranes that contain the embryo then fetus and amniotic fluid within the uterus. The trophoblast begins to produce human chorionic gonadotropin (hCG) as this helps prepare the endometrial surface for implantation by making structural changes known as decidualisation.[2] The trophoblast then implants into the endometrium (decidua). After this occurs, the syncytiotrophoblast (the outer layer of the trophoblast) forms finger-like projections called villi and invades the decidua to reach the maternal blood supply.[2] As the villi branch out and contain blood vessels of the developing embryo, gaseous exchange between the mother and embryo results.[2] This is the beginning of **placentation**, or development of the placenta (Fig. 22.2).

Uterus, cervix and vagina

The uterus is a smooth muscle organ that can spontaneously contract just like any other smooth muscle. The muscle fibres of the uterus grow and form more fibres in early pregnancy. By **term**, the muscle fibres have increased to three times their usual diameter and ten times their usual length.[3] Before pregnancy, the capacity of the uterus is about 10 mL but by the end of pregnancy it can hold 5 L.[4] Oestrogen promotes growth

of uterine muscle fibres whereas progesterone maintains the myometrium to remain quiescent (in a quiet state) to allow for development and growth of the fetus and placenta before reaching the end of pregnancy.[3] As the uterus grows, it forms two main structural compartments: the upper part comprising the top of the uterus (referred to as the fundus) and the body of the uterus; and the lower part, comprising the isthmus and cervix.

In a non-pregnant state, the cervix is a closed, rigid and collagen-dense structure. During pregnancy, the cervix acts as a barrier to infection. The collagen fibres form a rigid structure which help keep the fetus in the uterus before it is ready to be born.[5] Over the course of pregnancy, the cervix softens as the network of collagen fibres is reorganised,[6] and the cervix transforms from a rigid structure to an elastic tissue in preparation for birth.[3] Due to the action of progesterone the mucus that is secreted by the cells of the cervix (endocervical cells) becomes thicker and more viscous, forming a 'plug' known as the operculum or show, preventing ascending infection[3] that could be harmful to the fetus. The plug is released during labour when the cervix begins to open and change shape.

The changes that occur in the vagina are to prepare for birth. Oestrogen acts on the muscle layer of the vagina, leading to hypertrophy of the muscle and changing the connective tissue so that it is more elastic[3] to allow for birth of the baby. The vagina can change colour to a deep reddish purple (known as Jacquemier's sign) due to the increased vascularity and blood flow.[3] Oestrogen produces change to the epithelium too, increasing the rate that superficial cells are shed, which increases the amount of vaginal discharge.[3] The white discharge is known as leucorrhoea and is considered a normal physiological change.

Immune system

During pregnancy, the immune response is biased towards an enhancement of innate immunity (the immunity you are born with) and away from adaptive immunity (also known as acquired immunity). Regulation of innate immunity is influenced by the fetoplacental unit.[7] This is because a cell-mediated response from adaptive immunity could be harmful to the fetus and reject it, as the mechanisms that are essential to protect the mother have the potential to destroy the placenta and fetus. Although the fetal membranes separate the fetus from the mother, some trophoblastic cells break away and enter the maternal circulation during implantation.[3] The release of foreign particles from the embryo into the maternal system stimulates a systemic inflammatory response. Within the adaptive immune response the cell-mediated (T helper 1, or Th1) response is made less functional in pregnancy whereas the antibody-mediated (T helper 2, or Th2), response is enhanced.[5] Increased levels of oestrogens and progesterone are thought to be responsible for the altered immune function.[8] For the mother, this change can put her at increased risk of developing some infections, but prevents her body from rejecting the fetus. She is not considered to be immunosuppressed, but her immune response is altered—this resolves after the pregnancy ends.[8]

Cardiovascular system

During pregnancy, extensive physiological adaptations to the cardiovascular system must occur to accommodate the needs of the growing fetus. This involves a delicate balance between the needs of the fetus and what the mother's body can tolerate without it being functionally compromised. The changes are predominantly reversible and demonstrate how adaptable the body can be. The main reasons why the cardiovascular system must change are to promote the growth and development of the fetoplacental unit, to increase circulatory function to meet the demands of pregnancy and fetal growth, and to compensate for blood loss that normally occurs after birth of the baby.

Haematological changes

Total blood volume is made up of plasma volume, white blood cells, platelets and red blood cell volume. The volume of blood circulating around the body increases by 30–40% in pregnancy (approximately 1.5 L).[5] As the total blood volume increases in pregnancy, there is a disproportionate amount of plasma volume compared with the total amount of red blood cells in circulation (also known as red cell mass).[9] Plasma volume increases by 45–50% whereas red cell mass increases by only 20–30%.[5] This leads to dilution of the blood characterised by decreased red cell count, haematocrit and haemoglobin, resulting in physiological anaemia, which is a normal finding in a healthy pregnancy. However, there is an advantage to the increase in plasma volume: it helps the blood to flow more easily as its viscosity (thickness) is reduced, so there is less resistance to it travelling through the maternal veins and arteries. The mother benefits by reduced cardiac effort and the fetus benefits with increased placental perfusion.

Total blood volume increases throughout pregnancy in order to:
- meet the needs of the enlarged uterus and provide extra blood flow for placental perfusion
- supply the metabolic needs of the fetus
- provide extra perfusion for maternal organs

- protect against harmful effects of impaired venous return (the heart can only pump out the same volume that is returned to it)
- help counteract against adverse effects of possible excessive blood loss at birth
- counterbalance the effects of increased arterial and venous capacity.

Further changes within the haematological system include an increase in clotting factors. The purpose of this change is to protect the mother from excessive blood loss at birth and to maintain blood flow to the placenta.[2] An increase in coagulation factors VII and VIII,[10] combined with reduced plasma fibrinolytic activity, results in blood that will clot more easily. Plasma fibrinogen concentration (factor I) rises by up to 200% by term, helping prevent haemorrhage when the placenta separates from the side of the uterus. This clever design means that pregnant women are at an increased risk of thromboembolic disease. During pregnancy the haemostatic balance becomes more hypercoagulable due to the increase in plasma levels of clotting factors.[11] In venous thromboembolism (VTE), blood clots inappropriately in the body resulting in conditions such as deep vein thrombosis (DVT) and pulmonary embolism (PE), which are associated with significant morbidity and mortality.[11] Although the overall risk of venous thromboembolic disease in pregnancy is one to two women per 1000, the risk of VTE for pregnant women and soon after giving birth is much higher than for non-pregnant women of the same age.[11] Comparing women of the same age, pregnant women have five times the risk of VTE than non-pregnant women and up to sixty times the risk in the first three months after giving birth compared with non-pregnant women.[11]

Vasodilation

As blood volume increases, vasodilation occurs. Although it is not fully understood how the increase in blood volume occurs, it is thought that the increased vasculature of the placenta and uterus (which is quite vasodilated) is a contributing factor. However, this does not account for all of the volume increase. Hormones of pregnancy such as progesterone and oestrogen contribute to vasodilation. These hormones are associated with nitric oxide production and the enhancement of endothelial function, which activates the renin-angiotensin-aldosterone system (RAAS),[5] a physiological system that regulates blood pressure in the body. Renin is an enzyme situated in the juxtaglomerular kidney cells, which are sensitive to changes in blood flow and blood pressure. In a pregnant woman, this stimulates sodium and water retention, as its role is to maintain arterial blood pressure and electrolyte homeostasis. As vasodilation causes dilution of the maternal circulation, this initiates fluid and electrolyte retention via the RAAS; plasma and extracellular fluid volumes expand, and cardiac output increases as a result.

Cardiac output increases in the first two trimesters and by the end of the pregnancy it is 30–50% higher than pre-pregnancy levels.[12] This is mainly due to increased stroke volume and heart rate. Stroke volume is increased to pump the increased volume of blood around the body and the rate at which the heart pumps increases to increase efficiency. However, arterial blood pressure is reduced in pregnancy, and this is mainly due to the decrease in systemic vascular resistance, associated with vasodilation. Furthermore, a rise in maternal body temperature[13] of 0.2–0.4°C from the effects of progesterone and increased basal metabolic rate (BMR) leads to increased heat production, vasodilation and lowered peripheral vascular resistance. Decreased peripheral vascular resistance results in a decrease in blood pressure in early pregnancy, particularly diastolic blood pressure. This reduces by an average of 10–15 mmHg by 24 weeks gestation.[2]

Later in pregnancy the weight of the gravid (pregnant) uterus can occlude, or compress, the inferior vena cava and laterally displace the subrenal aorta when the mother lies flat on her back.[2] This is known as **supine hypotension**, as venous return to the heart is impaired, maternal cardiac output can be reduced by 10–30% and there may be a dramatic reduction in blood pressure.[14] This will significantly decrease the perfusion of blood through the uterus to the placenta, which can compromise the fetus. Most women can adequately compensate for this change by raising their heart rate and increasing systemic vascular resistance. Blood from the lower limbs can be diverted and return to the heart through the collateral circulation (an alternative circulation pathway from the pelvis to the thorax).[14] However, approximately 8% of women experience supine hypotensive syndrome,[14] which is characterised by bradycardia, hypotension, dizziness, light-headedness and nausea. When the woman is lying down, tilting her onto her left side, by placing a pillow or wedge under her right hip, can relieve this compression of the uterus on the inferior vena cava.

In summary, a healthy pregnancy is a high-flow, low-resistance haemodynamic state with a significant amount of haemodilution. Haematological changes are summarised in Table 22.1.

Heart

The rest of the cardiovascular system adapts to cope with these haematological changes. Due to the increase in blood volume, cardiac output, stroke volume and

TABLE 22.1
Physiological changes in the cardiovascular system during pregnancy

Parameter	Adaptation	Magnitude	Non-pregnant (average value)	Timing of peak/ average peak value
Oxygen consumption	Increase	20–30%	180 mL/min	Term
Total body water	Increase	6–8 L		Term
Plasma volume	Increase	45–50%	2600 mL	32–34 weeks; 3850 mL
Red cell mass	Increase	20–30%	1400 mL	Term 1650 mL
Total blood volume	Increase	30–50%	4000 mL	32 weeks; 5500 mL
Cardiac output	Increase	30–50%	4.9 L/min	28 weeks; 7 L/min
Stroke volume	Increase			20 weeks
Heart rate	Increase	10–20 bpm	75 bpm	Trimester 1; 90 bpm
Systemic vascular resistance	Decrease	21%	–	Trimester 2
Pulmonary vascular resistance	Decrease	35%	–	34 weeks
Diastolic blood pressure	Decrease, returning to normal by term	10–15 mmHg	–	24 weeks
Systolic blood pressure	Minimal, no decrease	5–10 mmHg	–	24 weeks
Serum colloid osmotic pressure	Decrease	10–15%	–	14 weeks

Source: Marshall J, Raynor M. Myles textbook for midwives, 16 ed. Sydney: Churchill Livingstone; 2014.

heart rate, the heart increases in size.[2] This is because the chambers in the heart enlarge due to increased ventricular wall muscle. In addition, the progressive increases in blood volume increase diastolic filling, which results in distension of the chambers. These structural changes to the heart mimic those seen in exercise-induced cardiac remodelling, often seen in elite athletes.[15] In addition to its increase in size, the heart is displaced upwards and slightly to the left by the diaphragm, which is pushed up by the growing uterus.

Placenta

The role of the placenta is to support, nourish and protect the growing fetus.[16] Fetal development is dependent on the transportation of nutrients and oxygen across the placenta;[17] this depends on the size and structure of the placenta, which steadily increases throughout pregnancy. Many of the cardiovascular changes in pregnancy are impacted by the effect of the placenta on the maternal circulation. Five layers of placental tissue separate the maternal and fetal circulations; these are known as the **placental membrane** or placental barrier.[5] For substances to pass from the maternal circulation to the fetal circulation they must pass through these five layers. Maternal blood flows to the uterus via the uterine arteries and into the uterine spiral arteries. The spiral arteries are normally tightly coiled arteries with thick muscular walls. During the early stages of pregnancy, they are remodelled by trophoblast cells so that the muscular walls are destroyed and the vessels become dilated, sac-like uteroplacental vessels that allow blood to flow through them easily without resistance.[4] These structural changes of the spiral arteries result in low pressures in this system. The rate of blood flow within the maternal side of the placenta increases from about 50 mL/min at 10 weeks gestation to 500–600 mL/min at term.[5]

Respiratory system

Anatomical and physiological changes also occur in the respiratory system to meet the increasing oxygen requirements and metabolic demands of the mother, fetus and placenta. Anatomically, the growing uterus changes abdominal size and shape, moving the diaphragm up to 4 cm above its usual position, and increasing the transverse diameter of the chest by 2 cm (Fig. 22.3).[3] As a result, the thoracic cavity decreases in size and the lungs have to become more efficient at gas exchange within that space. The amount of air moved into and out of the lungs (minute ventilation) increases due to an increase in tidal volume (the amount of air expired when breathing normally), usually without a change in the respiratory rate.[18] Nevertheless, even

without this change, women breathe more deeply, even at rest. Although vital capacity remains the same, inspiratory capacity increases. Vital capacity is the amount of air that can be expired after maximal inspiration, indicating the maximum amount of air that can enter and leave the lungs during respiration.[1] For the lungs to make these changes, the rib cage expands outwards and the flexibility of the chest wall increases.[2] These changes are mediated by the hormones progesterone and relaxin, which relax the muscles and cartilage of the thorax, making the ribcage more flexible.[3] When acting on the bronchial and tracheal smooth muscle, progesterone reduces airway resistance, thus reducing the work of breathing.[5] During pregnancy, progesterone enhances sensitivity to carbon dioxide in the respiratory centre and lowers the threshold for carbon dioxide levels.[5] This is most likely a contributing factor to the feeling of shortness of breath (dyspnoea) that is commonly experienced in pregnancy.

Changes also occur to the upper respiratory tract. Blood flow to the mucosa of the nasopharynx increases, and the area becomes more oedematous (swollen).[3] Increases in pregnancy hormones (such as progesterone), increased blood volume, glandular hypersecretion, oedema and increased phagocyte activity alter the mucosa of the oro- and nasopharynx, leading to engorgement.[19] Swelling of the airways due to pregnancy-induced changes has the potential to be hazardous in a clinical situation where a pregnant women requires intubation: the rate of failed intubations is seven to eight times higher in pregnancy.[19]

Urinary system

The kidneys receive approximately 25% of cardiac output, more than any other organ in the body.[3] Therefore, structural and physiological changes in the urinary system during pregnancy are directly related to cardiovascular system adaptations. In addition to alterations due to increased blood volume and cardiac output, renal vascular resistance decreases due to the relaxing effects of progesterone. The main changes that are displayed in clinical findings are sodium retention and increased extracellular volume.[3] This makes it difficult to assess renal function, as the parameters that are normally used to assess renal function cannot be applied in pregnancy.

Due to increased blood volume, cardiac output and systemic vasodilation in pregnancy, renal circulation vasodilates to increase renal plasma flow (RPF). This is also in response to excreting fetal waste, which enters the maternal circulation from the placenta. Like the heart, the kidneys also increase in size, lengthening and

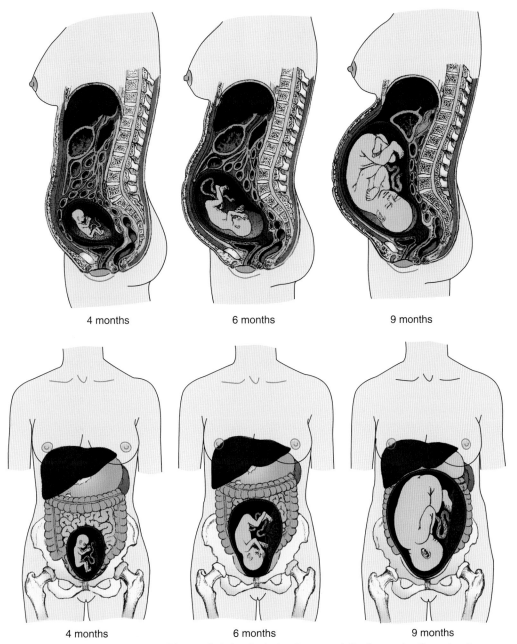

4 months 6 months 9 months

4 months 6 months 9 months

FIGURE 22.3 **Displacement of internal abdominal structures and diaphragm by the enlarging uterus at four, six and nine months of gestation.** (*Source:* Perry SE, Lowdermilk DL, Cashion K, Rhodes Alden K, Hockenberry MJ et al. Maternal child nursing care, 6 ed. Elsevier; 2018.)

increasing their volume by as much as 30%. Other structural changes are summarised in Table 22.2.

As with many changes in pregnancy, the changes to the urinary system are related to the effects of progesterone on smooth muscle.[3] The bladder and ureters need to adapt as the uterus increases in size, and they become displaced from their usual position in the pelvis. As the uterus grows it compresses and displaces the ureters from their usual position to a more lateral aspect in the mother's body.

TABLE 22.2
Structural changes in the urinary system during pregnancy

Organ	Change
Kidneys	Increase in size and length, mainly due to increased blood flow, vascular volume and interstitial space
Bladder	Capacity increases to 1 L; tone is decreased, leading to incompetence of vesicoureteric sphincters (may lead to reflux or urine); late in pregnancy bladder may be displaced
Glomeruli	Increase in size, but cell number remains the same
Renal calyces, pelvis and ureters	Dilation, lengthening and increased muscle tone; decreased peristalsis; late in pregnancy ureters become displaced and hold 25 times more urine (as much as 300 mL)

Source: Adapted from Rankin J. Physiology in childbearing with anatomy and related biosciences, 4 ed. Edinburgh: Elsevier; 2017.

TABLE 22.3
Physiological changes in the urinary system during pregnancy

Feature	Change
Renal blood flow	Increases by 35–60% by end of first trimester, with slight decrease at end of pregnancy
Tubular function	Retention of sodium and water; increased reabsorption of solutes, excretion of glucose, protein, urea, uric acid, water-soluble amino acids, calcium, hydrogen ions and phosphorus
Glomerular capillaries	Vasodilation in afferent and efferent capillaries
Glomerular filtration rate (GFR)	Increases by 40–50%
Renin-angiotensin-aldosterone system (RAAS)	All components increase; resistance to pressor effects of angiotensin II
Glucose	Values increase ten-fold
Amino acids	Protein excretion increases (values vary daily)

Source: Adapted from Rankin J. Physiology in childbearing with anatomy and related biosciences, 4 ed. Edinburgh: Elsevier; 2017.

Hydronephrosis (dilation of the renal pelvis) is a normal physiological adaptation of pregnancy.[3] Although the cause is not well understood, it is thought that a main contributor is compression of the ureters against the pelvic brim of the bony pelvis.[3] Outside of pregnancy this would be considered a pathological problem requiring investigation. Dilation of the renal pelvis and ureters and reduction in peristalsis starts as early as seven weeks gestation and is attributed to the effect of progesterone, a smooth muscle relaxant.[3] As the movement of urine from the kidneys slows, pregnant women are at increased risk of urinary tract infections (UTIs).[3] The ureters elongate and can develop curves, further contributing to urinary stasis and risk of UTIs.

As renal blood flow increases significantly within the kidneys, the glomerular filtration rate (GFR) increases. This means that a greater proportion of renal blood is filtered. This increase begins soon after conception and peaks around 9–16 weeks before stabilising.[3] The volume of urine produced in 24 hours is 25% higher in pregnancy.[3] As the GFR is increased, fluid and solutes in the tubules increase by 50–100%.[3] Tubular reabsorption therefore needs to increase to avoid excessive loss of sodium, glucose, chloride, potassium and water. However, due to the filtered load of metabolites being dramatically increased, tubular reabsorption is not able to fully compensate, leading to glucose and amino acids being

excreted in the urine. The tubules have a reduced ability to reabsorb glucose and this leads to glycosuria, or glucose in the urine, which is common among pregnant women. Proteinuria is also common among pregnant women due to increased excretion of amino acids. A value of 1+ on a protein dipstick is not considered abnormal in pregnancy.[3] Although proteinuria is not considered abnormal in isolation, when coupled with hypertension it may indicate a serious condition known as **preeclampsia**, which can put the woman and the fetus at risk.

As the volume of blood filtered through the kidneys increases, pregnant women experience increased frequency and urgency when emptying their bladder. Being on their feet throughout the day, coupled with decreased venous return in the lower limbs, means that when they lie in bed at night their body needs to reabsorb the accumulation of oedema from the lower extremities. This results in increased diuresis at night and the urine is more diluted.

Physiological changes to the urinary system are summarised in Table 22.3.

After giving birth, rapid and sustained diuresis occurs, especially in the first five days. The first day after giving birth is associated with glomerular hyperfiltration, with filtration increasing by 41% above normal levels, and by two weeks **postpartum** it is 20% above normal levels.[3] A urine output of 3000 mL and a single void of 500–1000 mL is considered normal during this period. Within three weeks fluid and electrolyte balance normalises. Most structural changes to the urinary system return to normal in six to eight weeks, but can take up to three months.

Gastrointestinal system

The gastrointestinal (GI) system undergoes significant changes in pregnancy as the mother's body meets the nutritional needs of the fetus as well as her own. Hormones of pregnancy often result in altered function of the GI system, causing much discomfort to the mother. These issues, although quite worrisome to the mother, resolve after the birth of her baby. Pregnancy is associated with increased appetite and consumption of food, but it is also a time to avoid certain foods that could contain bacteria harmful to the fetus.[20] Progesterone is a driving factor in the increased consumption of food as it is known to stimulate appetite.[5] Metabolic adaptations during pregnancy are important to: provide the fetus with adequate stores of energy for growth and development and transition to birth outside the uterus; meet maternal needs to cope with the physiological changes and adaptations of pregnancy; and provide enough energy and substrate stores for pregnancy, labour and lactation.[5]

Mouth

Gingival tissue contains oestrogen and progesterone receptors.[5] Oestrogen increases blood flow to the gums and accelerates the turnover of gum epithelial lining cells,[5] changing the consistency of connective tissue. As a result, the gums become swollen and spongy[3] and the mother is at increased risk of bleeding gums, gingivitis and periodontal disease. This can have a detrimental impact on pregnancy and infant outcomes such as preterm birth.[21] In addition, the electrolyte content and microorganism load alter as saliva becomes more acidic.[5] Some women experience the sensation of an excessive amount of saliva (called ptyalism) but this is rare.[5] Difficulties in swallowing are usually related to nausea and vomiting in the first trimester.

GI disturbances

Nausea and vomiting are common among pregnant women, with approximately 50–80% experiencing nausea and 50% experiencing vomiting.[22] Although commonly known as 'morning sickness' these pregnancy-related symptoms are not confined to the morning and can occur at any time during the day. They are commonly experienced in the first trimester, with a very small number of women experiencing them beyond 20 weeks gestation. Nausea and vomiting are associated with rising levels of hCG and oestrogens.[22]

Oesophagus, stomach and intestines

As pregnancy progresses and nausea and vomiting recede, up to 80% of women will experience the symptoms of heartburn in the third trimester,[3] although this can occur at any time during pregnancy. Heartburn is a burning sensation in the upper part of the digestive tract, including the throat.[23] The cause is related to progesterone function, which relaxes the lower oesophageal sphincter between the oesophagus and stomach. This is also described as decreased lower oesophageal sphincter pressure.[23] The lower oesophageal sphincter plays an important role as a pressure barrier, minimising gastro-oesophageal reflux from the stomach to the oesophagus.[5] Because the sphincter is more relaxed from progesterone, regurgitation of stomach acid can occur. The lower oesophageal sphincter's decreased responsiveness to pressure during pregnancy[5] may signal the loss of an important protective response. As intra-abdominal pressure increases as the uterus grows in size, this may contribute to heartburn.[23]

Within the stomach there is a delay in emptying of the stomach contents and a reduced secretion rate of gastric juices.[3] This is caused by the effect of progesterone decreasing gastric muscle tone and motility.[3] However, gastric emptying time remains the same.[5]

In response to reduced stores of iron in the maternal circulation, duodenal absorption of iron almost doubles late in pregnancy.[5] The decrease in intestinal motility assists with the absorption of nutrients such as iron and calcium, as nutrients and fluids remain in the intestinal lumen for longer than usual.[5] Progesterone is thought to enhance the absorption of calcium, sodium and water and the net secretion of potassium.[5] Water and sodium absorption in the large colon increase because of reduced motility and increased transit time in the large intestine.[5] As a result, stools are smaller due to lower water content. Decreased gastric muscle tone and motility in the stomach, along with prolonged small intestine transit time and increased water absorption from the colon, all contribute to many pregnant women experiencing constipation. In addition, the enlarging uterus acts as a mechanical obstruction to the intestines, further contributing to constipation.[24]

Metabolism

Changes to metabolic processes during pregnancy are essential in order to provide adequate nutrients for fetal growth and development.[5] Pregnancy is considered to be an anabolic state where food intake and appetite increase, and physical activity decreases.[5] Much of the weight gain in the first two trimesters is due to an accumulation of maternal fat and the increased volume of blood.[5] To make nutrients, in particular glucose, available to the growing fetus, the mother's body becomes increasingly insulin resistant.[25] This is facilitated by the hormone human placental lactogen (hPL). hPL has similar properties to growth hormones and prolactin as it stimulates growth of fetal tissue and maternal tissue,[4] in particular breast tissue in preparation for lactation.[2] hPL is secreted by the syncytiotrophoblast (the outer layer of the trophoblast) and helps regulate maternal carbohydrate, protein and lipid metabolism and fetal growth.[2] Along with oestrogen, progesterone and leptin, hPL alters glucose utilisation to increase the availability of glucose and amino acids to transfer to the fetus.[5]

LABOUR AND BIRTH

Labour is the three-stage process of regular and coordinated muscular contractions of the uterus that lead to effacement and dilation of the cervix, followed by expulsive contractions resulting in the birth of the baby and then the placenta.[26] During pregnancy, mild contractions or tightening of the uterine muscle occur, but are often unnoticed by the woman.[26] Strong, regular, rhythmic contractions are prevented by uterotonic inhibitors such as progesterone, relaxin, nitric oxide and prostacyclin.[26] The cells of the myometrium (the smooth muscle tissue of the uterus) change their structure in the last few weeks of pregnancy, enabling them to contract more strongly. The four main events responsible for these changes are: an increase in electrical activity; an increased responsiveness to the microenvironment; a change in the ratio of hormones; and an increase in ion channels on myometrial cells.[26] As the fetus matures and reaches the end of pregnancy the fetal hypothalamus stimulates release of corticotropin-releasing hormone (CRH) from the anterior pituitary gland.[3] This releases adrenocorticotropic hormone (ACTH), which causes the fetal adrenal gland to produce cortisol and dehydroepiandrosterone sulfate (DHEAS).[3] This is known as the fetal hypothalamus-pituitary-adrenal axis. Cortisol plays a role in maturing fetal organ systems to assist with adaptation to life outside the uterus, but it also converts progesterone to oestrogen, helping to trigger the onset of labour.[3]

For the fetus to be born successfully, the cervix needs to efface (shorten) and dilate (widen) to allow its passage from the uterus and through the vagina. As the cervix is a rigid structure, it needs to first undergo a process called **ripening**. At the end of pregnancy increasing levels of oestrogen relative to progesterone promote degradation of collagen in the cervix, helping it to soften.[26] The cervix and uterus interact with each other during labour. Stretching of the cervix stimulates local release of prostaglandin F2α and oxytocin from the posterior pituitary gland, which in turn increases uterine activity.[26] The role of **oxytocin** in labour is described as a positive feedback loop. This can be explained when looking at Ferguson's reflex, which is a neurohormonal reflex.[3] As uterine contractions push the fetus onto the cervix, and the cervix is stretched, messages are sent via neural pathways to the posterior pituitary gland to release oxytocin.[3] Stretch or dilation of the cervix and vagina is a strong stimulus for oxytocin to be secreted. During labour and birth, oxytocin is released in pulses, leading to contractions that dilate the cervix, resulting in more oxytocin secretion.

Uterine contractions commence in the fundus (top of the uterus) and spread across and downwards.[2] As well as regular contractions, the myometrium does not completely relax or lengthen after each contraction, rather it retains some shortening (known as retraction) (Fig. 22.4).[2] This means that the upper segment

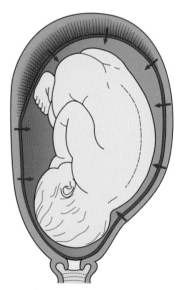

FIGURE 22.4 **Contraction and retraction of uterine muscle.** (*Source:* Adapted from Marshall J, Raynor M. Myles textbook for midwives, 16 ed. Sydney: Churchill Livingstone; 2014.)

gradually becomes shorter during labour, which in turn moves the fetus down through the pelvis. This assists with effacement and dilation of the cervix where the muscle fibres around the internal os (the inner part of the cervix) are drawn upwards as the upper segment of the uterus maintains retraction.[2] It is common in the first stage of labour for women to experience contractions every 2–3 minutes, lasting approximately 1 minute.[2] Labour commences when regular strong contractions begin to efface and dilate the cervix. It is usually classified as 'active' once the cervix has dilated approximately 3–4 cm.[26]

Other physiological changes that often occur in the first stage of labour include release of the operculum (show), the mucous plug in the cervix. In addition, as the pressure within the uterus increases, the membranes surrounding the fetus often rupture, releasing amniotic fluid.[2]

The second stage of labour commences when the cervix has been completely drawn up into the lower segment of the uterus, commonly described as fully dilated. This stage can last from a few minutes to up to 2 hours. Contractions continue, but the force of the contractions increases, and maternal behaviour changes, with many women experiencing an overwhelming urge to push.[2] With each contraction the superficial muscles of the pelvic floor stretch, especially the transverse perineal muscles, as the head of the fetus descends.[2] In between contractions, the head recedes, allowing the muscles to gradually thin. Once the head has crowned, it restitutes; that is, the head returns to its original position in alignment with the shoulders.[26] This is necessary because the fetal head and body must navigate their way through the pelvis taking advantage of the widest diameters (Fig. 22.5). Once the body of the baby is born, unless there are signs of breathing issues, the umbilical cord is clamped and cut within a few minutes.[27] Skin-to-skin contact between mother and baby at birth (and beyond) helps stimulate the production of oxytocin and prolactin,[3] assisting with lactation.

The third stage of labour is defined as the time from the baby being born until the placenta and membranes are delivered. During this stage, the myometrium contracts (under the influence of oxytocin), helping the placenta to shear off the side of the uterus (Fig. 22.6). This action also helps achieve haemostasis as the uterine blood vessels are constricted when the myometrium contracts.[28] A fibrin mesh forms to cover the placental site and control bleeding. This takes 5–10% of all the circulating fibrinogen,[2] which is why fibrinogen concentration increases during pregnancy.

BREASTFEEDING

The breasts are made up of milk-producing mammary glands,[1] a complex exocrine gland whose function is to produce, secrete and deliver milk to the baby.[29] Although most of the structures of the breast are formed before a female is born, the final stages of mammary development occur during pregnancy when breast size increases. In addition to breast growth during pregnancy, the nipples become more erect, and the areolae darken and enlarge,[30] which assists the baby to latch onto the breast after birth. **Lactogenesis** is the transition from pregnancy to lactation and occurs in two stages. In the first stage, the mammary glands develop the capacity to secrete milk.[30] During pregnancy, oestrogen, progesterone, prolactin and hPL induce the physiological transition of the mammary glands from branched tissues that do not secrete any substances to highly active secreting organs.[29] The mammary glands develop a vast network of ducts and alveoli, grouped into seven to 10 lobes resembling the branches of a tree.[29] In the third trimester of pregnancy, colostrum—which is high in protein and minerals and low in carbohydrates, fat and some vitamins (compared with mature breastmilk)—is secreted.[30] When babies are born, their intestines are sterile. Colostrum provides the first colonisation of the intestines and is very important as it delivers beneficial bacteria to the gut.[30] Breastfed babies have higher concentrations of lactobacilli and bifidobacteria,[30] beneficial bacteria.

After the baby has been born and the placenta delivered, progesterone levels decrease dramatically.[30] This triggers the second stage of lactogenesis. The epithelial cells that were differentiated during pregnancy to secrete milk begin to synthesise and transport components necessary for milk secretion.[29] Usually two to three days after the birth, there is an onset of copious milk secretion.[30] The milk ejection or let-down reflex (how milk is forced out of the breast) is regulated by the hormone oxytocin.[3] Sensory nerves in the nipple and areola convey information to the midbrain and hypothalamus via afferent fibres in the dorsal horn of the spinal cord when the baby starts suckling.[3] This results in the release of oxytocin from the posterior lobe of the pituitary gland.[3] Oxytocin contracts the myoepithelial cells situated around the milk-secreting glands to generate contractile force.[29] The release of oxytocin also assists with smooth muscle contraction, resulting in shortening and widening of the ducts to allow milk to flow.[3] This process follows the same positive feedback loop as described for the role of oxytocin in labour. The size of the breast does not determine the amount of synthesised milk; instead, it is the baby's ability to remove milk from the breast and the

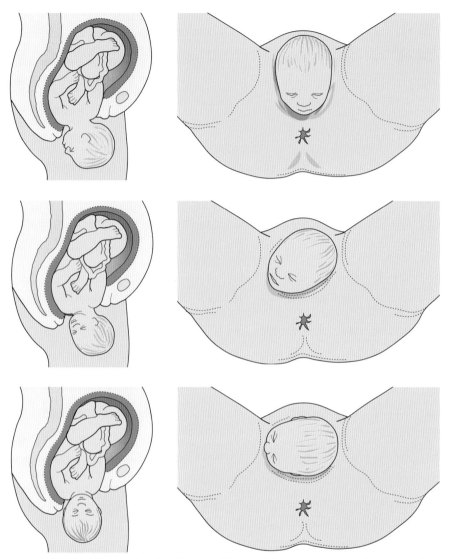

FIGURE 22.5 **Birth of the head and restitution.** (*Source:* Adapted from Marshall J, Raynor M. Myles textbook for midwives, 16 ed. Sydney: Churchill Livingstone; 2014.)

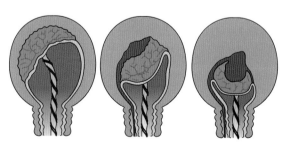

FIGURE 22.6 **The third stage of labour.** (*Source:* Adapted from Marshall J, Raynor M. Myles textbook for midwives, 16 ed. Sydney: Churchill Livingstone; 2014.)

baby's appetite that regulate milk supply.[30] This is commonly known as the **supply and demand principle of breastfeeding**.

The hormone prolactin plays a role in maintaining milk secretion and supply, as do metabolic hormones such as insulin and glucocorticoids.[29] Ongoing regulation of milk supply (**galactopoiesis**) is maintained by the removal of milk from the mammary glands by the baby.[29] A whey protein that inhibits the synthesis of milk constituent is present in breastmilk.[2] As this protein collects in the breast (when milk stores accumulate), this exerts a negative feedback control on the production of milk.[2] Therefore, when a baby feeds and removes the milk from the breast, this autocrine inhibitory factor is removed and more milk is produced.

In addition to providing nutrition for the baby that is dynamic and changes across the period of breastfeeding, lactation assists in returning the female body to its pre-pregnant state. As oxytocin is released to trigger milk let-down, it acts on the uterus to contract,[2] reducing blood loss in the postnatal period and returning the uterus to its original size and position in the pelvis.[3] Breastfeeding is thought to aid with postpartum weight loss by rapidly lowering maternal circulating glucose and triglycerides, reducing insulin secretion and mobilising adipose tissue stores.[31]

AGE-RELATED CHANGES TO FERTILITY

As a woman ages, her ability to conceive and produce offspring diminishes. The most common reason for this is the depletion of follicles from the ovary. The number of ovarian follicles is determined from birth and declines as the female ages. The quality of oocytes decreases as the number of follicles declines, resulting in lower rates of fertilisation and conception in older women and an

increased rate of early-pregnancy loss.[32] Follicle loss is accelerated from about 35 years of age as the reproductive cycle begins to cease, resulting in approximately 100 to 1000 follicles, compared with 1 million at birth.[32] As a female is born with a finite number of follicles, the time they are exposed to internal and environmental factors, oxidative stress and mitochondrial dysfunction can affect the number and quality of oocytes. Oxidative stress is understood to play a role in tissue ageing and affects cellular mechanisms. Additionally, DNA double-stranded breaks (DSBs) accumulate with age, and the repair mechanisms of DNA in oocytes are poorly activated, resulting in cell death.[32]

CONCLUSION

The female body undergoes major adaptations to maintain a pregnancy and support the growing fetus. Although many of these changes are dramatic, nearly all will resolve and the body returns to normal functioning after birth and lactation have ceased. Understanding what is considered normal in pregnancy will assist you in recognising what may not be normal during pregnancy.

CASE STUDY 22.1

Alyssa is a 31-year-old woman who is 32 weeks pregnant with her first baby. She is starting to feel fatigued after being at work all day and is finding it harder to get comfortable in bed at night. Her midwife has recommended that she sleep on her left side, as she might experience supine hypotension if she lies flat on her back.

Q1. Late in pregnancy, when the mother is in a supine position the weight of the gravid uterus compresses which major artery?

   a. Inferior vena cava
   b. Superior vena cava
   c. Femoral artery
   d. Carotid artery

Q2. The rate of blood flowing through the placenta increases from 50 mL/min at 10 weeks gestation to _____/min at 40 weeks gestation.

   a. 100–200 mL
   b. 200–300 mL
   c. 400–500 mL
   d. 500–600 mL

Q3. Physiological anaemia occurs during pregnancy because:

   a. plasma volume increases by 20–25% and red blood cells increase by 15%.
   b. plasma volume increases by 30–40% and red blood cells increase by 18–30%.
   c. plasma volume increases by 35–60% and red blood cells increase by 20–30%.
   d. plasma volume increases by 45–50% and red blood cells increase by 20–30%.

Q4. Explain why supine hypotension can occur at this stage of gestation.

Q5. What physical symptoms might Alyssa experience with supine hypotension?

CASE STUDY 22.2

Tara is 20 weeks pregnant and suffering from constipation. She is vegan and as a result her diet is high in plant-based fibre.

Q1. Late in pregnancy, duodenal absorption of iron:
   a. decreases due to the increasing demands on the woman from the placenta.
   b. decreases due to the increasing demands on the woman from the placenta.
   c. increases as a response to reduced stores of iron in the maternal circulation.
   d. remains the same.

Q2. Which hormone is thought to enhance absorption of calcium, sodium and water and net secretion of potassium in the intestines?
   a. Progesterone
   b. Human placental lactogen
   c. Oestrogen
   d. Relaxin

Q3. Approximately how many women experience heartburn during their pregnancy?
   a. 15%
   b. 35%
   c. 60%
   d. 80%

Q4. Outline the physiological changes to the gastrointestinal system that may account for Tara's constipation.

Q5. What else could contribute to constipation during pregnancy?

CASE STUDY 22.3

Pham is 26 weeks pregnant with her second baby. She attends the hospital clinic for a scheduled pregnancy check-up. Pham tells her midwife that she is waking up at night needing to empty her bladder. She says that during the day is fine, but at night she needs to go more frequently. Her midwife takes a routine urinalysis and informs Pham that she has glycosuria.

Q1. The kidneys receive approximately how much of total cardiac output?
   a. 10%
   b. 18%
   c. 25%
   d. 30%

Q2. Hydronephrosis, also known as dilation of the renal pelvis, is:
   a. a normal physiological adaptation of pregnancy due to the effects of progesterone.
   b. a normal physiological adaptation of pregnancy due to the effects of hPL.
   c. an abnormal physiological adaptation of pregnancy due to the effects of progesterone.
   d. an abnormal physiological adaptation of pregnancy that requires immediate investigation.

Q3. During the postpartum period, the mother experiences rapid and sustained diuresis, especially in the first five days after giving birth. This results in:
   a. glomerular hypofiltration, decreasing the normal filtration rate.
   b. glomerular hyperfiltration, increasing filtration by 41%.
   c. glomerular hyperfiltration, increasing filtration by 51%.
   d. a urine output of 1500 mL.

Q4. What structural changes to the urinary system experienced during pregnancy could explain glycosuria?

Q5. Explain the interaction between the urinary and cardiovascular systems causing Pham to have an increased need to urinate at night.

CASE STUDY 22.4

Sasha gave birth to her daughter Hannah three days ago. She is experiencing changes to her breasts, as they feel heavy and full and are leaking breastmilk. She is concerned about how much milk her baby is drinking, and whether she is getting enough. Her midwife explains how the volume of breastmilk is regulated.

Q1. Why is it important for the establishment of breastfeeding that all of the placental tissue is removed after the birth of the baby?

    a. The presence of placental tissue can make the breastmilk taste different to the baby.

    b. The high levels of progesterone produced by the placenta need to reduce so that lactogenesis II can begin.

    c. Progesterone levels need to remain high so that the second stage of lactogenesis can begin.

    d. Remnants of placental tissue prevent the production of oxytocin.

Q2. Why is it so important for Sasha's baby to have colostrum as her first feed?

    a. Colostrum is high in fat and keeps the baby full for longer.

    b. Colostrum contains high levels of protein important for the transition to life outside the uterus.

    c. Colostrum contains beneficial bacteria that colonise the sterile gut.

    d. Colostrum is high in carbohydrates which the baby can easily metabolise.

Q3. Breastfeeding helps reduce postpartum bleeding by:

    a. triggering the release of oxytocin, which contracts the uterus, reducing blood loss.

    b. triggering the release of oxytocin, which reduces levels of progesterone, reducing blood loss.

    c. the milk let-down reflex reduces blood flow to the uterus, reducing blood loss.

    d. helping to keep the circulating level of progesterone high, reducing blood loss.

Q4. What anatomical and physiological changes occurred in Sasha's body during pregnancy to prepare her for breastfeeding?

Q5. Explain the supply and demand principle in breast milk production.

REFERENCES

1. Patton KT, Thibodeau GA. Anatomy and physiology, 10 ed. St Louis: Elsevier; 2019.
2. Marshall J, Raynor M. Myles textbook for midwives, 16 ed. Sydney: Churchill Livingstone; 2014.
3. Rankin J. Physiology in childbearing with anatomy and related biosciences, 4 ed. Edinburgh: Elsevier; 2017.
4. Coad J, Dunstall M. Anatomy and physiology for midwives, 3 ed. Sydney: Churchill Livingstone; 2011.
5. Blackburn ST. Maternal, fetal and neonatal physiology: a clinical perspective, 4 ed. St Louis: Saunders; 2013.
6. Banos N, Perez-Moreno A, Migliorelli F, et al. Quantitative analysis of the cervical texture by ultrasound and correlation with gestational age. Fetal Diagn Ther 2017;41(4):265–72.
7. Racicot K, Mor G. Risks associated with viral infections during pregnancy. J Clin Invest 2017;127:1591–9.
8. Mathad JS, Gupta A. Pulmonary infections in pregnancy. Semin Respir Crit Care Med 2017;38(2):174–84.
9. Sun D, McLeod A, Gandhi S, et al. Anemia in pregnancy: a pragmatic approach. Obstet Gynecol Surv 2017;72(12):730–7.
10. Robinson S, Longmuir K, Pavord S. Haematology of pregnancy. Medicine (Baltimore) 2017;45(4):251–5.
11. Bain E, Wilson A, Tooher R, et al. Prophylaxis for venous thromboembolic disease in pregnancy and the early postnatal period. Cochrane Database Syst Rev 2014;(2): CD001689.
12. Rossberg N, Stangl K, Stangl V. Pregnancy and cardiovascular risk: a review focused on women with heart disease undergoing fertility treatment. Eur J Prev Cardiol 2016; 23(18):1953–61.
13. Charkoudian N, Hart ECJ, Barnes JN, et al. Autonomic control of body temperature and blood pressure: influences of female sex hormones. Clin Auton Res 2017;27(3): 149–55.
14. Humphries A, Stone P, Mirjalili SA. The collateral venous system in late pregnancy: a systematic review of the literature. Clin Anat 2017;30(8):1087–95.
15. Weiner RB, Baggish AL. Exercise-induced cardiac remodeling. Prog Cardiovasc Dis 2012;54(5):380–6.
16. Pavlicev M, Norwitz ER. Human parturition: nothing more than a delayed menstruation. Reprod Sci 2018;25(2):166–73.
17. Huang L, Fan L, Ding P, et al. The mediating role of placenta in the relationship between maternal exercise during pregnancy and full-term low birth weight. J Matern Fetal Neonatal Med 2018;31(12):1561–7.
18. Bonham CA, Patterson KC, Strek ME. Asthma outcomes and management during pregnancy. Chest 2018;153(2): 515–27.
19. Bobrowski RA. Pulmonary physiology in pregnancy. Clin Obstet Gynecol 2010;53(2):285–300.
20. National Health and Medical Research Council (NHMRC). Australian dietary guidelines. Canberra: National Health and Medical Research Council; 2013.

21. George A, Johnson M, Blinkhorn A, et al. Views of pregnant women in South Western Sydney towards dental care and an oral-health program initiated by midwives. Health Promot J Austr 2013;24(3):178–84.

22. Matthews A, Haas DM, O'Mathuna DP, et al. Interventions for nausea and vomiting in early pregnancy. Cochrane Database Syst Rev 2015;(9):CD007575.

23. Phupong V, Hanprasertpong T. Interventions for heartburn in pregnancy. Cochrane Database Syst Rev 2015;(9):CD007575.

24. Rungsiprakarn P, Laopaiboon M, Sangkomkamhang US, et al. Interventions for treating constipation in pregnancy. Cochrane Database Syst Rev 2015;(9):CD011448.

25. Wang Q, Würtz P, Auro K, et al. Metabolic profiling of pregnancy: cross-sectional and longitudinal evidence. BMC Med 2016;14(1):205.

26. Pairman S, Pincombe J, Thorogood C, et al. Midwifery: preparation for practice, 3 ed. Sydney: Elsevier; 2015.

27. World Health Organization. Guideline: delayed umbilical cord clamping for improved maternal and infant health and nutrition outcomes. Geneva: World Health Organization; 2014.

28. Sebghati M, Chandraharan E. An update on the risk factors for and management of obstetric haemorrhage. Womens Health (Lond) 2017;13(2):34–40.

29. Lee S, Kelleher SL. Biological underpinnings of breastfeeding challenges: the role of genetics, diet, and environment on lactation physiology. Am J Physiol Endocrinol Metab 2016;311(2):E405–22.

30. Wambach K, Riordan J. Breastfeeding and human lactation. 5th ed. Burlington, MA: Jones & Bartlett Learning; 2016.

31. Gunderson EP, Lewis CE, Lin Y, et al. Lactation duration and progression to diabetes in women across the childbearing years: the 30-year cardia study. JAMA Intern Med 2018;178(3):328–37.

32. Gore AC, Hall JE, Hayes FJ. Aging and reproduction. In: Plant TM, Zeleznik AJ, editors. Knobil and Neill's physiology of reproduction. 4th ed. Academic Press; 2015.

Index

Page numbers followed by "*f*" indicate
figures and "*t*" indicate tables.